Protein Is Essential to Life—and a Prime Player in Your Well-Being, Fitness, and Mood.

Here Is Your Chance to Put Protein to Work for You!

Thinking about eating more soy foods, using protein supplements, or snacking on energy bars? The nutrition experts help you to make the best use of each choice, find your own personalized protein factor, and maximize your health.

THE PROTEIN COUNTER

provides all the information you need about protein, plus 15,000 entries—alphabetized for quick, easy reference—giving the portion size, calorie, protein, carbohydrate, and fat values for each food. Everything you need is at your fingertips!

THE PROTEIN COUNTER
Should be packed in every gym bag!

Books by Annette B. Natow and Jo-Ann Heslin

The Antioxidant Vitamin Counter

Calcium Counts

The Calorie Counter (Second Edition)

The Carbohydrate, Sugar, and Fiber Counter

The Cholesterol Counter (Fifth Edition)

The Complete Food Counter

Count on a Healthy Pregnancy

The Diabetes Carbohydrate and Calorie Counter
(Second Edition)

Eating Out Food Counter

The Fat Attack Plan

The Fat Counter (Fifth Edition)

The Food Shopping Counter (Second Edition)

Get Skinny the Smart Way

The Healthy Heart Food Counter

Megadoses

The Most Complete Food Counter

No-Nonsense Nutrition for Kids

The Pocket Encyclopedia of Nutrition

The Pocket Fat Counter (Second Edition)

The Pocket Protein Counter

The Pregnancy Nutrition Counter

The Protein Counter (Second Edition)

The Sodium Counter

Published by POCKET BOOKS

THE
PROTEIN
COUNTER

2ND EDITION

Annette B. Natow, Ph.D., R.D.
and Jo-Ann Heslin, M.A., R.D.

POCKET BOOKS

New York   London   Toronto   Sydney   Singapore

POCKET BOOKS, a division of Simon & Schuster, Inc.
1230 Avenue of the Americas, New York, NY 10020

ISBN: 0-7434-6434-6

First Pocket Books printing of this revised edition February 2003

10 9 8 7 6 5 4 3 2 1

POCKET and colophon are registered trademarks of Simon & Schuster, Inc.

For information regarding special discounts for bulk purchases, please contact Simon & Schuster Special Sales at 1-800-456-6798 or business@simonandschuster.com

Cover design by Lisa Cohen

Printed in the U.S.A.

ANNETTE B. NATOW, PHD, RD, CDN and JO-ANN HESLIN, MA, RD, CDN are the authors of twenty-eight books on nutrition including *The Cholesterol Counter, The Fat Counter, The Complete Food Counter, The Carbohydrate, Fiber and Sugar Counter, Get Skinny The Smart Way* and *The Diabetes Carbohydrate and Calorie Counter,* (all available from Pocket Books) and two college textbooks. Both are former faculty members of Adelphi University and the State University of New York, Downstate Medical Center. They are editors of the Journal of Nutrition for the Elderly and serve as editorial board members for *Environmental Nutrition Newsletter* and are frequently quoted in the media.

For more information on other books by Annette B. Natow and Jo-Ann Heslin, go to www.thenutritionexperts.com.

To our families, who support us through every project:

Harry, Allen, Irene, Sarah, Meryl, Laura, Marty, George, Emily, Steven, Joe, Kristen, Brian, Karen, and John.

Acknowledgments

For graciously sharing their knowledge: Martin Lefkowitz, M.D., and Irene E. Rosenberg, M.D.; and for reading the book in its many stages of progress, Karen J. Nolan, M.Ed., exercise physiologist, University of Toledo.

For all her support and help, our agent, Nancy Trichter.

Without the tireless cooperation of Steven Natow, M.D., and Stephen Llano, *The Protein Counter*, second edition, would never have been completed.

And a special thank you to our editor, Micki Nuding.

*The fact that protein food is both a fuel
and a building material makes its place
in the diet confusing.*

MARY SWARTZ ROSE, PH.D.
Feeding the Family
The Macmillan Company, 1919

Contents

THE
PROTEIN
COUNTER

*Every day your body loses millions of cells.
They are used up, worn out, rubbed off, and are
even cut off, like your beard or fingernails.
You need protein to replace these cells.*

*Except for water, there is more protein in our
bodies than anything else. A 143 pound man
has over 25 pounds of it!*

Introduction

Protein is found in every cell, tissue, and substance in the body except for urine and bile. Our bodies contain many thousands of specific proteins, each one different and designed to do its special job. Bones, teeth, muscles, enzymes, skin, and blood all contain protein. Active tissues like muscles and glands are high in protein, while less active tissue, like fat, has less.

When you don't get enough protein to replace lost cells and maintain normal functions, your body will cannibalize its own tissues, and the body wastes away. That's why it is so important to get enough protein. But you should realize that excess protein is of no benefit to the body. It is simply used up for energy or converted to fat, which is stored. Changing the excess protein to energy or fat makes the liver and kidneys work overtime as they process it and get rid of the waste.

Protein is very important because it is:

- Necessary for life
- Necessary for growth
- Part of every cell in your body
- Needed to replace worn out cells
- Necessary to repair damaged tissue
- A major part of your immune system
- A major part of every enzyme
- A source of energy

You get protein from the food you eat. Foods like meat, milk, beans, vegetables, eggs, and grains contain protein which, in turn, supply amino acids. Your body uses amino acids as the building blocks to make the specific proteins it needs. All body proteins are made from about 20 different amino acids. These amino acids combine in different ways to make distinct kinds of protein, in the same way that different letters of the alphabet combine to form different words.

Almost all foods contain protein—some more, some less. Fruits have little protein compared to meat, milk, cheese, beans, grains, and vegetables. When you eat different foods, you get varying amounts of protein and varying amounts of the different amino acids they contain.

Of the 20 different amino acids found in food, 9 are essential. *These nine must be obtained directly from the food you eat.* The remaining 11 can be made in the body. This is one of the reasons why it's so important to eat a variety of foods. It guarantees you'll get all the different amino acids you need. For example, beans may be short in one of the essential amino acids, while rice and other grains have plenty of it. When you eat beans and rice together or even separately during the day, their amino acids pool together so that your body has a supply of all the amino acids needed to build cells.

Protein and Amino Acid Supplements

Throughout history, people have sought ways to improve their physical ability. Meat was believed to be good because it's animal muscle and builds body muscle. There are reports that as early as the sixth century B.C., a dedicated Greek wrestler, Milo of Crotona, ate 20 pounds of meat every day to build up his body. Athletes today are still looking for ways to enhance performance. Many believe, as Milo did, that extra meat or just more protein or even individual amino acids will increase their muscle size and strength. That simply isn't true. Eating more protein is not a shortcut to a strong, active body.

Extra protein, by itself, will not build muscles or improve performance. The only thing that builds muscle is working the muscle. Even though muscle is 22% protein, you need only 14 extra grams of protein a day to build a pound of muscle a week. Americans eat about twice as much protein as they need, which is more than enough to meet the need for muscle growth. Protein supplements are not necessary. They are expensive, and may not be any more effective than the intact proteins in foods.

Your body does not store excess protein. So when more protein calories are eaten than are needed, the extra is used for energy, or turned into fat and stored. Excess protein builds body fat, not muscle. Also, when you make your body change excess protein into fat or energy, you put a strain on the liver and kidneys. This extra workload may damage the organs. Getting rid of the waste formed from this process may also lead to calcium loss, gout (painful joints), and dehydration.

What About Protein Supplements?

Protein supplements are made from food proteins like dried milk, egg white, soy, or combinations of these. While there is no evidence that supplements are beneficial, they can be used to get lowfat protein when dieting or training. Other substitutes, such as tuna packed in water, skim milk, skinless chicken breast, hard cooked eggs, and egg substitutes, work just as well. They're also cheaper and you may enjoy them more.

> ✦ *Protein Point*
>
> Want to boost your morning protein? Add an egg white or ¼ cup of egg substitute to your breakfast scrambled egg.

What About Amino Acid Supplements?

Amino acids taken as supplements are popular for athletes and body builders as acceptable replacements for anabolic androgenic steroids. Certain amino acids are claimed to build muscles, aid fat loss, provide energy, and repair muscles.

Arginine and *ornithine* are taken to enhance growth hormone production. Arginine has been shown to increase growth hormone temporarily when taken at very high doses, but the increased hormone does not lead to increases in muscle mass or strength.

Leucine has been shown to enhance protein production. It does not seem to increase muscle mass or strength. Leucine, *isoleucine* and *valine*, a family of amino acids, are said to be the body's preferred energy source during endurance exercise. There is no evidence to support this claim.

Tryptophan is used by the body to make *serotonin*, a chemical that transmits nerve messages in the brain. Serotonin has a calming effect. It may make you feel sleepy and relieve pain. It also reduces appetite and carbohydrate craving. Tryptophan is considered by some to be a natural tranquilizer. Prescription drugs that raise serotonin levels are used to treat depression. Athletes use tryptophan to calm their jitters and improve their performance. Meals high in carbohydrate also increase tryptophan levels in the brain, causing a calming effect.

Lysine, another amino acid, is sometimes used to prevent and relieve canker sores, shingles, and herpes infections. Scientific evidence does not support this.

There is no evidence that taking amino acids will be of any benefit to athletes. Taking individual amino acids can cause imbalances in the body which have caused toxic effects in animals. Your body gets all the amino acids it needs from foods.

To sum up:

- Excess protein from protein powders or amino acid powders is not needed and may not be healthy.
- Individual amino acid supplements are not better than intact proteins found in foods.
- Converting excess protein to fat or using excess protein for energy may stress the liver and kidneys.
- Protein breakdown products are excreted in the urine, pulling a good deal of water and minerals from the body along with the waste.
- Protein and amino acid supplements may cause weight gain, dehydration, gout, and calcium loss.

✦ Protein Point

Research shows that a meal high in protein helps to keep you awake and alert, while a meal high in carbohydrate tends to make you sleepy.

Growth and Protein

During pregnancy, infancy, childhood, and adolescence, protein needs are high. In the first 6 months of life, infants need more than twice as much protein as adults. Premature infants need even more. During pregnancy, the body's protein need reflects the baby's growth rate, with the greatest need in the second half of pregnancy. During childhood and adolescence the need for protein gradually decreases until, by age 15 in females and 19 in males, the intake is at an adult level.

Repair and Protein

When the body is stressed in any way, physically or mentally, protein is lost. This increases the need for protein. When it's too hot or too cold, extra protein is needed. More protein is needed to replace nitrogen during heavy sweating. Exercise, fever, surgery, injury, infection, and broken bones all increase your protein need. Even emotional stress, like losing your job or taking an exam, causes protein loss. Extra protein is needed to make up for all these losses.

✦ *Protein Point*

Necessary Nitrogen

Protein is the body's source of nitrogen. You lose nitrogen every day in urine, feces, skin, hair, nails, and sweat. Nitrogen is replaced by protein foods.

Athletes and Protein

Athletes also need more protein. Although carbohydrate and fat are the major fuels used for energy, it is now accepted that protein is used for energy, too. That is why experts suggest more for athletes. The protein factor needed by athletes can be found in the table "Your Daily Protein Factor" on page 11.

Although you might not consider yourself an athlete, the number one public health message today is to be more active. Experts recommend 30 minutes of activity for everyone, every day.

Exercise helps keep the heart healthy, lowers cholesterol, strengthens immunity, improves balance, helps control weight, promotes mental health, enhances sexual desire and performance, helps relieve tension headaches, improves appearance, reduces stress, and increases your sense of well-being. Exercise can also lower the risk of developing diabetes, osteoporosis, and some cancers. In spite of all these benefits, not many Americans have incorporated regular exercise into their lives—only 20% exercise regularly, while 60% do nothing.

Energy Foods

Nutrition bars or energy bars have moved from health food stores into the supermarkets. They are a quick, portable energy source. They go by many names: protein bars, power bars, diet bars, energy bars, and meal replacement bars.

This is a hot new food category aimed not only at athletes but also targeted to women dieters, people on the go, and even those looking for a mental edge. Many bars are very sweet and are more like a candy than a healthy snack. Most include vitamins and minerals, often in high amounts. Others have added ingredients like amino acids and herbs. Read the ingredient label carefully when choosing bars as snacks or meal replacements. Cereal bars are better "energy bars" for children and pregnant women. In Part 1 of *The Protein Counter,* you'll find over 250 energy and cereal bar brands listed.

Many drinks are now energy enhanced, too. Those high in sugar and caffeine should be used only occasionally; these are not good fluid replacers. As with energy bars, read the ingredient list fully to make the best choices. Experts still recommend water as the "number 1" fluid replacement. Over 100 energy drinks are listed in *The Protein Counter*.

Vegetarians and Protein

Who are vegetarians? Almost everyone! Some eat no animal foods at all, others eat plant foods along with milk, eggs, and fish. Still others eat all of these foods plus poultry, but no red meat. Some make vegetarian choices some of the time but not all the time. Vegetarian eating has become part of the way we eat.

Diets that include animal foods provide plenty of protein. A completely plant-based diet that includes a variety of foods also provides all needed nutrients and protein. Peanut butter, nuts, beans, tofu, soy, meat substitutes, and grains are all excellent protein sources.

Looking at Labels

The Nutrition Facts Panel on labels gives you information about the amount of protein in a serving of food. It's given in grams and also as a percentage of the Daily Value (DV). The DV is based on the amount of protein recommended for a 2,000 calorie diet. This may be more or less than the amount of calories you usually eat. For example, the label of a can of solid white tuna in spring water shows that a 2-ounce serving (one quarter cup) has 15 grams of protein, which is 27% of the DV. When you are counting your protein intake, the number of grams is a more useful figure so that you can see how the food fits into your personal protein recommendation for the day.

When you look at the ingredient list on a label, you may see some unfamiliar words. A can of chicken broth may show, in addition to chicken broth, *hydrolyzed protein, wheat gluten* and *monosodium glutamate*. These ingredients are actually protein and add to the total protein in the food. The following list gives some examples of protein ingredients.

These Are Protein Too!

Casein	Protein hydrolysates
Corn gluten	Seitan (wheat gluten)
Egg whites	Skim milk powder
Gelatin	Soybean curd (tofu)
Gluten	Soy milk
Hydrolyzed plant protein (HPP)	Soy protein concentrate
Hydrolyzed vegetable protein (HVP)	Textured vegetable protein (TVP)
	Tofu
Isolated soy protein	Wheat gluten
Monosodium glutamate (MSG)	Whey

Your Protein Needs

How much protein you need each day depends on your weight, activity level, age, and overall health. You'll find the table "Your Daily Protein Factor" on page 11. Use this table and the 4 steps on pages 12–13 to figure out your individual protein needs.

Your Daily Protein Factor

Determine How Much Protein You Need Each Day

Age or Condition	Grams Protein per Kilogram of Target Weight
Teens	
Males	0.9
Females	0.8
Adults	0.8
Mature adults	1.0
Recreational athletes	0.8 to 1.0
Endurance athletes	1.2 to 1.8
Strength training	1.7 to 1.8
Strenuous exercise*	1.8 to 2.0
Mature athletes	1.0 to 1.5
Infections, fractures, fever, surgery	1.0 to 1.4
Severe trauma	1.5 to 2.5
Pregnancy	1.3 to 1.5
Breastfeeding	
1st six months	0.8 + 15 grams**
2nd six months	0.8 + 12 grams**

* daily exercise program of one hour or more
** add 15 or 12 grams of protein a day to the normal protein requirement
   of 0.8 per kilograms of weight

Figuring Out Your Daily Protein Requirement

1. Determine your daily protein factor.

Check the table "Your Daily Protein Factor," page 11, to determine the category that is right for you.

For example, if you are a recreational athlete, your protein factor is 0.8 to 1.0 grams of protein.

Your daily protein factor is: _____

2. Find your "target" weight.

Your protein requirement is based on your weight. Here is a simple way to determine your target weight.

Women: Give yourself 100 pounds for the first 5 feet of your height and add 5 pounds for each additional inch over 5 feet (or subtract 5 pounds for each inch under 5 feet).

For example, if you're 5 feet, 6 inches tall:

100 pounds (for the first 5 feet)
+30 pounds (6 additional inches × 5 pounds each)
130 pounds Target Weight

Men: Give yourself 106 pounds for the first 5 feet of your height and add 6 pounds for each additional inch over 5 feet.

For example, if you're 5 feet, 9 inches tall:

106 pounds (for the first 5 feet)
+54 pounds (9 additional inches × 6 pounds each)
160 pounds Target Weight

Add 10% for large body frame; subtract 10% for a small body frame. If you're not sure of your frame size, a large shoe size is a good predictor of a large frame.

> _____ pounds (for the first 5 feet)
> + _____ pounds (_____ additional inches
> × _____ pounds each)
> _____ pounds Target Weight

Your target weight: _____

3. Convert your weight in pounds to kilograms.

To determine your weight in kilograms, divide your weight in pounds by 2.2.

> _____ (your weight or target weight) ÷ 2.2 = _____
> weight in kilograms

— or —

The chart "Converting Weight in Pounds to Kilograms", page 14 can be used to complete this step.
Your weight in kilograms: _____

4. Setting your daily requirement for protein.

Multiply your protein factor (from Step #1) times your weight in kilograms (from Step #3).

For example, if you are a recreational athlete weighing 75 kilograms, your daily protein factor would be 0.8 to 1.0.

> 0.8 (protein factor) × 75 kilograms =
> 60 grams of protein/day
> 1.0 (protein factor) × 75 kilograms =
> 75 grams of protein/day

A recreational athlete weighing 75 kilograms should be eating a minimum 60 to 75 grams of protein each day.

_____ your protein factor × _____ weight in kilograms = _____ grams protein/day

Your daily protein requirement is: _____ grams of protein per day

Now that you know how many grams of protein you need each day, use *The Protein Counter* to select the best choices to meet your needs. If your situation changes—for example, if you get pregnant or you change your exercise program—simply use Steps 1 to 4 on pages 12 to 13 to recalculate your daily protein requirement.

Converting Weight in Pounds to Kilograms

Weight in Pounds	Weight in Kilograms
85	39
90	41
95	42
100	45
105	48
110	50
115	52
120	54
125	57
130	59
135	61
140	64

Weight in Pounds	Weight in Kilograms
145	66
150	68
155	70
160	73
165	75
170	77
175	79
180	82
185	84
190	86
195	88
200	91
210	93

Want to Know More?

Americans get an average of 15–17% of their calories each day from protein. That leaves 83–85% of calories remaining from fat and carbohydrate. The recommended intake of fat is 30–35% of total calories, leaving 48–55% of daily calories as carbohydrate.

Your daily intake of protein, carbohydrate, and fat calories should be:

protein	10–20%
carbohydrate	50–55%
fat	30–35%

You can individualize this, if you like, to decrease fat below 30% and increase protein or carbohydrate to fit your needs.

You may be wondering how to determine how many calories you need each day. Once you have figured your target weight, you can use this weight to get a good estimate of the amount of calories your need each day.

- If you are not very active, you'll need 12 calories a pound of your target weight.
- If you get at least a ½ hour of activity a day, you'll need 15 calories a pound of your target weight.
- If you do daily vigorous exercise, you'll need 18 or more calories a pound of your target weight.

For example, if you get at least ½ hour of activity a day and weigh 150 pounds:

150 pounds × 15 calories a pound = 2250 calories per day

Using the recommendations of 10–20% protein calories, 50–55% carbohydrate calories, and 30–35% fat calories, each day you should be eating:

your calories per day × 20% protein = protein calories each day
2250 calories per day × 20% = 450 protein calories each day

your calories per day × 50% carbohydrate = carbohydrate calories each day
2250 calories per day × 50% = 1125 carbohydrate calories each day

your calories per day × 30% fat = fat calories each day.
2250 calories per day × 30% = 675 fat calories

450 protein calories + 1125 carbohydrate
calories + 675 fat calories = 2250 calories each day

Whether you want to simply track your protein intake for the day or set up a complete eating plan that includes protein, fat, and carbohydrate, *The Protein Counter* is the best guide you can use.

Eat well—Stay Active—Be Well!

Using the Counter Section

The Protein Counter lists the calories, carbohydrate, fat, and protein content of 15,000 foods. Now you can check and compare the values in your favorite foods and, when necessary, choose substitutes before you shop or eat. This will help you make the right choices.

The counter section of the book is divided into two parts—Part 1: Brand Name, Nonbranded Foods and Take-out Foods, and Part 2: Restaurant Chains.

In Part 1 all foods are listed alphabetically, from abalone to zucchini. For each category, you will first find nonbranded (generic) foods listed in alphabetical order, followed by an alphabetical listing of brand name foods. The nonbranded listing will help you determine calorie, carbohydrate, fat, and protein values for foods when you aren't able to find your favorite brand. They will also help you evaluate store brands. Large categories are often divided into subcategories such as canned, fresh, frozen, and ready-to-eat, making it easier to find what you're looking for.

Because we all eat out so often, there are over 450 take-out foods listed in Part 1. These are found in the take-out subcategory throughout this section. Look there for foods you take out or order in, because these choices are not nutrition labeled.

In some cases, foods are grouped by category. For example, chow mein is found under the category ASIAN FOOD. Group categories include:

Asian Food   Page 27
    includes all types of Asian foods except
    egg rolls and sushi, which are found in
    separate categories

Deli Meats/Cold Cuts   Page 167
    includes all sandwich meats except
    chicken, ham, and turkey, which
    are found in separate categories

Dinner   Page 170
    includes all by brand name, except pasta
    dinners, which are found in a separate
    category

Liquor/Liqueur   Page 242
    includes all alcoholic beverages except
    beer, champagne, and wine, which are
    found in separate categories

Nutrition Supplements   Page 260
    includes all meal replacers and diet
    drinks, except energy bars and energy
    drinks, which are found in separate
    categories

Sandwiches   Page 331
    includes popular sandwich choices

Spanish Food   Page 364
> includes all types of Spanish and Mexi-
> can foods except salsa and tortillas, which
> are found in separate categories

In Part 2: Restaurant Chains, there are 53 national and regional restaurant, doughnut, ice cream, candy, and coffee chains listed.

Definitions

as prep (as prepared): refers to food that has been prepared according to package directions

lean and fat: describes meat with some fat on its edges that is not cut away before cooking, or poultry prepared with skin and fat as purchased

lean only: refers to lean meat, that is trimmed of all visible fat or poultry without skin

shelf stable: refers to prepared products found on the supermarket shelf that are ready-to-eat or be heated and do not require refrigeration

take-out: describes prepared dishes that you purchase ready-to-eat; those included serve as a guide to the calorie, carbohydrate, fat and protein values of similar products you may purchase

Abbreviations

avg	=	average
diam	=	diameter
fl	=	fluid
frzn	=	frozen
g	=	gram
in	=	inch
lb	=	pound
lg	=	large
med	=	medium
mg	=	milligram
oz	=	ounce
pkg	=	package
pt	=	pint
prep	=	prepared
qt	=	quart
reg	=	regular
sec	=	second
serv	=	serving
sm	=	small
sq	=	square
tbsp	=	tablespoon
tr	=	trace
tsp	=	teaspoon
w/	=	with
w/o	=	without
<	=	less than

Notes

Carbohydrate = Carb
    All carbohydrate values are given in grams (g).

Fat = Fat
    All fat values are given in grams (g).

Protein = Prot
    All protein values are given in grams (g).

tr (trace) = less than 1 gram of carbohydrate, fat,
        or protein.

Discrepancies in figures are due to rounding, product reformulation, and reevaluation. Labeling law allows rounding of values. Because much of our data is analysis data obtained directly from manufacturers, not from labels, our values may not always be exactly the same as label information because our data have not been rounded.

PART I

Brand Name, Nonbranded (Generic) & Take-Out Foods

> ✦ Protein Point
>
> *Protein* is derived from the Greek word *proteios*, which means "of prime importance."

FOOD	PORTION	CALS	PROT	FAT	CARB
ABALONE					
fresh fried	3 oz	161	17	6	9
ACEROLA JUICE					
juice	1 cup	51	1	1	12
ADZUKI BEANS					
canned sweetened	1 cup	702	11	tr	163
dried cooked	1 cup	294	17	tr	57
AKEE					
fresh	3.5 oz	223	5	20	5
ALE					
(see BEER AND ALE, MALT)					
ALFALFA					
(see also SPROUTS)					
sprouts	1 cup	40	1	tr	1
ALLIGATOR					
cooked	3 oz	126	28	2	0
ALMONDS					
almond butter honey & cinnamon	1 tbsp	96	3	8	4
almond butter w/ salt	1 tbsp	101	2	9	3
almond butter w/o salt	1 tbsp	101	2	10	3
almond meal	1 oz	116	11	5	8
almond paste	1 oz	127	3	8	12
jordan almonds	10 (1.4 oz)	190	4	7	28
praline	17 pieces (1.4 oz)	210	5	12	21
Lance					
Smoked	1 pkg (0.8 oz)	130	6	10	4
AMARANTH					
(see CEREAL, COOKIES)					
ANCHOVY					
canned in oil	5	42	6	2	0
canned in oil	1 can (1.6 oz)	95	13	4	0
fresh fillets	3 (0.4 oz)	21	2	1	tr
ANTELOPE					
roasted	3 oz	127	25	2	0
APPLE					
canned					
Del Monte					
Fruit Pleasures Pie Spiced Apples	½ cup (4.1 oz)	70	0	0	18
dried					
rings	10	155	1	tr	42
fresh					
Chiquita					
Apple	1 med (5.4 oz)	80	0	0	22
Cool Cut					
Apples & Caramel Dip	1 pkg (4.25 oz)	180	1	5	32

FOOD	PORTION	CALS	PROT	FAT	CARB
APPLE JUICE					
Apple & Eve					
100% Juice	8 fl oz	110	1	0	26
Cider	8 fl oz	110	1	0	27
Eden					
Organic Juice	8 oz	80	0	0	23
Ocean Spray					
100% Juice	8 oz	110	0	0	28
Snapple					
Snapple Apple	8 fl oz	120	0	0	30
Swiss Miss					
Hot Apple Cider Mix Low Calorie	1 serv	14	0	0	3
Veryfine					
100% Juice	1 bottle (10 oz)	150	0	0	38
APPLESAUCE					
Eden					
Organic	½ cup	50	0	0	15
Mott's					
Single-Serve Cinnamon	1 pkg (4 oz)	100	0	0	26
APRICOT JUICE					
nectar	1 cup	141	1	tr	36
APRICOTS					
canned					
Del Monte					
Halves Unpeeled Lite	½ cup (4.3 oz)	60	0	0	16
Orchard Select Halves Unpeeled	½ cup (4.4 oz)	80	0	0	21
dried					
halves	10	83	1	tr	22
fresh					
apricots	3	51	1	tr	12
ARROWHEAD					
fresh boiled	1 med (⅕ oz)	9	1	tr	2
ARTICHOKE					
canned					
Progresso					
Hearts	2 pieces (2.9 oz)	30	2	0	6
Hearts Marinated	2 pieces (1.1 oz)	170	0	5	2
fresh					
boiled	1 med (4 oz)	60	4	tr	13
hearts cooked	½ cup	42	3	tr	9
frozen					
cooked	1 pkg (9 oz)	108	7	1	22
ASIAN FOOD					
(*see also* DINNER, EGG ROLLS, PASTA, SUSHI)					
canned					
chow mein chicken	1 cup	95	7	tr	18

FOOD	PORTION	CALS	PROT	FAT	CARB
Chun King					
Beef Pepper Oriental BiPack	1 cup (8.8 oz)	98	10	2	13
Chow Mein Beef BiPack	1 cup (8.6 oz)	78	8	1	11
Chow Mein BiPack Chicken	1 cup (8.8 oz)	98	8	3	11
Chow Mein Pork BiPack	1 cup (8.6 oz)	78	7	2	9
Hot & Spicy Chicken BiPack	1 cup (8.6 oz)	98	8	3	11
Sweet & Sour Chicken BiPack	1 cup (8.9 oz)	161	7	2	29
La Choy					
Beef Pepper Oriental BiPack	1 cup (8.8 oz)	98	10	2	13
Chow Mein Beef BiPack	1 cup (8.6 oz)	78	8	1	11
Chow Mein Chicken BiPack	1 cup (8.9 oz)	98	8	3	11
Chow Mein Shrimp BiPack	1 cup (8.6 oz)	52	4	1	9
Main Entree Chow Mein Chicken	1 cup (9.3 oz)	80	8	4	6
Oriental Beef w/ Noodles BiPack	1 cup (8.8 oz)	156	18	3	18
Oriental Chicken w/ Noodles BiPack	1 cup (8.7 oz)	154	14	4	18
Sweet & Sour Chicken BiPack	1 cup (8.9 oz)	161	7	2	29
Teriyaki Chicken BiPack	1 cup (8.6 oz)	109	8	3	15
fresh					
wonton wrappers	1	23	1	tr	5
Azumaya					
Round Wraps	10	160	6	1	31
Square Wraps	6	160	6	1	31
Wrappers Large Square	3	170	7	1	35
Nasoya					
Won Ton Wrappers	8	160	6	1	31
frozen					
Banquet					
Fried Rice w/ Chicken & Egg Rolls	1 meal (8.5 oz)	330	12	9	51
Birds Eye					
Easy Recipe Creations Oriental Lo Mein as prep	2¼ cups (8.7 oz)	230	8	4	40
Easy Recipe Creations Sesame Ginger Teriyaki as prep	2¼ cups (8.7 oz)	140	6	2	24
Easy Recipe Creations Spicy Szechuan Cashews	2¼ cups (8.7 oz)	180	6	5	29

FOOD	PORTION	CALS	PROT	FAT	CARB
Green Giant					
Create A Meal LoMein Stir Fry as prep	1¼ cups (10 oz)	320	30	70	35
Create A Meal Sweet & Sour Stir Fry as prep	1¼ cups (10 oz)	290	27	7	29
Create A Meal Szechuan Stir Fry as prep	1¼ cups (10 oz)	340	28	15	22
Create A Meal Teriyaki Stir Fry as prep	1¼ cups (10 oz)	240	27	6	18
La Choy					
Beef Pepper Oriental	1 cup (7.1 oz)	151	8	1	30
Chow Mein Vegetable	1 cup (8.9 oz)	108	2	2	20
Lean Cuisine					
Everyday Favorites Oriental Style Dumplings	1 pkg (9 oz)	300	10	6	51
Everyday Favorites Teriyaki Stir Fry	1 pkg (10 oz)	290	18	4	45
Stouffer's					
Chicken Chow Mein w/ Rice	1 pkg (10.6 oz)	260	13	5	40
Tyson					
Chicken Fried Rice Kit w/ Sauce	1 pkg (14 oz)	440	27	6	69
Weight Watchers					
Smart Ones Chicken Chow Mein	1 pkg (9 oz)	200	12	2	34
Smart Ones Hunan Style Rice & Vegetables	1 pkg (10.34 oz)	280	7	0	45
Smart Ones King Pao Noodles & Vegetables	1 pkg (10 oz)	250	8	8	37
Smart Ones Spicy Szechaun Style Vegetables & Chicken	1 pkg (9 oz)	220	11	2	39
take-out					
buddha's delight w/ cellophane noodles fat choi jai	1 serv (7.6 oz)	211	7	4	44
cha siu bao steamed buns w/ chicken filling	1 (2.3 oz)	160	5	3	26
chicken teriyaki	¾ cup	399	30	27	7
chicken teriyaki w/ rice	1 serv (11 oz)	430	19	6	77
chop suey w/ beef & pork	1 cup	300	26	17	13
chop suey w/ pork	1 cup	375	19	29	29
chow mein chicken	1 cup	255	31	10	10
chow mein pork	1 cup	425	32	24	21
chow mein shrimp	1 cup	221	13	10	21
chow mein vegetable	1 serv (8 oz)	90	3	3	15

FOOD	PORTION	CALS	PROT	FAT	CARB
filipino chicken adobo	1 serv (15 oz)	555	33	26	45
fried rice	6.6 oz	249	4	6	48
fried rice w/ egg	6.7 oz	395	8	20	49
phad thai	1 serv (9.2 oz)	232	11	9	30
sesame seed paste bun	1 (2.5 oz)	220	5	6	39
shrimp chips	1¼ cups (1 oz)	140	2	6	19
shu mai chicken & vegetable dumplings	6 (3.6 oz)	160	10	5	18
spring roll	1 (3.5 oz)	112	12	2	37
sweet & sour pork	1 serv (8 oz)	250	6	8	37
sweet red bean bun	1 (2.5 oz)	130	4	1	38
szechuan chicken w/ lo mein	1 cup (5.3 oz)	190	10	1	35
wonton fried	½ cup (1 oz)	111	2	8	8
wonton soup	1 cup	205	16	3	26
ASPARAGUS					
canned					
spears	½ cup	24	3	1	3
Del Monte					
Cuts & Tips	½ cup (4.4 oz)	20	2	0	3
Spears Extra Long	½ cup (4.4 oz)	20	2	0	3
Spears Tender Young	½ cup (4.4 oz)	20	2	0	3
Tips Hand Selected	½ cup (4.4 oz)	20	2	0	3
Green Giant					
Cut Spears	½ cup (4.2 oz)	20	2	0	3
Cut Spears 50% Less Sodium	½ cup (4.2 oz)	20	2	0	3
Extra Long Spears	4.5 oz	20	2	0	3
Spears	4.5 oz	20	2	0	3
LeSueur					
Spears Extra Large	4.5 oz	20	2	0	3
S&W					
Green	6 pieces (4.5 oz)	15	2	0	4
fresh					
cooked	4 spears	14	2	tr	3
cooked	½ cup	22	2	tr	4
frozen					
cooked	4 spears	17	2	tr	3
cooked	1 pkg (10 oz)	82	9	1	14
Green Giant					
Harvest Fresh Cuts	⅔ cup (3 oz)	25	2	0	4
ATEMOYA					
fresh	½ cup	94	1	1	24
AVOCADO					
fresh	1	324	4	31	15
fresh mashed	1 cup	370	5	35	17
Chiquita					
Fresh	⅕ med (1 oz)	55	1	5	3

FOOD	PORTION	CALS	PROT	FAT	CARB
take-out					
guacamole	1 serv (2.2 oz)	105	1	10	5
BACON					
(see also BACON SUBSTITUTES)					
breakfast strips cooked	3 strips	156	10	12	tr
gammon lean & fat grilled	4.2 oz	274	35	15	0
pan fried	3 strips	109	6	9	tr
Black Label					
Center Cut cooked	3 slices (0.5 oz)	70	5	6	0
Cooked	2 slices (0.5 oz)	80	5	7	0
Low Salt cooked	2 slices (0.5 oz)	80	5	7	0
Health Is Wealth					
Uncured Sliced	2 slices (0.5 oz)	70	3	7	0
Hormel					
Bacon Bits	1 tbsp (7 g)	30	3	2	0
Bacon Pieces	1 tbsp (7 g)	25	3	2	0
Microwave cooked	2 slices (0.5 oz)	70	5	5	0
Old Smokehouse					
Cooked	2 slices (0.5 oz)	80	5	7	0
Oscar Mayer					
Bacon Bits	1 tbsp (0.2 oz)	25	3	2	0
Bacon Pieces	1 tbsp (0.2 oz)	25	2	2	0
Center Cut cooked	2 slices (0.4 oz)	70	4	5	0
Cooked	2 slices (0.5 oz)	70	4	6	0
Lower Sodium cooked	2 slices (0.5 oz)	70	5	5	1
Thick Cut cooked	1 slice (0.4 oz)	60	4	5	0
Range Brand					
Cooked	2 slices (0.7 oz)	100	7	9	0
Ready Crisp					
Fully Cooked	3 slices (0.5 oz)	70	4	6	0
Red Label					
Cooked	2 slices (0.5 oz)	80	5	7	0
BACON SUBSTITUTES					
bacon substitute	1 strip	25	1	2	1
Bac-Os					
Chips or Bits	1½ tbsp (7 g)	30	3	2	2
Lightlife					
Fakin' Bacon Bits	1 tsp	45	1	1	1
Smart Bacon	2 strips (0.8 oz)	45	6	2	2
Louis Rich					
Turkey Bacon	1 slice (0.5 oz)	35	2	3	0
Morningstar Farms					
Breakfast Strips	2 (0.5 oz)	60	2	5	2
Worthington					
Stripples	2 strips (0.5 oz)	60	2	5	2
BAGEL					
cinnamon raisin	1 (3½ in)	194	7	1	39

FOOD	PORTION	CALS	PROT	FAT	CARB
cinnamon raisin toasted	1 (3½ in)	194	7	1	39
egg	1 (3½ in)	197	8	2	38
egg toasted	1 (3½ in)	197	8	2	38
mini onion	1 (1.4 oz)	100	4	0	20
oat bran	1 (3½ in)	181	8	1	38
oat bran toasted	1 (3½ in)	181	8	1	38
onion	1 (3½ in)	195	8	1	38
plain	1 (3½ in)	195	8	1	38
plain toasted	1 (3½ in)	195	8	1	38
poppy seed	1 (3½ in)	195	8	1	38
Amy's Organic					
Cinnamon Raisin	1 (3.5 oz)	240	8	2	52
Plain	1 (3.5 oz)	230	8	2	48
Poppy Seed	1 (3.5 oz)	230	8	2	48
Sesame	1 (3.5 oz)	240	8	2	48
Otis Spunkmeyer					
Barnstormin' Blueberry	1 (3.6 oz)	250	10	3	50
Barnstormin' Cinnamon Raisin	1 (3.6 oz)	230	9	2	47
Barnstormin' Onion	1 (3.6 oz)	230	9	2	47
Barnstormin' Plain	1 (3.6 oz)	240	10	3	49
Pepperidge Farm					
Mini	1 (1.4 oz)	120	5	0	24
Plain	1 (3.5 oz)	290	11	1	60
Sara Lee					
Blueberry	1 (2.8 oz)	210	8	1	41
Cinnamon Raisin	1 (2.8 oz)	220	8	1	45
Egg	1 (2.8 oz)	210	7	1	44
Oat Bran	1 (2.8 oz)	210	8	1	42
Onion	1 (2.8 oz)	210	7	0	44
Plain	1 (2.8 oz)	210	8	1	43
Poppy Seed	1 (2.8 oz)	210	8	1	41
Sesame Seed	1 (2.8 oz)	210	8	2	42
Thomas'					
Everything	1 (3.6 oz)	300	10	4	56
Multi-Grain	1 (3.6 oz)	280	11	2	55
Plain	1 (3.6 oz)	280	10	2	56
Uncle B's					
Plain	1 (2.8 oz)	210	8	1	41
Wonder					
Blueberry	1 (3 oz)	210	7	1	43
Cinnamon Raisin	1 (3 oz)	210	8	1	42
Onion	1 (3 oz)	210	8	1	43
Plain	1 (3 oz)	210	8	1	43
Rye	1 (3 oz)	220	9	1	42
Wheat	1 (3 oz)	210	8	1	43
BAKING POWDER					
baking powder	1 tsp	2	0	0	1

FOOD	PORTION	CALS	PROT	FAT	CARB
BAKING SODA					
baking soda	1 tsp	0	0	0	0
BALSAM PEAR					
leafy tips cooked	½ cup	10	1	tr	2
leafy tips raw	½ cup	7	1	tr	1
pods cooked	½ cup	12	1	tr	3
BAMBOO SHOOTS					
canned sliced	1 cup	25	2	1	4
fresh	½ cup	21	2	tr	1
fresh cooked	½ cup	15	2	tr	2
BANANA					
banana chips	1 oz	147	1	10	17
fresh	1	105	1	tr	27
fresh mashed	1 cup	207	2	1	53
Chiquita					
Fresh	1 med (4.4 oz)	110	1	0	29
Rainforest Farms					
Slices Dried	5 slices (1.3 oz)	60	1	0	12
BARBECUE SAUCE					
(see also SAUCE)					
barbecue	1 cup	188	5	5	32
House Of Tsang					
Hong Kong	1 tbsp (0.6 oz)	10	0	0	2
Hunt's					
Honey Hickory	2 tbsp (1.2 oz)	54	1	tr	12
Mesquite	2 tbsp (1.2 oz)	40	1	tr	9
Open Range Original	2 tbsp (1.2 oz)	39	1	tr	9
Open Range Premier	2 tbsp (1.3 oz)	56	1	tr	13
Teriyaki	2 tbsp (1.2 oz)	46	1	tr	11
Kraft					
Char-Grill	2 tbsp (1.3 oz)	60	0	0	13
BARLEY					
flour	1 cup (5.2 oz)	511	15	2	110
malt flour	1 cup (5.7 oz)	585	17	3	127
pearled cooked	1 cup (5.5 oz)	193	4	1	44
pearled uncooked	1 cup (7 oz)	704	20	2	155
BARRACUDA					
fresh	3 oz	122	14	8	0
BASS					
freshwater raw	3 oz	97	16	3	0
sea cooked	3 oz	105	20	2	0
sea raw	3 oz	82	16	2	0
striped baked	3 oz	105	19	3	0
BEANS					
(see also individual names)					
canned					
baked beans plain	½ cup	118	6	1	26
baked beans vegetarian	½ cup	118	6	1	26

FOOD	PORTION	CALS	PROT	FAT	CARB
baked beans w/ beef	½ cup	161	8	5	22
baked beans w/ franks	½ cup	182	9	8	20
baked beans w/ pork	½ cup	133	7	2	25
baked beans w/ pork & sweet sauce	½ cup	140	7	2	26
baked beans w/ pork & tomato sauce	½ cup	123	7	1	24
refried beans	½ cup	134	8	1	23
B&M					
Barbeque Baked Beans	½ cup (4.6 oz)	210	8	1	42
Bush's					
Barbecue	½ cup (4.6 oz)	160	6	1	32
Maple Cured Bacon	½ cup (4.6 oz)	150	7	1	28
Vegetarian	½ cup (4.6 oz)	130	6	0	24
Chi-Chi's					
Refried	½ cup (4.2 oz)	100	5	1	18
Refried Beans Fat Free	½ cup (4.2 oz)	120	5	0	17
Refried Beans Vegetarian	½ cup (4.2 oz)	100	5	1	18
Eden					
Organic Baked w/ Sorghum & Mustard	½ cup (4.6 oz)	150	8	0	27
Gebhardt					
Chili	½ cup (4.6 oz)	134	7	1	31
Refried Jalapeno	½ cup (4.5 oz)	105	7	3	19
Refried No Fat	½ cup (4.5 oz)	92	7	tr	20
Refried Traditional	½ cup (4.5 oz)	109	6	3	20
Refried Vegetarian	½ cup (4.5 oz)	118	8	2	21
Green Giant					
Pork And Beans w/ Tomato Sauce	½ cup (4.5 oz)	120	5	1	23
Spicy Chili	½ cup (4.5 oz)	110	6	1	20
Three Bean Salad	½ cup (4.2 oz)	90	3	0	20
Health Valley					
Honey Baked	½ cup	110	7	0	25
Honey Baked No Salt	½ cup	110	7	0	25
Hormel					
Beans & Wieners	1 can (7.5 oz)	290	11	12	34
Hunt's					
Big John's Beans & Fixin's	½ cup (4.7 oz)	127	7	4	23
Homestyle Country Kettle	½ cup (4.6 oz)	152	7	2	31
Homestyle Special Recipe	½ cup (4.7 oz)	185	7	3	36
Mix & Serve	½ cup (4.7 oz)	125	2	3	30
Pork & Beans	½ cup (4.6 oz)	157	6	5	27
Pork & Beans	½ cup (4.5 oz)	130	6	1	28
Kid's Kitchen					
Microwave Meals Beans & Weiners	1 cup (7.5 oz)	310	13	13	37

FOOD	PORTION	CALS	PROT	FAT	CARB
Open Range					
Ranch	½ cup (4.4 oz)	124	6	3	23
Pringles					
Vegetarian	1 cup (7.9 oz)	250	11	1	48
Rosarita					
3 Bean Recipe Bacon & Jalapeno	½ cup (4.6 oz)	117	8	2	22
3 Bean Recipe Chiles & Chicken	½ cup (4.6 oz)	115	7	1	22
3 Bean Recipe Chilies & Chorizo	½ cup (4.6 oz)	111	8	2	19
3 Bean Recipe Onions & Peppers	½ cup (4.6 oz)	104	7	1	20
Fiesta Beans Bacon & Jalapenos	½ cup (4.6 oz)	117	8	2	22
Fiesta Beans Chicken & Chilies	½ cup (4.6 oz)	115	7	1	22
Fiesta Beans Chilies & Chorizo	½ cup (4.6 oz)	110	8	2	19
Fiesta Beans Onions & Peppers	½ cup (4.6 oz)	104	8	1	20
Refried Bacon	½ cup (4.5 oz)	116	6	3	19
Refried Green Chile	½ cup (4.5 oz)	110	6	3	20
Refried Low Fat Black	½ cup (4.5 oz)	107	8	1	23
Refried Nacho Cheese	½ cup (4.5 oz)	108	8	2	19
Refried No Fat	½ cup (4.5 oz)	120	7	0	28
Refried No Fat Green Chiles & Lime	½ cup (4.5 oz)	101	8	tr	22
Refried No Fat w/ Zesty Salsa	½ cup (4.5 oz)	105	6	tr	24
Refried Onion	½ cup (4.5 oz)	114	6	3	21
Refried Spicy	½ cup (4.5 oz)	118	7	3	22
Refried Traditional	½ cup (4.5 oz)	108	5	1	19
Refried Vegetarian	½ cup (4.5 oz)	237	15	5	42
S&W					
Barbecue Beans Ranch Recipe	½ cup (4.5 oz)	100	6	2	25
Taco Bell					
Home Originals Fat Free Refried Beans	½ cup (4.6 oz)	110	7	0	21
Home Originals Fat Free Refried Beans w/ Mild Chilies	½ cup (4.5 oz)	110	7	0	20
Home Originals Refried Beans	½ cup (4.7 oz)	140	5	3	23
Van Camp					
Baked Fat Free	½ cup (4.6 oz)	132	6	tr	29

FOOD	PORTION	CALS	PROT	FAT	CARB
Baked Original	½ cup (4.7 oz)	143	7	1	29
Baked Southern Style Sauteed Onion	½ cup (4.8 oz)	145	6	1	35
Baked Sweet Hickory & Bacon	1 can (4.8 oz)	143	6	1	32
Beanee Weenee BBQ	1 cup (7.7 oz)	290	14	12	36
Beanee Weenee Baked	1 cup (9.1 oz)	410	18	14	58
Beanee Weenee Microwave	1 cup (7.5 oz)	260	14	11	29
Beanee Weenee Original	1 cup (9.1 oz)	320	16	14	35
Beanee Weenee Zestful	1 cup (7.7 oz)	300	14	12	40
Brown Sugar	½ cup (4.6 oz)	170	7	3	31
Pork And Beans	½ cup (4.6 oz)	110	6	2	23
Vegetarian	½ cup (4.6 oz)	110	6	1	23
frozen					
Natural Touch					
Nine Bean Loaf	1 in slice (3 oz)	160	8	8	13
mix					
Melting Pot					
Terrazza Napoli Mixed Beans	1 cup	200	9	2	41
take-out					
baked beans	½ cup	190	7	6	27
barbecue beans	3.5 oz	120	4	tr	26
four bean salad	3.5 oz	100	4	tr	20
refried beans	½ cup	43	2	2	5
three bean salad	¾ cup	230	5	11	31
BEAN SPROUTS					
(*see* ALFALFA, SPROUTS)					
BEAR					
simmered	3 oz	220	28	11	0
BEAVER					
roasted	3 oz	140	30	6	0
simmered	3 oz	141	23	5	0
BEECHNUTS					
dried	1 oz	164	2	14	10
BEEF					
(*see also* BEEF DISHES, VEAL)					
canned					
corned beef	3 oz	85	10	5	0
Armour					
Chopped Beef	2 oz	170	7	15	2
Corned Beef	2 oz	120	15	7	1
Potted Meat	1 can (3 oz)	120	12	7	0
Tripe	3 oz	90	18	2	0
Hormel					
Corned Beef	2 oz	120	15	7	0
Cubed Beef	½ cup (4.9 oz)	130	25	3	0
Potted Meat	4 tbsp (2 oz)	100	7	8	0

FOOD	PORTION	CALS	PROT	FAT	CARB
Treet					
Luncheon Loaf	2 oz	130	6	11	3
Luncheon Loaf 50% Less Fat	2 oz	110	6	8	4
dried					
Armour					
Sliced	7 slices (1 oz)	60	8	2	2
Hormel					
Pillow Pack	10 slices (1 oz)	45	8	1	0
fresh					
bottom round lean & fat trim 0 in Choice roasted	3 oz	172	24	8	0
bottom round lean & fat trim 0 in Select braised	3 oz	171	27	6	0
bottom round lean & fat trim 0 in Select roasted	3 oz	150	24	24	0
bottom round lean & fat trim 0 in braised	3 oz	193	26	26	0
bottom round lean & fat trim ¼ in Choice braised	3 oz	241	24	15	0
bottom round lean & fat trim ¼ in Choice roasted	3 oz	221	22	14	0
bottom round lean & fat trim ¼ in Select braised	3 oz	220	25	13	0
bottom round lean & fat trim ¼ in Select roasted	3 oz	199	23	11	0
brisket flat half lean & fat trim 0 in braised	3 oz	183	26	8	0
brisket flat half lean & fat trim ¼ in braised	3 oz	309	21	24	0
brisket point half lean & fat trim 0 in braised	3 oz	304	20	24	0
brisket point half lean & fat trim ¼ in braised	3 oz	343	19	29	0
brisket whole lean & fat trim 0 in braised	3 oz	247	23	17	0
brisket whole lean & fat trim ¼ in braised	3 oz	327	27	27	0
chuck arm pot roast lean & fat trim 0 in braised	3 oz	238	25	14	0
chuck arm pot roast lean & fat trim ¼ in braised	3 oz	282	23	20	0
chuck blade roast lean & fat trim 0 in braised	3 oz	284	23	21	0
chuck blade roast lean & fat trim ¼ in braised	3 oz	293	23	22	0

FOOD	PORTION	CALS	PROT	FAT	CARB
corned beef brisket cooked	3 oz	213	15	16	tr
eye of round lean & fat trim 0 in Choice roasted	3 oz	153	24	5	0
eye of round lean & fat trim 0 in Select roasted	3 oz	137	24	4	0
eye of round lean & fat trim ¼ in Choice roasted	3 oz	205	23	12	0
eye of round lean & fat trime ¼ in Select roasted	3 oz	184	23	10	0
flank lean & fat trim 0 in braised	3 oz	224	23	14	0
flank lean & fat trim 0 in broiled	3 oz	192	22	11	0
ground extra lean broiled medium	3 oz	217	22	14	0
ground extra lean broiled well done	3 oz	225	24	14	0
ground extra lean fried medium	3 oz	216	21	14	0
ground extra lean fried well done	3 oz	224	24	14	0
ground extra lean raw	4 oz	265	21	19	0
ground lean broiled medium	3 oz	231	21	16	0
ground lean broiled well done	3 oz	238	24	15	0
ground regular broiled medium	3 oz	246	20	18	0
ground regular broiled well done	3 oz	248	23	17	0
ground low-fat w/ carrageenan raw	4 oz	160	20	7	tr
porterhouse steak lean & fat trim ¼ in Choice broiled	3 oz	260	21	19	0
porterhouse steak lean only trim ¼ in Prime broiled	3 oz	185	24	9	0
rib eye small end lean & fat trim 0 in Choice broiled	3 oz	261	21	19	0
rib large end lean & fat trim 0 in roasted	3 oz	300	20	24	0
rib large end lean & fat trim ¼ in broiled	3 oz	295	18	24	0
rib large end lean & fat trim ¼ in roasted	3 oz	310	19	25	0

FOOD	PORTION	CALS	PROT	FAT	CARB
rib small end lean & fat trim 0 in broiled	3 oz	252	21	18	0
rib small end lean & fat trim ¼ in broiled	3 oz	285	20	22	0
rib small end lean & fat trim ¼ in roasted	3 oz	295	19	24	0
rib whole lean & fat trim ¼ in Choice broiled	3 oz	306	19	25	0
rib whole lean & fat trim ¼ in Choice roasted	3 oz	320	19	27	0
rib whole lean & fat trim ¼ in Prime roasted	3 oz	348	19	30	0
rib whole lean & fat trim ¼ in Select broiled	3 oz	274	19	21	0
rib whole lean & fat trim ¼ in Select roasted	3 oz	286	19	23	0
shank crosscut lean & fat trim ¼ in Choice simmered	3 oz	224	26	12	0
short loin top loin lean & fat trim 0 in Choice broiled	3 oz	193	23	10	0
short loin top loin lean & fat trim 0 in Choice broiled	1 steak (5.4 oz)	353	43	19	0
short loin top loin lean & fat trim 0 in Select broiled	1 steak (5.4 oz)	309	44	14	0
short loin top loin lean & fat trim ¼ in Choice braised	3 oz	253	22	18	0
short loin top loin lean & fat trim ¼ in Choice broiled	1 steak (6.3 oz)	536	46	38	0
short loin top loin lean & fat trim ¼ in Prime broiled	1 steak (6.3 oz)	582	46	43	0
short loin top loin lean & fat trim ¼ in Select broiled	1 steak (6.3 oz)	473	46	31	0
short loin top loin lean only trim 0 in Choice broiled	1 steak (5.2 oz)	311	43	14	0
short loin top loin lean only trim ¼ in Choice broiled	1 steak (5.2 oz)	314	42	15	0
shortribs lean & fat Choice braised	3 oz	400	18	36	0
t-bone steak lean & fat trim ¼ in Choice broiled	3 oz	253	21	18	0
t-bone steak lean only trim ¼ in Choice broiled	3 oz	182	24	9	0
tenderloin lean & fat trim 0 in Select broiled	3 oz	194	23	11	0
tenderloin lean & fat trim ¼ in Choice broiled	3 oz	259	21	19	0

FOOD	PORTION	CALS	PROT	FAT	CARB
tenderloin lean & fat trim ¼ in Choice roasted	3 oz	288	20	22	0
tenderloin lean & fat trim ¼ in Choice broiled	3 oz	208	23	12	0
tenderloin lean & fat trim ¼ in Prime broiled	3 oz	270	21	20	0
tenderloin lean & fat trim ¼ in Select roasted	3 oz	275	21	21	0
tenderloin lean only trim 0 in Select broiled	3 oz	170	24	7	0
tenderloin lean only trim ¼ in Choice broiled	3 oz	188	24	10	0
tenderloin lean only trim ¼ in Select broiled	3 oz	169	24	7	0
tip round lean & fat trim 0 in Choice roasted	3 oz	170	24	8	0
tip round lean & fat trim 0 in Select roasted	3 oz	158	24	6	0
tip round lean & fat trim ¼ in Choice roasted	3 oz	210	23	13	0
tip round lean & fat trim ¼ in Prime roasted	3 oz	233	22	15	0
tip round lean & fat trim ¼ in Select roasted	3 oz	191	23	10	0
top round lean & fat trim 0 in Choice braised	3 oz	184	30	6	0
top round lean & fat trim 0 in Select braised	3 oz	170	30	5	0
top round lean & fat trim ¼ in Choice braised	3 oz	221	29	11	0
top round lean & fat trim ¼ in Choice broiled	3 oz	190	26	9	0
top round lean & fat trim ¼ in Choice fried	3 oz	235	28	13	0
top round lean & fat trim ¼ in Prime broiled	3 oz	195	26	9	0
top round lean & fat trim ¼ in Select braised	3 oz	175	26	7	0
top round lean & fat trim ¼ in Select braised	3 oz	199	29	8	0
top sirloin lean & fat trim 0 in Choice broiled	3 oz	194	25	10	0
top sirloin lean & fat trim 0 in Select broiled	3 oz	166	25	6	0
top sirloin lean & fat trim ¼ in Choice broiled	3 oz	228	23	14	0
top sirloin lean & fat trim ¼ in Choice fried	3 oz	277	24	19	0

FOOD	PORTION	CALS	PROT	FAT	CARB
top sirloin lean & fat trim ¼ in Select broiled	3 oz	208	24	12	0
tripe raw	4 oz	111	16	4	0
Organic Valley					
Extra Lean Ground	3 oz	130	18	6	0
Extra Lean Patties	1 (3.2 oz)	130	19	6	0
frozen					
patties broiled medium	3 oz	240	21	17	0
ready-to-eat					
Alpine Lace					
Roast Beef 97% Fat Free	2 oz	70	13	2	1
Boar's Head					
Corned Beef Brisket	2 oz	80	12	4	0
Eye Round Pepper Seasoned	2 oz	90	14	3	0
Italian Style Oven Roasted Top Round	2 oz	80	12	2	2
Roast Beef Cajun	2 oz	80	14	3	0
Top Round Deluxe	2 oz	90	14	3	0
Top Round Oven Roasted No Salt Added	2 oz	90	14	3	0
Tyson					
Beef Strips Seasoned	1 serv (3 oz)	140	20	6	1
take-out					
roast beef medium	2 oz	70	12	2	0
roast beef rare	2 oz	70	12	2	0
BEEF DISHES					
canned					
corned beef hash	3 oz	155	10	10	9
Armour					
Corned Beef Hash	1 cup (8.3 oz)	440	19	30	23
Corned Beef Hash w/ Peppers & Onions	1 cup (8.3 oz)	270	19	30	23
Roast Beef Hash	1 cup (8.4 oz)	400	20	25	23
Roast Beef In Gravy	½ cup (4.6 oz)	150	25	4	3
Stew	1 cup (8.6 oz)	220	8	12	21
Dinty Moore					
Meatball Stew	1 cup (8.4 oz)	250	13	15	17
Sliced Potatoes & Beef	1 can (7.5 oz)	230	10	9	28
Stew	1 cup (8.3 oz)	230	11	14	16
Hormel					
Beef Goulash	1 can (7.5 oz)	230	13	11	19
Roast Beef w/ Gravy	2 oz	60	11	2	1
Mary Kitchen					
Corned Beef Hash	1 cup (8.3 oz)	410	21	27	22
Corned Beef Hash 50% Reduced Fat	1 cup (8.3 oz)	280	19	12	25

FOOD	PORTION	CALS	PROT	FAT	CARB
Roast Beef Hash	1 cup (8.3 oz)	390	21	24	22
Sausage Hash	1 cup (8.3 oz)	410	20	27	23
frozen					
Banquet					
Sandwich Toppers Creamed Chipped Beef	1 pkg (4 oz)	120	7	6	8
Sandwich Toppers Gravy & Salisbury Steak	1 pkg (5 oz)	210	9	16	8
Sandwich Toppers Gravy & Sliced Beef	1 pkg (4 oz)	70	8	2	5
mix					
Hamburger Helper					
BBQ Beef as prep	1 cup	320	21	10	37
Beef Pasta as prep	1 cup	270	20	10	26
Beef Romanoff as prep	1 cup	280	20	10	27
Beef Stew as prep	1 cup	260	18	10	26
Beef Taco as prep	1 cup	280	19	10	31
Beef Teriyaki as prep	1 cup	290	18	10	34
Cheddar & Broccoli as prep	1 cup	350	22	15	33
Cheddar Melt as prep	1 cup	310	20	12	31
Cheddar'n Bacon as prep	1 cup	330	23	15	27
Cheeseburger Macaroni as prep	1 cup	360	23	16	33
Cheesy Hashbrowns as prep	1 cup	400	21	19	39
Cheesy Italian as prep	1 cup	320	22	14	28
Cheesy Shells as prep	1 cup	330	21	15	30
Chili Macaroni as prep	1 cup	290	20	10	30
Fettuccine Alfredo as prep	1 cup	300	20	13	26
Four Cheese Lasagne as prep	1 cup	330	21	14	31
Italian Parmesan w/ Rigatoni as prep	1 cup	300	20	11	31
Lasagne as prep	1 cup	270	19	10	29
Meat Loaf as prep	⅕ loaf	270	24	14	11
Meaty Spaghetti & Cheese as prep	1 cup	290	20	10	30
Mushroom & Wild Rice as prep	1 cup	310	20	12	30
Nacho Cheese as prep	1 cup	320	22	13	30
Pizza Pasta w/ Cheese Topping as prep	1 cup	280	19	10	31
Pizzabake as prep	⅙ pie	270	17	10	28
Potatoes Au Gratin as prep	1 cup	280	18	13	25
Potatoes Stroganoff as prep	1 cup	250	17	11	23
Reduced Sodium Cheddar Spirals as prep	1 cup	300	20	13	27

FOOD	PORTION	CALS	PROT	FAT	CARB
Reduced Sodium Italian Herby as prep	1 cup	270	19	10	29
Reduced Sodium Southwestern Beef as prep	1 cup	300	20	10	32
Rice Oriental as prep	1 cup	280	18	10	32
Salisbury as prep	1 cup	270	19	10	26
Spaghetti as prep	1 cup	270	19	10	27
Stroganoff as prep	1 cup	320	21	13	30
Swedish Meatballs as prep	1 cup	290	19	14	25
Three Cheeses as prep	1 cup	340	21	15	32
Zesty Italian as prep	1 cup	300	20	10	32
Zesty Mexican as prep	1 cup	280	19	10	31
ready-to-eat					
Thomas E. Wilson					
Roast Beef In Brown Gravy	1 serv + gravy (3.5 oz)	160	22	6	3
shelf-stable					
Dinty Moore					
Microwave Cup Corned Beef Hash	1 pkg (7.5 oz)	350	19	22	19
Microwave Cup Hearty Burger Stew	1 pkg (7.5 oz)	240	12	13	19
Microwave Cup Stew	1 pkg (7.5 oz)	190	11	10	15
Hormel					
Microcup Meals Stew	1 cup (7.5 oz)	190	11	10	15
Lunch Bucket					
Beef Stew	1 pkg (7.5 oz)	170	6	9	17
TastyBite					
Beef Roganjosh	1 pkg (9.5 oz)	270	18	15	19
Meatballs Vindaloo	1 pkg (9.5 oz)	270	12	18	17
take-out					
beef bouriguignon	1 serv (7 oz)	254	23	16	3
bubble & squeak	5 oz	186	2	13	16
bulgoghi korean grilled beef	1 serv (5.2 oz)	256	23	15	5
cornish pasty	1 (8 oz)	847	20	52	79
greek moussaka	1 serv (8.5 oz)	450	24	33	12
irish stew	1 cup (7 oz)	280	23	16	10
kebab indian	1 (5.4 oz)	553	47	40	2
kheena	6.7 oz	781	34	71	1
koftas	5	280	18	22	3
samosa	2 (4 oz)	652	6	62	20
shepherds pie	1 serv (7 oz)	282	16	16	20
steak & kidney pie w/ top crust	1 slice (5 oz)	400	21	26	23
stew	6 oz	208	17	13	6

FOOD	PORTION	CALS	PROT	FAT	CARB
stew w/ vegetables	1 cup	220	16	11	15
stroganoff	¾ cup	260	14	19	43
swiss steak	4.6 oz	214	23	9	10
toad in the hole	1 (4.7 oz)	383	10	29	23
BEEFALO					
roasted	3 oz	160	26	5	0
BEER AND ALE					
alcohol free beer	7 fl oz	50	1	tr	11
ale brown	10 oz	77	1	0	8
ale pale	10 oz	88	1	0	12
beer regular	12 oz can	146	1	0	13
lager	10 oz	80	1	0	4
pilsener lager beer	7 fl oz	85	1	tr	13
stout	10 oz	102	1	0	6
BEET JUICE					
juice	7 oz	72	2	0	16
BEETS					
canned					
harvard	½ cup	89	1	tr	22
pickled	½ cup	75	1	tr	19
sliced	½ cup	27	1	tr	6
Del Monte					
Pickled Crinkle Style Sliced	½ cup (4.5 oz)	80	1	0	19
Sliced	½ cup (4.3 oz)	35	1	0	8
Whole	½ cup (4.3 oz)	35	1	0	8
Green Giant					
Sliced	½ cup (4.2 oz)	35	1	0	8
Sliced No Salt Added	½ cup (4.2 oz)	35	1	0	8
Whole	½ cup (4.2 oz)	35	1	0	8
LeSueur					
Baby Whole	½ cup (4.3 oz)	35	1	0	8
S&W					
Julienne	½ cup (4.3 oz)	30	1	0	7
Pickled Sliced	1 oz	15	0	0	4
Sliced	½ cup (4.3 oz)	30	1	0	7
Whole Small	½ cup (4.3 oz)	30	1	0	7
fresh					
greens cooked	½ cup	20	2	tr	4
sliced cooked	½ cup (3 oz)	38	1	tr	9
whole cooked	2 (3.5 oz)	44	2	tr	10
whole raw	2 (5.7 oz)	70	3	tr	16
BEVERAGES					

(*see* BEER AND ALE, CHAMPAGNE, COFFEE, DRINK MIXERS, ENERGY DRINKS, FRUIT DRINKS, ICED TEA, LIQUOR/LIQUEUR, MALT, MILKSHAKE, SODA, TEA/HERBAL TEA, WATER, WINE, WINE COOLER)

FOOD	PORTION	CALS	PROT	FAT	CARB
BISCUIT					
mix					
buttermilk	1 (2 oz)	191	4	7	28

FOOD	PORTION	CALS	PROT	FAT	CARB
Bisquick					
Buttermilk	½ cup	150	2	6	21
Cheese Garlic	½ cup	160	2	7	22
Cinnamon Swirl	½ cup	150	2	4	30
Mix	⅓ cup (1.4 oz)	160	3	6	25
Reduced Fat	⅓ cup	140	3	3	27
Kentucky Kernel					
Biscuit	¼ cup (1 oz)	171	3	5	28
ready-to-eat					
oatcakes	2 (4 oz)	115	3	5	16
refrigerated					
buttermilk	1 (1 oz)	98	2	4	14
plain	1 (1 oz)	98	2	4	14
1869 Brand					
Buttermilk	1 (1.1 oz)	100	2	5	12
Hungry Jack					
Butter Tastin' Flaky	1 (1.2 oz)	100	2	5	14
Cinnamon & Sugar	1 (1.2 oz)	110	2	4	17
Flaky	1 (1.2 oz)	100	2	5	14
Flaky Buttermilk	1 (1.2 oz)	100	2	5	14
Pillsbury					
Big Country Butter Tastin'	1 (1.2 oz)	100	2	4	13
Big Country Buttermilk	1 (1.2 oz)	100	2	4	14
Big Country Southern Style	1 (1.2 oz)	100	2	4	14
Buttermilk	1 (2.2 oz)	150	4	2	29
Country	1 (2.2 oz)	150	4	2	29
Grands Blueberry	1 (2.1 oz)	210	4	9	29
Grands Butter Tastin'	1 (2.1 oz)	200	4	10	24
Grands Buttermilk	1 (2.1 oz)	200	4	10	24
Grands Buttermilk Reduced Fat	1 (2.1 oz)	190	4	7	27
Grands Extra Rich	1 (2.1 oz)	220	4	12	25
Grands Flaky	1 (2.1 oz)	200	4	9	25
Grands Golden Corn	1 (1.2 oz)	210	4	10	26
Grands HomeStyle	1 (2.1 oz)	210	4	10	25
Grands Southern Style	1 (2.1 oz)	200	4	10	24
Southern Style Flaky	1 (1.2 oz)	100	2	5	14
Tender Layer Buttermilk	1 (2.2 oz)	160	4	5	27
take-out					
buttermilk	1 (2 oz)	212	4	10	27
plain	1 (35 g)	276	4	34	13
tea biscuit	1 (3 oz)	210	5	3	30
w/ egg	1 (4.8 oz)	316	11	20	24
w/ egg & bacon	1 (5.2 oz)	458	17	31	29
w/ egg & ham	1 (6.7 oz)	442	20	27	30
w/ egg & sausage	1 (6.3 oz)	581	19	39	41
w/ egg & steak	1 (5.2 oz)	410	18	28	21
w/ egg cheese & bacon	1 (5.1 oz)	477	16	31	33

FOOD	PORTION	CALS	PROT	FAT	CARB
w/ ham	1 (4 oz)	386	13	18	44
w/ sausage	1 (4.4 oz)	485	12	32	40
w/ steak	1 (4.9 oz)	455	13	26	44
BISON					
roasted	3 oz	122	24	2	0
BLACK BEANS					
canned					
Eden					
Organic	½ cup (4.6 oz)	100	7	0	18
Green Giant					
Black Beans	½ cup (4.5 oz)	50	6	0	18
Progresso					
Black Beans	½ cup (4.6 oz)	110	7	1	17
dried					
cooked	1 cup	227	15	1	41
mix					
Bean Cuisine					
Pasta & Beans Mediterranean Black Beans & Fusilli	1 serv	210	7	1	30
BLACKBERRIES					
canned in heavy syrup	½ cup	118	2	tr	30
fresh	½ cup	37	1	tr	9
unsweetened frzn	1 cup	97	2	1	24
BLACKEYE PEAS					
canned					
w/pork	½ cup	199	7	4	40
Eden					
Organic	½ cup (4.6 oz)	90	6	1	16
Green Giant					
Blackeye Peas	½ cup (4.4 oz)	90	6	0	16
dried					
cooked	1 cup	198	13	1	36
Hurst					
HamBeens California w/ Ham	1 serv	120	8	1	22
frozen					
Birds Eye					
Blackeye Peas	½ cup (2.8 oz)	110	7	1	21
BLINTZE					
Golden					
Cheese	1 (2.1 oz)	80	6	2	13
take-out					
cheese	1 (2.7 oz)	160	5	9	15
BLUEBERRIES					
canned in heavy syrup	1 cup	225	2	1	56
fresh	1 cup	82	1	1	20
unsweetened frzn	1 cup	78	1	1	19
Tree Of Life					
Organic	1 cup (5 oz)	80	1	0	20

FOOD	PORTION	CALS	PROT	FAT	CARB
BLUEFIN					
fillet baked	4.1 oz	186	30	6	0
BLUEFISH					
fresh baked	3 oz	135	22	5	0
BOAR					
wild roasted	3 oz	136	24	4	0
BOK CHOY					
(*see* CABBAGE)					
BONITO					
fresh	3 oz	117	20	4	0
BORAGE					
fresh chopped cooked	3½ oz	25	2	1	4
BOTTLED WATER					
(*see* WATER)					
BOYSENBERRIES					
in heavy syrup	1 cup	226	3	tr	57
unsweetened frzn	1 cup	66	1	tr	16
BRAINS					
beef pan-fried	3 oz	167	11	13	0
beef simmered	3 oz	136	9	11	0
lamb braised	3 oz	124	11	9	0
lamb fried	3 oz	232	14	19	0
pork braised	3 oz	117	10	8	0
veal braised	3 oz	115	10	8	0
veal fried	3 oz	181	12	14	0
Armour					
Pork Brains In Milk Gravy	⅔ cup (5.5 oz)	150	16	5	10
BRAN					
corn	1 cup (2.7 oz)	170	6	1	65
oat	½ cup (1.6 oz)	116	8	3	31
oat cooked	½ cup (3.8 oz)	44	4	1	13
rice	½ cup (2.1 oz)	187	8	12	29
wheat	½ cup (2 oz)	63	5	1	19
Hodgson Mill					
Oat	¼ cup (1.4 oz)	120	6	3	23
Quaker					
Oat Bran	½ cup (1.4 oz)	150	7	3	25
BRAZIL NUTS					
dried unblanched	1 oz	186	4	19	4
BREAD					
(*see also* BAGEL, BISCUIT, BREADSTICK, CROISSANT, ENGLISH MUFFIN, MUFFIN, ROLL, SCONE)					
canned					
boston brown	1 slice (1.6 oz)	88	2	1	20
frozen					
Marie Callender's					
Cornbread & Honey Butter	1 piece + butter	210	2	11	28
Original Garlic	1 piece	190	4	8	23

FOOD	PORTION	CALS	PROT	FAT	CARB
Parmesan & Romano Garlic	1 piece	200	5	10	23
New York					
Garlic	1 slice (2 oz)	190	3	8	27
Garlic Reduced Fat	1 slice (2 oz)	160	4	4	29
Texas Garlic Toast	1 in slice (1.4 oz)	160	3	9	17
Pepperidge Farm					
Garlic	1 slice (1.8 oz)	170	5	10	15
Garlic Sourdough 30% Reduced Fat	1 slice (1.8 oz)	170	6	7	22
Monterey Jack Jalapeno Cheese	1 slice (2 oz)	145	5	11	22
Mozzeralla Garlic Cheese	1 slice (2 oz)	201	6	10	21
mix					
cornbread	1 piece (2 oz)	189	4	6	29
Hodgson Mill					
European Cheese & Herb	¼ cup (1.2 oz)	130	5	1	21
Honey Whole Wheat	¼ cup (1.2 oz)	120	5	1	22
ready-to-eat					
baguette whole wheat	2 oz	140	6	0	29
challah	1 slice (2 oz)	160	3	3	29
cracked wheat	1 slice	65	2	1	12
egg	1 slice (1.4 oz)	115	4	2	19
french	1 slice (1 oz)	78	3	1	15
french	1 loaf (1 lb)	1270	43	18	230
gluten	1 slice	47	2	tr	8
italian	1 loaf (1 lb)	1255	41	4	256
italian	1 slice (1 oz)	81	3	1	15
navajo fry	1 (10.5 in diam)	527	11	15	85
navajo fry	1 (5 in diam)	296	6	9	48
oat bran	1 slice	71	3	1	12
oat bran reduced calorie	1 slice	46	2	1	10
oatmeal	1 slice	73	2	1	13
oatmeal reduced calorie	1 slice	48	2	1	10
pita	1 reg (2 oz)	165	5	1	33
pita	1 sm (1 oz)	78	3	tr	16
pita whole wheat	1 reg (2 oz)	170	6	2	35
pita whole wheat	1 sm (1 oz)	76	3	1	16
protein	1 slice	47	2	tr	8
pumpernickel	1 slice	80	3	1	15
raisin	1 slice	71	2	1	14
rice bran	1 slice	66	1	1	12
rye	1 slice	83	3	1	16
rye reduced calorie	1 slice	47	2	1	9
seven grain	1 slice	65	3	1	12
sourdough	1 slice (1 oz)	78	3	1	15
vienna	1 slice (1 oz)	78	3	1	15

FOOD	PORTION	CALS	PROT	FAT	CARB
wheat reduced calorie	1 slice	46	2	1	10
wheat berry	1 slice	65	2	1	12
wheat bran	1 slice	89	3	1	17
wheat germ	1 slice	74	3	1	14
white	1 slice	67	2	1	12
white reduced calorie	1 slice	48	2	1	10
white toasted	1 slice	67	2	1	13
white cubed	1 cup	80	2	1	15
whole wheat	1 slice	70	3	1	13
Arnold					
Bran'nola Country Oat	1 slice (1.3 oz)	110	4	2	20
Country Buttermilk	1 slice (1.3 oz)	110	4	2	20
Country Wheat	1 slice (1.3 oz)	100	4	2	19
Natural 100% Whole Wheat	1 slice (1.3 oz)	90	4	1	16
Raisin Cinnamon	1 slice (1 oz)	80	2	2	15
Bread Du Jour					
French	3 in slice (2 oz)	140	5	1	26
Damascus					
Pita	1 (2 oz)	130	6	0	29
Pita Whole Wheat	1 (2 oz)	160	6	0	32
Wraps Honey Wheat	½ wrap (2 oz)	130	5	0	28
Wraps Plain	½ wrap (2 oz)	130	5	0	29
Wraps Spinach	1 (2 oz)	280	10	0	56
Wraps Tomato	1 12-inch (4 oz)	240	10	0	58
Home Pride					
Wheat	1 slice (1 oz)	80	2	1	14
La Mexicana					
Wraps Chocolate	1 (1.3 oz)	120	4	3	18
Wraps Southwestern Mild Chili	1 (1.3 oz)	120	4	4	18
Wraps Spinach	1 (1.3 oz)	120	4	4	18
Wraps Tomato Basil	1 (1.3 oz)	120	4	4	18
Milton's					
Healthy Multi-Grain	1 slice (1.4 oz)	110	3	1	24
Pepperidge Farm					
Apple Cinammon	1 slice (1 oz)	80	4	2	15
Deli Swirl Rye & Pump	1 slice (1.1 oz)	80	3	1	15
Farmhouse Hearty White	1 slice (1.5 oz)	110	5	2	20
Farmhouse Sourdough	1 slice (1.5 oz)	110	4	2	20
Natural Whole Grain Whole Wheat	1 slice (1.2 oz)	90	4	1	16
Natural Whole Grain Honey Oat	1 slice (1.2 oz)	90	4	2	15
Sandwich Pocket Wheat	1 (2 oz)	160	6	1	30
Sandwich Pocket White	1 (2 oz)	150	6	1	30
Swirl Cinnamon	1 slice (1 oz)	90	2	3	15
Swirl Raisin Cinnamon	1 slice (1 oz)	80	3	2	14

FOOD	PORTION	CALS	PROT	FAT	CARB
Stroehmann					
100% Whole Wheat	1 slice (1.3 oz)	90	5	1	17
D'Italiano Italian No Seeds	1 slice (1 oz)	80	2	1	15
D'Italiano Italian Seeded	1 slice (1 oz)	80	2	1	15
Family White	1 slice (0.8 oz)	65	2	1	13
Homestyle Split Top Wheat	1 slices (0.8 oz)	60	2	0	13
Homestyle Split Top White	1 slice (0.8 oz)	65	2	1	12
Honey Cracked Wheat	1 slice (1.2 oz)	80	3	1	16
King White	1 slice (0.8 oz)	65	2	1	13
Potato	1 slice (1.2 oz)	100	3	2	19
Ranch White	1 slice (0.8 oz)	65	2	1	13
Rye	1 slice (1.1 oz)	80	3	1	15
Rye w/ Caraway	1 slice (1.1 oz)	80	3	1	15
Twelve Grain	1 slice (1.2 oz)	90	3	1	17
TastyBite					
Nan Kontos Massala	½ loaf (1.4 oz)	120	7	3	15
Nan Kontos Onion	½ loaf (1.4 oz)	120	7	4	15
Nan Kontos Roghani	½ loaf (1.4 oz)	125	4	3	19
Nan Kontos Tandoori	½ loaf (1.4 oz)	120	4	3	19
Roti Kontos Missy	½ loaf (1.4 oz)	125	5	4	18
Valley Lahvosh					
Valley Wraps	1 (1 oz)	100	4	1	19
refrigerated					
Pillsbury					
Crusty French Loaf	⅕ loaf (2.2 oz)	150	5	2	27
Grands Wheat	1 (2.1 oz)	200	4	8	27
take-out					
chapatis as prep w/ fat	1 bread (1.6 oz)	95	3	2	18
chapatis as prep w/o fat	1 (2½ oz)	141	5	1	31
cornbread	2 in x 2 in (1.4 oz)	107	4	2	18
cornstick	1 (1.3 oz)	101	2	4	13
focaccia onion	1 piece (4.6 oz)	282	6	10	43
focaccia rosemary	1 piece (3.5 oz)	251	6	7	40
focaccia tomato olive	1 piece (4.7 oz)	270	6	8	42
garlic bread	2 slices (2 oz)	190	3	8	27
irish soda bread	1 slice (2 oz)	174	4	3	34
naan	1 bread (3.5 oz)	286	7	9	43
papadums fried	2 (1.5 oz)	81	4	4	9
paratha	1 bread (2.1 oz)	201	4	10	23
BREAD COATING					
Don's Chuck Wagon					
Chicken Baking Mix	¼ cup (1 oz)	95	3	0	21
Fish & Chips Mix	¼ cup (1 oz)	100	3	0	21
Fish Mix	¼ cup (1 oz)	95	4	0	21
Mushroom Batter Mix	¼ cup (1 oz)	95	3	0	21
Onion Ring Mix	¼ cup (1 oz)	100	3	0	21
Seafood Bake & Fry Mix	¼ cup (1 oz)	95	2	0	21

FOOD	PORTION	CALS	PROT	FAT	CARB
Luzianne					
Cajun Chicken Coating Mix	2 tbsp (1 oz)	100	3	1	20
Oven Fry					
Extra Crispy For Chicken	⅛ pkg (0.5 oz)	60	2	1	10
Extra Crispy For Pork	⅛ pkg (0.5 oz)	60	2	2	11
Shake 'N Bake					
Classic Italian Chicken or Pork	⅛ pkg (0.4 oz)	40	1	1	7
Hot & Spicy Chicken or Pork	⅛ pkg (0.4 oz)	40	1	1	7
Original For Chicken	⅛ pkg (0.4 oz)	40	1	1	7
Original For Fish	¼ pkg (0.7 oz)	80	2	2	14
Original For Pork	⅛ pkg (0.4 oz)	45	1	1	8
BREAD MACHINE MIX					
Fleischmann's					
Apple Cinnamon	⅛ loaf	160	5	1	32
Cinnamon Raisin	⅛ loaf	160	5	1	33
Country White	⅛ loaf (1.6 oz)	170	6	3	31
Cranberry Orange	⅛ loaf	150	2	2	33
Honey Oatmeal	⅛ loaf	160	5	1	33
Italian Herb	⅛ loaf	160	5	2	29
Sourdough	⅛ loaf	150	5	2	29
Stoneground Wheat	⅛ loaf	160	5	1	32
BREADCRUMBS					
dry	1 cup	426	14	6	78
dry seasonsed	1 cup (4 oz)	441	17	3	85
fresh	⅔ cup	76	4	1	14
Progresso					
Garlic & Herb	¼ cup (1 oz)	100	4	2	18
Italian Style	¼ cup (1 oz)	110	4	2	20
Parmesan	¼ cup (1 oz)	100	4	2	17
Plain	¼ cup (1 oz)	110	4	2	19
BREADFRUIT					
fresh	¼ small	99	1	tr	26
seeds cooked	1 oz	48	2	1	9
seeds raw	1 oz	54	2	2	8
seeds roasted	1 oz	59	2	tr	11
BREADNUTTREE SEEDS					
dried	1 oz	104	2	tr	23
BREADSTICKS					
onion poppyseed	1	64	2	1	11
plain	1 sm	25	1	1	4
plain	1	41	1	1	7
Bread Du Jour					
Original	1 (1.9 oz)	130	5	1	25
Sourdough	1 (1.9 oz)	130	5	1	25
New York					
Garlic Soft	1 (1.5 oz)	140	3	4	23

FOOD	PORTION	CALS	PROT	FAT	CARB
Pillsbury					
Soft	1 (1.4 oz)	110	3	2	19
Soft Garlic & Herb	1 (2.1 oz)	180	4	7	25
Stella D'Oro					
Garlic	1 (0.4 oz)	40	1	1	7
Grissini Style Fat Free	3 (0.5 oz)	60	2	0	12
Original	1 (0.4 oz)	45	1	1	7
Potato 'N Onion	1 (0.4 oz)	45	1	1	8
Roasted Garlic	1 (0.4 oz)	45	1	1	8
Sesame	1 (0.4 oz)	50	1	3	7
Snack Stix Cracked Pepper	4 (0.5 oz)	70	2	2	11
Snack Stix Salted	4 (0.5 oz)	70	2	2	11
Sodium Free	1 (0.4 oz)	45	1	1	7
Wheat	1 (0.3 oz)	40	1	1	6

BREAKFAST BAR
(*see* CEREAL BARS, ENERGY BARS)

BREAKFAST DRINKS
(*see also* ENERGY DRINKS, NUTRITION SUPPLEMENTS)

FOOD	PORTION	CALS	PROT	FAT	CARB
Carnation					
Instant Breakfast Vanilla as prep w/ skim milk	1 serv	220	13	1	39
Instant Breakfast Vanilla as prep w/ whole milk	1 serv	280	13	8	39

BROAD BEANS

FOOD	PORTION	CALS	PROT	FAT	CARB
canned	1 cup	183	14	1	32
dried cooked	1 cup	186	13	1	33
fresh cooked	3½ oz	56	5	tr	10

BROCCOFLOWER

FOOD	PORTION	CALS	PROT	FAT	CARB
fresh raw	½ cup (1.8 oz)	16	1	tr	3

BROCCOLI

FOOD	PORTION	CALS	PROT	FAT	CARB
fresh					
chinese broccoli (gai lan) cooked	1 cup (3.1 oz)	19	1	1	3
chopped cooked	½ cup	22	2	tr	4
frozen					
chopped cooked	½ cup	25	3	tr	5
spears cooked	½ cup	25	3	tr	5
spears cooked	10 oz pkg	69	8	tr	13
Amy's Organic					
Pocket Sandwich Broccoli & Cheese	1 (4.5 oz)	270	8	10	37
Birds Eye					
Florets	1 cup (3 oz)	25	2	0	4
In Cheese Sauce	½ cup (4 oz)	70	3	4	7
Green Giant					
Butter Sauce	4 oz	50	2	2	7
Cheese Sauce	⅔ cup (3.9 oz)	70	3	3	9
Chopped	¾ cup (2.8 oz)	25	2	0	4

FOOD	PORTION	CALS	PROT	FAT	CARB
Cuts	1 cup (2.9 oz)	25	2	0	4
Harvest Fresh Cut	⅔ cup (3.2 oz)	25	2	0	4
Harvest Fresh Spears	3.5 oz	25	2	0	4
Select Florets	1⅓ cups (2.9 oz)	25	2	0	4
Select Spears	3 oz	25	2	0	4
Health Is Wealth					
Broccoli Munchees	2 (1 oz)	60	2	2	10
Stouffer's					
Au Gratin	1 serv (4 oz)	100	5	4	10
Tree Of Life					
Cuts	1 cup (3.1 oz)	25	2	0	4
BROWNIE					
frozen					
Greenfield					
Fat Free Homestyle	1 (1.3 oz)	110	2	0	27
Otis Spunkmeyer					
Blue Yonder w/ Walnuts	1 (2 oz)	230	3	10	34
Weight Watchers					
Brownie A La Mode	1 (3.14 oz)	190	5	4	33
Double Fudge Brownie Parfait	1 (5.3 oz)	190	6	3	39
home recipe					
plain	1 (0.8 oz)	112	2	7	12
w/nuts	1 (0.8 oz)	95	1	6	11
mix					
plain	1 (1.2 oz)	139	1	7	20
plain low calorie	1 (0.8 oz)	84	1	2	16
Betty Crocker					
Chocolate Chunk as prep	1	180	1	9	25
Dark Chocolate Fudge as prep	1	170	1	7	24
Dark Chocolate w/ Syrup as prep	1	170	2	7	25
Fudge as prep	1	170	1	7	23
German Chocolate Coconut Pecan Filling as prep	1	200	1	8	29
Hot Fudge as prep	1	170	2	8	23
Original as prep	1	180	1	6	27
Peanut Butter as prep	1	180	3	8	23
Stir'n Bake w/ Mini Kisses as prep	1 serv	220	2	7	38
Turtle w/ Caramel & Pecans as prep	1	170	1	8	25
Walnut as prep	1	180	2	9	23
No Pudge!					
Cappuccino Fudge	1	100	2	0	21
Mint Fudge	½ cup	100	2	0	21
Original Fudge	1	100	2	0	21
Raspberry Fudge	1	100	2	0	21

FOOD	PORTION	CALS	PROT	FAT	CARB
Sweet Rewards					
Low Fat Fudge as prep	1	130	2	3	27
Reduced Fat Supreme as prep	1	140	2	3	27
ready-to-eat					
plain	1 sm (1 oz)	115	1	5	18
plain	1 lg (2 oz)	227	3	9	36
w/ nuts	1 (1 oz)	100	1	4	16
Dolly Madison					
Fudge	1 (3 oz)	330	3	11	54
Entenmann's					
Little Bites	3 (2.2 oz)	290	3	16	37
Ultimate Fudge	1 (1.6 oz)	220	3	13	27
Greenfield					
Blondie Fat Free Apple Spice	1 (1.3 oz)	110	2	0	26
Health Valley					
Bar w/ Fudge Filling	1 bar	110	3	0	26
Hostess					
Brownie Bites	3 (1.3 oz)	170	2	9	21
Fudge	1 (3 oz)	330	3	11	54
Light	1 (1.4 oz)	140	1	3	28
Lance					
Fudge Nut	1 (2.25 oz)	340	3	13	56
Little Debbie					
Brownie Lights	1 (2 oz)	190	3	3	39
Brownie Loaves	1 (2.1 oz)	260	3	15	31
Fudge	1 pkg (2.1 oz)	270	2	13	39
Tastykake					
Fudge Walnut	1 (3 oz)	370	5	17	52
Tom's					
Fudge Nut	1 pkg (2.5 oz)	300	3	13	45
refrigerated					
Toll House					
Brownie Dough	½ pkg (1.5 oz)	180	2	7	26
take-out					
plain	1 2 in sq (2.1 oz)	243	3	10	39
BRUSSELS SPROUTS					
fresh					
cooked	½ cup	30	2	tr	7
cooked	1 sprout	8	1	tr	2
frozen					
cooked	½ cup	33	3	tr	6
Birds Eye					
Brussels Sprouts	11 sprouts	35	3	0	7
Green Giant					
Butter Sauce	⅔ cup (3.6 oz)	60	3	2	9

FOOD	PORTION	CALS	PROT	FAT	CARB
BUCKWHEAT					
groats roasted cooked	1 cup (5.9 oz)	647	6	1	34
groats roasted uncooked	1 cup (5.7 oz)	567	19	4	123
BUFFALO					
water buffalo roasted	3 oz	111	23	2	0
BULGUR					
cooked	1 cup (6.3 oz)	151	7	tr	34
uncooked	1 cup (4.9 oz)	479	17	2	106
Hodgson Mill					
Bulgur w/ Soygrits	¼ cup (1.4 oz)	120	6	1	24
BURBOT (FISH)					
fresh baked	3 oz	98	65	1	0
BURDOCK ROOT					
cooked	1 cup	110	3	tr	26
BUTTER					
(*see also* BUTTER BLENDS, BUTTER SUBSTITUTES, MARGARINE)					
stick	1 stick (4 oz)	813	1	92	tr
whipped	4 oz	542	1	61	tr
Breakstone's					
Salted	1 tbsp (0.5 oz)	100	0	11	0
Hotel Bar					
Stick	1 tbsp (0.5 oz)	100	0	11	0
Keller's					
European	1 tbsp (0.5 oz)	100	0	11	0
Land O Lakes					
Salted	1 tbsp (0.5 oz)	100	0	11	0
Ultra Creamy Salted	1 tbsp (0.5 oz)	110	0	12	0
Organic Valley					
Butter	1 tbsp (0.5 oz)	100	0	11	0
Unsalted	1 tbsp (0.5 oz)	110	0	12	0
BUTTER BEANS					
canned					
Green Giant					
Butter Beans	½ cup (4.5 oz)	90	6	0	16
Van Camp					
Butter Beans	½ cup (4.6 oz)	110	8	1	22
frozen					
Birds Eye					
Speckled	½ cup (2.7 oz)	100	6	0	20
BUTTER BLENDS					
(*see also* BUTTER, BUTTER SUBSTITUTES, MARGARINE)					
stick	1 stick	811	1	91	1
Brummel & Brown					
Spread Made w/ Yogurt	1 tbsp (0.5 oz)	50	0	5	0
BUTTERFISH					
baked	3 oz	159	19	9	0
fillet baked	1 oz	47	6	3	0

FOOD	PORTION	CALS	PROT	FAT	CARB
BUTTERNUTS					
dried	1 oz	174	7	16	3
BUTTERSCOTCH					
Nestle					
Morsels	1 tbsp	80	0	4	9
CABBAGE					
(*see also* COLESLAW)					
chinese bok choy shredded cooked	½ cup	10	1	tr	2
chinese pak-choi raw shredded	½ cup	5	1	tr	1
chinese pe-tsai raw shredded	1 cup	12	1	tr	2
chinese pe-tsai shredded cooked	1 cup	16	2	tr	3
danish raw	1 head (2 lbs)	228	13	2	49
danish raw shredded	½ cup (1.2 oz)	9	1	tr	2
danish shredded cooked	½ cup (2.6 oz)	17	1	tr	3
green raw	1 head (2 lbs)	228	12	2	49
green raw shredded	½ cup (1.2 oz)	9	1	tr	2
green shredded cooked	½ cup (2.6 oz)	17	1	tr	3
napa cooked	1 cup (3.8 oz)	13	1	tr	2
red shredded cooked	½ cup	16	1	tr	3
savoy raw shredded	½ cup	10	1	tr	2
savoy shredded cooked	½ cup	18	1	tr	4
take-out					
korean kimchee	½ cup	22	2	tr	4
stuffed cabbage	1 (6 oz)	373	25	22	18
sweet & sour red cabbage	4 oz	61	1	3	8
CACTUS					
napoles fresh sliced	½ cup (1.5 oz)	7	1	tr	1
pricklypear fresh	1 cup (5.3 oz)	56	2	1	13
CAKE					
(*see also* BROWNIE, CAKE MIX, COOKIE, DANISH PASTRY, DOUGHNUT, PIE)					
angelfood	1 cake (11.9 oz)	876	20	3	197
angelfood home recipe	1/12 cake (1.9 oz)	142	4	tr	32
apple crisp home recipe	1 recipe 6 serv (29.6 oz)	1377	15	31	273
battenburg cake	1 slice (2 oz)	204	3	10	28
boston cream pie frzn	1/8 cake (3.2 oz)	232	2	8	40
carrot w/ cream cheese icing home recipe	1 cake 10 in diam	6175	63	328	775
cheesecake	1/8 cake (2.8 oz)	256	4	18	20
cheesecake	1 cake 9 in diam	3350	60	213	317
cheesecake home recipe	1/12 cake (4.5 oz)	456	9	9	32
cherry fudge w/ chocolate frosting	1/8 cake (2.5 oz)	187	2	9	27

FOOD	PORTION	CALS	PROT	FAT	CARB
chocolate cupcake creme filled w/ frosting home recipe	1 (1.8 oz)	188	2	7	30
chocolate w/o frosting home recipe	2 layers (39.9 oz)	4067	60	172	608
chocolate w/o frosting home recipe	½₂ cake (3.3 oz)	340	5	14	51
coffeecake creme-filled chocolate frosting home recipe	⅛ cake (3.2 oz)	298	5	10	49
coffeecake crumb topped cinnamon home recipe	½₂ cake (2.1 oz)	240	4	12	30
coffeecake fruit	⅛ cake (1.8 oz)	156	3	5	26
cream puff shell home recipe	1 (2.3 oz)	239	6	17	15
crumpet	1 (2.3 oz)	131	4	1	31
devil's food cupcake w/ chocolate frosting	1	120	2	4	20
devil's food w/ creme filling	1 (1 oz)	105	1	4	17
eccles cake	1 slice (2 oz)	285	2	16	36
eclair	1 (1.4 oz)	149	2	10	15
eclair home recipe	1 (3 oz)	262	6	16	24
fruitcake	1 piece (1.5 oz)	139	1	4	27
fruitcake dark home recipe	1 cake 7½ in x 2¼ in	5185	74	228	738
jelly roll lemon filled	1 slice (3 oz)	210	3	2	48
madeira cake	1 slice (1 oz)	98	1	4	15
pound	1 cake 8½ x 3½ x 3 in	1935	26	94	257
pound	½₀ cake (1 oz)	117	2	6	15
pound fat free	1 cake (12 oz)	961	18	4	208
pound cake home recipe	1 loaf 8½ in x 3½ in	1935	33	94	265
sheet cake w/ white frosting home recipe	1 cake 9 in sq	4020	37	129	694
sheet cake w/o frosting home recipe	⅑ cake	315	4	12	48
sheet cake w/o frosting home recipe	1 cake 9 in sq	2830	35	108	434
shortcake home recipe	1 (2.3 oz)	225	4	9	32
sour cream pound	½₀ cake (1 oz)	117	1	5	16
sponge	½₂ cake (1.3 oz)	110	2	1	23
sponge home recipe	½₂ cake (2.2 oz)	140	3	2	27
sponge cake dessert shell	1 (0.8 oz)	75	2	1	16
sponge w/ creme filling	1 (1.5 oz)	155	1	5	27
tiramisu	1 cake (4.4 lbs)	5732	101	421	439
toaster pastry apple	1 (1¾ oz)	204	2	5	37
toaster pastry blueberry	1 (1¾ oz)	204	2	5	37

FOOD	PORTION	CALS	PROT	FAT	CARB
toaster pastry brown sugar cinnamon	1 (1¾ oz)	206	3	7	34
toaster pastry cherry	1 (1¾ oz)	204	2	5	37
toaster pastry strawberry	1 (1¾ oz)	204	2	5	37
treacle tart	1 slice (2.5 oz)	258	3	10	42
vanilla slice	1 slice (2½ oz)	248	3	13	30
white w/ coconut frosting home recipe	¹⁄₁₂ cake (3.9 oz)	399	5	12	71
white w/o frosting home recipe	¹⁄₁₂ cake (2.6 oz)	264	4	9	42
white w/ white frosting	¹⁄₁₆ cake	260	3	9	42
white w/ white frosting	1 cake 9 in diam	4170	43	148	670
yellow w/ chocolate frosting	⅛ cake (2.2 oz)	242	2	11	36
yellow w/ chocolate frosting	1 cake 9 diam	3895	40	175	620
yellow w/o frosting home recipe	2 layers (28.7 oz)	2947	43	119	433
yellow w/o frosting home recipe	¹⁄₁₂ cake (2.4 oz)	245	4	10	36
Baby Watson					
Cheesecake	1 slice (3 oz)	260	4	18	19
Carousel					
New York Cheese Cake	1 cake (3 oz)	250	4	19	16
Dolly Madison					
Angel Food	1 slice (2.1 oz)	160	3	2	34
Apple Crumb	1 (1.6 oz)	160	2	5	28
Banana Dream Flip	1 (3.5 oz)	390	3	16	59
Bear Claw	1 (2.75 oz)	270	5	10	40
Carrot	1 (4 oz)	360	4	8	67
Chocolate Snack Squares	1 (1.6 oz)	210	2	10	28
Cinnamon Buttercrumb	1 (1.6 oz)	170	2	6	28
Cinnamon Buttercrumb Low Fat	1 (1.5 oz)	140	1	2	29
Cinnamon Stix	1 (1.3 oz)	170	1	9	21
Creme Cakes	2 (1.9 oz)	210	1	8	32
Cupcakes Chocolate	1 (2 oz)	210	2	7	35
Cupcakes Spice	1 (2 oz)	230	2	10	33
Dunkin' Stix	1 (1.3 oz)	170	1	9	20
Frosty Angel	1 (3.5 oz)	330	4	6	65
Holiday Cupcakes	1 (1.9 oz)	180	1	3	35
Honey Bun	1 (3.7 oz)	440	6	25	49
Koo Koos	1 (1.8 oz)	200	1	9	29
Mini Coconut Loaf	1 (3.5 oz)	350	3	10	62
Mini Pound Cake	1 (3.2 oz)	310	5	11	48
Raspberry Square	1 (1.8 oz)	190	1	8	28
Sweet Roll Apple	1 (2.2 oz)	200	3	6	33
Sweet Roll Cherry	1 (2.2 oz)	210	3	6	34
Sweet Roll Cinnamon	1 (2.2 oz)	230	3	7	36
Texas Cinnamon Bun	1 (4.2 oz)	440	7	15	69

FOOD	PORTION	CALS	PROT	FAT	CARB
Zingers Devil's Food	2 (2.6 oz)	270	2	8	46
Zingers Lemon	1 (1.4 oz)	150	1	6	22
Zingers Raspberry	1 (1.4 oz)	150	1	6	22
Zingers Yellow	2 (2.5 oz)	280	2	8	50
Drake's					
Coffee Cake Low Fat	1 (1.1 oz)	110	1	2	21
Mini Coffee Cakes	4 (1.83 oz)	220	3	9	33
Yodel's	1 (1 oz)	150	2	9	16
Dutch Mill					
Dessert Shells Chocolate Covered	1 (0.5 oz)	80	1	5	8
Entenmann's					
Apple Puffs	1 (3 oz)	270	2	13	37
Cupcakes Light Chocolate Creme Filled	1 (2 oz)	160	1	0	39
Hot Cross Buns	1 (2.3 oz)	230	4	7	37
Stollen Fruit	⅛ cake (2 oz)	210	3	7	34
Greenfield					
Blondie Fat Free Chocolate Chip	1 (1.3 oz)	110	2	0	27
Hostess					
Angel Food	⅛ cake (2 oz)	160	3	2	33
Chocodiles	1 (1.6 oz)	240	2	11	33
Chocolicious	1 (1.6 oz)	190	1	7	30
Coffee Crumb	1 (1.1 oz)	130	1	5	19
Crumb Cake Light	1 (1 oz)	100	1	2	18
Cupcakes Chocolate	1 (1.8 oz)	180	2	6	30
Cupcakes Orange	1 (1.5 oz)	160	1	5	27
Cupcakes Light Chocolate	1 (1.6 oz)	140	2	2	29
Ding Dongs	2 (2.7 oz)	360	3	19	44
Ho Ho's	2 (2 oz)	250	2	12	34
Honey Bun Glazed	1 (2.7 oz)	320	4	19	34
Honey Bun Iced	1 (3.4 oz)	410	5	24	42
Shortcake Dessert Cups	1 (1 oz)	100	1	2	17
Sno Balls	1 (1.8 oz)	180	1	5	31
Suzy Q's	1 (2 oz)	230	2	9	35
Sweet Roll Cherry	1 (2.2 oz)	210	3	6	34
Sweet Roll Cinnamon	1 (2.2 oz)	230	3	7	36
Twinkies	1 (1.5 oz)	150	1	5	25
Twinkies Light	1 (1.5 oz)	130	1	2	27
Jell-O					
Dessert Delights Cheesecake	1 bar (1.4 oz)	160	2	7	20
Dessert Delights Chocolate Fudge Pudding	1 bar (1.4 oz)	150	2	6	23
Kellogg's					
Pop-Tarts Apple Cinnamon	1 (1.8 oz)	210	2	6	37
Pop-Tarts Blueberry	1 (1.8 oz)	210	2	5	36

FOOD	PORTION	CALS	PROT	FAT	CARB
Pop-Tarts Brown Sugar Cinnamon	1 (1.8 oz)	210	3	6	35
Pop-Tarts Cherry	1 (1.8 oz)	200	2	5	37
Pop-Tarts Chocolate Graham	1 (1.8 oz)	210	3	6	35
Pop-Tarts Frosted Apple Cinnamon	1 (1.8 oz)	190	2	3	39
Pop-Tarts Frosted Blueberry	1 (1.8 oz)	200	2	5	37
Pop-Tarts Frosted Brown Sugar Cinnamon	1 (1.8 oz)	210	3	7	34
Pop-Tarts Frosted Cherry	1 (1.8 oz)	200	2	5	38
Pop-Tarts Frosted Chocolate Vanilla Creme	1 (1.8 oz)	200	3	5	37
Pop-Tarts Frosted Chocolate Fudge	1 (1.8 oz)	200	3	5	37
Pop-Tarts Frosted Grape	1 (1.8 oz)	200	2	5	38
Pop-Tarts Frosted Raspberry	1 (1.8 oz)	210	2	5	37
Pop-Tarts Frosted S'mores	1 (1.8 oz)	200	3	6	36
Pop-Tarts Frosted Strawberry	1 (1.8 oz)	200	2	5	38
Pop-Tarts Frosted Wild Berry	1 (2 oz)	210	2	5	39
Pop-Tarts Frosted Wild Watermelon	1 (2 oz)	210	2	5	39
Pop-Tarts Low Fat Blueberry	1 (1.8 oz)	190	2	3	39
Pop-Tarts Low Fat Cherry	1 (1.8 oz)	190	2	3	39
Pop-Tarts Low Fat Frosted Brown Sugar Cinnamon	1 (1.8 oz)	190	2	3	39
Pop-Tarts Low Fat Frosted Chocolate Fudge	1 (1.8 oz)	190	3	3	39
Pop-Tarts Low Fat Frosted Strawberry	1 (1.8 oz)	190	2	3	39
Pop-Tarts Low Fat Strawberry	1 (1.8 oz)	190	2	3	39
Pop-Tarts Strawberry	1 (1.8 oz)	200	2	5	37
Lance					
Dunking Sticks	1 (2.75 oz)	180	2	10	22
Fig Cake	½ piece (2.1 oz)	110	1	2	21
Fig Cake Fat Free	½ piece (2.1 oz)	100	1	0	22
Honey Bun	1 (3 oz)	330	4	13	47
Pecan Twirls	1 pkg (2 oz)	220	3	9	32
Swiss Rolls	1 (2.5 oz)	170	1	9	23
Little Debbie					
Angel Cakes Lemon	1 (1.6 oz)	130	2	1	29
Angel Cakes Raspberry	1 (1.6 oz)	130	2	1	29
Banana Nut Loaves	1 (1.9 oz)	220	2	10	31

FOOD	PORTION	CALS	PROT	FAT	CARB
Banana Twins	1 (2.2 oz)	250	2	10	39
Be My Valentine Chocolate	1 (2.2 oz)	280	2	13	38
Be My Valentine Vanilla	1 (2.2 oz)	290	2	14	38
Blueberry Loaves	1 (2 oz)	220	3	10	29
Chocolate Chip	1 (2.4 oz)	310	2	15	41
Christmas Tree Cake	1 pkg (1.5 oz)	190	1	10	26
Coconut Creme	1 (1.7 oz)	210	1	10	30
Coffee Cake Apple	1 (2.1 oz)	230	2	7	39
Cupcake Creme Filled Chocolate	1 (1.6 oz)	180	2	9	26
Cupcake Creme Filled Orange	1 (1.7 oz)	210	1	10	29
Cupcake Creme Filled Strawberry	1 (1.7 oz)	210	1	10	29
Devil Cremes	1 (1.6 oz)	190	1	8	29
Devil Squares	1 (2.2 oz)	270	2	13	39
Easter Basket Cake Chocolate	1 (2.4 oz)	300	3	14	40
Easter Basket Cake Vanilla	1 (2.5 oz)	320	2	10	43
Fall Party Cake Chocolate	1 (2.4 oz)	290	2	14	42
Fall Party Cake Vanilla	1 (2.5 oz)	310	2	15	44
Fancy Cakes	1 (2.4 oz)	300	1	15	42
Frosted Fudge	1 (1.5 oz)	200	2	10	25
Golden Cremes	1 (1.5 oz)	150	1	5	26
Holiday Cake Roll Cherry Creme	1 (2.1 oz)	260	2	12	37
Holiday Snack Cake Chocolate	1 (2.4 oz)	300	3	14	41
Holiday Snack Cake Vanilla	1 (2.5 oz)	320	2	15	41
Honey Bun	1 (1.8 oz)	220	3	13	24
Pecan Spinwheels	1 (1 oz)	110	1	4	16
Snack Cake Chocolate	1 (2.5 oz)	310	2	15	44
Strawberry Shortcake Roll	1 (2.1 oz)	230	1	8	41
Swiss Rolls	1 (2.1 oz)	270	2	12	38
Zebra Cakes	1 (2.6 oz)	330	2	16	45
Marie Callender's					
Cobbler Apple	1 serv (4.25 oz)	370	2	20	45
Cobbler Berry	1 serv (4.25 oz)	370	3	21	41
Cobbler Cherry	1 serv (4.25 oz)	380	3	19	50
Cobbler Peach	1 serv (4.25 oz)	380	3	18	47
Natural Touch					
Toaster Square Blueberry	1 (2.8 oz)	180	6	2	33
Toaster Squares Date Walnut	1 (2.8 oz)	200	6	3	36
Nature's Choice					
Toaster Pastries Fat Free Apple Cinnamon	1 (1.9 oz)	180	3	0	41

FOOD	PORTION	CALS	PROT	FAT	CARB
Toaster Pastries Fat Free Blueberry	1 (1.9 oz)	180	3	0	41
Toaster Pastries Fat Free Raspberry	1 (1.9 oz)	180	3	0	41
Toaster Pastries Fat Free Strawberry	1 (1.9 oz)	180	3	0	41
Toaster Pastries Low Fat Cherry	1 (1.9 oz)	180	3	3	36
Toaster Pastries Low Fat Frosted Blueberry	1 (1.9 oz)	190	3	2	42
Toaster Pastries Low Fat Frosted Chocolate	1 (1.9 oz)	200	3	3	42
Toaster Pastries Low Fat Frosted Cinnamon	1 (1.9 oz)	190	3	2	42
Toaster Pastries Low Fat Frosted Strawberry	1 (1.9 oz)	190	3	2	42
Toaster Pastries Low Fat Peach Apricot	1 (1.9 oz)	180	3	3	36
Pepperidge Farm					
Apple Turnover	1 (3.1 oz)	330	4	14	48
Blueberry Turnovers	1 (3.1 oz)	340	4	16	45
Cherry Turnover	1 (3.1 oz)	320	4	13	46
Large Layer Chocolate Fudge	⅛ cake (2.4 oz)	260	3	11	31
Large Layer Coconut	⅛ cake (2.4 oz)	260	2	11	35
Large Layer Vanilla	⅛ cake (2.4 oz)	250	2	11	35
Mini Turnover Apple	1 (1.4 oz)	140	2	8	15
Mini Turnover Cherry	1 (1.4 oz)	140	2	8	16
Mini Turnover Strawberry	1 (1.4 oz)	140	2	7	18
Peach Turnover	1 (3.1 oz)	340	4	15	47
Raspberry Turnovers	1 (3.1 oz)	330	4	14	47
Philadelphia					
Snack Bars Classic Cheesecake	1 (1.5 oz)	200	2	13	17
Pillsbury					
Apple Turnovers	1 (2 oz)	170	2	8	23
Cherry Turnovers	1 (2 oz)	180	2	8	24
Sara Lee					
Cheesecake 25% Reduced Fat	¼ cake (4.2 oz)	310	9	13	40
Cheesecake Cherry Cream	¼ cake (4.7 oz)	350	6	12	55
Cheesecake Chocolate Chip	¼ cake (4.2 oz)	410	8	21	47
Cheesecake French	⅙ cake (3.9 oz)	350	5	21	24
Cheesecake French Strawberry	⅙ cake (4.3 oz)	320	4	14	43
Cheesecake Strawberry Cream	¼ cake (4.7 oz)	330	6	12	49
Coffee Cake Butter Streusel	⅙ cake (1.9 oz)	220	4	12	25

FOOD	PORTION	CALS	PROT	FAT	CARB
Coffee Cake Crumb	⅛ cake (2 oz)	220	3	9	32
Coffee Cake Pecan	⅙ cake (1.9 oz)	230	4	12	24
Coffee Cake Raspberry	⅙ cake (1.9 oz)	220	3	8	27
Coffee Cake Reduced Fat Cheese	⅙ cake (1.9 oz)	180	3	6	28
Layer Cake Coconut	⅛ cake (2.8 oz)	260	2	14	33
Layer Cake Double Chocolate	⅛ cake (2.8 oz)	260	3	13	33
Layer Cake Fudge Golden	⅛ cake (2.8 oz)	260	2	13	34
Layer Cake German Chocolate	⅛ cake (2.9 oz)	280	3	14	35
Layer Cake Vanilla	⅛ cake (2.8 oz)	260	2	14	32
Original Cheesecake	¼ cake (4.2 oz)	350	7	18	39
Pound Cake All Butter	¼ cake (2.7 oz)	320	4	16	38
Pound Cake Chocolate Swirl	¼ cake (2.9 oz)	330	5	16	42
Pound Cake Family Size	⅙ cake (2.7 oz)	310	4	17	36
Pound Cake Reduced Fat	¼ cake (2.7 oz)	280	4	11	42
Pound Cake Strawberry Swirl	¼ cake (2.9 oz)	290	4	11	44
Strawberry Shortcake	⅛ cake (2.5 oz)	180	2	7	27
SnackWell's					
Streusal Squares Apple Cinnamon	1 (1.5 oz)	150	1	3	31
Streusal Squares Cherry	1 (1.5 oz)	150	1	3	31
Tastykake					
Banana Creamie	1 (1.5 oz)	170	1	7	25
Bear Claw Apple	1 (3 oz)	280	4	7	50
Bear Claw Cinnamon	1 (3 oz)	300	5	8	53
Big Texas	1 (3 oz)	300	5	9	51
Breakfast Bun Chocolate Raisin	1 (3.2 oz)	330	5	8	59
Bunny Trail Treats	1 (1.3 oz)	150	1	6	25
Chocolate Creamie	1 (1.5 oz)	180	1	8	25
Chocolate Krimpies	2 (2.2 oz)	240	3	10	38
Coffee Roll Glazed	1 (3 oz)	300	5	9	51
Coffee Roll Vanilla	1 (3.2 oz)	320	5	9	56
Cupcakes	2 (2.1 oz)	200	2	5	37
Cupcakes Butter Cream Cream Filled Iced	2 (2.2 oz)	240	2	8	40
Cupcakes Chocolate CreamFilled Iced	2 (2.2 oz)	230	2	8	39
Cupcakes Low Fat Chocolate Cream Filled	2 (2.2 oz)	200	3	3	42
Cupcakes Low Fat Vanilla Cream Filled	2 (2.2 oz)	190	2	2	42
Cupid Kake	1 (1.3 oz)	150	1	6	25
Honey Bun Glazed	1 (3.2 oz)	350	5	17	47
Honey Bun Iced	1 (3.2 oz)	350	5	17	47

FOOD	PORTION	CALS	PROT	FAT	CARB
Junior Chocolate	1 (3.3 oz)	330	4	12	54
Junior Coconut	1 (3.3 oz)	310	3	8	54
Junior Koffee Kake	1 (2.5 oz)	270	3	9	42
Junior Pound Kake	1 (3 oz)	320	5	13	45
Kandy Kakes Chocolate	3 (2 oz)	250	2	13	35
Kandy Kakes Coconut	2 (2.7 oz)	330	3	18	43
Kandy Kakes Peanut Butter	2 (1.3 oz)	190	3	9	21
Koffee Kake Cream Filled	2 (2 oz)	240	2	10	35
Koffee Kake Low Fat Apple	2 (2 oz)	170	2	2	34
Koffee Kake Low Fat Lemon	2 (2 oz)	180	2	3	36
Koffee Kake Low Fat Raspberry	2 (2 oz)	170	2	2	36
Kreepy Kakes	2 (2.2 oz)	240	2	8	38
Kreme Krimpies	2 (2 oz)	230	2	9	34
Krimpets Butterscotch Iced	2 (2 oz)	210	2	5	38
Krimpets Jelly Fillled	2 (2 oz)	190	2	3	38
Krimpets Strawberry	2 (2 oz)	210	2	5	37
Kringle Kake	1 (1.3 oz)	150	1	6	25
Santa Snacks	2 (2.2 oz)	240	2	8	38
Sparkle Kake	1 (1.3 oz)	150	1	6	25
Tasty Tweets	2 (2.2 oz)	240	2	8	38
Tropical Delight Coconut	2 (2 oz)	190	3	9	26
Tropical Delight Guava	2 (2 oz)	190	2	7	30
Tropical Delight Papaya	2 (2 oz)	200	2	7	32
Tropical Delight Pineapple	2 (2 oz)	200	2	7	32
Vanilla Creamie	1 (1.5 oz)	190	1	9	25
Witchy Treat	1 (1.3 oz)	150	1	6	24
Tom's					
Honey Bun	1 pkg (3 oz)	360	4	20	41
Honey Bun Jelly Filled	1 pkg (4 oz)	490	6	29	52
Marble Pound	1 pkg (2.5 oz)	300	4	16	35
Texas Cinnamon Roll	1 pkg (4 oz)	360	7	6	71
Tortuga					
Cayman Island Rum Cake	1 piece (2 oz)	194	2	9	27
Weight Watchers					
Chocolate Raspberry Royale	1 (3.5 oz)	190	4	3	38
Chocolate Eclair	1 (2.1 oz)	150	2	4	25
Danish Coffee Cake Apple Cinnamon	1 piece (1.9 oz)	160	3	3	30
Danish Coffee Cake Cheese	1 piece (1.9 oz)	160	4	3	29
Danish Coffee Cake Raspberry	1 piece (1.9 oz)	160	4	3	30
Double Fudge	1 piece (2.75 oz)	190	4	4	36
French Style Cheesecake	1 piece (3.9 oz)	170	7	4	28
New York Style Cheesecake	1 piece (2.5 oz)	150	6	5	21
Strawberry Parfait Royale	1 (5.24 oz)	180	5	2	35
Triple Chocolate Eclair	1 (2.14 oz)	160	3	5	25

FOOD	PORTION	CALS	PROT	FAT	CARB
take-out					
angelfood	1/12 cake (1 oz)	73	2	tr	16
apple crisp	1/2 cup (5 oz)	230	37	5	46
baklava	1 oz	126	2	9	10
boston cream pie	1/6 cake (3.3 oz)	293	4	12	43
cannoli w/ cannoli cream	1	369	6	21	42
carrot w/ cream cheese icing	1/12 cake (3.9 oz)	484	5	29	52
cheesecake w/ cherry topping	1/12 cake (5 oz)	359	6	23	33
chocolate w/ chocolate frosting	1/8 cake (2.2 oz)	235	3	11	35
coffeecake cheese	1/6 cake (2.7 oz)	258	5	12	38
coffeecake crumb topped cheese	1/6 cake (2.7 oz)	258	5	12	38
coffeecake crumb topped cinnamon	1/9 cake (2.2 oz)	263	4	15	29
cream puff w/ custard filling	1 (4.6 oz)	336	9	20	30
french apple tart	1 (3.5 oz)	302	4	15	37
fruitcake	1/36 cake (2.9 oz)	302	3	10	54
gingerbread	1/9 cake (2.6 oz)	264	3	12	36
panettone	1/12 cake (2.9 oz)	300	6	12	43
petit fours	2 (0.9 oz)	120	1	7	15
pineapple upside down	1/9 cake (4 oz)	367	4	14	58
pound fat free	1 oz	80	2	tr	17
pound cake	1 slice (1 oz)	120	2	5	15
sacher torte	1 slice (2.2 oz)	240	4	11	30
sheet cake w/ white frosting	1/9 cake	445	4	14	77
strudel apple	1 piece (2½ oz)	195	2	8	29
tiramisu	1 piece (5.1 oz)	409	7	30	31
trifle w/ cream	6 oz	291	4	16	34
yellow w/ vanilla frosting	1/8 cake (2.2 oz)	239	2	9	38
CAKE ICING					
vanilla as prep w/ butter home recipe	1 recipe (20.1 oz)	1972	4	24	448
Betty Crocker					
Rich & Creamy Dark Chocolate	2 tbsp (1.3 oz)	130	1	6	23
CAKE MIX					
(*see also* CAKE)					
angelfood	10 in cake (20.9 oz)	1535	36	2	350
angelfood	1/12 cake (1.8 oz)	129	3	tr	29
carrot w/o frosting	2 layers (29.6 oz)	2886	43	133	395
carrot w/o frosting	1/12 cake (2.5 oz)	239	4	11	33
cheesecake no-bake	1/8 cake (3.5 oz)	271	6	13	35
chocolate pudding type w/o frosting	1/12 cake (2.7 oz)	270	4	14	34
chocolate pudding type w/o frosting	2 layers (32.4 oz)	3234	43	172	409

FOOD	PORTION	CALS	PROT	FAT	CARB
chocolate w/o frosting	2 layers (26.8 oz)	2393	44	92	384
chocolate w/o frosting	⅟₁₂ cake (2.3 oz)	198	4	8	32
chocolate w/o frosting low sodium	⅟₁₀ cake (1.3 oz)	116	1	3	23
coffeecake crumb topped cinnamon	⅛ cake (2 oz)	178	3	5	30
devil's food w/o frosting	⅟₁₂ cake (2.3 oz)	198	4	8	32
devil's food w/ chocolate frosting	⅟₁₆ cake	235	3	8	40
devil's food w/ chocolate frosting	1 cake 9 in diam	3755	49	136	645
fudge w/o frosting	⅟₁₂ cake (2.3 oz)	198	4	8	32
german chocolate pudding type w/ coconut nut frosting	⅟₁₂ cake (3.9 oz)	404	4	21	55
gingerbread	⅑ cake (2.4 oz)	207	3	7	34
gingerbread	1 cake 8 in sq	1575	18	39	291
lemon w/o frosting no sugar low sodium	⅟₁₀ cake (1.3 oz)	118	1	3	23
marble pudding type w/o frosting	⅟₁₂ cake (2.6 oz)	253	3	12	35
marble pudding type w/o frosting	2 layers (30.6 oz)	3021	36	148	412
white pudding type w/o frosting	2 layers (29 oz)	2915	30	123	427
white pudding type w/o frosting	⅟₁₂ cake (2.4 oz)	244	3	10	36
white w/o frosting	⅟₁₂ cake (2.2 oz)	190	3	5	34
white w/o frosting	2 layer cake (26 oz)	2265	30	57	410
white w/o frosting no sugar low sodium	⅟₁₀ cake (1.3 oz)	118	1	3	23
yellow pudding-type w/o frosting	⅟₁₂ cake (2.6 oz)	257	3	12	35
yellow pudding-type w/o frosting	2 layers (31 oz)	3084	40	139	421
yellow w/ chocolate frosting	⅟₁₆ cake	235	3	8	40
yellow w/o frosting	⅟₁₂ cake (2.2 oz)	202	3	6	34
yellow w/o frosting	2 layers (26.5 oz)	2415	35	71	411
yellow w/ chocolate frosting	1 cake 9 in diam	3895	40	175	620
Betty Crocker					
Angel Food Fat Free	⅟₁₂ cake	140	3	0	32
Angel Food Fat Free Confetti as prep	⅟₁₂ cake	150	3	0	34
Cheesecake Chocolate Chip as prep	⅛ cake	410	3	28	32
Cheesecake Original as prep	⅛ cake	400	2	27	30

FOOD	PORTION	CALS	PROT	FAT	CARB
Cheesecake Strawberry Swirl as prep	⅛ cake	380	2	25	32
Pineapple Upside Down as prep	⅛ cake	420	2	14	64
Quick Bread Banana	¹⁄₁₂ cake	170	2	7	25
Quick Bread Cinnamon Streusel as prep	¹⁄₁₄ cake	180	3	7	26
Quick Bread Cranberry Orange as prep	¹⁄₁₂ cake	170	2	6	29
Quick Bread Lemon Poppy Seed as prep	¹⁄₁₂ cake	170	2	7	25
Stir'n Bake Carrot Cake w/ Cream Cheese Frosting as prep	⅛ cake	260	2	7	46
Stir'n Bake Coffee Cake w/ Cinnamon Streusel as prep	⅛ cake	230	2	2	36
Stir'n Bake Devils Food w/ Chocolate Frosting as prep	⅛ cake	240	2	7	42
Stir'n Bake Yellow w/ Chocolate Frosting as prep	⅛ cake	240	2	7	43
SuperMoist Butter Pecan as prep	¹⁄₁₂ cake	240	1	10	35
SuperMoist Butter Yellow as prep	¹⁄₁₂ cake	260	2	11	36
SuperMoist Carrot as prep	¹⁄₁₀ cake	320	2	15	42
SuperMoist Cherry Chip as prep	¹⁄₁₀ cake	300	2	13	41
SuperMoist Chocolate Fudge as prep	¹⁄₁₂ cake	270	2	12	35
SuperMoist Golden Vanilla as prep	¹⁄₁₂ cake	240	1	10	35
SuperMoist Lemon as prep	¹⁄₁₂ cake	240	1	10	35
SuperMoist Milk Chocolate as prep	¹⁄₁₂ cake	240	2	10	34
SuperMoist Pineapple as prep	¹⁄₁₂ cake	250	1	7	25
SuperMoist Spice as prep	¹⁄₁₂ cake	240	1	10	36
SuperMoist Strawberry as prep	¹⁄₁₂ cake	250	1	10	35
SuperMoist White as prep	¹⁄₁₂ cake	230	2	14	34
SuperMoist White Light as prep	¹⁄₁₀ cake	210	2	3	43
Bisquick					
Mix	⅓ cup (1.4 oz)	160	3	6	25
Reduced Fat	⅓ cup (1.4 oz)	140	3	3	27

FOOD	PORTION	CALS	PROT	FAT	CARB
Dromedary					
Date Bread	1/11 cake (2 oz)	190	2	7	29
Date Nut Roll	1/2 in slice	80	1	2	13
Gingerbread	1 piece (2 in x 2 in)	100	1	2	19
Pound	1/2 in slice	150	2	6	21
Duncan Hines					
Angel Food as prep	1/12 pkg (1.3 oz)	140	4	0	31
Butter Recipe Golden as prep	1/12 cake	320	3	16	42
Cupcake Yellow as prep	1	180	1	0	29
Dark Chocolate Fudge as prep	1/12 cake	290	4	15	34
Devil's Food Moist Deluxe as prep	1/12 cake (1.5 oz)	290	4	15	34
Fudge Marble Moist Deluxe as prep	1/12 cake (1.5 oz)	250	3	17	36
Lemon Supreme Moist Deluxe	1/12 cake (1.5 oz)	250	3	17	36
White Moist Deluxe as prep	1/12 cake	190	3	6	34
Yellow Moist Deluxe as prep	1/12 cake (1.5 oz)	250	3	17	36
Yellow Moist Deluxe as prep	1/12 cake	250	3	11	36
Estee					
Chocolate as prep	1/5 cake	190	2	4	36
White as prep	1/5 cake	200	2	4	38
Hodgson Mill					
Gingerbread Whole Wheat	1/4 cup (1 oz)	110	2	0	24
Jell-O					
No Bake Cherry Cheesecake as prep	1/8 cake (4.8 oz)	340	5	12	52
No Bake Double Layer Chocolate as prep	1/8 cake (4.4 oz)	260	4	12	34
No Bake Double Layer Cookies And Creme as prep	1/8 cake (4.5 oz)	390	5	19	51
No Bake Double Layer Lemon as prep	1/8 cake (4.4 oz)	260	4	12	36
No Bake Homestyle Cheesecake as prep	1/8 cake (4.6 oz)	360	7	15	50
No Bake Peanut Butter Cup as prep	1/8 cake (3.8 oz)	380	5	23	41
No Bake Reduced Fat Strawberry Swirl Cheesecake as prep	1/8 cake (4 oz)	250	7	6	44
No Bake Strawberry Cheesecake as prep	1/8 cake (4.8 oz)	340	5	12	52
Real Cheesecake as prep	1/8 cake (4.6 oz)	360	7	16	47

FOOD	PORTION	CALS	PROT	FAT	CARB
Sweet Rewards					
Reduced Fat White as prep	1/12 cake	180	2	3	36
Reduced Fat Yellow as prep	1/12 cake	200	2	5	37
CALABAZA					
fresh	1/2 cup	32	1	tr	8
CALZONE					
take-out					
cheese	1 (12 oz)	1020	48	54	86
CANADIAN BACON					
grilled	1 pkg (6 oz)	257	34	12	2
Boar's Head					
Canadian Bacon	2 oz	70	12	3	1
Hormel					
Sandwich Style	3 slices (2 oz)	70	10	3	0
Oscar Mayer					
Canadian Bacon	2 slices (1.6 oz)	50	8	2	0
Yorkshire Farms					
Uncured	3 oz	100	17	4	9
CANADIAN BACON SUBSTITUTES					
Yves					
Canadian Veggie Bacon	1 serv (2 oz)	80	17	1	1
CANDY					
(*see also* CHEWING GUM, MARSHMALLOW)					
caramels	1 pkg (2.5 oz)	271	3	6	55
caramels chocolate	1 bar (2.3 oz)	231	1	2	56
carob bar	1 (3.1 oz)	453	11	28	42
crisped rice bar almond	1 bar (1 oz)	130	2	6	18
crisped rice bar chocolate chip	1 bar (1 oz)	115	4	4	21
dark chocolate	1 oz	150	1	10	16
fondant chocolate coated	1 lg (1.2 oz)	128	1	3	28
fruit pastilles	1 tube (1.4 oz)	101	2	0	25
marzipan	1 oz	128	3	7	15
milk chocolate	1 bar (1.55 oz)	226	3	14	26
milk chocolate crisp	1 bar (1.45 oz)	203	3	11	28
milk chocolate w/ almonds	1 bar (1.45 oz)	215	4	14	22
nougat nut cream	0.5 oz	49	1	4	8
peanut bar	1 (1.4 oz)	209	6	14	19
peanuts chocolate covered	1 cup (5.2 oz)	773	19	50	74
peanuts chocolate covered	10 (1.4 oz)	208	5	13	20
pretzels chocolate covered	1 oz	130	2	5	20
pretzels chocolate covered	1 (0.4 oz)	50	1	2	8
sesame crunch	1 oz	146	3	9	14
sesame crunch	20 pieces (1.2 oz)	181	4	12	18
sweet chocolate	1 bar (1.45 oz)	201	2	14	25
sweet chocolate	1 oz	143	1	10	17
100 Grand					
Bar	1 bar (1.5 oz)	200	2	8	30

FOOD	PORTION	CALS	PROT	FAT	CARB
5th Avenue					
Snack Size	1 bar (0.58)	80	1	4	10
Andes					
Chocolate Covered Mint Patties	1 (0.5 oz)	60	0	1	13
Baby Ruth					
Bar	1 bar (2.1 oz)	270	4	13	36
Fun Size	1 bar (1 oz)	130	3	6	17
Barricini					
Dark Chocolate Raspberry Creme Shells	1 piece (0.3 oz)	47	0	3	5
Bittyfinger					
Bars	2	170	2	7	27
Body Smarts					
Chocolate Peanut Crunch	2 bars (1.8 oz)	210	5	6	34
Butterfinger					
BB's	1 pkg (1.7 oz)	230	2	9	33
Bar	1 (2.1 oz)	270	3	11	42
Fun Size	1 bar	100	1	4	15
Cape Cod Provisions					
Cranberry Bog Frogs	3 pieces (1.9 oz)	250	3	12	34
Carmello					
Snack Size	1 (0.66 oz)	90	1	4	12
Charms					
Blow Pop	1 (0.6 oz)	70	0	0	17
Chunky					
Bar	1 (1.4 oz)	210	3	11	24
Crunch					
Fun Size	4 bars	210	2	11	26
Del Monte					
Radical Raizins Cinnamon	1 pkg (0.7 oz)	70	0	0	18
Radical Raizins Rainbow	1 pkg (0.7 oz)	70	0	0	18
Estee					
Caramels Vanilla & Chocolate	5	115	1	5	26
Dark Chocolate	½ bar (1.4 oz)	200	2	14	23
Milk Chocolate	½ bar (1.4 oz)	230	4	17	17
Milk Chocolate w/ Almonds	½ bar (1.4 oz)	230	4	17	16
Milk Chocolate w/ Crisp Rice	½ bar (1.2 oz)	370	7	26	29
Milk Chocolate w/ Fruit & Nuts	½ bar (1.4 oz)	220	4	16	18
Mint Chocolate	½ bar (1.4 oz)	200	2	14	23
Peanut Brittle	⅓ box (1.3 oz)	160	3	9	28
Peanut Butter Cups	5	200	5	12	19
Sugar Free Fruit Gum Drops	23	80	0	0	36
Sugar Free Gourmet Jelly Beans	26	70	0	0	24
Sugar Free Gummy Apple Rings	5	70	0	0	28

FOOD	PORTION	CALS	PROT	FAT	CARB
Sugar Free Licorice Gum Drops	11	90	1	0	36
Favorite Brands					
Candy Corn	24 pieces (1.4 oz)	150	0	0	37
Circus Peanuts	5 pieces (1.6 oz)	160	1	0	39
Gummallo Apple Ring	5 pieces (1.4 oz)	120	2	0	27
Gummallo Peach Ring	5 pieces (1.4 oz)	120	2	0	27
Gummi Bears	18 pieces (1.4 oz)	130	2	0	30
Gummi Dinos	7 pieces (1.3 oz)	120	2	0	28
Gummi Worms	4 pieces (1.4 oz)	130	2	0	29
Neon Worms	4 pieces (1.4 oz)	120	2	0	28
Sour Gummi Bears	16 pieces (1.4 oz)	110	2	0	26
Sour Gummi Worms	4 pieces (1.6 oz)	130	2	0	29
Godiva					
Chocolatier Dark Chocolate w/ Raspberry	1 bar (1.5 oz)	220	2	11	28
Chocolatier Milk Chocolate	1 bar (1.5 oz)	230	3	13	26
Mochaccino Mousse	2 pieces (1.25 oz)	210	2	15	17
Truffles Assorted	2 pieces (1.5 oz)	220	2	13	24
Goetze's					
Cow Tales	1 pkg (1 oz)	110	1	3	20
Goobers					
Peanuts	1 pkg (1.38 oz)	210	4	13	20
Haviland					
Chocolate Covered Thin Mints	6 (1.5 oz)	170	1	5	33
Hershey					
Amazin'Fruit Gummy Candy	1 snack pkg (0.7 oz)	60	1	0	15
Bar	1 (0.6 oz)	100	2	6	9
Candy-Coated Milk Chocolate Eggs	4 pieces	90	1	5	12
Cookies 'n' Mint	1 bar (0.6 oz)	90	1	5	11
Kisses	1	25	0	2	3
Milk Chocolate	1 bar (0.6 oz)	90	1	5	10
Milk Chocolate w/ Almonds	1 bar (0.6 oz)	100	2	6	9
PayDay Snack Size	1 (0.66 oz)	90	2	5	11
Pot Of Gold Solitaires	5 pieces	90	2	6	8
ReeseSticks Snack Size	2 pieces (1.2 oz)	190	3	11	19
Sweet Escapes Chocolate Toffee Crisp	1 bar (0.66 oz)	80	1	4	12
Sweet Escapes Peanut Butter Crispy	1 bar (0.7 oz)	70	1	3	12
Jolly Rancher					
Lollipops All Flavors	1 (0.6 oz)	60	0	0	16
Just Born					
Hot Tamales	1 pkg (2.1 oz)	220	0	0	55
Mike and Ike Berry Fruits	1 pkg (2.1 oz)	220	0	0	55
Mike and Ike Original	1 pkg (1.2 oz)	220	0	0	55

[handwritten:] Good & Plenty Licorice candy 130 cal = 13 pcs or 10 cal each

FOOD	PORTION	CALS	PROT	FAT	CARB
Kit Kat					
Bar	1 (0.56 oz)	80	1	4	10
Krackel					
Bar	1 (0.6 oz)	90	1	5	11
Lance					
Chocolaty Peanut Bar	1 (2 oz)	290	9	15	32
K-Nuts	4 pieces (1.5 oz)	240	4	15	23
Peanut Bar	1 (1.75 oz)	270	10	15	23
Whistle Pop	1 (0.67 oz)	70	0	0	19
Lifesavers					
Gummi Shapes Barnum's Animals	1 pkg (0.8 oz)	70	1	0	18
Lindt					
Truffles Milk Chocolate	3 pieces (1.3 oz)	210	2	17	15
Milk Duds					
Snack Size	4 boxes (1.3 oz)	160	1	6	26
Necco					
Bridge Mix	¼ cup (1.5 oz)	180	2	9	27
Chocolate Covered Raisins	30 pieces (1.5 oz)	170	1	7	30
Malted Milk Balls	11 pieces (1.5 oz)	180	1	6	28
SkyBar	1 bar (1.5 oz)	190	2	9	28
Nestle					
Buncha Crunch	1 pkg (1.4 oz)	90	2	10	26
Crunch	1 bar (1.55 oz)	230	2	12	29
Crunch Disk	1 (1.2 oz)	180	2	9	22
Crunchkins	5 pieces	190	2	10	24
Jingles Milk Chocolate Butterfinger	5 pieces	180	2	8	26
Jingles Milk Chocolate Crunch	7 pieces	220	2	11	28
Jingles White Crunch	7 pieces	230	3	14	24
Milk Chocolate	1 bar (1.45 oz)	220	2	13	26
Nesteggs Milk Chocolate Butterfinger	5 pieces	210	3	10	28
Nesteggs Milk Chocolate Crunch	5 pieces	190	2	10	24
Nesteggs White Crunch	7 pieces	230	3	14	24
Treasures Butterfinger	3 pieces	180	2	9	24
Treasures Crunch	4 pieces (1.4 oz)	210	2	11	26
Treasures Peanut Butter	4 pieces	250	4	17	23
Turtles	2 pieces (1.2 oz)	160	2	9	20
Turtles Bite Size	1 piece (0.4 oz)	50	1	2	6
White Crunch	1 bar (1.4 oz)	220	3	13	23
Newman's Own					
Organic Peanut Butter Cups Dark Chocolate	3 pieces (1.2 oz)	180	3	12	18
Organic Peanut Butter Cups Milk Chocolate	3 pieces (1.2 oz)	180	4	12	18

FOOD	PORTION	CALS	PROT	FAT	CARB
Organic Peppermint Cups	3 pieces (1.2 oz)	180	2	12	20
Oh Henry!					
Bar	1 (1.8 oz)	120	2	5	16
Palmer					
Milk Chocolate Lollipop	1 (0.9 oz)	130	1	7	16
Pez					
Candy	1 roll (0.3 oz)	35	0	0	9
Planters					
Original Peanut Bar	1 pkg (1.6 oz)	230	6	14	22
Raisinets					
Candy	1 pkg (1.58 oz)	200	2	8	31
Fun Size	3 pkg (1.7 oz)	200	2	8	43
Reese's					
Eggs	1 (0.6 oz)	90	2	5	9
FastBreak	1 bar (2 oz)	270	5	13	34
Nutrageous	1 (0.6 oz)	90	2	5	9
Pieces	25 (0.7 oz)	100	3	4	12
ReeseSticks Peanut Butter	2 pieces (1.2 oz)	190	3	11	19
Rokeach					
Cotton Candy	2 cups (1 oz)	110	0	0	28
Russell Stover					
Peanut Butter & Grape Jelly	1 piece (0.8 oz)	100	2	6	10
Peanut Butter & Red Raspberry Cups	2 (1.2 oz)	140	3	9	14
Pecan Delights	1 pkg (1.8 oz)	250	3	17	22
Pecan Roll	1 (1.75 oz)	260	3	18	23
S'mores	3 (1.4 oz)	210	2	12	22
Sugar Free Peanut Butter Cups	4 pieces (1.3 oz)	200	5	13	17
Sugar Free Pecans & Caramel	2 pieces (1.2 oz)	170	2	12	17
Simply Lite					
Sugar Free Lil'l Bits Chocolately	36 pieces (1.4 oz)	130	3	5	28
Sugar Free Lil'l Bits Peanut Buttery	36 pieces (1.4 oz)	140	4	5	26
Sugar Free Patteez	5 pieces (1.3 oz)	110	1	3	29
Smucker's					
Fruit Fillers Strawberry	1 pkg (0.9 oz)	80	1	0	19
Snickers					
Cruncher	3 fun size (1.4 oz)	230	4	13	25
Sno Caps					
Candies	1 pkg (2.3 oz)	300	2	13	48
Steel's					
Salt Water Taffy Assorted	3 pieces (1 oz)	90	0	1	22
Swedish Fish					
Original	19 pieces (1.4 oz)	160	0	0	39

FOOD	PORTION	CALS	PROT	FAT	CARB
Symphony					
Bar	1 (0.6 oz)	100	1	6	10
W/ Almonds & Chocolate Chips	1 bar (0.6 oz)	90	1	6	9
Tobler					
Orange Dark Chocolate	5 pieces (1.5 oz)	240	2	13	28
Tom's					
Jelly Beans	1 pkg (2.25 oz)	230	0	0	58
Twix					
Caramel	1 fun size (0.5 oz)	80	1	4	10
Twizzlers					
Cherry	1 pieces	35	0	0	9
Licorice	1 piece	35	0	0	9
Pull'n'Peel Cherry	1 piece (1 oz)	90	1	0	19
Strawberry	1 piece	35	0	0	9
Whatchamacallit					
Bar	1 (0.58 oz)	80	1	4	10
Whitman's					
Snoopy Treats Caramel Peanuts Milk Chocolate	1 snack size (1.4 oz)	80	2	5	24
York					
Chocolate Covered Peppermint Bites	15 pieces (1 oz)	150	1	3	31
Peppermint Patty	1 (0.49 oz)	50	0	1	11
CANTALOUPE					
dried	3.5 pieces (1.4 oz)	140	0	0	34
fresh cubed	1 cup	57	1	tr	13
fresh half	½	94	2	1	22
CARDOON					
fresh cooked	3½ oz	22	1	tr	5
CARIBOU					
roasted	3 oz	142	25	4	0
CAROB					
carob mix as prep w/ whole milk	9 oz	195	8	8	23
flour	1 cup	185	5	1	92
CARP					
fresh	3 oz	108	15	5	0
fresh cooked	3 oz	138	19	6	0
fresh cooked	1 fillet (6 oz)	276	39	12	0
roe raw	1 oz	37	7	tr	tr
CARROT JUICE					
canned	6 oz	73	2	tr	17
CARROTS					
canned					
S&W					
Julienne	½ cup (4.3 oz)	30	1	0	5

FOOD	PORTION	CALS	PROT	FAT	CARB
Sliced	½ cup (4.3 oz)	30	1	0	5
Whole Small	½ cup (4.3 oz)	30	1	0	5
fresh					
raw	1 (2.5 oz)	31	1	tr	7
raw shredded	½ cup	24	1	tr	6
slices cooked	½ cup	35	1	tr	8
Dole					
Shredded	1 cups (3 oz)	40	1	0	9
frozen					
slices cooked	½ cup	26	1	tr	6
CASABA					
cubed	1 cup	45	2	tr	11
fresh	⅒	43	1	tr	10
CASHEWS					
cashew butter w/o salt	1 tbsp	94	3	8	4
dry roasted salted	1 oz	163	4	13	9
dry roasted w/ salt	18 nuts (1 oz)	160	4	13	9
oil roasted	1 oz	163	5	14	8
oil roasted salted	1 oz	163	5	14	8
Frito Lay					
Salted	1 oz	180	5	15	7
Lance					
Cashews	1 pkg (1⅛ oz)	200	6	16	8
CATFISH					
channel breaded & fried	3 oz	194	15	11	7
channel raw	3 oz	99	15	4	0
CATSUP					
(*see* KETCHUP)					
CAULIFLOWER					
fresh					
cooked	½ cup (2.2 oz)	14	1	tr	3
flowerets cooked	3 (2 oz)	12	1	tr	2
flowerets raw	3 (2 oz)	14	1	tr	3
green cooked	1½ cup (3.2 oz)	29	3	tr	6
green raw	1 head 7 in diam (18 oz)	158	15	2	31
green raw	1 cup (2.2 oz)	20	2	tr	4
green raw floweret	1 (0.9 oz)	8	1	tr	2
raw	½ cup (1.8 oz)	13	1	tr	3
frozen					
cooked	½ cup	17	1	tr	3
Green Giant					
Cheese Sauce	½ cup (3.5 oz)	60	2	3	8
Florets	1 cup (2.8 oz)	25	2	0	4
CAVIAR					
black	1 oz	71	7	5	1
black	1 tbsp	40	4	3	1

FOOD	PORTION	CALS	PROT	FAT	CARB
red	1 tbsp	40	4	3	1
red	1 oz	71	7	5	1
CELERIAC					
fresh cooked	3½ oz	25	1	tr	6
raw	½ cup	31	1	tr	7
CELERY					
diced cooked	½ cup	13	1	tr	3
CELTUCE					
raw	3½ oz	22	1	tr	4
CEREAL					
bran flakes	¾ cup (1 oz)	90	4	1	22
corn flakes	1¼ cup (1 oz)	110	2	tr	24
corn flakes low sodium	1 cup (0.9 oz)	100	2	tr	22
corn grits white regular & quick as prep w/ water & salt	¾ cup (6.4 oz)	109	3	tr	24
corn grits white regular or quick as prep	¾ cup (6.4 oz)	109	3	tr	24
corn grits yellow regular & quick as prep w/ water & salt	¾ cup (6.4 oz)	109	3	tr	24
corn grits yellow regular & quick not prep	1 cup (5.5 oz)	579	14	2	124
crispy rice	1 cup (1 oz)	111	2	tr	25
crispy rice low sodium	1 cup (0.9 oz)	105	1	tr	23
farina as prep w/ water	¾ cup (6.1 oz)	88	2	tr	19
farina not prep	1 tbsp (0.4 oz)	40	1	tr	9
granola	½ cup (2.1 oz)	285	9	15	32
oatmeal instant w/ cinnamon & spice as prep w/ water	1 pkg (5.6 oz)	177	5	2	35
oatmeal instant w/ raisins & spice as prep w/ water	1 cup (5.5 oz)	161	4	2	32
oatmeal instant w/ bran & raisins as prep w/ water	1 pkg (6.8 oz)	158	5	2	30
oatmeal istant as prep w/ water	1 cup (8.2 oz)	138	6	2	24
oatmeal regular & quick as prep w/ water	¾ cup (6.1 oz)	149	5	2	19
oatmeal regular & quick not prep	⅓ cup (0.9 oz)	104	4	2	18
oatmeal instant cooked w/o salt	1 cup	145	6	2	25
oatmeal quick cooked w/o salt	1 cup	145	6	2	25

FOOD	PORTION	CALS	PROT	FAT	CARB
oatmeal regular cooked w/o salt	1 cup	145	6	2	25
puffed rice	1 cup (0.5 oz)	56	1	tr	13
puffed wheat	1 cup (0.4 oz)	44	2	tr	10
shredded mini wheats	1 cup (1.1 oz)	107	3	1	24
shredded wheat rectangular	1 biscuit (0.8 oz)	85	3	tr	19
shredded wheat round	2 biscuits (1.3 oz)	136	4	1	31
sugar-coated corn flakes	¾ cup (1 oz)	110	1	1	26
whole wheat hot natural as prep w/ water	¾ cup (6.4 oz)	113	4	1	25
Albers					
Hominy Quick Grits uncooked	¼ cup	140	3	1	31
Alpen					
Corn Flakes	1 serv (1 oz)	110	2	tr	25
No Salt No Sugar	1 serv (2 oz)	200	7	3	34
Regular	1 serv (2 oz)	200	7	3	37
Barbara's Bakery					
Apple Cinnamon O's	¾ cup	110	3	1	24
Bite Size Shredded Oats	1¼ cups (2 oz)	220	6	3	46
Cinnamon Puffins	1¼ cup (2 oz)	100	2	1	26
Cocoa Crunch Stars	1 cup (1 oz)	110	2	1	26
Frosted Corn Flakes	1 cup (1 oz)	110	2	1	27
Fruit Juice Sweetened Breakfast O's	1 cup (1 oz)	120	5	2	22
Fruit Juice Sweetened Brown Rice Crisps	1 cup (1 oz)	120	2	1	25
Fruit Juice Sweetened Corn Flakes	1 cup (1 oz)	110	2	0	26
GrainShop	⅔ cup (1 oz)	90	3	1	24
Honey Crunch Stars	1 cup (1 oz)	110	2	0	26
Honey Nut Toasted O's	¾ cup	120	3	2	23
Organic Fruity Punch	1 cup (1 oz)	110	2	1	26
Organic Soy Essence	¾ cup (1 oz)	100	3	1	25
Puffins	¾ cup (0.9 oz)	90	2	1	23
Shredded Spoonfuls	¾ cup (1.1 oz)	110	5	2	23
Shredded Wheat	2 biscuits (1.4 oz)	140	4	1	31
General Mills					
Basic 4	1 cup (1.9 oz)	200	4	2	42
Boo Berry	1 cup (1 oz)	120	1	1	27
Cheerios	1 cup (1 oz)	110	3	2	22
Cheerios Apple Cinnamon	¾ cup (1 oz)	120	2	2	25
Cheerios Frosted	1 cup (1 oz)	120	2	1	25
Cheerios Honey Nut	1 cup (1 oz)	120	3	2	24
Cheerios Multi Grain	1 cup (1 oz)	110	3	1	24
Cheerios Team	1 cup (1 oz)	120	2	1	25
Chex Corn	1 cup (1 oz)	110	2	0	26

FOOD	PORTION	CALS	PROT	FAT	CARB
Chex Honey Nut	¾ cup	120	1	1	26
Chex Morning Mix Cinnamon	1 pkg (1.1 oz)	130	2	4	24
Chex Morning Mix Fruit & Nut	1 pkg (1.1 oz)	180	2	4	24
Chex Morning Mix Honey Nut	1 pkg (1.1 oz)	130	2	4	24
Chex Multi-Bran	1 cup (2 oz)	200	4	2	49
Chex Rice	1¼ cup (1.1 oz)	120	2	0	27
Cinnamon Grahams	¾ cup (1 oz)	120	1	1	26
Cinnamon Toast Crunch	¾ cup (1 oz)	130	1	4	24
Cocoa Puffs	1 cup (1 oz)	120	1	1	26
Cookie Crisp	1 cup (1 oz)	120	1	1	26
Count Chocula	1 cup (1 oz)	120	1	1	26
Country Corn Flakes	1 cup (1 oz)	120	2	0	26
Fiber One	½ cup (1 oz)	60	2	1	24
Franken Berry	1 cup (1 oz)	120	1	1	27
French Toast Crunch	¾ cup (1 oz)	120	1	1	26
Gold Medal Raisin Bran	1⅓ cups (1.9 oz)	170	5	2	41
Golden Grahams	¾ cup (1 oz)	120	1	1	25
Harmony	1¼ cups (1.9 oz)	200	5	4	44
Honey Nut Clusters	1 cup (1.9 oz)	210	4	3	46
Kaboom	1¼ cup (1 oz)	120	2	1	24
Kix	1⅓ cup (1 oz)	120	2	1	26
Kix Berry Berry	¾ cup (1 oz)	120	1	2	26
Lucky Charms	1 cup (1 oz)	120	2	1	25
Nature Valley Low Fat Fruit Granola	⅔ cup (1.9 oz)	210	4	3	44
Newquick	¾ cup (1 oz)	120	1	2	25
Oatmeal Crisp Almond	1 cup (1.9 oz)	220	5	5	42
Oatmeal Crisp Apple Cinnamon	1 cup (1.9 oz)	210	5	2	45
Oatmeal Crisp Raisin	1 cup (1.9 oz)	210	5	2	44
Para Su Familia Cinnamon Stars	1 cup (1 oz)	120	1	1	28
Para Su Familia Fruitis	1 cup (1 oz)	120	1	1	25
Para Su Familia Raisin Bran	1¼ cups (2 oz)	170	5	2	41
Raisin Nut Bran	¾ cup (1.9 oz)	200	4	4	41
Reese's Puffs	¾ cup	130	2	3	23
Snack'N Dash Cinnamon Toast Crunch	1 pkg (1.2 oz)	140	2	4	27
Snack'N Dash Honey Nut Cheerios	1 pkg (1 oz)	110	3	1	23
Snack'N Dash Lucky Charms	1 pkg (1 oz)	110	2	1	24
Sunrise Organic	¾ cup (1 oz)	110	1	1	26
Total Brown Sugar & Oat	¾ cup (1 oz)	110	2	1	23
Total Corn Flakes	1⅓ cup (1 oz)	110	2	0	24

FOOD	PORTION	CALS	PROT	FAT	CARB
Total Raisin Bran	1 cup (1.9 oz)	170	4	1	41
Total Whole Grain	¾ cup (1 oz)	110	2	1	23
Trix	1 cup (1 oz)	120	1	1	27
Wheat Hearts	¼ cup (1.3 oz)	130	5	1	26
Wheaties	1 cup (1 oz)	110	3	1	24
Wheaties Energy Crunch	1 cup (1.9 oz)	210	6	3	42
Wheaties Frosted	¾ cup (1 oz)	110	1	1	27
Wheaties Raisin Bran	1 cup (1.9 oz)	180	4	1	45
Grainfield's					
Brown Rice	1 serv (1 oz)	110	3	1	24
Crisp Rice	1 serv (1 oz)	112	3	tr	25
Raisin Bran	1 serv (1 oz)	90	2	2	20
Wheat Flakes	1 serv (1 oz)	100	3	1	20
Health Valley					
10 Bran O's Apple Cinnamon	¾ cup	100	3	0	23
Bran w/ Apples & Cinnamon	¾ cup	160	5	0	41
Golden Flax	½ cup	190	6	3	38
Granola 98% Fat Free Date Almond	⅔ cup	180	5	1	43
Healthy Crunches & Flakes Almond	¾ cup	130	3	0	31
Healthy Crunches & Flakes Apple Cinnamon	¾ cup	130	3	0	31
Healthy Crunches & Flakes Honey Crunch	¾ cup	130	3	0	31
Hot Cereal Cups Amazing Apple!	1 pkg	220	9	2	43
Hot Cereal Cups Banana Gone Nuts	1 pkg	240	10	3	45
Hot Cereal Cups Maple Madness!	1 pkg	240	9	2	47
Hot Cereal Cups Terrific 10 Grain!	1 pkg	220	12	3	41
Oat Bran O'S	¾ cup	100	3	0	23
Organic Amaranth Flakes	¾ cup	100	3	0	24
Organic Blue Corn Bran Flakes	¾ cup	100	3	0	24
Organic Bran w/ Raisin	¾ cup	160	5	0	40
Organic Fiber 7 Flakes	¾ cup	100	3	0	24
Organic Healthy Fiber Flakes	¾ cup	100	3	0	23
Organic Oat Bran Flakes	¾ cup	100	3	0	24
Organic Oat Bran Flakes w/ Raisins	¾ cup	110	3	0	26
Puffed Honey Sweetened Corn	1 cup	110	2	0	28

FOOD	PORTION	CALS	PROT	FAT	CARB
Puffed Honey Sweetened Crisp Brown Rice	1 cup	110	1	0	28
Raisin Bran Flakes	1¼ cup	190	5	0	47
Real Oat Bran	½ cup	200	6	3	34
Healthy Choice					
Almond Crunch w/ Raisins	1 cup (2 oz)	210	5	3	46
Golden Multi-Grain Flakes	¾ cup (1.1 oz)	110	3	0	26
Toasted Brown Sugar Squares	1 cup (2 oz)	190	5	1	44
Hodgson Mill					
Cracked Wheat	¼ cup (1.4 oz)	110	4	1	26
Multi Grain w/ Flaxseed & Soy	⅓ cup (1.4 oz)	160	7	3	25
Kashi					
Breakfast Pilaf as prep	½ cup (4.9 oz)	170	6	3	30
Go Apple Spice	½ cup (4.9 oz)	270	7	3	56
Go Banana Almond	½ cup (4.9 oz)	280	7	4	57
Go Berry Tart	½ cup (4.9 oz)	260	7	3	55
Go Blueberry Bliss	½ cup (4.9 oz)	260	7	3	55
Go Cherry Vanilla	½ cup (4.9 oz)	260	7	3	54
Go Just Peachy	½ cup (4.9 oz)	260	7	3	54
GoLean	¾ cup (1.4 oz)	120	8	1	28
Good Friends	¾ cup (1 oz)	90	3	1	24
Honey Puffed	1 cup (1 oz)	120	3	1	25
Medley	½ cup (1 oz)	100	4	1	20
Pillows Apple	¾ cup (1.9 oz)	200	3	1	45
Pillows Chocolate	¾ cup (1.9 oz)	200	3	1	45
Pillows Strawberry Crisp	¾ cup (1.9 oz)	200	3	1	46
Puffed	1 cup (0.9 oz)	70	3	tr	13
Kellogg's					
All-Bran	½ cup (1.1 oz)	80	4	1	24
All-Bran Bran Buds	⅓ cup (1 oz)	80	3	1	24
All-Bran Extra Fiber	½ cup (0.9 oz)	50	3	1	20
Apple Jacks	1 cup (1.2 oz)	120	2	0	30
Cocoa Frosted Flakes	¾ cup (1.1 oz)	120	1	0	28
Cocoa Krispies	¾ cup (1.1 oz)	120	1	1	27
Complete Oat Bran Flakes	¾ cup (1 oz)	110	4	1	23
Complete Wheat Bran Flakes	¾ cup (1 oz)	90	3	1	23
Corn Flakes	1 cup (1 oz)	100	2	0	24
Corn Pops K-Sentials	1 oz	100	1	0	25
Cracklin' Oat Bran	¾ cup (1.7 oz)	190	4	7	35
Crispix	1 cup (1 oz)	110	2	0	25
Froot Loops K-Sentials	1 oz	100	2	1	24
Frosted Flakes	¾ cup (1.1 oz)	120	1	0	28
Granola Low Fat	½ cup (1.7 oz)	190	4	3	39
Honey Crunch Corn Flakes	¾ cup (1.1 oz)	120	2	1	26

FOOD	PORTION	CALS	PROT	FAT	CARB
Just Right Crunchy Nuggets	1 cup (2 oz)	210	4	2	46
Just Right Fruit & Nut	1 cup (2.1 oz)	220	4	2	49
Low Fat w/ Raisins	⅔ cup (2.1 oz)	220	5	3	47
Mini-Wheat Frosted	1 cup (1.8 oz)	180	5	1	41
Mini-Wheat Strawberry Squares	¾ cup (1.8 oz)	170	4	1	40
Mini-Wheats Apple Cinnamon Squares	¾ cup (1.9 oz)	180	4	1	44
Mini-Wheats Blueberry Squares	¾ cup (1.9 oz)	180	4	1	43
Mini-Wheats Frosted Bite Size	24 pieces (2.1 oz)	200	6	1	48
Mini-Wheats Raisin Squares	¾ cup (1.9 oz)	180	5	1	42
Mueslix Apple & Almond Crunch	¾ cups (1.9 oz)	200	5	5	39
Mueslix Raisin & Almond	⅔ cup (1.9 oz)	200	5	3	41
Nutri-Grain Almond Raisin	1¼ cup (1.7 oz)	180	4	3	38
Nutri-Grain Golden Wheat	¾ cup (1 oz)	100	3	1	23
Product 19	1 cup (1 oz)	100	2	0	25
Raisin Bran	1 cup (2.1 oz)	200	6	2	47
Rice Krispies	1¼ cup (1.2 oz)	120	2	0	29
Rice Krispies Razzle Dazzle	¾ cup (1 oz)	110	1	0	25
Rice Krispies Treats	¾ cup (1 oz)	120	1	2	26
Smacks	¾ cup (1 oz)	100	2	1	24
Smart Start	1 cup (1.8 oz)	180	3	1	43
Special K	1 cup (1.1 oz)	110	6	0	21
Lundberg					
Purely Organic Hot'n Creamy Rice	⅓ cup	190	4	2	43
Morning Traditions					
Banana Nut Crunch	1 cup (2 oz)	250	5	6	43
Blueberry Morning	1¼ cup (1.9 oz)	220	4	3	43
Cranberry Almond Crunch	1 cup (1.9 oz)	220	4	3	44
Great Grains Crunchy Pecan	⅔ cup (1.9 oz)	220	5	6	38
Great Grains Raisins Dates & Pecans	⅔ cup (1.9 oz)	210	4	5	39
Nabisco					
100% Bran	⅓ cup (1 oz)	80	4	1	23
Frosted Shredded Wheat Bite Size	1 cup (1.8 oz)	190	4	1	44
Honey Nut Shredded Wheat Bite Size	1 cup (1.8 oz)	200	5	2	43
Original Shredded Wheat	2 biscuits (1.6 oz)	160	5	1	38
Original Shredded Wheat 'N Bran	1¼ cup (2.1 oz)	200	7	1	47
Original Shredded Wheat Spoon Size	1 cup (1.7 oz)	170	5	1	41

FOOD	PORTION	CALS	PROT	FAT	CARB
Post					
Alpha-Bits	1 cup (1 oz)	130	3	2	27
Alpha-Bits Marshmallow	1 cup (1 oz)	120	2	1	25
Bran Flakes	¾ cup (1 oz)	100	3	1	24
Cocoa Pebbles	¾ cup (1 oz)	120	1	1	26
Fruit & Fibre Dates Raisins & Walnuts	1 cup (1.9 oz)	210	4	3	42
Fruit & Fibre Peaches Raisins & Almonds	1 cup (1.9 oz)	210	4	3	42
Golden Crisp	¾ cup (1 oz)	110	1	0	25
Grape-Nuts	¾ cup (1 oz)	100	3	1	24
Grape-Nuts Flakes	¾ cup (1 oz)	100	3	1	24
Honey Bunches Of Oats	¾ cup (1 oz)	120	2	2	25
Honey Bunches Of Oats w/ Almonds	¾ cup (1.1 oz)	130	3	3	24
Honeycomb	1⅓ cups (1 oz)	110	2	1	26
Post Toasties	1 cup (1 oz)	100	2	0	24
Raisin Bran	1 cup (2 oz)	190	4	1	47
Selects Blueberry Morning	¾ cup (1.3 oz)	140	2	2	30
Waffle Crisp	1 cup (1 oz)	130	2	3	24
Quaker					
Instant Grits Original	1 pkg (1 oz)	100	2	0	22
Multigrain	½ cup (1.4 oz)	130	5	2	29
Oatmeal Instant	1 pkg (1 oz)	100	4	2	19
Oatmeal Instant Apples & Cinnamon	1 pkg (1.2 oz)	130	3	2	27
Oatmeal Instant Bananas & Cream	1 pkg (1.2 oz)	130	3	3	26
Oatmeal Instant Blueberries & Cream	1 pkg (1.2 oz)	130	3	3	26
Oatmeal Instant Cinnamon & Spice	1 pkg (1.6 oz)	170	4	2	35
Oatmeal Instant Kid's Choice Chocolate Chip Cookie	1 pkg (1.5 oz)	160	4	3	32
Oatmeal Instant Kid's Choice Cookie'n Cream	1 pkg (1.5 oz)	160	4	3	31
Oatmeal Instant Kid's Choice Fruity Marshmallow	1 pkg (1.4 oz)	150	4	2	31
Oatmeal Instant Kid's Choice Oatmeal Raisin Cookie	1 pkg (1.5 oz)	160	3	2	32
Oatmeal Instant Kid's Choice Radical Raspberry	1 pkg (1.4 oz)	150	4	3	29
Oatmeal Instant Kid's Choice S'mores	1 pkg (1.5 oz)	160	4	3	32
Oatmeal Instant Kid's Choice Strawberries'n Stuff	1 pkg (1.4 oz)	150	3	2	30

FOOD	PORTION	CALS	PROT	FAT	CARB
Oatmeal Instant Kid's Choice Twisted Strawberry Banana	1 pkg (1.4 oz)	150	3	2	31
Oatmeal Instant Maple & Brown Sugar	1 pkg (1.5 oz)	160	4	2	32
Oatmeal Instant Peaches & Cream	1 pkg (1.2 oz)	140	3	3	27
Oatmeal Instant Raisin & Spice	1 pkg (1.5 oz)	150	3	2	33
Oatmeal Instant Raisin Date & Walnut	1 pkg (1.3 oz)	140	3	3	27
Oatmeal Instant Strawberries & Cream	1 pkg (1.2 oz)	140	3	3	27
Oatmeal Nutrition for Women Golden Brown Sugar	1 pkg (1.6 oz)	170	5	2	33
Oatmeal Quick'n Hearty Microwave	1 pkg (1 oz)	110	4	2	19
Oatmeal Quick'n Hearty Microwave Apple Spice	1 pkg (1.6 oz)	170	4	2	35
Oatmeal Quick'n Hearty Microwave Brown Sugar Cinnamon	1 pkg (1.5 oz)	150	4	2	31
Oatmeal Quick'n Hearty Microwave Cinnamon Double Raisin	1 pkg (1.6 oz)	170	4	2	35
Oatmeal Quick'n Hearty Microwave Honey Bran	1 pkg (1.4 oz)	150	4	2	30
Oats Old Fashion	½ cup (1.4 oz)	150	5	3	27
Oats Quick	½ cup (1.4 oz)	150	5	3	27
Oats Steel Cut	½ cup (1.4 oz)	150	5	3	27
Whole Wheat Hot Natural	½ cup (1.4 oz)	130	5	1	30
Sunbelt					
Berry Basic	½ cup (1.9 oz)	220	6	6	40
Granola Banana Nut	½ cup (1.9 oz)	250	5	9	37
Granola Cinnamon Raisins	½ cup (1.9 oz)	200	5	3	42
Granola Fruit & Nut	½ cup (1.9 oz)	240	4	7	40
Muesli 5 Whole Grains	½ cup (1.9 oz)	210	4	2	44
Uncle Sam					
Cereal	1 cup (1.9 oz)	190	7	1	38
Weetabix					
Cereal	2 biscuits (1.2 oz)	100	3	1	21
Wheatena					
Cereal	⅓ cup (1.4 oz)	150	5	1	33

CEREAL BARS

(*see also* ENERGY BARS, NUTRITION SUPPLEMENTS)

chewy raisin	1 (1 oz)	127	2	5	19
granola	1 (1 oz)	134	3	7	18
granola almond	1 (1 oz)	140	2	7	18

FOOD	PORTION	CALS	PROT	FAT	CARB
granola chocolate chip	1 (1 oz)	124	2	5	20
granola peanut	1 (1 oz)	136	3	6	18
granola peanut butter	1 (1 oz)	137	3	7	18
granola chewy	1 (1 oz)	126	2	5	19
granola chewy chocolate chip	1 (1 oz)	119	2	5	10
granola chewy chocolate chip graham & marshmallow	1 (1 oz)	121	2	4	20
granola chewy chocolate coated chocolate chip	1 (1 oz)	132	2	7	18
granola chewy chocolate coated peanut butter	1 (1 oz)	144	3	9	15
granola chewy nut & raisin	1 (1 oz)	129	2	6	18
granola chewy peanut butter	1 (1 oz)	121	3	5	18
granola chewy peanut butter & chocolate chip	1 (1 oz)	122	3	6	18
Barbara's Bakery					
Nature's Choice Apple Cinnamon	1 bar (1.3 oz)	120	2	2	27
Nature's Choice Blueberry	1 bar (⅓ oz)	120	2	2	27
Nature's Choice Cherry	1 bar (1.3 oz)	120	2	2	27
Nature's Choice Granola Carob Chip	1 bar (0.7 oz)	80	2	2	16
Nature's Choice Granola Cinnamon & Raisin	1 bar (0.7 oz)	80	2	2	16
Nature's Choice Granola Oats 'N Honey	1 bar (0.7 oz)	80	2	2	15
Nature's Choice Granola Peanut Butter	1 bar (0.7 oz)	80	2	3	14
Nature's Choice Raspberry	1 bar (1.3 oz)	120	2	2	27
Nature's Choice Strawberry	1 bar (1.3 oz)	120	2	2	27
Nature's Choice Triple Berry	1 bar (1.3 oz)	120	2	2	27
Dolly Madison					
Apple	1 (1.3 oz)	120	1	2	25
Blueberry	1 (1.3 oz)	120	1	2	25
Raspberry	1 (1.3 oz)	120	1	2	24
Strawberry	1 (1.3 oz)	120	1	2	24
Entenmann's					
Apple Cinnamon	1 (1.3 oz)	140	1	3	25
Blueberry	1 (1.3 oz)	140	1	3	25
Oatmeal Apple Cinnamon	1 (1.3 oz)	140	1	3	27
Oatmeal Apple Raisin	1 (1.3 oz)	140	1	3	27
Raspberry	1 (1.3 oz)	140	1	3	27
Strawberry	1 (1.3 oz)	140	1	3	25

FOOD	PORTION	CALS	PROT	FAT	CARB
Estee					
Rice Crunchie Chocolate	1 (0.7 oz)	50	1	0	15
Rice Crunchie Chocolate Chip	1 (0.7 oz)	50	1	0	15
Rice Crunchie Peanut Butter	1 (0.7 oz)	60	1	1	15
Rice Crunchie Vanilla	1 (0.7 oz)	60	1	0	14
General Mills					
Milk 'N Cereal Bars Chex	1 bar (1.6 oz)	160	6	4	26
Milk 'N Cereal Bars Cinnamon Toast Crunch	1 bar (1.6 oz)	180	6	4	30
Glenny's					
Chocolate Crunch Creamy Low Fat	1 bar (1.75 oz)	190	3	3	36
Chocolate Crunch Roasted Peanut	1 bar (1.75 oz)	200	4	4	36
Chocolate Crunch Toasted Almond	1 bar (1.75 oz)	200	4	4	36
Health Valley					
98% Fat Free Raisin Cinnamon	⅔ cup	180	5	1	43
98% Fat Free Tropical	⅔ cup	180	5	1	43
Blueberry	1	140	2	0	35
Breakfast Bakes Apple Cinnamon	1 bar	110	2	0	26
Breakfast Bakes California Strawberry	1 bar	110	2	0	26
Breakfast Bakes Mountain Blueberry	1 bar	110	2	0	26
Breakfast Bakes Red Raspberry	1 bar	110	2	0	26
Chocolate Chip	1	140	2	0	35
Crisp Rice Bars Apple Cinnamon	1	110	1	0	26
Crisp Rice Bars Orange Date	1	110	1	0	26
Crisp Rice Bars Tropical Fruit	1	110	1	0	26
Date Almond	1	140	2	0	35
Fiber 7 Flakes w/ Strawberry	1 bar	110	2	0	26
O's Almond	¾ cup	120	3	0	26
O's Apple Cinnamon	¾ cup	120	3	0	26
O's Honey Crunch	¾ cup	120	3	0	26
Oat Bran Flakes w/ Blueberry	1 bar	110	2	0	26
Raisin	1	140	2	0	35
Raisin Bran Flakes w/ Apple Raisin	1 bar	110	2	0	26

FOOD	PORTION	CALS	PROT	FAT	CARB
Raspberry	1	140	2	0	35
Strawberry	1	140	2	0	35
Hershey's					
Crispy Rice Snacks Peanut Butter	1 bar (0.5 oz)	60	1	2	9
Hostess					
Apple	1 (1.3 oz)	120	1	2	25
Banana Nut	1 (1.3 oz)	120	2	2	25
Blueberry	1 (1.3 oz)	120	1	2	25
Raspberry	1 (1.3 oz)	120	1	2	24
Strawberry	1 (1.3 oz)	120	1	2	24
Kellogg's					
Nutri-Grain Apple Cinnamon	1 (1.3 oz)	140	2	3	27
Nutri-Grain Blueberry	1 (1.3 oz)	140	2	3	27
Nutri-Grain Cherry	1 (1.3 oz)	140	2	3	27
Nutri-Grain Mixed Berry	1 (1.3 oz)	140	2	3	27
Nutri-Grain Peach	1 (1.3 oz)	140	2	3	27
Nutri-Grain Raspberry	1 (1.3 oz)	140	2	3	27
Nutri-Grain Strawberry	1 (1.3 oz)	140	2	3	27
Nutri-Grain Twists Low Fat Apple Cinnamon	1 (1.3 oz)	140	1	3	27
Nutri-Grain Twists Low Fat Banana Strawberry	1 (1.3 oz)	140	1	3	26
Nutri-Grain Twists Low Fat Strawberry Blueberry	1 (1.3 oz)	140	1	3	27
Rice Krispies Treats	1 (0.8 oz)	90	1	2	18
Rice Krispies Treats Cocoa	1 (0.8 oz)	100	1	4	16
Rice Krispies Treats Peanut Butter Chocolate	1 (0.8 oz)	110	2	4	16
Kudos					
Chocolate Coated Chocolate Chip	1	120	1	5	20
Chocolate Coated Peanut Butter	1	90	1	3	17
Snickers	1	100	1	4	16
With M&M's	1	90	1	3	17
Little Debbie					
Raspberry	1 (1.3 oz)	130	1	3	28
S'mores Granola Treats	1 (1 oz)	130	2	5	21
Strawberry	1 (1.3 oz)	130	1	3	28
Nabisco					
Nutter Butter Granola Bar	1 (1 oz)	120	2	8	21
Oreo Granola Bar	1 (1 oz)	120	2	4	21
Nature Valley					
Low Fat Chewy Orchard Blend	1 bar (1 oz)	110	2	2	22
Nature's Choice					
Carob Chip	1 bar (0.7 oz)	80	2	3	16

FOOD	PORTION	CALS	PROT	FAT	CARB
Cinnamon & Raisin	1 bar (0.7 oz)	80	2	2	16
Fat Free Apple	1 bar (1.3 oz)	110	2	0	27
Fat Free Blueberry	1 bar (1.3 oz)	110	2	0	27
Fat Free Cranberry	1 bar (1.3 oz)	110	2	0	27
Fat Free Peach	1 bar (1.3 oz)	110	2	0	27
Fat Free Raspberry	1 bar (1.3 oz)	110	2	0	27
Fat Free Strawberry	1 bar (1.3 oz)	110	2	0	27
Low Fat Triple Berry	1 bar (1.3 oz)	130	2	2	28
Low Fat Very Cherry	1 bar (1.3 oz)	130	2	2	28
Oats 'n Honey	1 bar (0.7 oz)	80	2	2	15
Peanut Butter	1 bar (0.7 oz)	80	2	3	14
Nutri-Grain					
Fruit-full Squares Apple	1 (1.7 oz)	180	3	4	35
Fruit-full Squares Banana	1 (1.7 oz)	190	3	5	35
Fruit-full Squares Cinnamon Raisin	1 (1.7 oz)	180	3	4	35
Quaker					
Chewy Chocolate Chip	1 (1 oz)	120	2	4	21
Chewy Cookies 'n Cream	1 (1 oz)	110	2	3	22
Chewy Peanut Butter Chocolate Chunk	1 (1 oz)	120	2	3	20
Chewy Graham Slam Chocolate Chip	1 (1 oz)	110	2	2	22
Chewy Graham Slam Peanut Butter	1 (1 oz)	110	2	2	22
Chewy Low Fat Chocolate Chunk	1 (1 oz)	110	2	2	22
Chewy Low Fat Oatmeal Raisin	1 (1 oz)	110	1	2	22
Chewy Low Fat S'mores	1 (1 oz)	110	1	2	22
Fruit & Oatmeal Apple Cinnamon	1 (1.3 oz)	130	1	3	26
Fruit & Oatmeal Low Fat Cherry Cobbler	1 (1.3 oz)	140	2	3	26
Fruit & Oatmeal Low Fat Strawberry	1 (1.3 oz)	140	2	3	26
Fruit & Oatmeal Low Fat Strawberry Banana	1 (1.3 oz)	130	1	3	26
Fruit & Oatmeal Low Fat Strawberry Cheesecake	1 (1.3 oz)	130	2	3	26
SnackWell's					
Country Fruit Medley	1 (1.3 oz)	130	1	3	27
Fat Free Apple Cinnamon	1 (1.3 oz)	120	1	0	28
Fat Free Blueberry	1 (1.3 oz)	120	1	0	28
Fat Free Strawberry	1 (1.3 oz)	120	1	0	28
Hearty Fruit'n Grain Crisp Autumn Apple	1 (1.3 oz)	130	1	3	25

FOOD	PORTION	CALS	PROT	FAT	CARB
Hearty Fruit'n Grain Mixed Berry	1 (1.3 oz)	120	1	3	25
Hearty Fruit'n Grain Orchard Cherry	1 (1.3 oz)	130	1	5	26
Sunbelt					
Apple	1 (1.3 oz)	130	1	3	28
Blueberry	1 (1.3 oz)	130	1	3	28
Chewy Granola Almond	1 (1 oz)	130	2	7	17
Chewy Granola Apple Cinnamon	1 (1.2 oz)	140	2	3	28
Chewy Granola Chocolate Chip	1 (1.2 oz)	160	2	7	23
Chewy Granola Oatmeal Raisin	1 (1.2 oz)	130	2	3	27
Chewy Granola Oats & Honey	1 (1 oz)	120	2	5	19
Granola Fudge Dipped Chocolate Chip	1 (1.5 oz)	200	2	10	27
Granola Fudge Dipped Macaroon	1 (1.4 oz)	190	2	10	24
Weight Watchers					
Apple Cinnamon	1 (1 oz)	100	1	2	21
Blueberry	1 (1 oz)	100	1	2	21
Raspberry	1 (1 oz)	100	1	2	21
CHAYOTE					
fresh cooked	1 cup	38	1	1	8
raw cut up	1 cup	32	1	tr	7
CHEESE					
(*see also* CHEESE DISHES, CHEESE SUBSTITUTES, COTTAGE CHEESE, CREAM CHEESE, NEUFCHATEL)					
beaufort	1 oz	115	8	9	tr
bel paese	1 oz	112	7	9	0
blue	1 oz	100	6	8	1
brick	1 oz	105	7	8	1
brie	1 oz	95	8	8	tr
cacio di roma sheep's milk cheese	1 oz	130	8	10	0
caerphilly	1.4 oz	150	9	13	0
camembert	1 oz	85	6	7	tr
cantal	1 oz	105	7	9	tr
caraway	1 oz	107	7	8	1
chabichou	1 oz	95	6	8	tr
chaource	1 oz	83	5	7	tr
cheddar	1 oz	114	7	9	tr
cheddar low fat	1 oz	49	9	2	1
cheddar shredded	1 cup	455	28	37	1
cheshire	1 oz	110	7	9	1
colby	1 oz	112	7	9	1

FOOD	PORTION	CALS	PROT	FAT	CARB
comte	1 oz	114	8	9	tr
coulommiers	1 oz	88	6	7	tr
crottin	1 oz	105	6	9	tr
derby	1.4 oz	161	10	14	0
edam	1 oz	101	7	8	tr
emmentaler	1 oz	115	8	9	tr
feta	1 oz	75	4	6	1
fontina	1 oz	110	7	9	tr
frais	1.6 oz	51	3	3	3
gjetost	1 oz	132	3	8	12
goat fresh	1 oz	23	1	2	tr
goat hard	1 oz	128	9	10	1
goat semisoft	1 oz	103	6	8	1
goat soft	1 oz	76	5	6	tr
gorgonzola	1 oz	107	5	9	tr
gouda	1 oz	101	7	8	1
gruyere	1 oz	117	8	9	tr
lancashire	1.4 oz	149	9	12	0
leicester	1.4 oz	160	10	14	0
limburger	1 oz	93	8	8	tr
lymeswold	1.4 oz	170	6	16	tr
maroilles	1 oz	97	6	8	tr
monterey	1 oz	106	7	9	tr
morbier	1 oz	99	7	8	tr
muenster	1 oz	104	7	9	tr
parmesan grated	1 tbsp (5 g)	23	2	2	tr
parmesan hard	1 oz	111	10	7	1
picodon	1 oz	99	6	8	tr
pimento	1 oz	106	6	9	tr
pont l'eveque	1 oz	86	6	7	tr
port du salut	1 oz	100	7	8	tr
provolone	1 oz	100	7	8	1
pyrenees	1 oz	101	6	8	tr
quark 20% fat	1 oz	33	4	1	1
quark 40% fat	1 oz	48	3	3	1
quark made w/ skim milk	1 oz	22	4	tr	1
queso anego	1 oz	106	6	9	1
queso asadero	1 oz	101	6	8	1
queso chichuahua	1 oz	106	6	8	2
queso fresco	1 oz	41	4	2	1
queso manchego	1 oz	107	8	8	tr
queso panela	1 oz	74	6	5	1
raclette	1 oz	102	7	8	tr
reblochon	1 oz	88	6	7	tr
romadur 40% fat	1 oz	83	7	6	tr
romano	1 oz	110	9	8	1
roquefort	1 oz	105	6	9	1
rouy	1 oz	95	7	8	tr

FOOD	PORTION	CALS	PROT	FAT	CARB
saint marcellin	1 oz	94	5	8	tr
saint nectaire	1 oz	97	6	8	tr
saint paulin	1 oz	85	7	6	tr
sainte maure	1 oz	99	6	8	tr
selles sur cher	1 oz	93	5	8	tr
stilton blue	1.4 oz	164	9	14	0
stilton white	1.4 oz	145	8	13	0
swiss	1 oz	107	8	8	1
tilsit	1 oz	96	7	7	1
tome	1 oz	92	6	7	tr
triple creme	1 oz	113	3	11	tr
vacherin	1 oz	92	5	8	tr
wensleydale	1.4 oz	151	9	13	0
whey cheese	1 oz	126	4	8	9
yogurt cheese	1 oz	80	6	7	0
Alouette					
Garlic & Herbs	2 tbsp (0.8 oz)	70	1	7	1
Alpine Lace					
American Jalapeno Peppers	1 slice (1 oz)	80	6	6	2
American Less Fat Less Sodium White	1 slice (1 oz)	50	6	6	2
American Less Fat Less Sodium Yellow	1 slice (1 oz)	80	6	6	2
Cheddar Reduced Fat	1 slice (1 oz)	70	8	5	1
Colby Reduced Fat	1 slice (1 oz)	80	9	5	1
Fat Free Parmesan	2 tsp (5 g)	10	1	0	0
Feta Reduced Fat	1 oz	50	5	3	1
Feta Reduced Fat Sun Dried Tomato & Basil	1 oz	50	5	3	1
Goat Reduced Fat	1 oz	40	2	3	tr
Mozzarella Reduced Fat	1 oz	70	8	3	1
Muenster Reduced Sodium	1 slice (1 oz)	100	7	9	1
Provolone Smoked Reduced Fat	1 slice (1 oz)	70	9	5	1
Swiss Reduced Fat	1 slice (1 oz)	90	8	6	1
Boar's Head					
American	1 oz	100	6	9	1
Baby Swiss	1 oz	110	7	9	tr
Canadian Cheddar	1 oz	110	7	10	0
Double Glouster Yellow	1 oz	110	7	10	0
Havarti	1 oz	110	6	10	0
Havarti w/ Dill	1 oz	110	6	10	0
Havarti w/ Jalapeno	1 oz	110	6	10	0
Lacey Swiss	1 oz	90	9	6	0
Longhorn Colby	1 oz	110	7	9	tr
Monterey Jack	1 oz	100	6	9	0
Monterey Jack w/ Jalapeno	1 oz	100	6	9	0

FOOD	PORTION	CALS	PROT	FAT	CARB
Mozzarella	1 oz	90	6	7	tr
Muenster	1 oz	100	6	8	0
Muenster Low Sodium	1 oz	100	6	8	0
Provolone Picante Sharp	1 oz	100	7	8	1
Swiss	1 oz	110	8	8	tr
Swiss No Salt Added	1 oz	110	8	8	tr
Breakstone's					
Ricotta	¼ cup (2.2 oz)	110	7	8	3
Cabot					
Cheddar	1 oz	110	7	9	tr
Cheddar Five Peppercorn	1 oz	110	7	9	tr
Cheddar Mediterranean	1 oz	110	7	9	tr
Cheddar Sundried Tomato Basil	1 oz	110	7	9	tr
Cheddar Toasted Onion & Chive	1 oz	110	7	9	tr
Cheddar Light 50% Reduced Fat	1 oz	70	8	5	1
Cheddar Light 50% Reduced Fat Jalapeno	1 oz	70	8	5	1
Cheddar Light 50% Reduced Fat Tomato Basil	1 oz	70	8	5	1
Cheddar Light 75% Reduced Fat	1 oz	60	9	3	1
Dehydrated Cheddar Powder	2 tsp (5 g)	25	1	2	1
Monterey Jack	1 oz	110	7	9	tr
Cedar Grove					
Marble Colby	1 oz	110	7	9	0
Organic Tomato Basil Cheddar	1 oz	110	7	9	0
Cheez Whiz					
Light	2 tbsp (1.2 oz)	80	6	3	6
Cracker Barrel					
Baby Swiss	1 oz	110	7	9	0
Cheddar Extra Sharp	1 oz	120	6	10	0
Cheddar Marbled Sharp	1 oz	110	7	9	tr
Cheddar New York Aged	1 oz	120	6	10	0
Cheddar Sharp	1 oz	120	6	10	0
Cheddar Vermont Sharp	1 oz	110	7	9	tr
Reduced Fat Cheddar Extra Sharp	1 oz	90	7	6	tr
Reduced Fat Cheddar Sharp	1 oz	90	7	6	tr
Reduced Fat Cheddar Vermont Sharp	1 oz	90	7	6	tr

FOOD	PORTION	CALS	PROT	FAT	CARB
Whipped Spreadable Cream Cheese & Extra Sharp Cheddar	2 tbsp (0.9 oz)	80	3	8	tr
Whipped Spreadable Cream Cheese & Sharp Cheddar	2 tbsp (0.9 oz)	80	3	8	tr
Whipped Spreadable Cream Cheese & Sharp Cheddar w/ Herbs	2 tbsp (0.9 oz)	80	3	8	tr
Di Giorno					
Parmesan Grated	2 tsp (5 g)	25	2	2	0
Parmesan Shredded	2 tsp (5 g)	20	2	2	0
Romano Grated	2 tsp (5 g)	25	2	2	0
Romano Shredded	2 tsp (5 g)	20	2	2	0
Fleurs De France					
Brie	3.5 oz	311	21	25	tr
Friendship					
Farmer	2 tbsp (1 oz)	50	5	3	0
Handi-Snacks					
Cheez'n Breadsticks	1 pkg (1.1 oz)	120	4	6	12
Cheez'n Crackers	1 pkg (1.1 oz)	110	3	7	9
Cheez'n Pretzels	1 pkg (1 oz)	100	4	5	11
Mozzarella String Cheese	1 piece (1 oz)	80	7	6	0
Nacho Stix'n Cheez	1 pkg (1.1 oz)	110	4	6	11
Hollow Road Farms					
Sheep's Milk	1 oz	45	3	3	1
Kraft					
Cheddar Extra Sharp	1 oz	120	6	10	0
Cheddar Medium	1 oz	110	7	9	tr
Cheddar Mild	1 oz	110	7	9	tr
Cheddar Sharp	1 oz	120	6	10	0
Cheddary Melts Medium Cheddar	1 oz	110	5	9	2
Cheddary Melts Mild Cheddar	1 oz	110	5	9	2
Cheddary Melts Shreds Medium Cheddar	¼ cup (1.1 oz)	120	6	9	2
Cheddary Melts Shreds Mild Cheddar	¼ cup (1.1 oz)	120	6	9	2
Cheese Food w/ Garlic	1 oz	90	5	7	2
Cheese Food w/ Jalapeno Peppers	1 oz	90	5	7	2
Colby	1 oz	110	7	9	tr
Colby Monterey Jack	1 oz	110	7	9	0
Deluxe American	1 oz	100	6	9	tr
Deluxe American White	1 oz	100	6	9	tr
Deluxe Singles American	1 (1 oz)	110	6	9	tr
Deluxe Singles American	1 (0.7 oz)	70	4	6	tr

FOOD	PORTION	CALS	PROT	FAT	CARB
Deluxe Singles Pimento	1 (1 oz)	100	6	8	tr
Deluxe Singles Swiss	1 (1 oz)	90	6	7	0
Deluxe Singles Swiss	1 slice (0.7 oz)	70	5	5	0
Free Shredded Cheddar	¼ cup (0.9 oz)	40	9	0	1
Free Shredded Mozzarella	¼ cup (1 oz)	45	9	0	2
Grated Parmesan	2 tsp (5 g)	20	2	2	0
Grated Romano	2 tsp (5 g)	20	2	2	0
Marbled Cheddar Mild	1 oz	110	7	9	tr
Marbled Cheddar & Monterey Jack	1 oz	110	7	9	tr
Marbled Cheddar & Whole Milk Mozzarella	1 oz	100	6	8	tr
Marbled Colby Monterey Jack	1 oz	110	7	9	0
Monterey Jack	1 oz	110	6	9	0
Monterey Jack w/ Jalapeno Peppers	1 oz	110	7	9	tr
Mozzarella Part Skim Low Moisture	1 oz	80	8	5	tr
Mozzarella String Cheese Low Moisture Part Skim	1 piece (1 oz)	80	7	6	0
Pizza Shredded Four Cheese	¼ cup (0.9 oz)	90	6	7	tr
Pizza Shredded Mozzarella & Cheddar	⅓ cup (1.1 oz)	120	7	9	1
Pizza Shredded Mozzarella & Provolone w/ Smoke Flavor	¼ cup (0.9 oz)	90	6	7	tr
Reduced Fat Cheddar Mild	1 oz	90	7	6	tr
Reduced Fat Cheddar Sharp	1 oz	90	7	6	tr
Reduced Fat Colby	1 oz	80	7	6	0
Reduced Fat Monterey Jack	1 oz	80	7	6	tr
Shredded Cheddar Medium	¼ cup (0.9 oz)	100	6	8	tr
Shredded Cheddar Mild	¼ cup (0.9 oz)	100	6	8	tr
Shredded Cheddar Sharp	1 oz (0.9 oz)	110	6	9	tr
Shredded Cheddar & Monterey Jack	¼ cup (0.9 oz)	100	6	8	tr
Shredded Colby & Monterey Jack	¼ cup (0.9 oz)	100	6	8	tr
Shredded Hearty Italian	⅓ cup (1.1 oz)	100	7	8	2
Shredded Italian Style Classic Garlic	⅓ cup (1.1 oz)	100	7	8	2
Shredded Italian Style Mozzarelle & Parmesan	⅓ cup (1.1 oz)	100	7	8	1
Shredded Lower Fat Cheddar Mild	¼ cup (0.9 oz)	80	7	6	tr
Shredded Lower Fat Cheddar Sharp	¼ cup (0.9 oz)	80	7	6	tr

FOOD	PORTION	CALS	PROT	FAT	CARB
Shredded Lower Fat Colby & Monterey Jack	¼ cup (0.9 oz)	80	7	5	tr
Shredded Lower Fat Mozzarella	⅓ cup (1.1 oz)	80	9	5	tr
Shredded Lower Fat Pizza Cheese	⅓ cup (1.1 oz)	90	9	6	1
Shredded Mexican Style Cheddar & Monterey Jack	⅓ cup (1.1 oz)	120	7	10	tr
Shredded Mexican Style Cheddar & Monterey Jack w/ Jalapeno Peppers	⅓ cup (1.1 oz)	120	7	10	tr
Shredded Mexican Style Four Cheese	⅓ cup (1.1 oz)	120	7	10	tr
Shredded Mexican Style Taco Cheese	⅓ cup (1.1 oz)	120	7	10	1
Shredded Monterey Jack	¼ cup (0.9 oz)	100	6	8	tr
Shredded Parmesan	2 tsp (5 g)	20	2	2	0
Shredded Part Skim Mozzarella	¼ cup (1.1 oz)	90	8	6	tr
Shredded Swiss	¼ cup (0.9 oz)	100	7	8	tr
Shredded Whole Milk Mozzarella	¼ cup (1.1 oz)	100	7	8	1
Shredded Finely Cheddar Mild	¼ cup (1.1 oz)	120	7	10	tr
Shredded Finely Cheddar Sharp	¼ cup (1.1 oz)	120	7	10	tr
Shredded Finely Colby & Monterey Jack	¼ cup (1 oz)	110	7	9	tr
Shredded Finely Lower Fat Cheddar Mild	⅓ cup (1.1 oz)	100	8	7	1
Shredded Finely Lower Fat Cheddar Sharp	⅓ cup (1.1 oz)	100	8	7	1
Shredded Finely Part Skim Mozzarella	¼ cup (1.1 oz)	90	8	6	tr
Shredded Finely Swiss	¼ cup (0.9 oz)	110	7	8	tr
Singles American	1 (1.2 oz)	110	6	8	3
Singles American	1 (0.7 oz)	60	3	5	2
Singles American	1 (0.6 oz)	60	3	5	2
Singles Mild Mexican	1 (0.7 oz)	70	4	5	2
Singles Monterey	1 slice (0.7 oz)	70	4	5	2
Singles Pimento	1 (0.7 oz)	60	4	5	1
Singles Reduced Fat American	1 (0.7 oz)	50	5	3	2
Singles Reduced Fat American White	1 (0.7 oz)	50	4	3	2
Singles Sharp	1 slice (0.7 oz)	70	4	6	tr
Singles Swiss	1 slice (0.7 oz)	70	4	5	1
Singles Nonfat American	1 (0.7 oz)	30	4	0	3

FOOD	PORTION	CALS	PROT	FAT	CARB
Singles Nonfat American White	1 (0.7 oz)	30	4	0	3
Singles Nonfat Sharp Cheddar	1 (0.7 oz)	35	5	0	3
Singles Nonfat Swiss	1 slice (0.7 oz)	30	5	0	3
Slices Cheddar Mild	1 (1 oz)	110	7	9	tr
Slices Colby	1 (1.6 oz)	180	11	14	tr
Slices Part Skim Mozzarella	1 (1.6 oz)	130	12	8	tr
Slices Part Skim Mozzarella	1 (1.5 oz)	120	12	8	tr
Slices Provolone Smoke Flavor	1 (1.5 oz)	150	11	11	tr
Slices Swiss	1 (1.5 oz)	170	12	13	tr
Slices Swiss	1 (1.3 oz)	150	10	12	tr
Slices Swiss	1 (0.8 oz)	90	6	7	0
Slices Swiss	1 (1.6 oz)	180	12	14	tr
Slices Swiss Aged	1 (1.5 oz)	170	12	13	tr
Slices Deli-Thin Part Skim Mozzarella	1 (1 oz)	80	8	5	tr
Slices Deli-Thin Swiss	1 (0.8 oz)	90	6	7	0
Slices Deli-Thin Swiss Aged	1 (0.8 oz)	90	6	7	0
Slices Reduced Fat Swiss	1 (1.3 oz)	130	11	9	tr
Spread Bacon	2 tbsp (1.1 oz)	90	5	8	tr
Spread Olive & Pimento	2 tbsp (1.1 oz)	70	2	6	3
Spread Pimento	2 tbsp (1.1 oz)	80	2	6	3
Spread Pineapple	2 tbsp (1.1 oz)	70	2	5	4
Spread Roka Brand Blue	2 tbsp (1.1 oz)	90	5	8	tr
Swiss	1 oz	110	8	9	0
Land O Lakes					
American	1 slice (0.7 oz)	80	4	6	1
American Jalapeno	1 slice (0.6 oz)	70	3	6	1
American Light	1 oz	70	7	5	2
American Reduced Salt	1 oz	110	6	9	tr
American Sharp	2 slices (1 oz)	100	5	9	1
American & Swiss	1 slice (0.6 oz)	70	4	5	1
Baby Swiss	1 oz	110	6	9	0
Chedarella	1 oz	100	7	8	0
Cheddar	1 oz	100	6	9	tr
Cheddar Extra Sharp	1 oz	110	6	8	tr
Cheddar Sharp	1 oz	110	7	9	tr
Cheese Spread Golden Velvet	1 oz	80	5	6	2
Colby	1 oz	110	7	9	tr
Jalapeno Light	1 oz	70	7	4	1
Monterey Jack	1 oz	110	6	8	tr
Monterey Jack Hot Pepper	1 oz	110	6	8	tr
Mozzarella	1 oz	80	7	6	tr
Muenster	1 oz	100	6	8	0
Parmesan Grated	1 tbsp	35	3	4	0

FOOD	PORTION	CALS	PROT	FAT	CARB
Provolone	1 oz	100	7	8	tr
Swiss	1 oz	110	8	8	tr
Swiss Light	1 oz	80	9	4	tr
Light N'Lively					
Singles American	1 (0.7 oz)	45	5	3	2
Old English					
American Sharp	1 slice (1 oz)	100	6	9	tr
Organic Valley					
Aged Swiss Unpasteurized	1 oz	100	8	8	tr
Cheddar Reduced Fat Low Sodium	1 oz	90	8	6	1
Cheddar Sharp & Mild	1 oz	110	7	9	1
Cheddar Sharp & Mild Unpasteurized	1 oz	110	7	9	1
Colby	1 oz	110	7	9	1
Colby Unpasteurized	1 oz	110	7	9	1
Farmer Reduced Fat	1 oz	90	7	6	1
Feta	1 oz	90	6	7	0
Monterey Jack	1 oz	100	6	8	1
Monterey Jack Reduced Fat	1 oz	80	8	5	1
Mozzarella Part Skim	1 oz	80	8	5	1
Muenster	1 oz	100	6	8	1
Pepper Jack	1 oz	110	6	9	1
Provolone	1 oz	100	7	8	1
String Part Skim	1 oz	80	8	5	1
Wisconsin Raw Milk Cheese	1 oz	100	6	8	1
Polly-O					
String Lite	1 piece (1 oz)	60	7	3	tr
President					
Feta Fat Free	1 oz	30	6	0	2
Rouge Et Noir					
Breakfast	1 oz	86	5	7	1
Brie	1 oz	86	5	7	1
Camembert	1 oz	86	5	7	1
Schloss	1 oz	86	5	7	1
Sargento					
Blue Crumbled	¼ cup (1 oz)	100	6	8	1
Cheddar	1 slice (1 oz)	110	6	9	1
Cheddar Shredded	¼ cup (1 oz)	110	6	9	1
Cheese For Nachos & Tacos Shredded	¼ cup (1 oz)	110	6	9	1
Cheese For Pizza Shredded	¼ cup (1 oz)	90	7	6	0
Cheese For Tacos Shredded	¼ cup (1 oz)	110	6	9	1
Colby	1 slice (1 oz)	110	6	9	0
Colby-Jack Shredded	¼ cup (1 oz)	110	6	9	tr
Jarlsberg	1 slice (1.2 oz)	120	9	9	1

FOOD	PORTION	CALS	PROT	FAT	CARB
Monterey Jack	1 slice (1 oz)	100	6	9	0
Monterey Jack Shredded	¼ cup (1 oz)	100	6	9	0
MooTown Snackers Cheddar	1 piece (0.8 oz)	100	5	8	1
MooTown Snackers Cheddar Mild Light	1 piece (0.8 oz)	60	7	4	tr
MooTown Snackers Cheese & Pretzels	1 pkg (0.9 oz)	90	3	3	12
MooTown Snackers Colby-Jack	1 piece (0.8 oz)	90	5	8	tr
MooTown Snackers Pizza Cheese & Sticks	1 pkg (1 oz)	100	3	4	13
MooTown Snackers String	1 piece (0.8 oz)	70	6	5	tr
MooTown Snackers String Light	1 piece (0.8 oz)	60	7	3	tr
Mozzarella	1 slice (1.5 oz)	130	11	9	2
Mozzarella Shredded	¼ cup (1 oz)	80	7	6	1
Muenster	1 slice (1 oz)	100	6	9	tr
Parmesan Grated	1 tbsp (5 g)	25	2	2	0
Parmesan Shredded	¼ cup (1 oz)	110	9	7	1
Parmesan & Romano Shredded	¼ cup (1 oz)	110	9	7	1
Parmesan & Romano Grated	1 tbsp (5 g)	25	2	2	0
Pizza Double Cheese Shredded	¼ cup (1 oz)	90	7	6	1
Preferred Light Cheddar Mild Shredded	¼ cup (1 oz)	70	8	5	tr
Preferred Light Cheese For Tacos Shredded	¼ cup (1 oz)	70	8	5	tr
Preferred Light Mozzarella	1 slice (1.5 oz)	90	11	5	0
Preferred Light Mozzarella Shredded	¼ cup (1 oz)	70	8	3	tr
Preferred Light Swiss	1 slice (1 oz)	80	9	4	tr
Provolone	1 slice (1 oz)	100	7	8	0
Recipe Blend 4 Cheese Mexican Shredded	¼ cup (1 oz)	110	6	9	tr
Recipe Blend 6 Cheese Italian Shredded	¼ cup (1 oz)	90	7	7	0
Ricotta Light	¼ cup (2.2 oz)	60	5	3	3
Ricotta Old Fashioned	¼ cup (2.2 oz)	90	7	6	3
Ricotta Part-Skim	¼ cup (2.2 oz)	80	7	5	2
Swiss	1 slice (0.7 oz)	80	6	6	0
Swiss Shredded	¼ cup (1 oz)	110	8	8	0
Swiss Wafer Thin	2 slices (1 oz)	110	5	9	0
Sorrento					
Mozzarella Part Skim Jalapeno	1 oz	80	8	5	1

FOOD	PORTION	CALS	PROT	FAT	CARB
Tree Of Life					
Cheddar 33% Reduced Fat Organic Milk	1 oz	90	8	6	1
Colby	1 oz	110	7	9	1
Colby Organic Milk	1 oz	120	7	10	1
Farmer Part-Skim Organic Milk	1 oz	90	7	6	1
Jalapeno Organic Milk	1 oz	110	6	9	1
Monterey Jack 35% Reduced Fat Organic Milk	1 oz	80	8	5	1
Monterey Jack Organic Milk	1 oz	100	6	8	1
Mozzarella Organic Milk	1 oz	80	8	5	1
Muenster Organic Milk	1 oz	100	6	8	1
Provolone	1 oz	100	7	8	1
Velveeta					
Light	1 oz	60	5	3	3
Shredded	¼ cup (1.3 oz)	130	8	9	3
Shredded Mild Mexican w/ Jalapeno Pepper	¼ cup (1.3 oz)	120	8	9	3
Spread	1 oz	90	5	6	3
Spread Hot Mexican	1 oz	90	5	6	3
Spread Mild Mexican	1 oz	90	5	6	3
Weight Watchers					
Cheddar Mild Yellow	1 oz	80	8	5	1
Cheddar Sharp Yellow	1 oz	80	8	5	1
Fat Free Grated Italian Topping	1 tbsp	20	2	0	2
Fat Free Reduced Sodium Yellow	2 slices (0.75 oz)	30	5	0	3
Fat Free Sharp Cheddar	2 slices (0.75 oz)	30	5	0	3
Fat Free Swiss	2 slices (0.75 oz)	30	5	0	2
Fat Free White	2 slices (0.75 oz)	30	5	0	3
Fat Free Yellow	2 slices (0.75 oz)	30	5	0	3
Wholesome Valley					
Organic American Reduced Fat	1 slice (0.7 oz)	50	4	3	2
CHEESE DISHES					
frozen					
Banquet					
Mozzeralla Nuggets	6	260	9	18	19
Health Is Wealth					
Mozzarella Sticke	2 (1.3 oz)	120	5	5	14
Stouffer's					
Welsh Rarebit	½ cup (2.5 oz)	120	5	9	5
home recipe					
welsh rarebit as prep w/ 1 white toast	1 slice	228	8	16	14

FOOD	PORTION	CALS	PROT	FAT	CARB
take-out					
cheese omelette as prep w/ 2 eggs	1 (6.8 oz)	519	31	44	tr
fondue	½ cup (3.8 oz)	247	15	15	4
souffle	1 serv (7 oz)	504	23	38	18
CHEESE SUBSTITUTES					
mozzarella	1 oz	70	3	3	7
Sargento					
Cheddar Shredded	¼ cup (1 oz)	90	5	7	2
Mozzarella Shredded	¼ cup (1 oz)	80	6	6	tr
Yves					
Good Slice American	1 slice (0.7 oz)	35	4	2	0
Good Slice Cheddar	1 slice (0.7 oz)	35	4	2	1
Good Slice Jalapeno Jack	1 slice (0.7 oz)	35	4	2	0
Good Slice Mozzarella	1 slice (0.7 oz)	30	4	2	0
Good Slice Swiss	1 slice (0.7 oz)	35	4	2	1
CHERIMOYA					
fresh	1	515	7	2	131
CHERRIES					
canned					
sour in heavy syrup	½ cup	232	2	tr	60
sour in light syrup	½ cup	189	2	tr	49
sour water packed	1 cup	87	2	tr	22
sweet in heavy syrup	½ cup	107	1	tr	27
sweet in light syrup	½ cup	85	1	tr	22
sweet juice pack	½ cup	68	1	tr	17
sweet water pack	½ cup	57	1	tr	15
Del Monte					
Dark Pitted In Heavy Syrup	½ cup (4.2 oz)	100	1	0	24
fresh					
sour	1 cup	51	1	tr	13
sweet	10	49	1	1	11
Chiquita					
Cherries	21	90	2	1	22
frozen					
sour unsweetened	1 cup	72	1	1	17
sweet sweetened	1 cup	232	3	tr	58
CHERRY JUICE					
Eden					
Montmorency Juice	8 oz	140	1	1	33
Juicy Juice					
Drink	1 box (4.23 oz)	70	0	0	17
Drink	1 box (8.5 oz)	140	0	0	34
Kool-Aid					
Black Cherry Drink as prep w/ sugar	1 serv (8 oz)	100	0	0	25
Bursts Cherry Drink	1 (7 oz)	100	0	0	25
Splash Drink	1 serv (8 oz)	110	0	0	29

FOOD	PORTION	CALS	PROT	FAT	CARB
Sugar Free Drink Mix as prep	1 serv (8 oz)	5	0	0	0
Mott's					
Cherry	1 box (8 oz)	120	0	0	31
Ocean Spray					
Black Cherry Blast	8 oz	140	0	0	33
Veryfine					
Juice-Ups	8 fl oz	130	0	0	33
CHESTNUTS					
chinese cooked	1 oz	44	1	tr	10
chinese dried	1 oz	103	2	tr	23
chinese raw	1 oz	64	1	tr	14
chinese roasted	1 oz	68	1	tr	15
cooked	1 oz	37	1	tr	8
creme de marrons	1 oz	73	1	tr	18
dried peeled	1 oz	105	1	1	22
japanese dried	1 oz	102	1	tr	23
japanese raw	1 oz	44	1	tr	10
japanese roasted	1 oz	57	1	tr	13
roasted	2 to 3 (1 oz)	70	1	1	15
roasted	1 cup	350	5	3	76
CHEWING GUM					
bubble gum	1 block (8 g)	27	0	0	8
stick	1 (3 g)	10	0	0	3
Aquafresh					
Peppermint	2 pieces	5	0	0	2
Arm & Hammer					
Dental Care Spearmint or Peppermint	2 pieces (2.5 g)	5	0	0	2
Dentyne					
Ice Peppermint	2 pieces (3 g)	5	0	0	2
Lance					
Big Red Cinnamon	1 piece (3 g)	10	0	0	2
Double Bubble	1 piece (7 g)	25	0	0	6
Double Mint	1 piece (3 g)	10	0	0	2
Winterfresh					
Stick	1 stick (3 g)	10	0	0	2
CHIA SEEDS					
dried	1 oz	134	5	7	14
CHICKEN					
(*see also* CHICKEN DISHES, CHICKEN SUBSTITUTES, DINNER, HOT DOGS)					
canned					
chicken spread	1 tbsp	25	2	2	1
chicken spread	1 oz	55	4	3	2
chicken spread barbeque flavored	1 oz	55	4	3	2
w/ broth	1 can (5 oz)	234	31	11	0
w/ broth	½ can (2.5 oz)	117	15	6	0

FOOD	PORTION	CALS	PROT	FAT	CARB
fresh					
broiler/fryer back w/ skin batter dipped & fried	½ back (2.5 oz)	238	16	16	7
broiler/fryer back w/ skin floured & fried	1.5 oz	146	12	9	3
broiler/fryer back w/ skin roasted	1 oz	96	8	7	0
broiler/fryer back w/ skin stewed	½ back (2.1 oz)	158	14	11	0
broiler/fryer back w/o skin fried	½ back (2 oz)	167	17	9	3
broiler/fryer breast w/ skin batter dipped & fried	½ breast (4.9 oz)	364	35	18	13
broiler/fryer breast w/ skin batter dipped & fried	2.9 oz	218	21	11	8
broiler/fryer breast w/ skin roasted	½ breast (3.4 oz)	193	29	8	0
broiler/fryer breast w/ skin roasted	2 oz	115	17	5	0
broiler/fryer breast w/ skin stewed	½ breast (3.9 oz)	202	30	8	0
broiler/fryer breast w/o skin fried	½ breast (3 oz)	161	29	4	tr
broiler/fryer breast w/o skin roasted	½ breast (3 oz)	142	27	3	0
broiler/fryer breast w/o skin stewed	2 oz	86	17	2	0
broiler/fryer dark meat w/ skin batter dipped & fried	5.9 oz	497	36	31	16
broiler/fryer dark meat w/ skin floured & fried	3.9 oz	313	30	19	4
broiler/fryer dark meat w/ skin roasted	3.5 oz	256	26	16	0
broiler/fryer dark meat w/ skin stewed	3.9 oz	256	26	16	0
broiler/fryer dark meat w/o skin fried	1 cup (5 oz)	334	41	16	4
broiler/fryer dark meat w/o skin roasted	1 cup (5 oz)	286	38	14	0
broiler/fryer dark meat w/o skin stewed	1 cup (5 oz)	269	36	13	0
broiler/fryer dark meat w/o skin stewed	3 oz	165	22	8	0
broiler/fryer drumstick w/ skin batter dipped & fried	1 (2.6 oz)	193	16	11	6
broiler/fryer drumstick w/ skin floured & fried	1 (1.7 oz)	120	13	7	1

FOOD	PORTION	CALS	PROT	FAT	CARB
broiler/fryer drumstick w/ skin roasted	1 (1.8 oz)	112	14	6	0
broiler/fryer drumstick w/ skin stewed	1 (2 oz)	116	14	6	0
broiler/fryer drumstick w/o skin fried	1 (1.5 oz)	82	12	3	0
broiler/fryer drumstick w/o skin roasted	1 (1.5 oz)	76	12	2	0
broiler/fryer drumstick w/o skin stewed	1 (1.6 oz)	78	13	3	0
broiler/fryer leg w/ skin batter dipped & fried	1 (5.5 oz)	431	34	26	14
broiler/fryer leg w/ skin floured & fried	1 (3.9 oz)	285	30	16	3
broiler/fryer leg w/ skin roasted	1 (4 oz)	265	30	15	0
broiler/fryer leg w/ skin stewed	1 (4.4 oz)	275	30	16	0
broiler/fryer leg w/o skin fried	1 (3.3 oz)	195	27	9	1
broiler/fryer leg w/o skin roasted	1 (3.3 oz)	182	26	8	0
broiler/fryer leg w/o skin stewed	1 (3.5 oz)	187	26	8	0
broiler/fryer light meat w/ skin batter dipped & fried	4 oz	312	27	17	11
broiler/fryer light meat w/ skin floured & fried	2.7 oz	192	24	9	1
broiler/fryer light meat w/ skin roasted	2.8 oz	175	23	9	0
broiler/fryer light meat w/ skin stewed	3.2 oz	181	9	9	0
broiler/fryer light meat w/o skin fried	1 cup (5 oz)	268	46	8	1
broiler/fryer light meat w/o skin roasted	1 cup (5 oz)	242	43	6	0
broiler/fryer light meat w/o skin stewed	1 cup (5 oz)	223	40	6	0
broiler/fryer neck w/ skin stewed	1 (1.3 oz)	94	7	7	0
broiler/fryer neck w/o skin stewed	1 (.6 oz)	32	4	1	0
broiler/fryer skin batter dipped & fried	from ½ chicken (6.7 oz)	748	20	55	44
broiler/fryer skin batter dipped & fried	4 oz	449	12	33	26
broiler/fryer skin floured & fried	from ½ chicken (2 oz)	281	24	24	5

FOOD	PORTION	CALS	PROT	FAT	CARB
broiler/fryer skin floured & fried	1 oz	166	6	14	3
broiler/fryer skin roasted	from ½ chicken (2 oz)	254	11	23	0
broiler/fryer skin stewed	from ½ chicken (2.5 oz)	261	11	24	0
broiler/fryer thigh w/ skin batter dipped & fried	1 (3 oz)	238	19	14	8
broiler/fryer thigh w/ skin floured & fried	1 (2.2 oz)	162	17	9	2
broiler/fryer thigh w/ skin roasted	1 (2.2 oz)	153	16	10	0
broiler/fryer thigh w/ skin stewed	1 (2.4 oz)	158	16	10	0
broiler/fryer thigh w/o skin fried	1 (1.8 oz)	113	15	5	1
broiler/fryer thigh w/o skin roasted	1 (1.8 oz)	109	13	6	0
broiler/fryer thigh w/o skin stewed	1 (1.9 oz)	107	14	5	0
broiler/fryer w/ skin floured & fried	½ chicken (11 oz)	844	90	47	10
broiler/fryer w/ skin fried	½ chicken (16.4 oz)	1347	81	81	44
broiler/fryer w/ skin roasted	½ chicken (10.5 oz)	715	82	41	0
broiler/fryer w/ skin stewed	½ chicken (11.7 oz)	730	82	42	0
broiler/fryer w/ skin neck & giblets batter dipped & fried	1 chicken (2.3 lbs)	2987	235	180	93
broiler/fryer w/ skin neck & giblets roasted	1 chicken (1.5 lbs)	1598	183	90	tr
broiler/fryer w/ skin neck & giblets stewed	1 chicken (1.6 lbs)	1625	184	93	tr
broiler/fryer w/o skin fried	1 cup	307	43	13	2
broiler/fryer w/o skin roasted	1 cup (5 oz)	266	41	10	0
broiler/fryer w/o skin stewed	1 oz	54	7	3	0
broiler/fryer w/o skin stewed	1 cup (5 oz)	248	38	9	0
broiler/fryer wing w/ skin batter dipped & fried	1 (1.7 oz)	159	10	11	5
broiler/fryer wing w/ skin floured & fried	1 (1.1 oz)	103	8	7	1
broiler/fryer wing w/ skin roasted	1 (1.2 oz)	99	9	7	0
broiler/fryer wing w/ skin stewed	1 (1.4 oz)	100	9	7	0

FOOD	PORTION	CALS	PROT	FAT	CARB
capon w/ skin neck & giblets roasted	1 chicken (3.1 lbs)	3211	402	165	1
cornish hen w/ skin roasted	1 hen (8 oz)	595	51	42	0
cornish hen w/o skin & bone roasted	1 hen (3.8 oz)	144	25	4	0
cornish hen w/o skin & bone roasted	½ hen (2 oz)	72	13	2	0
cornish hen w/ skin roasted	½ hen (4 oz)	296	25	21	0
roaster dark meat w/o skin roasted	1 cup (5 oz)	250	33	12	0
roaster light meat w/o skin roasted	1 cup (5 oz)	214	38	6	0
roaster w/ skin neck & giblets roasted	1 chicken (2.4 lbs)	2363	257	140	1
roaster w/ skin roasted	½ chicken (1.1 lbs)	1071	115	64	0
roaster w/o skin roasted	1 cup (5 oz)	469	9	28	0
stewing dark meat w/o skin stewed	1 cup (5 oz)	361	39	21	0
stewing w/ skin neck & giblets stewed	1 chicken (1.3 lbs)	1636	157	107	tr
stewing w/ skin stewed	½ chicken (9.2 oz)	744	70	49	0
stewing w/ skin stewed	6.2 oz	507	34	34	0
Perdue					
Boneless Skinless Breasts Cooked	3 oz	110	25	2	0
Boneless Breast Roasted Garlic Herb	1 piece (3 oz)	90	18	1	3
Breaded Breast Strips Barbecue	3 oz	120	12	1	16
Breaded Breast Strips Hot & Spicy	3 oz	110	12	1	13
Breaded Breast Strips Original	3 oz	120	14	1	14
Burger Cooked	1 (3 oz)	160	17	10	0
Chicken Breast Seasoned Italian Cooked	1 piece (3 oz)	90	18	1	3
Chicken Breast Seasoned Lemon Pepper Cooked	1 piece (3 oz)	90	18	1	3
Chicken Breast Seasoned Teriyaki Cooked	1 piece (3 oz)	90	18	1	3
Ground Cooked	3 oz	170	18	11	0
Ground Breast Cooked	3 oz	80	19	1	0
Honey Rotisserie Dark Meat	3 oz	200	12	16	1
Honey Rotisserie White Meat	3 oz	140	19	8	1
Oven Stuffer Dark Meat Roasted	3 oz	210	18	15	0

FOOD	PORTION	CALS	PROT	FAT	CARB
Oven Stuffer Drumstick Roasted	1 (3.6 oz)	190	22	11	0
Oven Stuffer White Meat Roasted	3 oz	170	21	9	0
Oven Stuffer Wingette Roasted	3 (3.4 oz)	220	21	15	0
Seasoned Roasting Chicken Toasted Garlic Dark Meat	3 oz	190	16	14	1
Seasoned Roasting Chicken Toasted Garlic White Meat	3 oz	160	19	9	1
Seasoned Strips Parmesan Garlic cooked	3 oz	100	20	2	2
Seasoned Strips Savory Classic cooked	3 oz	90	19	1	1
Seasoned Strips Spicy Fiesta cooked	3 oz	140	16	7	3
Split Breast Cooked	1 piece (6.8 oz)	370	48	20	0
Thin Sliced Breast Rosemary Garlic Thyme	1 piece (3 oz)	90	20	2	1
Thin Sliced Breast Tomato Herb	1 piece (3 oz)	90	20	2	1
Whole Dark Meat cooked	3 oz	150	17	16	0
Whole White Meat Cooked	3 oz	170	21	10	0
Wings Roasted	2 (3.2 oz)	210	19	15	0
Tyson					
Broth Marinated Breast Filet	1 (4.7 oz)	140	26	4	0
Broth Marinated Drums	2 (4 oz)	140	17	7	0
Broth Marinated Thighs	1 (4.9 oz)	380	17	34	1
Broth Marinated Wings	4 pieces (4.2 oz)	240	20	18	0
Chicken Broccoli & Cheese	1 piece (5.9 oz)	320	20	16	23
Chicken Stuffed w/ Wild Rice & Mushroom	1 piece (5.9 oz)	300	23	12	25
Cordon Bleu	1 piece (5.9 oz)	350	25	17	24
Cornish Hen	1 serv (4 oz)	180	18	12	0
Kiev	1 piece (5.9 oz)	460	20	32	24
Wampler					
Breast Tenders	4 oz	130	27	2	0
frozen					
Banquet					
Breast Nuggets	7	280	13	20	11
Breast Patties Grilled Honey BBQ	1	110	13	5	3
Breast Patties Grilled Honey Mustard	1	120	13	5	5
Breast Tenders Our Original	3	250	12	15	15

FOOD	PORTION	CALS	PROT	FAT	CARB
Breast Tenders Southern	3 pieces	260	12	16	16
Country Fried	1 serv (3 oz)	270	14	18	13
Fat Free Baked Breast Patties	1	100	9	0	15
Fried Our Original	1 serv (3 oz)	280	14	18	15
Honey BBQ Skinless Fried	1 serv (3 oz)	230	18	13	9
Hot 'n Spicy Fried	1 serv (3 oz)	260	14	18	13
Nuggets Our Original	6	270	14	19	12
Nuggets Southern Fried	5	270	12	18	16
Patties Our Original	1	190	7	14	10
Patties Southern Fried	1	190	8	12	10
Skinless Fried	1 serv (3 oz)	220	18	13	7
Smokehouse Big Wings	2 (0.6 oz)	200	14	17	4
Southern Fried	1 serv (3 oz)	280	14	18	15
Wings Firehouse Big	2	190	14	14	1
Wings Honey BBQ	4	380	31	24	15
Wings Hot & Spicy	4 pieces	280	18	20	9
Country Skillet					
Bites	5	270	12	16	18
Breast Tenders	3	240	11	14	16
Chunks	5	270	12	18	18
Fried	3 oz	270	14	18	13
Nuggets	10	280	14	17	16
Patties	1	190	9	12	12
Southern Fried Chunks	5	270	11	18	17
Southern Fried Patties	1	190	9	12	12
Health Is Wealth					
Nuggets	4 (3 oz)	150	14	6	9
Patties	1 (3 oz)	150	13	6	9
Tenders	3 (3 oz)	130	14	3	11
Kid Cuisine					
Dino Mite Nuggets	4 pieces	300	11	23	10
Radical Racin' Nuggets w/ Cheese	4 pieces	300	11	23	12
Weaver					
Breast Strips	3 pieces (3.3 oz)	210	14	11	13
Breast Tenders	5 pieces (3 oz)	220	14	15	8
Croquettes	1 serv (3.5 oz)	290	11	18	22
Dutch Frye Nuggets	5 pieces (3.3 oz)	280	14	20	12
Honey Battered Tenders	5 pieces (2.9 oz)	230	12	15	12
Hot Wings Buffalo Style	3 pieces (2.7 oz)	190	18	13	0
Mini Drums Crispy	5 pieces (3.3 oz)	250	14	16	14
Nuggets	4 pieces (2.7 oz)	210	11	15	9
Patties	1 (2.6 oz)	180	10	11	10
Rondelet	1 (2.6 oz)	170	10	10	10
Rondelet Dutch Frye	1 (2.6 oz)	230	11	16	10
Rondelet Italian	1 (2.6 oz)	210	10	14	12

FOOD	PORTION	CALS	PROT	FAT	CARB
ready-to-eat					
chicken roll light meat	1 pkg (6 oz)	271	33	13	4
chicken roll light meat	2 oz	90	11	4	1
poultry salad sandwich spread	1 tbsp (13 g)	109	2	2	1
poultry salad sandwich spread	1 oz	238	3	4	2
Banquet					
Fat Free Baked Breast Tenders	3	120	13	0	16
Boar's Head					
Breast Hickory Smoked	2 oz	60	11	1	tr
Breast Oven Roasted	2 oz	50	11	1	tr
Breast Bar B Q Sauce Basted	2 oz	60	11	1	3
Butterball					
Crispy Baked Breasts Italian Style Herb	1 piece (0.5 oz)	190	17	6	16
Crispy Baked Breasts Lemon Pepper	1 piece (0.5 oz)	200	16	7	16
Crispy Baked Breasts Original	1 piece (0.5 oz)	180	16	6	16
Crispy Baked Breasts Parmesan	1 piece (0.5 oz)	200	17	7	16
Crispy Baked Breasts Southwestern	1 piece (0.5 oz)	170	17	6	13
Tenders Baked Breast	3 pieces	170	14	6	15
Tenders Hickory Smoked Grilled	4 pieces + sauce	160	17	5	12
Tenders Oriental Grilled	4 pieces + sauce	160	17	5	12
Carl Buddig					
Chicken Sliced	1 pkg (2.5 oz)	110	12	7	1
Lean Slices Honey Smoked Breast	1 pkg (2.5 oz)	70	12	1	3
Lean Slices Roasted Breast	1 pkg (2.5 oz)	60	13	1	1
Chicken By George					
Cajun	1 breast (4 oz)	130	21	4	3
Caribbean Grill	1 breast (4 oz)	150	22	4	8
Garlic & Herb	1 breast (4 oz)	120	21	3	3
Italian Bleu Cheese	1 breast (4 oz)	130	20	5	2
Lemon Herb	1 breast (4 oz)	120	20	3	3
Lemon Oregano	1 breast (4 oz)	130	20	4	3
Mesquite Barbecue	1 breast (4 oz)	130	21	3	5
Mustard Dill	1 breast (4 oz)	140	20	5	2
Roasted	1 breast (4 oz)	110	20	3	1
Teriyaki	1 breast (4 oz)	130	21	3	6
Tomato Herb w/ Basil	1 breast (4 oz)	140	20	5	5

FOOD	PORTION	CALS	PROT	FAT	CARB
Louis Rich					
Carving Board Classic Baked	2 slices (1.6 oz)	45	9	1	2
Carving Board Grilled	2 slices (1.6 oz)	45	9	1	2
Deli-Thin Oven Roasted Breast	4 slices (1.8 oz)	50	10	1	1
Oven Roasted Deluxe Breast	1 slice (1 oz)	30	5	1	1
Oscar Mayer					
Free Oven Roasted Breast	4 slices (1.8 oz)	45	10	0	1
Perdue					
Breast Cutlets Homestyle	1 (2.9 oz)	110	14	1	12
Breast Cutlets Italian Style	1 (2.9 oz)	120	15	2	11
Breast Filets In Barbecue Sauce	1 piece + 3 tbsp sauce (5.9 oz)	200	24	1	24
Breast Strips In Garlic & Herb Sauce	1 serv (5 oz)	100	18	1	4
Breast Strips In Marinara Sauce	1 serv (5 oz)	120	18	3	5
Breast Strips In Teriyaki Sauce	1 serv (5 oz)	190	20	1	26
Carved Breast Honey Roasted	½ cup (2.5 oz)	100	18	2	2
Carved Breast Original Roasted	½ cup (2.5 oz)	90	19	2	1
Cutlets Cooked	1 (3.5 oz)	220	15	11	15
Nuggets	5 (3.4 oz)	210	15	11	15
Nuggets Chicken & Cheese	5 (3.4 oz)	230	15	13	15
Short Cuts Italian	½ cup (2.5 oz)	100	19	3	0
Short Cuts Lemon Pepper	½ cup (2.5 oz)	100	19	3	1
Short Cuts Southwestern	½ cup (2.5 oz)	100	18	3	1
Tyson					
Breaded Breast Chunks	6 pieces (2.9 oz)	230	9	16	13
Breaded Breast Fillet	2 pieces (2.8 oz)	180	12	8	15
Breaded Breast Pattie	1 (2.6 oz)	190	11	12	9
Breaded Breast Tenders	5 pieces (3 oz)	220	14	15	8
Breaded Chicken Chunks	6 pieces (3 oz)	220	13	14	11
Chick'n Quick Chick'n Cheddar	1 patty (2.6 oz)	220	11	14	12
Chicken Bits Southern Fried	6 pieces (2.9 oz)	260	11	19	11
Chicken Strips	1 serv (3 oz)	90	20	1	0
Chicken Strips Southwestern	1 serv (3 oz)	110	18	3	2
Country Fried Chicken Fritter	5 pieces (2.9 oz)	260	11	18	13
Drumsticks Hot BBQ Style	2 (3.5 oz)	160	22	7	3
Glazed Grilled Breast Pattie	1 (2.7 oz)	120	12	7	1
Grilled Chicken Pattie	1 (2.9 oz)	170	13	12	1

FOOD	PORTION	CALS	PROT	FAT	CARB
Nuggets Breaded White Meat	6 pieces (2.9 oz)	250	11	18	12
Patties Southern Fried	1 (2.9 oz)	260	11	19	11
Roasted Drumsticks	3 (5.6 oz)	320	44	15	2
Roasted Drumsticks w/o Skin	2 (3.3 oz)	140	22	5	1
Roasted Half Chicken	1 serv (3 oz)	160	16	11	1
Roasted Whole Chicken	1 serv (3 oz)	160	16	11	1
Roasted Breast Boneless w/o Skin	1 (3.7 oz)	130	26	3	1
Roasted Breast Half w/o Skin	1 (4.3 oz)	150	30	3	1
Roasted Half Breast w/ Skin	1 (5.1 oz)	260	34	13	1
Roasted Half Chicken w/o Skin	1 serv (3 oz)	120	17	6	1
Roasted Tabasco Wings	3 (3 oz)	190	16	13	1
Roasted Thigh w/ Skin	1 (3.6 oz)	270	19	21	1
Roasted Thighs w/o Skin	1 (2.9 oz)	150	19	8	1
Roll White Meat	2 oz	90	10	6	0
Southern Fried Breaded Breast Pattie	1 (2.6 oz)	180	11	12	8
Southern Fried Breast Fillets	2 pieces (3.4 oz)	210	15	11	14
Southern Fried Chunks	6 pieces (2.9 oz)	260	11	19	11
Tenders Breaded Honey Battered	5 pieces (2.9 oz)	230	12	15	12
Tenders Breaded Pattie	3 pieces (3.2 oz)	100	13	0	11
Thick'n Crispy Pattie	1 (2.6 oz)	200	10	14	10
Wings BBQ	3 pieces (3.2 oz)	200	19	13	2
Wings Hot N'Spicy	4 (3.2 oz)	210	18	14	1
Wings Teriyaki	4 pieces (3.4 oz)	190	21	12	2
Wings Of Fire	4 pieces (3.4 oz)	220	20	15	1
take-out					
oven roasted breast of chicken	2 oz	60	11	1	0

CHICKEN DISHES

(*see also* CHICKEN SUBSTITUTES, DINNER)

canned

FOOD	PORTION	CALS	PROT	FAT	CARB
Bumble Bee					
Chicken Salad	1 pkg (3.5 oz)	230	10	10	25
Dinty Moore					
Noodles & Chicken	1 can (7.5 oz)	180	7	8	19
Stew	1 cup (8.5 oz)	220	12	11	16
mix					
Chicken Skillet Helper					
Stir-Fried Chicken as prep	1 cup	270	18	9	30

FOOD	PORTION	CALS	PROT	FAT	CARB
Hamburger Helper					
Reduced Sodium Cheddar Spirals Chicken Recipe as prep	1 cup	240	20	6	27
Reduced Sodium Italian Herb Chicken Recipe as prep	1 cup	200	19	2	29
Reduced Sodium Southwestern Beef Chicken Recipe as prep	1 cup	220	20	3	32
Tyson					
Mandarin Wrap Kit	1½ wraps (14.6 oz)	630	30	15	92
ready-to-eat					
salad low fat	⅓ cup	90	8	2	9
Wampler					
Cacciatore	1 cup	260	30	9	10
Fajitas	1 cup	210	23	7	13
Salad	⅓ cup	200	9	14	9
Salad Lite	⅓ cup	130	9	7	9
Smokey Barbecue Chicken	1 cup	430	42	15	31
Sweet-n-Sour	1 cup	250	20	4	35
shelf-stable					
Dinty Moore					
Microwave Cup Chicken & Dumpling	1 pkg (7.5 oz)	200	15	6	21
Microwave Cup Stew	1 pkg (7.5 oz)	180	10	8	18
Lunch Bucket					
Chicken Fiesta	1 pkg (7.5 oz)	160	6	2	30
Dumplings'n Chicken	1 pkg (7.5 oz)	140	5	5	21
TastyBite					
Chicken Moglai	1 pkg (9.5 oz)	300	21	16	20
take-out					
boneless breaded & fried w/ barbecue sauce	6 pieces (4.6 oz)	330	17	18	25
boneless breaded & fried w/ honey	6 pieces (4 oz)	339	17	18	27
boneless breaded & fried w/ mustard sauce	6 pieces (4.6 oz)	323	17	17	21
boneless breaded & fried w/ sweet & sour sauce	6 pieces (4.6 oz)	346	17	18	29
breast & wing breaded & fried	2 pieces (5.7 oz)	494	36	30	20
chicken & dumplings	¾ cup	256	23	12	12
chicken & noodles	1 cup	365	22	18	26
chicken a la king	1 cup	470	27	34	12
chicken cacciatore	¾ cup	394	33	24	9
chicken pie w/ top crust	1 slice (5.6 oz)	472	19	31	32
drumstick breaded & fried	2 pieces (5.2 oz)	430	30	27	16

FOOD	PORTION	CALS	PROT	FAT	CARB
groundnut stew hkatenkwan	1 serv (15.7 oz)	576	38	40	18
jamaican jerk wings	4 wings (9.9 oz)	709	57	51	3
sancocho de pollo dominican chicken stew	1 serv	702	71	30	34
thigh breaded & fried	2 pieces (5.2 oz)	430	30	27	16
CHICKEN SUBSTITUTES					
Health Is Wealth					
Buffalo Wings	3 pieces (2.2 oz)	100	10	2	11
Chicken-Free Nuggets	3 pieces (2.25 oz)	90	10	1	11
Chicken-Free Patties	1 (3 oz)	120	14	2	15
Loma Linda					
Chicken Supreme Mix not prep	⅓ cup (0.9 oz)	90	15	1	6
Chik Nuggets	5 pieces (3 oz)	240	12	16	13
Fried Chik'n w/ Gravy	2 pieces (2.8 oz)	160	12	10	4
Morningstar Farms					
Chik Nuggets	4 pieces (3 oz)	160	13	4	17
Chik Patties	1 (2.5 oz)	150	9	6	15
Meatless Buffalo Wings	5 pieces (3 oz)	200	13	9	16
Quorn					
Cutlets	1 (3.5 oz)	200	10	8	20
Nuggets	3-4 pieces (3 oz)	180	8	8	18
Patties	1 patty (2.6 oz)	160	8	7	12
Tenders	1 cup (3 oz)	90	12	2	8
Worthington					
Chic-Ketts	2 slices (1.9 oz)	120	13	7	2
Chicken Sliced or Roll	2 slices (2 oz)	80	9	5	1
Chicken Sliced	2 slices (2 oz)	80	9	5	1
ChikStiks	1 (1.6 oz)	110	9	7	3
CrispyChik Patties	1 (2.5 oz)	150	8	6	15
Cutlets	1 slice (2.1 oz)	70	11	1	3
Diced Chik	¼ cup (1.9 oz)	40	7	0	1
FriChik	2 pieces (3.2 oz)	120	10	8	1
FriChik Low Fat	2 pieces (3 oz)	80	10	3	2
Golden Croquettes	4 pieces (3 oz)	210	14	10	14
Yves					
Veggie Chicken Burgers	1 (3 oz)	120	17	3	6
CHICKPEAS					
canned					
chickpeas	1 cup	285	12	3	54
Green Giant					
Garbanzo	½ cup (4.4 oz)	110	6	2	18
Progresso					
Chick Peas	½ cup (4.6 oz)	120	5	3	20
Garbanzo	½ cup (4.4 oz)	110	6	2	18
dried					
cooked	1 cup	269	15	4	45

FOOD	PORTION	CALS	PROT	FAT	CARB
CHICORY					
greens raw chopped	½ cup	21	2	tr	4
root raw	1 (2.1 oz)	44	1	tr	11
roots raw cut up	½ cup (1.6 oz)	33	1	tr	8
CHILI					
chili w/ beans	1 cup	286	15	14	30
Amy's Organic					
Whole Meals Chili & Cornbread	1 pkg (10.5 oz)	320	11	6	59
Armour					
Chili No Beans	1 cup (8.7 oz)	390	14	29	18
Chili w/ Beans Western Style	1 cup (8.8 oz)	370	14	22	29
Chili w/ Beans	1 cup (8.9 oz)	370	13	21	33
Chili w/ Beans Hot	1 cup (8.9 oz)	370	13	21	33
Vienna Sausage & Chili	1 cup (8.7 oz)	410	14	27	27
Carroll Shelby's					
Original Texas Chili Kit	2 tbsp	60	2	1	12
Chef Boyardee					
Chili Mac	½ can (7 oz)	260	10	11	30
Chili Man					
Seasoning Mix	1 tbsp (7 g)	25	1	1	4
Del Monte					
Sauce	1 tbsp (0.6 oz)	20	0	0	5
Gebhardt					
Chili Quik Seasoning	1 tbsp (0.3 oz)	43	1	1	8
Plain	1 cup (9.4 oz)	232	7	19	11
With Beans	1 cup (9.4 oz)	322	15	15	32
Health Valley					
Burrito	1 cup	160	13	1	28
Enchilada	1 cup	160	13	1	28
Fajita	1 cup	80	7	0	15
In A Cup Black Bean Mild	¾ cup	120	10	1	21
In A Cup Texas Style Spicy	¾ cup	120	10	1	21
Vegetarian Lentil Mild	1 cup	160	13	1	28
Vegetarian Lentil No Salt	1 cup	80	7	0	14
Vegetarian Mild	1 cup	160	13	1	28
Vegetarian Mild No Salt	1 cup	160	13	1	28
Vegetarian Spicy	1 cup	160	13	1	28
Vegetarian Spicy No Salt	1 cup	160	13	1	28
Vegetarian w/ 3 Beans Mild	1 cup	160	13	1	28
Vegetarian w/ Black Beans Mild	1 cup	160	13	1	28
Vegetarian w/ Black Beans Spicy	1 cup	160	13	1	28
Healthy Choice					
Bowls Chili & Cornbread	1 meal (9.5 oz)	350	21	8	49
Hormel					
Chunky w/ Beans	1 cup (8.7 oz)	270	18	7	34

FOOD	PORTION	CALS	PROT	FAT	CARB
Hot No Beans	1 cup (8.3 oz)	210	16	9	17
Hot w/ Beans	1 cup (8.7 oz)	270	18	7	33
Microcup Meals Chili Mac	1 cup (7.5 oz)	200	11	9	17
Microcup Meals Hot w/ Beans	1 cup (7.3 oz)	220	15	6	27
Microcup Meals No Beans	1 cup (7.3 oz)	190	14	8	15
Microcup Meals w/ Beans	1 cup (7.3 oz)	220	15	6	27
No Beans	1 cup (8.3 oz)	210	16	9	17
Turkey No Beans	1 cup (8.3 oz)	190	24	3	17
Turkey w/ Beans	1 cup (8.7 oz)	210	17	3	30
Vegetarian	1 cup (8.7 oz)	200	12	1	38
With Beans	1 cup (8.7 oz)	270	18	7	33
Hunt's					
Chili Beans	½ cup (4.5 oz)	87	6	1	17
Chili Sauce	2 tbsp (1.2 oz)	35	1	tr	8
Hurst					
HamBeens Chili Beans	1 serv	130	8	1	22
Instant India					
Chili Ginger Paste	2 tbsp (1 oz)	90	1	7	6
Just Rite					
With Beans	1 cup (9 oz)	379	18	27	31
Lean Cuisine					
Everyday Favorites Three Bean Chili w/ Rice	1 pkg (10 oz)	250	11	6	37
Lunch Bucket					
Chili w/ Beans	1 pkg (7.5 oz)	260	12	12	25
Manwich					
Homestyle Fixins	½ cup (4.6 oz)	84	6	1	19
Marie Callender's					
Chili & Cornbread	1 meal (16 oz)	560	27	21	67
Natural Choice					
Organic Vegan Three Bean	½ cup (4.6 oz)	140	9	1	24
Natural Touch					
Vegetarian	1 cup (8.1 oz)	170	18	1	21
Nature's Entree					
Texas Chili	1 pkg (12 oz)	320	26	7	43
Open Range					
Plain	1 cup (8.8 oz)	353	18	26	19
With Beans	1 cup (9 oz)	281	17	16	25
Stouffer's					
With Beans	1 pkg (8.75 oz)	270	15	10	29
Ultimate					
No Beans Hot	1 cup (8.7 oz)	420	20	30	18
Turkey w/ Beans	1 cup (8.7 oz)	260	17	9	28
W/ Beans	1 cup (8.7 oz)	320	18	16	25
W/ Beans Hot	1 cup (8.7 oz)	320	18	16	25
Van Camp					
Beanee Weenee Chilee	1 cup (7.7 oz)	240	14	12	27

FOOD	PORTION	CALS	PROT	FAT	CARB
Chili w/ Beans	1 cup (8.9 oz)	350	19	21	28
Mexican Style Chili Beans	½ cup (4.6 oz)	110	7	2	21
Wampler					
Turkey	1 cup	250	23	7	22
Wick Fowler's					
2 Alarm Chili Kit	3 tbsp	60	2	2	10
False Alarm Chili Kit	2 tbsp	50	2	2	9
Wolf Brand					
Plain	7.5 oz	330	25	22	10
Worthington					
Chili	1 cup (8.1 oz)	290	19	15	21
Low Fat	1 cup (8.1 oz)	170	18	1	21
Yves					
Veggie Chili	1 pkg (10.5 oz)	230	21	1	37
take-out					
con carne w/ beans	8.9 oz	254	25	8	22

CHILI PEPPERS
(*see* PEPPERS)

CHINESE CABBAGE
(*see* CABBAGE)

CHINESE FOOD
(*see* ASIAN FOOD)

CHIPS
(*see also* POPCORN, PRETZELS, SNACKS)

FOOD	PORTION	CALS	PROT	FAT	CARB
barbecue	1 bag (7 oz)	971	15	64	105
barbecue	1 oz	139	2	9	15
corn	1 oz	153	2	10	16
corn	1 bag (7 oz)	1067	13	66	113
corn barbecue	1 oz	148	2	9	16
corn barbecue	1 bag (7 oz)	1036	14	65	111
corn cones	1 oz	145	2	8	18
corn cones nacho	1 oz	152	2	9	17
corn onion	1 oz	142	2	6	19
potato	1 bag (8 oz)	1217	16	79	120
potato	1 oz	152	2	10	15
potato cheese	1 oz	140	2	8	16
potato cheese	1 bag (6 oz)	842	14	46	98
potato light	1 oz	134	2	6	19
potato light	1 bag (6 oz)	801	12	35	114
potato sour cream & onion	1 oz	150	2	10	15
potato sour cream & onion	1 bag (7 oz)	1051	16	67	102
potato sticks	½ cup (0.6 oz)	94	1	6	10
potato sticks	1 oz	148	2	10	15
potato sticks	1 pkg (1 oz)	148	2	10	15
taco	1 oz	136	2	7	18
taco	1 bag (8 oz)	1089	18	55	143
taro	1 oz	141	1	7	19
taro	10 (0.8 oz)	115	1	6	16

FOOD	PORTION	CALS	PROT	FAT	CARB
tortilla	1 oz	142	2	7	18
tortilla	1 bag (7.5 oz)	1067	15	56	134
tortilla nacho	1 oz	141	2	7	18
tortilla nacho	1 bag (8 oz)	1131	18	58	142
tortilla nacho light	1 oz	126	3	4	20
tortilla nacho light	1 bag (6 oz)	757	15	26	122
tortilla ranch	1 oz	139	2	7	18
tortilla ranch	1 bag (7 oz)	969	15	47	128
Barbara's Bakery					
Potato	1¼ cup (1 oz)	150	2	10	15
Potato No Salt Added	1¼ cups (1 oz)	150	2	10	15
Potato Ripple	1¼ cup (1 oz)	150	2	10	15
Potato Yogurt & Green Onion	1¼ cup (1 oz)	150	2	9	15
Tortilla Blue Corn	15 chips (1 oz)	140	3	7	16
Tortilla Blue Corn No Salt	15 chips (1 oz)	140	3	7	16
Tortilla Pinta Salsa	15 chips (1 oz)	130	2	6	19
Bruno & Luigi's					
Pasta Chips Garlic & Herb	1 oz	117	4	1	23
Cape Cod					
Potato Golden Russet	1 pkg (0.5 oz)	70	1	4	8
Chester's					
Flamin'Hot	1 oz	140	2	8	17
Salsa	1 oz	140	2	7	18
Doritos					
3D's Cooler Ranch	27 (1 oz)	140	2	6	18
3D's Nacho Cheesier	27 (1 oz)	140	2	7	17
Cooler Ranch	12 (1 oz)	140	2	7	18
Flamin' Hot	11 (1 oz)	140	2	7	17
Nacho Cheesier	11 (1 oz)	140	2	7	17
Salsa Verde	12 (1 oz)	150	2	7	20
Smokey Red	12 (1 oz)	150	2	7	21
Spicy Nacho	12 (1 oz)	140	2	6	18
Toasted Corn	13 (1 oz)	140	2	7	18
Wow Nacho Cheesier	1 pkg (0.75 oz)	70	2	1	13
Durangos					
Tortilla	15 (1 oz)	150	2	7	20
Eden					
Brown Rice Chips	1 oz	150	2	7	19
Sea Vegetable Chips	1 oz	140	1	5	23
Fritos					
Chili Cheese	31 (1 oz)	160	2	10	16
Corn Chips BBQ	29 (1 oz)	150	2	9	16
Corn Chips King Size	12 (1 oz)	150	2	10	16
Corn Chips Sabrositas Flamin' Hot	30 (1 oz)	150	2	9	16
Corn Chips Sabrositas Lime'N Chile	28 (1 oz)	150	2	9	17

FOOD	PORTION	CALS	PROT	FAT	CARB
Corn Chips Wild N'Mild Ranch	28 (1 oz)	160	2	10	15
Original	32 (1 oz)	160	2	10	15
Scoops	11 (1 oz)	160	2	10	17
Texas Grill Honey BBQ	15 (1 oz)	150	2	9	16
Guiltless Gourmet					
Tortilla Baked Chili Lime	18 (1 oz)	110	2	2	22
Tortilla Baked Mucho Nacho	18 (1 oz)	110	2	2	22
Tortilla Baked Organic Blue Corn	18 (1 oz)	110	3	2	22
Tortilla Baked Picante Ranch	18 (1 oz)	110	2	2	22
Tortilla Baked Red Corn	18 (1 oz)	110	2	2	22
Tortilla Baked Spicy Black Bean	18 (1 oz)	110	3	2	22
Tortilla Baked Sweet White Corn	18 (1 oz)	110	3	2	22
Tortilla Baked Yellow Corn	18 (1 oz)	110	2	2	22
Tortilla Baked Yellow Corn Unsalted	18 (1 oz)	110	3	1	22
Herr's					
Potato	1 oz	140	2	8	16
Tortilla Restaurant Style White Corn	10 chips (1 oz)	140	3	6	18
Lance					
BBQ	22 (1 oz)	160	2	10	15
Cajun	15 (1 oz)	150	2	10	14
Corn Chips	39 (1.25 oz)	200	2	11	14
Corn Chips Hot BBQ	35 (1.25 oz)	210	2	13	20
Hot Fries	1 pkg (0.9 oz)	140	2	10	11
Mesquite BBQ	22 (1 oz)	150	2	10	15
Potato	23 (1 oz)	160	2	10	15
Ripple	15 (1 oz)	160	1	11	14
Salt & Vinegar	22 (1 oz)	160	2	10	14
Sour Cream & Onion	22 (1 oz)	160	2	10	15
Tortilla Fiesta Salsa Triangles	16 (1 oz)	140	2	7	18
Tortilla Nacho Mini Round	46 (½5 oz)	180	3	9	21
Tortilla Nacho Triangles	15 (1 oz)	140	2	14	18
Lay's					
Adobadas	16 (1 oz)	170	2	10	18
Baked KC Masterpiece BBQ	11 (1 oz)	120	2	3	22
Baked Original	11 (1 oz)	110	2	2	23
Baked Roasted Herb	12 (1 oz)	130	2	3	25
Baked Sour Cream & Onion	12 (1 oz)	120	2	2	21
Classic	20 (1 oz)	150	2	10	15
Deli Style Hot N'Tangy BBQ	18 (1 oz)	150	2	10	16

FOOD	PORTION	CALS	PROT	FAT	CARB
Deli Style Jalapeno	17 (1 oz)	150	2	10	16
Deli Style Original	17 (1 oz)	140	1	10	16
Deli Style Salt & Vinegar	16 (1 oz)	90	1	10	16
Flamin' Hot	17 pieces (1 oz)	150	2	10	16
KC Masterpiece BBQ	15 (1 oz)	150	2	10	15
Onion & Garlic	19 (1 oz)	150	2	9	16
Salt & Vinegar	17 pieces (1 oz)	150	2	10	15
Sour Cream & Onion	17 pieces (1 oz)	160	2	11	12
Toasted Onion & Cheese	17 pieces (1 oz)	160	2	10	14
Wavy Au Gratin	13 (1 oz)	150	2	10	14
Wavy Original	11 pieces (1 oz)	160	2	10	15
Wavy Ranch	11 (1 oz)	160	2	11	14
Wow Mesquite BBQ	20 (1 oz)	75	2	0	17
Wow Original	20 (1 oz)	75	2	0	18
Wow Original	1 pkg (0.75 oz)	55	1	0	13
Wow Sour Cream & Chive	19 (1 oz)	80	2	0	17
Old Dutch Foods					
Potato	12–15 chips (1 oz)	150	2	8	16
Potato BBQ	12–15 chips (1 oz)	150	2	9	15
Potato BBQ Ripple	12–15 chips (1 oz)	150	2	9	16
Potato Cajun Ripple	12–15 chips (1 oz)	150	2	10	15
Potato Cheddar & Sour Cream Ripple	12–15 chips (1 oz)	160	2	9	16
Potato Cheddar & Sour Cream Ripples	12–15 chips (1 oz)	150	2	9	15
Potato Dill	12–15 chips (1 oz)	140	2	8	16
Potato Dutch Crunch	15–20 chips (1 oz)	130	2	6	18
Potato French Onion Ripple	12–15 chips (1 oz)	150	2	10	15
Potato Jalapeno & Cheddar Dutch Crunch	15–20 chips (1 oz)	130	2	6	17
Potato Jalapeno Cheese	12–15 chips (1 oz)	150	2	9	16
Potato Mesquite BBQ Dutch Crunch	15–20 chips (1 oz)	130	2	6	19
Potato Onion & Garlic	12–15 chips (1 oz)	140	2	8	16
Potato Outback Spicy BBQ	12–15 chips (1 oz)	150	2	10	15
Potato Ripples	12–15 chips (1 oz)	150	2	9	15
Potato Salt & Vinegar Dutch Crunch	15–20 chips (1 oz)	130	0	6	18
Potato Sour Cream & Onion	12–15 chips (1 oz)	150	2	9	15
Tortilla Bite Size White Corn	20 chips (1 oz)	150	2	8	18
Tortilla Nacho Cheese	15 chips (1 oz)	150	2	7	19
Tortilla Restaurant Style White	9 chips (1 oz)	140	2	7	20
Tostados White Corn	11 chips (1 oz)	140	2	7	20
Tostados Yellow	11 chips (1 oz)	140	2	6	21
Pita-Snax					
Cheddar Cheese	34 (1 oz)	110	3	2	21

FOOD	PORTION	CALS	PROT	FAT	CARB
Chili & Lime	34 (1 oz)	120	3	2	20
Cinnamon	34 (1 oz)	120	3	2	22
Dill Ranch	34 (1 oz)	120	3	2	21
Garlic	34 (1 oz)	120	3	2	22
Lightly Salted	34 (1 oz)	110	3	1	22
Pringles					
BBQ	14 chips (1 oz)	150	2	10	15
Cheese & Onion	14 chips (1 oz)	160	1	11	15
Cheez-ums	14 chips (1 oz)	150	2	10	14
Original	14 chips (1 oz)	160	2	11	15
Pizzalicious	14 chips (1 oz)	160	1	11	14
Ranch	14 chips (1 oz)	150	2	10	15
Salt & Vinegar	14 chips (1 oz)	160	1	11	15
Sour Cream & Onion	14 chips (1 oz)	160	2	10	15
Robert's American Gourmet					
Spirulina Spirals	1 oz	120	2	2	22
Ruffles					
Baked	10 (1 oz)	110	2	2	23
Baked Cheddar & Sour Cream	9 (1 oz)	120	2	3	21
Buffalo Style	11 chips (1 oz)	160	2	10	16
Cheddar & Sour Cream	11 chips (1 oz)	160	2	10	14
French Onion	11 (1 oz)	150	2	10	15
MC Masterpiece Mesquite BBQ	11 (1 oz)	150	1	10	15
Original	12 chips (1 oz)	150	2	10	14
Ranch	13 (1 oz)	150	2	9	15
Reduced Fat	16 (1 oz)	130	2	7	18
The Works	12 (1 oz)	160	2	11	14
Wow Cheddar & Sour Cream	15 (1 oz)	75	3	0	16
Wow Original	17 (1 oz)	75	2	0	17
Santitas					
100% White Corn	6 (1 oz)	130	2	6	19
Restaurant Style Chips	7 (1 oz)	130	2	6	19
Restaurant Style Strips	10 (1 oz)	130	2	6	19
Snyder's Of Hanover					
BBQ Rib	1 oz	140	2	7	17
Barbeque Corn	1.5 oz	230	3	14	22
Cheddar Bacon	1 oz	150	2	6	20
Corn Chips	1.5 oz	230	3	15	22
Grilled Steak & Onion	1 oz	140	2	6	20
Hot Buffalo	1 oz	150	2	7	20
Kosher Dill	1 oz	140	2	6	20
No Salt	1 oz	140	2	6	19
Potato	1 oz	140	2	6	19
Ripple	1 oz	140	2	6	18
Salt & Vinegar	1 oz	140	2	6	19

FOOD	PORTION	CALS	PROT	FAT	CARB
Sausage Pizza	1 oz	150	2	6	20
Sour Cream & Onion	1 oz	150	2	7	19
Tasty Veggie Potato Chips	1 oz	150	3	6	20
Tortilla Nacho	1 oz	140	2	7	19
Tortilla No Salt Yellow Corn	1 oz	140	2	6	19
Tortilla White Corn	1 oz	140	2	6	20
Tortilla Yellow Corn	1 oz	140	2	6	19
Tortilla Yellow Corn Mini	1 oz	160	2	8	20
Soya King					
Soy Mongolian BBQ	23 chips (1 oz)	140	1	7	19
Soy Original	23 chips (1 oz)	140	1	7	19
Soy Sour Cream & Onion	23 chips (1 oz)	140	1	7	19
Soy Taco	23 chips (1 oz)	140	1	7	19
Sunchips					
French Onion	13 (1 oz)	140	2	7	18
Harvest Cheddar	13 (1 oz)	140	2	6	19
Original	14 (1 oz)	140	2	6	19
Torengos					
Chips	13 chips (1 oz)	140	2	9	15
Tostitos					
Baked Bite Size	20 (1 oz)	110	3	1	24
Baked Bite Size Salsa & Cream Cheese	16 (1 oz)	120	2	3	21
Baked Original	13 (1 oz)	110	3	1	21
Bite Size	15 (1 oz)	140	2	8	17
Crispy Rounds	13 (1 oz)	150	2	8	17
Nacho Style	6 (1 oz)	140	2	6	19
Restaurant Style	7 (1 oz)	140	2	6	19
Restaurant Style Hint Of Lime	6 (1 oz)	140	2	6	19
Santa Fe Gold	7 (1 oz)	140	2	6	19
Wow Original	6 (1 oz)	90	2	1	20
Tyson					
Tortilla Salted	13 (1 oz)	150	2	7	20
Tortilla Yellow Corn Salted	13 (1 oz)	150	2	7	20
Utz					
Baked Crisps	12 (1 oz)	110	2	2	23
Carolina Barbeque	20 (1 oz)	150	2	9	14
Cheddar & Sour Cream	20 (1 oz)	160	2	10	14
Corn Chips	24 (1 oz)	160	2	10	16
Corn Chips Barbecue	24 (1 oz)	160	2	10	16
Grandma	20 (1 oz)	140	2	8	14
Grandma BBQ	20 (1 oz)	140	2	8	15
Home Style Kettle	20 (1 oz)	140	2	8	14
Home Style Kettle BBQ	20 (1 oz)	140	2	8	15
Kettle Classics Crunchy	20 (1 oz)	150	2	9	15
Kettle Classics Crunchy Mesquite BBQ	20 (1 oz)	150	2	9	15

FOOD	PORTION	CALS	PROT	FAT	CARB
No Salt Added	20 (1 oz)	150	2	9	14
Onion & Garlic	20 (1 oz)	150	2	9	14
Potato	20 (1 oz)	150	2	9	14
Reduced Fat BBQ	22 (1 oz)	140	2	6	19
Reduced Fat Ripple	24 (1 oz)	140	2	7	18
Ripple	20 (1 oz)	150	2	10	14
Ripple Sour Cream & Onion	20 (1 oz)	160	2	10	14
Ripple Barbeque	20 (1 oz)	150	2	10	14
Salt'N Vinegar	20 (1 oz)	150	2	9	14
The Crab Chip	20 (1 oz)	150	2	9	14
Tortilla Black Bean & Salsa	13 (1 oz)	150	2	7	19
Tortilla Low Fat Baked	10 (1 oz)	120	2	2	24
Tortilla Nacho	13 (1 oz)	150	2	8	19
Tortilla Restaurant Style	6 (1 oz)	140	2	7	18
Tortilla Spicy Nacho	13 (1 oz)	150	2	8	19
Tortilla White Corn	12 (1 oz)	140	2	7	18
Wavy	20 chips (1 oz)	150	2	9	14
Yes! Fat Free	20 (1 oz)	75	2	0	17
Yes! Fat Free Barbeque	20 (1 oz)	75	2	0	16
Yes! Fat Free Ripple	20 (1 oz)	75	2	0	17
Wow					
Tortilla Nacho Cheese	11 (1 oz)	90	2	1	18
CHITTERLINGS					
pork cooked	3 oz	258	9	24	0
CHOCOLATE					
(*see also* CANDY, CAROB, COCOA, ICE CREAM TOPPINGS, MILK DRINKS)					
baking					
baking	1 oz	145	3	15	8
grated unsweetened	1 cup (4.6 oz)	690	14	73	37
liquid unsweetened	1 oz	134	3	14	10
squares unsweetened	1 square (1 oz)	148	3	16	8
Baker's					
Bittersweet	½ square (0.5 oz)	70	1	6	7
German's Sweet	2 squares (0.5 oz)	60	1	4	8
Semi-Sweet	½ square (0.5 oz)	70	1	5	8
Unsweetened	½ square (0.5 oz)	70	2	7	4
White	½ square (0.5 oz)	80	1	5	8
Nestle					
Choco Bake	½ oz	80	1	8	5
Premier White Bar	½ oz	80	1	5	8
Semi-Sweet Bar	½ oz	70	<1	4	9
Unsweetened Bar	½ oz	80	2	7	4
chips					
milk chocolate	1 cup (6 oz)	862	12	52	100
semisweet	1 cup (6 oz)	804	7	50	106
semisweet	60 pieces (1 oz)	136	1	9	18
Baker's					
Real Milk Chocolate	½ oz	70	1	4	9

FOOD	PORTION	CALS	PROT	FAT	CARB
Real Semi-Sweet	½ oz	60	1	4	9
Semi-Sweet	½ oz	70	0	4	10
Hershey					
Milk Chocolate	1 tbsp (0.5 oz)	80	1	5	9
Mini Kisses For Baking	11 pieces (0.5 oz)	80	1	5	9
Premier White Milk Chips	1 tbsp (0.5 oz)	80	1	4	9
Skor English Toffee Baking Bits	1 tbsp (0.5 oz)	70	0	5	7
Toll House					
Mint-Chocolate	2 tbsp (1.5 oz)	130	1	3	25
Semi-Sweet	2 tbsp (1.5 oz)	130	1	4	24
mix					
powder	2–3 heaping tsp	75	1	1	20
powder as prep w/ whole milk	9 oz	226	9	9	31
Quik					
Chocolate Powder	2 tbsp (0.8 oz)	90	1	1	19
Chocolate Powder No Sugar	2 tbsp (0.4 oz)	40	1	1	7
CHOCOLATE MILK					
(see CHOCOLATE, COCOA, MILK DRINKS, MILKSHAKE)					
CHOCOLATE SYRUP					
chocolate fudge	1 tbsp (0.7 oz)	73	1	3	12
chocolate fudge	1 cup (11.9 oz)	1176	15	46	200
syrup	1 cup	653	6	3	177
syrup	2 tbsp	82	1	tr	22
syrup as prep w/ whole milk	9 oz	232	9	9	34
Hershey					
Lite	2 tbsp (1.2 oz)	50	0	0	12
Syrup	2 tbsp (1.4 oz)	100	1	0	24
Quik					
Chocolate	2 tbsp (1.3 oz)	100	1	1	23
Smucker's					
Plate Scapers Chocolate	2 tbsp	100	1	5	23
Toll House					
Mint Chocolate	2 tbsp (1.5 oz)	130	1	3	25
Semi-Sweet	2 tbsp (1.5 oz)	130	1	4	24
CHUTNEY					
coconut	¼ cup	74	1	7	4
CILANTRO					
fresh	1 cup (1.6 oz)	11	1	tr	2
CINNAMON					
sticks	0.5 oz	39	1	tr	8
CISCO					
smoked	3 oz	151	14	10	0
smoked	1 oz	50	5	3	0

FOOD	PORTION	CALS	PROT	FAT	CARB
CLAMS					
canned					
liquid only	1 cup	6	1	tr	tr
meat only	1 cup	236	41	3	8
meat only	3 oz	126	22	2	4
Bumble Bee					
Baby	2 oz	50	9	1	2
Progresso					
Creamy Clam Sauce	½ cup (4.2 oz)	110	5	6	8
Minced	¼ cup (2.1 oz)	25	4	0	2
Red Clam Sauce	½ cup (4.4 oz)	60	4	1	8
White Clam Sauce	½ cup (4.4 oz)	150	9	10	5
fresh					
cooked	3 oz	126	22	2	4
cooked	20 sm	133	23	2	5
raw	9 lg (6.3 oz)	133	23	2	5
raw	20 sm (6.3 oz)	133	23	2	5
frozen					
Mrs. Paul's					
Microwave Fried Clams	2.5 oz	260	8	15	23
take-out					
breaded & fried	20 sm	379	27	21	19
COCOA					
(see also CHOCOLATE)					
hot cocoa	1 cup	218	9	9	26
mix as prep w/ water	7 oz	103	3	1	23
mix w/ equal as prep w/ water	7 oz	48	4	tr	9
powder unsweetened	1 tbsp (5 g)	11	1	1	3
powder unsweetened	1 cup (3 oz)	197	17	12	47
Carnation					
Hot Cocoa 70 Calorie	1 pkg (0.7 oz)	70	3	0	15
Hot Cocoa Double Chocolate Meltdown	1 pkg (1.2 oz)	150	2	4	27
Hot Cocoa Fat Free Raspberry	1 pkg (0.3 oz)	30	2	0	4
Hot Cocoa Fat Free w/ Marshmallows	1 pkg (0.4 oz)	45	7	0	10
Hot Cocoa Lactose Free	1 pkg (1 oz)	120	1	2	25
Hot Cocoa Marshmallow Blizzard	1 pkg (1.5 oz)	180	2	2	39
Hot Cocoa Milk Chocolate	3 tbsp (1 oz)	110	2	1	24
Hot Cocoa Rich Chocolate	3 tbsp (1 oz)	110	1	1	24
Hot Cocoa Rich Chocolate Fat Free	1 pkg (0.3 oz)	25	2	0	4
Hot Cocoa Rich Chocolate No Sugar Added	3 tbsp (0.5 oz)	50	4	0	8

FOOD	PORTION	CALS	PROT	FAT	CARB
Hot Cocoa Rich Chocolate w/ Marshmallows	3 tbsp (1 oz)	110	1	1	24
Hershey					
Cocoa	1 tbsp (5 g)	20	1	1	3
European Cocoa	1 tbsp (5 g)	20	1	1	3
Nestle					
Cocoa	1 tbsp	15	1	1	3
Hot Cocoa Rich Chocolate	1 pkg (1 oz)	110	1	1	24
Hot Cocoa Rich w/ Marshmallows	1 pkg (1 oz)	110	1	1	24
Swiss Miss					
Hot Cocoa And Cream	1 serv	153	2	5	25
Hot Cocoa Chocolate Sensation	1 serv	148	2	4	27
Hot Cocoa Diet	1 serv	22	2	tr	4
Hot Cocoa Fat Free	1 serv	52	4	tr	9
Hot Cocoa Fat Free Marshmallow Lovers	1 serv	65	3	tr	13
Hot Cocoa Lite	1 serv	76	2	1	18
Hot Cocoa Marshmallow Lovers	1 serv	142	2	3	27
Hot Cocoa Milk Chocolate	1 serv	118	1	3	22
Hot Cocoa Milk Chocolate No Sugar Added	1 serv	55	2	1	10
Hot Cocoa Milk Chocolate w/ Marshmallows	1 serv	118	1	3	22
Hot Cocoa Rich Chocolate	1 serv	110	2	2	23
Hot Cocoa White Chocolate	1 serv	109	3	1	21
Hot Cocoa w/ Marshmallows No Sugar Added	1 serv	56	3	1	10
Premiere Hot Cocoa Almond Mocha	1 serv	144	2	3	28
Premiere Hot Cocoa English Toffee	1 serv	142	2	2	29
Premiere Hot Cocoa Raspberry Truffle	1 serv	144	2	3	28
Premiere Hot Cocoa Suisse Truffle	1 serv	142	2	2	28
Rich Hot Cocoa No Sugar Added	1 serv	54	2	1	10
Sidewalk Cafe Cappuccino	1 serv	119	3	4	18
Sidewalk Cafe Cinnamon	1 serv	126	3	4	21
Sidewalk Cafe French Vanilla	1 serv	121	3	4	19
Sidewalk Cafe Mocha	1 serv	120	3	4	20
Weight Watchers					
Hot Cocoa Mix as prep	1 pkg	70	6	0	7

FOOD	PORTION	CALS	PROT	FAT	CARB
COCONUT					
coconut water	1 cup	46	2	tr	9
cream canned	1 cup	568	8	52	25
cream canned	1 tbsp	36	1	3	2
dried sweetened flaked	7 oz pkg	944	7	64	95
dried sweetened flaked	1 cup	351	2	24	35
dried sweetened flaked canned	1 cup	341	3	24	32
dried sweetened shredded	7 oz pkg	997	6	71	95
dried sweetened shredded	1 cup	466	2	33	44
dried toasted	1 oz	168	2	13	13
dried unsweetened	1 oz	187	2	18	7
fresh	1 piece (1.5 oz)	159	2	15	7
fresh shredded	1 cup	283	3	27	12
milk canned	1 cup	445	5	48	6
milk frozen	1 cup	486	4	50	13
Baker's					
Angel Flake	1 tbsp (0.5 oz)	70	1	5	6
Angel Flake (canned)	2 tbsp (0.5 oz)	70	1	6	6
Premium Shred	2 tbsp (0.5 oz)	70	1	5	6
COD					
atlantic canned	3 oz	89	19	1	0
atlantic canned	1 can (11 oz)	327	71	3	0
atlantic dried	3 oz	246	53	2	0
atlantic fresh cooked	3 oz	89	19	1	0
atlantic fresh cooked	1 fillet (6.3 oz)	189	41	2	0
atlantic fresh raw	3 oz	70	15	1	0
pacific fresh baked	3 oz	95	21	1	0
roe canned	1 oz	34	6	1	tr
roe baked w/ butter & lemon juice	1 oz	36	6	1	tr
roe raw	1 oz	37	7	tr	tr
roe tarama	3.5 oz	547	8	55	6
COFFEE					
(*see also* COFFEE BEVERAGES, COFFEE SUBSTITUTES)					
instant					
Nescafe					
French Vanilla	1 tsp (2 g)	5	0	0	1
French Vanilla Decaf	1 tsp (2 g)	5	0	0	1
Hazelnut	1 tsp (2 g)	5	0	0	1
Irish Creme	1 tsp (2 g)	5	0	0	1
With Chicory	1 tsp (2 g)	5	0	0	1
regular					
roasted beans	1 oz	64	4	4	18
Nescafe					
Cafe Mocha	1 can (10 oz)	140	3	3	27
Caffe Latte	1 can (10 oz)	130	3	3	22
Caffe Latte Decaffeinated	1 can (10 oz)	130	3	3	22

FOOD	PORTION	CALS	PROT	FAT	CARB
Espresso Cafe Latte	1 pkg (0.6 oz)	70	3	2	10
Espresso Cafe Mocha	1 pkg (1 oz)	110	3	3	20
Espresso Cappuccino	1 pkg (0.6 oz)	80	3	3	11
Espresso Roast	1 can (10 oz)	90	1	1	21
French Vanilla	1 can (10 oz)	150	4	4	25
Hazelnut	1 can (10 oz)	130	3	3	22
take-out					
cafe au lait	1 cup (8 fl oz)	77	4	4	6
cappuccino	1 cup (8 fl oz)	77	4	4	6
coffee con leche	1 cup (8 fl oz)	77	4	4	6
irish coffee	1 serv (9 fl oz)	107	1	3	3
latte w/ skim milk	13 oz	88	8	tr	12
latte w/ whole milk	13 oz	152	8	8	12
mocha	1 mug (9.6 fl oz)	202	3	15	17
COFFEE BEVERAGES					
(*see also* COFFEE SUBSTITUTES)					
french mix as prep	7 oz	57	1	3	7
mocha mix as prep	7 oz	51	1	2	8
Arizona					
Iced Latte Supreme	8 oz	110	3	2	21
Iced Mocha Latte	8 oz	110	4	2	21
Chock full o'Nuts					
New York Cappuccino French Vanilla	1 pkg (0.9 oz)	90	2	2	19
New York Cappuccino Hazelnut	1 pkg. (0.9 oz)	90	2	2	19
Coffee House USA					
All Flavors	1 bottle (9.5 oz)	100	4	4	29
Gehl's					
Iced Cappuccino	1 can (11 oz)	190	11	2	33
General Foods					
International Coffee Sugar Free Fat Free Suisse Mocha as prep	1 serv (8 oz)	25	0	0	5
International Coffees Sugar Free Fat Free Decaffeinated French Vanilla	1 serv (8 oz)	25	0	0	5
International Coffees Sugar Free Fat Free Decaffeinated Suisse Mocha	1 serv (8 oz)	25	0	0	5
International Coffees Sugar Free Fat Free French Vanilla Cafe as prep	1 serv (8 oz)	25	0	0	5
Maxwell House					
Cafe Cappuccino Amaretto as prep	1 serv (8 oz)	90	1	1	19

FOOD	PORTION	CALS	PROT	FAT	CARB
Cafe Cappuccino Decaffeinated Mocha as prep	1 serv (8 oz)	100	2	3	17
Cafe Cappuccino Decaffeinated Vanilla as prep	1 serv (8 oz)	90	1	1	19
Cafe Cappuccino Irish Cream as prep	1 serv (8 oz)	90	1	1	19
Cafe Cappuccino Mocha as prep	1 serv (8 oz)	100	2	3	17
Cafe Cappuccino Sugar Free Mocha as prep	1 serv (8 oz)	60	1	3	7
Iced Cappuccino as prep w/ 2% milk	1 serv (8 oz)	180	8	5	27
Silk					
Coffee Soylatte	1 bottle (11 oz)	220	7	5	38
COFFEE SUBSTITUTES					
powder as prep w/ milk	6 oz	121	6	6	10
Natural Touch					
Kaffree Roma	1 tsp (2 g)	10	0	0	2
Roma Cappuccino	3 tbsp (0.4 oz)	50	1	3	5
Postum					
Instant Coffee Flavor as prep	1 serv (8 oz)	10	0	0	3
Instant as prep	1 serv (8 oz)	10	0	0	3
COFFEE WHITENERS					
(*see also* MILK SUBSTITUTES)					
Silk					
Creamer	1 tbsp	15	0	1	1
Creamer French Vanilla	1 tbsp	20	0	1	3
Creamer Hazelnut	1 tbsp	15	0	1	1
COLESLAW					
home recipe					
coleslaw w/ dressing	¾ cup	147	1	11	13
take-out					
coleslaw w/ dressing	½ cup	42	1	2	7
vinegar & oil coleslaw	3.5 oz	150	1	9	16
COLLARDS					
fresh cooked	½ cup	17	1	tr	4
frzn chopped cooked	½ cup	31	3	tr	6
Birds Eye					
Chopped Greens frzn	1 cup (3.1 oz)	30	2	0	2
COOKIES					
(*see also* BROWNIE, CAKE, DOUGHNUT, PIE)					
home recipe					
chocolate chip as prep w/ butter	1 (0.42 oz)	78	1	5	9

FOOD	PORTION	CALS	PROT	FAT	CARB
chocolate chip as prep w/ margarine	1 (0.56 oz)	78	1	5	9
oatmeal	1 (0.5 oz)	67	1	3	10
oatmeal w/ raisins	1 (0.52 oz)	65	1	2	10
peanut butter	1 (0.7 oz)	95	2	5	12
shortbread as prep w/ butter	1 (0.38 oz)	60	1	4	6
shortbread as prep w/ margarine	1 (0.38 oz)	60	1	4	6
sugar as prep w/ butter	1 (0.49 oz)	66	1	3	8
sugar as prep w/ margarine	1 (0.49 oz)	66	1	3	8
mix					
chocolate chip	1 (0.56 oz)	79	1	4	10
oatmeal	1 (0.6 oz)	74	1	3	10
oatmeal raisin	1 (0.6 oz)	74	1	3	10
Betty Crocker					
Chocolate Peanut Butter as prep	1 bar	180	2	9	25
Date Bar as prep	1 bar	150	1	6	23
Oatmeal as prep	2	150	2	6	22
GoldnBrown					
Fat Free	1 (1.1 oz)	120	2	0	27
ready-to-eat					
animal	11 crackers (1 oz)	126	2	4	21
animal crackers	1 box (2.4 oz)	299	4	9	51
australian anzac biscuit	1	98	1	3	17
chocolate chip	1 (0.4 oz)	48	1	2	7
chocolate chip	1 box (1.9 oz)	233	3	12	36
chocolate chip low fat	1 (0.25 oz)	45	1	2	7
chocolate chip soft-type	1 (0.5 oz)	69	1	4	9
chocolate w/ creme filling	1 (0.35 oz)	47	1	2	7
chocolate w/ creme filling chocolate coated	1 (0.60 oz)	82	1	5	11
chocolate w/ creme filling sugar free low sodium	1 (0.35 oz)	46	1	2	7
chocolate w/ extra creme filling	1 (0.46 oz)	65	1	3	9
chocolate wafer cookie crumbs	½ cup (5.9 oz)	728	11	25	120
cream cheese	1 (1.1 oz)	141	2	9	14
digestive biscuits plain	2	141	2	7	21
fig bars	1 (0.56 oz)	56	1	1	11
fudge	1 (0.73 oz)	73	1	1	17
graham	1 squares (0.24 oz)	30	1	1	5
graham chocolate covered	1 (0.49 oz)	68	1	3	9
graham honey	1 (0.24 oz)	30	1	1	5
hermits	1 (1 oz)	117	2	5	18
jumbles coconut	1 (1 oz)	121	1	7	13
ladyfingers	1 (0.38 oz)	40	1	1	7

FOOD	PORTION	CALS	PROT	FAT	CARB
macaroons	1 (0.8 oz)	97	1	3	17
madeleines	1 (0.8 oz)	86	2	5	10
marshmallow chocolate coated	1 (0.46 oz)	55	1	2	9
marshmallow pie chocolate coated	1 (1.4 oz)	165	2	7	26
molasses	1 (0.5 oz)	65	1	2	11
neapolitan tri-color cookie	1 (0.6 oz)	79	1	5	8
oatmeal	1 (0.52 oz)	71	1	4	9
oatmeal	1 (0.6 oz)	81	1	3	12
oatmeal soft-type	1 (0.5 oz)	61	1	2	10
oatmeal raisin	1 (0.6 oz)	81	1	3	12
oatmeal raisin soft-type	1 (0.5 oz)	61	1	2	10
peanut butter sandwich	1 (0.5 oz)	67	1	3	9
peanut butter sandwich sugar free low sodium	1 (0.35 oz)	54	1	3	5
peanut butter soft-type	1 (0.5 oz)	69	1	4	9
pinenut cookies	1 (1.1 oz)	134	4	9	11
raisin soft-type	1 (0.5 oz)	60	1	2	10
reginette queen'a biscuit	1 (0.8 oz)	86	2	3	13
shortbread	1 (0.28 oz)	40	1	2	5
shortbread pecan	1 (0.49 oz)	79	1	5	8
spritz	1 (0.4 oz)	42	1	2	6
sugar	1 (0.52 oz)	72	1	3	10
sugar low sugar sodium free	1 (0.24 oz)	30	1	1	5
toll house original	1 (0.8 oz)	105	2	6	13
zeppole	1 (0.8 oz)	78	1	6	6
Alternative Baking					
Vegan Chocolate Chip	1 serv (2.5 oz)	280	3	10	46
Vegan Expresso Chocolate Chip	1 serv (2 oz)	230	3	9	35
Vegan Lemon	1 serv (2.25 oz)	250	3	7	42
Vegan Oatmeal	1 serv (2.25 oz)	250	5	10	35
Vegan Peanut Butter	1 serv (2.25 oz)	270	5	10	40
Vegan Pumpkin	1 serv (2 oz)	200	2	6	35
Vegan Wheat Free Choco Cherry Chunk	1 serv (1.75 oz)	190	3	6	32
Vegan Wheat Free Hula Nut	1 serv (1.75 oz)	190	6	6	29
Vegan Wheat Free P-nut Fudge Fusion	1 serv (1.75 oz)	190	4	7	29
Vegan Wheat Free Snickerdoodle	1 serv (1.75 oz)	170	3	3	35
Amay's					
Chinese Style Almond	1 (0.5 oz)	80	1	4	10
Archway					
Alpine Fudge	1 (1.3 oz)	160	1	6	24

FOOD	PORTION	CALS	PROT	FAT	CARB
Carrot Cake	1 (1 oz)	130	1	5	19
Chocolate Chip Sugar Free	1 (0.8 oz)	110	1	5	16
Coconut Macaroon	2 (1.4 oz)	180	1	11	21
Devils Food Chocolate Drop Fat Free	1 (0.7 oz)	60	1	0	15
Dutch Cocoa	1 (0.9 oz)	100	1	4	18
Fruit & Honey Bar	1 (0.9 oz)	110	1	3	19
Ginger Snaps	5 (1 oz)	120	1	5	20
Homestyle Chocolate Chip	3 (1 oz)	130	1	7	17
Iced Spice	1 (1 oz)	120	1	5	19
Oatmeal	1 (0.9 oz)	100	1	4	16
Oatmeal Apple Filled	1 (0.9 oz)	90	1	3	16
Oatmeal Pecan	1 (0.9 oz)	110	1	4	16
Oatmeal Raisin Bran	1 (0.9 oz)	100	1	3	18
Oatmeal Raspberry Fat Free	1 (1.1 oz)	100	1	0	23
Oatmeal Sugar Free	1 (0.8 oz)	110	1	5	16
Oatmeal Raisin	1 (0.9 oz)	100	1	4	17
Oatmeal Raisin Fat Free	1 (1.1 oz)	100	1	0	24
Old Dutch Apple	1 (0.9 oz)	110	1	4	18
Peanut Butter	1 (1 oz)	150	2	9	16
Peanut Butter Fudge	1 (1.3 oz)	220	3	13	23
Peanut Butter Sugar Free	1 (0.8 oz)	110	2	6	14
Pecan Crunch	3 (1.2 oz)	180	2	10	20
Raspberry Filled	1 (0.8 oz)	90	1	4	15
Rocky Road	1 (0.8 oz)	110	1	5	16
Rocky Road Sugar Free	1 (0.8 oz)	100	1	5	15
Shortbread Sugar Free	1 (0.8 oz)	110	1	5	16
Strawberry Filled	1 (0.8 oz)	90	1	3	15
BP Gourmet					
Biscotti Fat Free Cinnamon Crunch	6 (1 oz)	110	2	0	24
Biscotti Fat Free Vanilla Crunch	4 (1 oz)	80	2	0	18
Chocolate Fudge Chip Sugar Free	5 (1 oz)	100	1	6	13
Dreams Chocolate	7 (1 oz)	120	2	3	21
Dreams Fat Free Chocolate Fudge	13 (1 oz)	100	2	0	25
Dreams Fat Free Vanilla	19 (1 oz)	100	2	0	25
Tangos Fat Free Chocolate Fudge Chip	4 (1 oz)	100	2	0	23
Bahlsen					
Afrika	8 (1.1 oz)	170	2	10	17
Butter Leaves	7 (1 oz)	140	2	7	19
Choco Leibniz	2 (1 oz)	140	2	7	18
Choco Star Dark Chocolate	3 (1.1 oz)	170	2	12	16
Choco Star Milk Chocolate	3 (1.1 oz)	180	2	12	16
Chocolate Hearts	4 (1 oz)	160	2	9	18

FOOD	PORTION	CALS	PROT	FAT	CARB
Delice	6 (1 oz)	140	2	6	19
Deloba	4 (0.9 oz)	130	2	5	19
Hanover Waffelin	5 (1 oz)	160	1	10	16
Hit Chocolate Vanilla Filled	2 (1 oz)	140	2	8	18
Hit Vanilla Chocolate Filled	2 (1 oz)	140	2	7	19
Kipferl	4 (1 oz)	150	2	9	16
Leibniz	6 (1 oz)	130	2	4	23
Nuss Dessert	3 (1.1 oz)	180	2	11	19
Probiers	6 (1.1 oz)	150	2	6	21
Twingo	6 (1.1 oz)	170	2	11	18
Waffeletten	4 (1 oz)	160	2	9	18
Baker's Harvest					
Animal	12 (0.9 oz)	130	2	3	22
Chocolate Graham	2 (0.9 oz)	130	2	3	24
Cinnamon Grahams	2 (0.9 oz)	130	1	5	19
Cinnamon Grahams Low Fat	2 (0.9 oz)	110	2	2	22
Graham	2 (0.9 oz)	120	1	4	21
Graham Low Fat	2 (0.9 oz)	110	2	2	22
Iced Oatmeal	1 (0.6 oz)	70	1	3	11
Pecan Shortbread	1 (0.5 oz)	80	1	5	10
Vanilla Wafers	7 (1.1 oz)	150	1	6	22
Barbara's Bakery					
Apple Cinnamon Bars Fat Free Whole Wheat	1 (0.7 oz)	60	1	0	14
Chocolate Chip	1 (0.6 oz)	80	1	4	10
Double Dutch Chocolate	1 (0.6 oz)	80	1	4	10
Nature's Choice Coconut Almond	1 bar (1 oz)	120	2	5	20
Nature's Choice Expresso Bean	1 bar (1 oz)	120	2	3	22
Nature's Choice Lemon Yogurt	1 bar (1 oz)	120	2	4	22
Nature's Choice Roasted Peanut	1 bar (1 oz)	130	3	5	20
Old Fashioned Oatmeal	1 (0.6 oz)	70	1	3	11
Raspberry Bars Fat Free Wheat Free Raspberry	1 (0.7 oz)	60	1	0	15
Snackimals Chocolate Chip	8 (1 oz)	120	2	5	18
Snackimals Oatmeal Wheat Free	8 (1 oz)	120	2	5	19
Snackimals Vanilla	8 (1 oz)	120	2	5	19
Traditional Blueberry Low Fat	1 (0.7 oz)	60	1	1	14
Traditional Fig Low Fat	1 (0.7 oz)	60	1	1	14
Traditional Shortbread	1 (0.6 oz)	80	1	4	10
Bed & Breakfast					
Cranberry Orange Oatmeal	1 (0.8 oz)	110	1	5	17

FOOD	PORTION	CALS	PROT	FAT	CARB
Enrobed Shortbread	2 (1.4 oz)	190	2	9	24
Fruit Center Key Lime	2 (1.1 oz)	140	1	6	22
Fruit Center Raspberry	2 (1.1 oz)	140	1	6	22
Beigel's					
Black & White	1 (1 oz)	100	1	3	18
Breaktime					
Coconut	1 (0.3 oz)	35	1	1	5
Oatmeal	1 (0.3 oz)	35	1	1	5
Brent & Sam's					
Chocolate Chip Pecan	2 (0.5 oz)	80	1	5	9
Chocolate Chips	2 (0.5 oz)	70	1	4	10
Bud's Best					
Caco Creme	7 (1 oz)	140	2	6	21
Chocolate Chip	6 (1 oz)	140	2	6	19
French Vanilla	7 (1 oz)	150	2	6	20
Oatmeal	6 (1 oz)	130	2	5	20
Cafe					
Cinnamony Twists Chocolate Chip	1 (0.5 oz)	40	0	2	7
Sugar Free California Almond	4 (1 oz)	110	2	4	17
Twists Cinnamony	1 (0.3 oz)	40	0	2	7
Carr's					
Ginger Lemon Cremes	2 (1 oz)	140	1	7	19
Carriage Trade					
Finnish Ginger Snaps	3	60	2	7	21
Chortles					
Cookies	½ pkg. (1 oz)	125	1	3	23
Cookie Lover's					
Chocolate Chip	1 (0.8 oz)	90	1	4	16
Creme Supremes	2 (0.9 oz)	120	1	5	18
Creme Supremes Mint	2 (0.9 oz)	120	1	5	18
Grahams	2 (1 oz)	100	2	1	22
Grahams Cinnamon	2 (1 oz)	110	2	1	24
Peanut Butter	1 (0.8 oz)	100	2	4	16
Shortbread	1 (0.8 oz)	120	2	7	13
Dare					
Blueberry Cheesecake	1 (0.6 oz)	90	1	5	11
Butter Shortbread	1 (0.5 oz)	63	1	4	7
Butter Creme	1 (0.6 oz)	85	1	4	11
Carrot Cake	1 (0.6 oz)	92	1	5	11
Chocolate Chip	1 (0.5 oz)	77	1	4	9
Chocolate Fudge	1 (0.7 oz)	97	1	5	13
Cinnamon Danish	1 (0.4 oz)	47	1	2	7
Coconut Creme	1 (0.7 oz)	99	1	5	12
French Creme	1 (0.5 oz)	80	1	5	8
Harvest From The Rain Forest	1 (0.5 oz)	70	1	4	7

FOOD	PORTION	CALS	PROT	FAT	CARB
Key Lime Creme	1 (0.6 oz)	86	1	4	12
Lemon Creme	1 (0.7 oz)	95	1	5	13
Maple Leaf Creme	1 (0.6 oz)	83	1	4	12
Maple Walnut Fudge	1 (0.7 oz)	99	1	5	13
Milk Chocolate Fudge	1 (0.7 oz)	99	1	5	12
Oatmeal Raisin	1 (0.4 oz)	59	1	3	8
Sun Maid Raisin Oatmeal	1 (0.5 oz)	52	1	3	8
De Beukelaer					
Pirouline	8 (1 oz)	130	3	4	23
Pirouline Viennese Wafers	1 (1 oz)	150	1	7	20
Delacre					
Chocosprits	1 (0.6 oz)	90	1	5	11
Marquisettes	3 (0.9 oz)	140	2	7	17
Roules d'Or	4 (1 oz)	180	1	8	19
Dunkaroos					
Chocolate Chip w/ Chocolate Frosting	1 pkg (1 oz)	120	1	5	20
Cinnamon Graham w/ Vanilla Frosting & Sprinkles	1 pkg (1 oz)	130	1	5	21
Cookies'n Creme	1 pkg (1 oz)	120	1	5	20
Dutch Mill					
Chocolate Chip	3 (1.1 oz)	160	1	10	18
Coconut Macaroons	3 (1 oz)	120	1	7	14
Oatmeal Raisin	3 (1 oz)	130	2	6	18
Eddyleon					
Jelly Graham Raspberry	1 (0.9 oz)	134	1	8	15
Pudding Cookies	1 (0.9 oz)	134	1	6	15
Entenmann's					
Little Bites Chocolate Chip	8 (1.8 oz)	240	2	12	33
Soft Baked Chocolate Chip	1 (0.7 oz)	100	1	5	13
Soft Baked Double Chocolate Chip	1 (0.7 oz)	100	1	5	14
Soft Baked Milk Chocolate Chip	1 (0.7 oz)	100	1	5	13
Soft Baked Original Chocolate Chip	3 (1 oz)	150	1	7	20
Soft Baked White Chocolate Macadamia Nut	1 (0.7 oz)	100	1	6	12
Soft Baked Light Chocolately Chip	2 (1 oz)	120	1	4	21
Soft Baked Light Oatmeal Raisin	2 (1 oz)	100	2	0	23
Estee					
Chocolate Chip	4	150	2	7	21
Coconut	4	140	2	6	19
Fig Bars	2	100	1	1	23

FOOD	PORTION	CALS	PROT	FAT	CARB
Fudge	4	150	2	7	19
Lemon Thins	4	140	2	6	19
Oatmeal Raisin	4	130	2	5	19
Sandwich Chocolate	3	160	2	6	24
Sandwich Original	3	160	2	6	24
Sandwich Peanut Butter	3	160	4	7	22
Sandwich Vanilla	3	160	2	5	25
Shortbread	4	130	2	4	22
Sugar Free Chocolate Chip	3	110	2	4	22
Sugar Free Chocolate Walnut	3	110	2	4	22
Sugar Free Coconut	3	110	2	4	22
Sugar Free Grahams Chocolate	2	110	3	2	27
Sugar Free Grahams Cinnamon	2	90	3	2	18
Sugar Free Grahams Old Fashion	2	90	3	2	17
Sugar Free Lemon	3	110	2	3	22
Sugar Free Wafer Banana Split	5	155	1	9	22
Sugar Free Wafer Chocolate	5	150	1	9	19
Sugar Free Wafer Chocolate Peanut Butter Caramel	5	150	1	8	22
Sugar Free Wafer Lemon Creme	5	150	1	8	22
Sugar Free Wafer Peanut Butter Creme	5	150	1	8	22
Sugar Free Wafer Vanilla	5	150	1	8	21
Sugar Free Wafer Vanilla Strawberry	5	150	1	8	22
Vanilla Thins	4	140	2	6	19
Falcone's					
Sorrentini	1 (1 oz)	100	2	4	16
Famous Amos					
Butter Shortie	1 (0.5 oz)	80	1	5	9
Chocolate Chip	4 (1 oz)	140	2	7	18
Chocolate Chip & Pecan	4 (1 oz)	140	1	8	18
Chocolate Chip Toffee	4 (1 oz)	130	1	6	18
Chocolate Creme Sandwich	3 (1.2 oz)	140	2	6	22
Chunky Chocolate Chip	1 (0.5 oz)	70	1	4	9
Fat Free Fig Bar	2 (1 oz)	90	1	0	21
Fat Free Strawberry Fruit Bar	2 (1 oz)	90	1	0	22
Fig Bar	2 (1.1 oz)	120	1	3	22
Oatmeal Chocolate Chip Walnut	4 (1 oz)	140	2	7	16
Oatmeal Raisin	4 (1 oz)	130	2	6	20

FOOD	PORTION	CALS	PROT	FAT	CARB
Oatmeal Macaroon Creme Sandwich	3 (1.2 oz)	160	2	7	23
Peanut Butter Chocolate Chunk	1 (0.5 oz)	80	1	5	9
Peanut Butter Creme Sandwich	3 (1.2 oz)	160	4	8	19
Pecan Shortie	1 (0.5 oz)	80	1	5	9
Vanilla Creme Sandwich	3 (1.2 oz)	160	2	7	24
Frookie					
Animal Frackers	14 (1 oz)	130	2	5	18
Chocolate Chip Wheat & Gluten Free	3 (1.1 oz)	140	1	5	23
Double Chocolate Wheat & Gluten Free	3 (1.1 oz)	130	1	4	23
Dream Creams Strawberry	4 (1 oz)	140	2	8	18
Dream Creams Vanilla	4 (1 oz)	140	2	8	18
Funky Monkeys Chocolate	16 (1 oz)	120	2	4	20
Funky Monkeys Vanilla	16 (1 oz)	120	2	4	20
Graham Cinnamon	2 (1 oz)	100	2	3	17
Graham Honey	2 (1 oz)	110	2	3	18
Lemon Wafers	8 (1 oz)	110	2	0	26
Old Fashioned Ginger Snaps	8 (1 oz)	120	1	2	24
Organic Chocolate Chip	3 (1.1 oz)	150	2	7	20
Organic Double Chocolate Chip	3 (1.1 oz)	140	2	6	20
Organic Iced Lemon	3 (1.3 oz)	165	2	6	27
Organic Oatmeal Raisin	3 (1.1 oz)	140	2	5	22
Peanut Butter Chunk Wheat & Gluten Free	3 (1.1 oz)	140	3	5	21
Sandwich Chocolate	2 (0.7 oz)	100	1	4	14
Sandwich Lemon	2 (0.7 oz)	100	1	4	14
Sandwich Peanut Butter	2 (0.7 oz)	100	1	4	14
Sandwich Vanilla	2 (0.7 oz)	100	1	4	14
Shortbread	5 (1 oz)	130	2	5	20
Vanilla Wafers	8 (1 oz)	110	2	0	26
General Henry					
Fruit Bars Apple	1 (0.6 oz)	60	1	1	13
Fruit Bars Blueberry	1 (0.6 oz)	60	1	1	12
Fruit Bars Fig	1 (0.6 oz)	60	1	1	12
Girl Scout					
Apple Cinnamon Reduced Fat	3 (1 oz)	120	2	5	18
Lemon Drops	3 (1.2 oz)	160	2	8	20
Samoas	2 (1 oz)	160	2	9	17
Striped Chocolate Chip	3 (1.2 oz)	180	2	10	20
Tagalongs	2 (0.9 oz)	150	3	10	13
Thin Mints	4 (1 oz)	140	1	8	18
Trefoils	5 (1.1 oz)	160	2	8	20

FOOD	PORTION	CALS	PROT	FAT	CARB
Godiva					
Biscotti Dipped In Milk Chocolate	1 (0.9 oz)	120	2	6	15
Golden Grahams Treats					
Chocolate Chunk	1 bar (0.8 oz)	90	1	3	17
Honey Graham	1 bar (0.8 oz)	90	1	2	17
King Size Chocolate Chunk	1 bar (1.6 oz)	190	2	5	35
King Size Honey Graham	1 bar (1.6 oz)	180	1	4	36
Gourmet					
Chocolate Chip	2 (1.1 oz)	160	2	9	19
Lemon Creme	2 (1.4 oz)	210	1	10	27
Oatmeal Raisin	2 (0.9 oz)	120	2	6	15
Peanut Butter Chip	2 (1 oz)	150	3	8	17
Raspberry Center	2 (1.1 oz)	140	1	5	21
Grandma's					
Chocolate Chip	1 (1.4 oz)	190	2	9	25
Fudge Chocolate Chip	1 (1.4 oz)	170	1	7	26
Fudge Sandwich	3	180	2	5	31
Fudge Vanilla Sandwich	3	120	1	4	21
Mini Fudge	9	150	2	7	21
Mini Peanut Butter	9	150	2	7	21
Mini Vanilla	9	150	2	7	22
Oatmeal Raisin	1 (1.4 oz)	160	1	6	26
Old Time Molasses	1 (1.4 oz)	160	2	4	29
Peanut Butter	1 (1.4 oz)	190	2	9	22
Peanut Butter Chocolate Chip	1 (1.4 oz)	190	4	9	23
Peanut Butter Sandwich	5	210	3	10	28
Rich N'Chewy	1 pkg	270	2	12	39
Vanilla Sandwich	3	180	2	5	32
Vanilla Sandwich	5	210	2	10	30
Handi-Snack					
Cookie Jammers Cookies & Fruit Spread	1 pkg (1.3 oz)	130	1	3	26
Health Valley					
Apple Spice	3	100	2	0	24
Apricot Delight	3	100	2	0	24
Biscotti Amaretto	2	120	3	3	23
Biscotti Chocolate	2	120	3	3	23
Biscotti Fruit & Nut	2	120	3	3	23
Cheesecake Bars Blueberry	1 bar	160	3	2	34
Cheesecake Bars Raspberry	1 bar	160	3	2	34
Cheesecake Bars Strawberry	1 bar	160	3	2	34
Chips Double Chocolate	3	100	3	0	24

FOOD	PORTION	CALS	PROT	FAT	CARB
Chips Old Fashioned	3	100	3	0	24
Chips Original	3	100	3	0	24
Chocolate Fudge Center	2	70	2	0	25
Chocolate Sandwich Bar Bavarian Creme	1 bar	150	3	0	35
Chocolate Sandwich Bars Caramel Creme	1 bar	150	3	0	35
Chocolate Sandwich Bars Vanilla Creme	1 bar	150	3	0	35
Date Delight	3	100	2	0	24
Graham Amaranth	8	100	4	0	23
Graham Oat Bran	8	100	4	0	30
Graham Original Amaranth	6	120	3	3	22
Hawaiian Fruit	3	100	2	0	24
Jumbo Apple Raisin	1	80	2	0	19
Jumbo Raisin Raisin	1	80	2	0	19
Jumbo Raspberry	1	80	2	0	19
Marshmallow Bars Chocolate Chip	1	90	1	0	22
Marshmallow Bars Old Fashioned	1	90	1	0	22
Marshmallow Bars Tropical Fruit	1	90	1	0	22
Oat Bran Fruit Bars Raisin Cinnamon	1 bar	160	3	1	34
Raisin Oatmeal	3	100	2	0	24
Raspberry Fruit Center	1	70	2	0	18
Tarts Baked Apple Cinnamon	1	150	3	0	35
Tarts California Strawberry	1	150	3	0	35
Tarts Chocolate Fudge	1	150	3	0	35
Tarts Cranberry Apple	1	150	3	0	35
Tarts Mountain Blueberry	1	150	3	0	35
Tarts Red Raspberry	1	150	3	0	35
Tarts Sweet Red Cherry	1	150	3	0	35
Hellema					
Almond	1 pkg (0.6 oz)	90	1	5	9
Hershey					
Cripsy Rice Snacks Peanut Butter	1 (0.6 oz)	70	1	3	10
Joseph's					
Almond Sugar Free	2 (0.9 oz)	100	1	5	14
Chocolate Chip Sugar Free	2 (0.9 oz)	100	1	5	15
Chocolate Walnut Sugar Free	2 (0.9 oz)	100	1	6	14
Coconut Sugar Free	2 (0.9 oz)	105	1	5	14
Lemon Sugar Free	2 (0.9 oz)	95	1	4	15
Oatmeal Raisin Sugar Free	2 (0.9 oz)	100	2	5	15

FOOD	PORTION	CALS	PROT	FAT	CARB
Peanut Butter Sugar Free	2 (0.9 oz)	95	2	5	13
Pecan Shortbread Sugar Free	2 (0.9 oz)	100	1	5	14
Keebler					
Animal Crackers Chocolate Chip	7 (1 oz)	130	2	5	22
Animal Crackers Ernie's	1 box	250	<4	9	41
Animal Crackers Iced	6 (1.1 oz)	150	2	5	24
Animal Crackers Sprinkled	6 (1.1 oz)	150	<2	5	24
Butter	5 (1.1 oz)	150	<2	6	22
Cookie Stix Butter	5 (1.2 oz)	160	<2	6	22
Cookie Stix Chocolate Chip	4 (0.9 oz)	130	<2	5	19
Cookie Stix Rainbow	5 (1.2 oz)	150	<2	6	23
Droxies	3 (1.1 oz)	140	<2	6	21
Droxies Reduced Fat	3 (1.1 oz)	140	<2	5	23
E.L. Fudge Fudge w/ Fudge Filling	2 (0.9 oz)	120	<2	6	17
E.L. Fudge w/ Peanut Butter Filling	2 (0.9 oz)	120	<2	6	16
Fudge Shoppe Fudge Sticks Peanut Butter	3 (1 oz)	150	<2	8	18
Ginger Snaps	5 (1.1 oz)	150	<2	6	24
Graham Cinnamon Crisp	8 (1 oz)	140	2	5	22
Graham Cinnamon Crisp Low Fat	8 (1 oz)	110	2	2	24
Graham Honey	8 (1.1 oz)	150	2	6	21
Graham Honey Low Fat	8 (1.1 oz)	120	2	2	26
Graham Original	8 (1 oz)	130	2	3	23
Oatmeal Country Style	2 (0.8 oz)	120	<2	5	17
Snack Size Chips Deluxe	1 pkg (2 oz)	300	3	16	36
Snack Size Chips Deluxe Chocolate Lovers	1 pkg (2 oz)	280	3	15	36
Snack Size Mini Fudge Stripes	1 pkg (2 oz)	280	3	14	38
Snack Size Rainbow Chips Deluxe	1 pkg (2 oz)	290	3	16	36
Snack Size Sandies w/ Pecans	1 pkg (2 oz)	300	3	17	33
Snackin' Grahams Cinnamon	21 (1 oz)	130	<2	3	23
Snackin' Grahams Honey	23 (1 oz)	130	<2	4	22
Soft Batch Homestyle Chocolate Chunk	1 (0.9 oz)	130	1	7	17
Soft Batch Homestyle Double Chocolate	1 (0.9 oz)	130	1	7	17
Soft Batch Homestyle Oatmeal Raisin	1 (0.9 oz)	130	1	5	20
Sugar Wafers Peanut Butter	4 (1.1 oz)	170	<3	9	19

FOOD	PORTION	CALS	PROT	FAT	CARB
Vanilla Wafers Reduced Fat	8 (1.1 oz)	130	<2	4	25
Vienna Fingers	2 (1 oz)	140	2	6	21
Vienna Fingers Lemon	2 (1 oz)	140	2	6	21
Knott's Berry Farm					
Shortbread Apricot	3 (1 oz)	120	2	5	17
Shortbread Boysenberry	3 (1 oz)	120	2	5	17
Shortbread Raspberry	3 (1 oz)	120	2	5	17
LU					
Le Bastogne	2 (0.8 oz)	120	1	5	18
Le Chocolatiers	3 (1 oz)	150	1	8	17
Le Dore	4 (1 oz)	140	2	6	21
Le Fondant	4 (1.1 oz)	170	1	10	19
Le Palmier	4 (1.2 oz)	180	2	10	20
Le Petit Beurre	4 (1.2 oz)	150	3	4	25
Le Petit Ecolier Dark Chocolate	2 (0.9 oz)	130	2	6	17
Le Petit Ecolier Hazelnut Milk Chocolate	2 (0.9 oz)	130	2	7	16
Le Petit Ecolier Milk Chocolate	2 (0.9 oz)	130	1	6	17
Le Pim's Orange	2 (0.9 oz)	90	1	3	17
Le Pim's Raspberry	2 (0.9 oz)	90	1	3	17
Le Raisin Dore	4 (1.2 oz)	160	2	7	23
Le Truffe Coconut	4 (1.2 oz)	190	1	12	17
Le Truffe Praline Chocolate	4 (1.2 oz)	170	2	9	20
Les Varietes	3 (0.9 oz)	140	1	7	17
La Choy					
Fortune	4 (1 oz)	112	2	tr	26
Lance					
Apple Bar Fat Free	1 (1.75 oz)	160	1	0	38
Apple Oatmeal Bar	1 (1.8 oz)	190	2	6	32
Big Town Banana	1 pkg (2 oz)	250	3	10	37
Big Town Chocolate	1 pkg (2 oz)	250	3	8	40
Big Town Vanilla	1 pkg (2 oz)	250	3	11	37
Choc-O-Lunch	1 pkg (1.5 oz)	200	3	8	31
Choc-O-Mint	1 pkg (1¼ oz)	190	2	9	24
Coated Graham	1 pkg (1.3 oz)	190	3	8	25
Fig Bar	1 (1.75 oz)	180	2	4	34
Fudge Chocolate Chip	1 (2 oz)	130	2	5	19
Gourmet Chocolate Chip	1 (2 oz)	130	2	6	18
Lem-O-Lunch	1 pkg (3.4 oz)	240	3	11	32
Lemon Nekot	1 pkg (1.5 oz)	210	3	10	28
Nut-O-Lunch	1 pkg (3.3 oz)	240	6	11	29
Oatmeal	1 (2 oz)	130	2	6	18
Oatmeal Creme	1 (2 oz)	240	3	10	35
Peanut Butter	1 (2 oz)	140	4	8	14

FOOD	PORTION	CALS	PROT	FAT	CARB
Peanut Butter Creme Wafer	1 pkg (1.5 oz)	230	4	12	26
Van-O-Lunch	1 pkg (1.5 oz)	210	2	8	31
Larzaroni					
Arancelli	8 (1 oz)	160	3	8	19
Calypso	3 (1 oz)	150	2	8	18
Limonelli	5 (1 oz)	140	2	8	16
Malaika	5 (1 oz)	158	3	9	17
Nanette	4 (1.2 oz)	170	3	9	20
Okla	3 (1 oz)	186	3	10	21
Oskar	10 (1 oz)	150	2	9	18
Samba	5 (1 oz)	160	3	10	14
Velieri	3 (0.9 oz)	120	2	5	17
Little Debbie					
Apple Flips	1 (1.2 oz)	150	1	5	24
Caramel Bars	1 (1.2 oz)	160	1	8	22
Cherry Cordials	1 (1.3 oz)	170	1	8	23
Coconut Rounds	1 (1.2 oz)	150	1	7	23
Cookie Wreaths	1 (0.6 oz)	100	1	5	12
Easter Puffs	1 (1.2 oz)	140	1	6	24
Fig Bars	1 (1.5 oz)	150	1	4	31
Fudge Delights	1 (1.1 oz)	110	1	2	24
Fudge Rounds	1 (1.2 oz)	140	1	6	23
German Chocolate Ring	1 (1 oz)	140	1	8	18
Ginger	1 (0.7 oz)	90	1	3	15
Jelly Creme Pies	1 (1.2 oz)	160	1	7	23
Marshmallow Crispy Bar	1 (1.3 oz)	140	2	4	26
Marshmallow Supremes	1 (1.1 oz)	130	1	5	22
Marshmallow Pie Banana	1 pkg (1.5 oz)	180	2	6	30
Marshmallow Pie Chocolate	1 (1.4 oz)	160	1	6	27
Nutty Bar	1 (2 oz)	310	5	18	32
Oatmeal Raisin	1 (1.3 oz)	160	2	7	25
Oatmeal Creme Pie	1 (1.3 oz)	170	1	7	26
Oatmeal Delights	1 (1.1 oz)	110	2	2	24
Oatmeal Lights	1 (1.3 oz)	130	2	3	29
Peanut Butter Bars	1 (1.9 oz)	270	4	15	32
Peanut Butter & Jelly Oatmeal Pie	1 (1.1 oz)	130	2	5	22
Peanut Clusters	1 (1.4 oz)	190	3	11	23
Pumpkin Delights	1 (1.2 oz)	150	1	5	24
Raisin Creme Pie	1 (1.2 oz)	140	1	5	23
Star Crunch	1 (1.1 oz)	140	0	6	22
Sugar Free Chocolate Chip	3 (1.1 oz)	140	2	7	21
Sugar Free Oatmeal	6 (1.1 oz)	120	2	4	23
Yo-Yo's	1 (1.2 oz)	130	1	6	21
Milk Lunch Brand					
New England Biscuits	4 (1.1 oz)	140	2	5	24
MoonPie					
Chocolate	1 (2.75 oz)	330	4	10	56

FOOD	PORTION	CALS	PROT	FAT	CARB
Mini Banana	1 (1.2 oz)	152	3	5	26
Mini Chocolate	1 (1.2 oz)	152	3	5	26
Mini Vanilla	1 (1.2 oz)	152	3	5	26
Mother's					
Almond Shortbread	3	180	2	11	19
Checkerboard Wafers	8	150	1	8	20
Chocolate Chip	2	160	2	8	20
Chocolate Chip Angel	3	180	2	9	21
Chocolate Chip Parade	4	130	1	5	19
Circus Animals	6	140	1	6	20
Classic Assortments	2	140	1	7	18
Cocadas	5	150	2	7	20
Cookie Parade	4	140	1	7	18
Dinosaur Grrrahams	2	130	2	3	24
Double Fudge	2	180	2	9	24
English Tea	2	180	2	7	26
Flaky Flix Fudge	2	140	1	7	17
Flaky Flix Vanilla	2	140	1	8	17
Gaucho Peanut Butter	2	190	3	10	22
Iced Oatmeal	2	130	2	4	22
Iced Raisin	2	180	1	8	24
MLB Double Header Duplex	3	170	2	8	23
Macaroon	2	150	1	8	18
Marias	3	170	2	6	28
Oatmeal	2	110	1	5	17
Oatmeal Chocolate Chip	2	120	2	5	19
Oatmeal Raisin	5	150	2	7	20
Oatmeal Walnut Chocolate Chip	2	130	2	6	17
Rainbow Wafers	8	150	1	8	20
Striped Shortbread	3	170	2	8	22
Sugar	2	140	1	6	19
Taffy	2	180	2	8	25
Triplet Assortment	2	140	1	7	18
Vanilla Wafers	6	150	2	6	24
Wallops Boysenberry	1	80	1	2	15
Wallops Honey Crust Fig	1	80	1	2	15
Wallops Honey Graham Fig	1	80	1	2	15
Wallops Mixed Berry	1	80	1	2	15
Wallops Peach Apricot	1	80	1	2	15
Wallops Raspberry	1	80	1	2	15
Wallops Strawberry	1	80	1	2	15
Walnut Fudge	2	130	1	7	16
Zoo Pals	14	140	2	5	23
Mrs. Alison's					
Coconut Bar	2 (1 oz)	130	2	6	19
Creme Wafers	5 (1.1 oz)	170	1	10	21
Duplex Sandwich	3 (1 oz)	130	1	5	20

FOOD	PORTION	CALS	PROT	FAT	CARB
Ginger Snaps	4 (1 oz)	130	2	3	23
Jelly Tops	5 (1 oz)	140	2	7	18
Lemon Creme	3 (1 oz)	130	1	5	21
Macaroons	2 (1 oz)	140	2	7	18
Pecan	2 (1 oz)	140	2	7	19
Shortbread	5 (1 oz)	120	2	5	19
Vanilla Sandwich	3 (1 oz)	130	1	5	21
Murray's					
Sugar Free Double Fudge	3 (1.2 oz)	140	2	6	23
Sugar Free Ginger Snap	6 (1 oz)	110	2	4	21
Sugar Free Peanut Butter	6 (1 oz)	130	3	7	17
Sugar Free Vanilla Sandwich Creme	3 (1 oz)	120	1	5	21
Sugar Free Vanilla Wafers	9 (1.1 oz)	120	2	4	23
Nabisco					
Barnum's Animal Crackers	10 (1 oz)	130	2	4	23
Barnum's Animal Crackers Chocolate	10 (1 oz)	130	2	4	23
Cafe Cremes Cappuccino	2 (1.1 oz)	160	1	8	22
Cafe Cremes Vanilla	2 (1.1 oz)	160	1	7	22
Cafe Cremes Vanilla Fudge	2 (1.1 oz)	200	2	10	27
Cameo	2 (1 oz)	130	1	5	21
Chips Ahoy!	3 (1.1 oz)	160	2	8	21
Chips Ahoy! Chewy	3 (1.3 oz)	170	1	8	24
Chips Ahoy! Munch Size	6 (1.1 oz)	160	2	8	21
Chips Ahoy! Reduced Fat	3 (1.1 oz)	140	2	5	22
Family Favorites Iced Oatmeal	1 (0.6 oz)	80	1	3	12
Family Favorites Oatmeal	1 (0.6 oz)	80	1	3	12
Famous Chocolate Wafers	5 (1.1 oz)	140	2	4	24
Grahams	4 (1 oz)	120	2	3	22
Honey Maid Chocolate	8 (1 oz)	120	2	3	22
Honey Maid Cinnamon Grahams	8 (1 oz)	120	2	3	23
Honey Maid Honey Grahams	8 (1 oz)	120	2	3	22
Honey Maid Low Fat Cinnamon Grahams	8 (1 oz)	110	2	2	23
Honey Maid Low Fat Grahams	8 (1 oz)	110	2	2	23
Honey Maid Oatmeal Crunch	8 (1 oz)	120	2	3	22
Lorna Doone	4 (1 oz)	140	2	7	19
Mallomars	2 (0.9 oz)	120	1	5	17
Marshmallow Twirls	1 (1 oz)	130	1	6	20
Mystic Mint	1 (0.5 oz)	90	1	5	11
National Arrowroot	1 (5 g)	20	0	1	4
Newton Fat Free Fig	2 (1 oz)	90	1	0	22

FOOD	PORTION	CALS	PROT	FAT	CARB
Newtons Fig	2 (1.1 oz)	110	1	3	22
Newtons Fat Free Apple	2 (1 oz)	90	1	0	21
Newtons Fat Free Cobblers Apple Cinnamon	1 (0.8 oz)	70	1	0	17
Newtons Fat Free Cobblers Peach Apricot	1 (0.8 oz)	70	1	0	17
Newtons Fat Free Cranberry	2 (1 oz)	100	1	0	22
Newtons Fat Free Raspberry	2 (1 oz)	100	1	0	23
Newtons Fat Free Strawberry	2 (1 oz)	90	1	0	21
Nilla Wafers	8 (1.1 oz)	140	1	5	24
Nilla Wafers Chocolate Reduced Fat	8 (1 oz)	110	2	2	23
Nilla Wafers Reduced Fat	8 (1 oz)	120	1	2	24
Nutter Butter Bites	10 (1 oz)	150	3	7	20
Nutter Butter Chocolate Peanut Butter Sandwich	2 (1 oz)	130	2	5	19
Nutter Butter Peanut Butter Sandwich	2 (1 oz)	130	2	6	19
Old Fashioned Ginger Snaps	4 (1 oz)	120	1	3	22
Oreo	3 (1.2 oz)	160	1	7	23
Oreo Double Stuff	2 (1 oz)	140	1	7	19
Oreo Halloween	2 (1 oz)	140	1	7	19
Pecanz	1 (0.5 oz)	90	1	5	9
Pinwheels Chocolate Marshmallow	1 (1 oz)	130	1	5	21
Rugrats Chocolate Frosted	8 (1.1 oz)	150	1	5	24
Rugrats Vanilla Frosted	8 (1.1 oz)	150	1	6	24
Social Tea	6 (1 oz)	120	2	4	20
Sweet Crispers Chocolate	18 (1.1 oz)	130	2	3	25
Sweet Crispers Chocolate Chip	18 (1.1 oz)	130	2	3	23
Teddy Grahams Chocolate	24 (1 oz)	130	2	5	22
Teddy Grahams Chocolately Chip	24 (1 oz)	130	2	5	23
Teddy Grahams Cinnamon	24 (1 oz)	130	2	4	23
Teddy Grahams Honey	24 (1 oz)	130	2	4	23
Nestle					
Flipz Crunchy Graham White Fudge Chocolate	8 (1 oz)	140	2	6	19
Newman's Own					
Fig Newman's Organic	2 (1.3 oz)	120	2	0	28
Nonni's					
Biscotti Cioccalati	1 (1 oz)	130	2	5	19
Biscotti Decadence	1 (1.1 oz)	130	2	5	19

FOOD	PORTION	CALS	PROT	FAT	CARB
Biscotti Original	1 (1 oz)	100	2	4	15
Biscotti Paradiso	1 (1.1 oz)	130	2	6	19
NutraBalance					
Fibre Oatmeal Raisin	1 (0.7 oz)	80	1	4	13
Protein Fortified	1 (2 oz)	260	7	14	28
ReNeph Spice	1 (2 oz)	210	9	7	29
Old Brussels					
Ginger Crisps	2 (0.9 oz)	140	2	4	23
Old London					
Coffee Toppers Chocolate Creme	3 (0.5 oz)	70	1	3	9
Coffee Toppers Vanilla Creme	3 (0.5 oz)	70	1	4	9
Olde World					
Pizzelle Almond	3 (1 oz)	90	2	4	12
Pizzelle Anise	3 (1 oz)	90	2	4	12
Pizzelle Chocolate	3 (1 oz)	100	2	5	11
Pizzelle Lemon	3 (1 oz)	90	2	4	12
Pizzelle Vanilla	3 (1 oz)	90	2	4	12
Otis Spunkmeyer					
Butter Sugar	1 med (1.3 oz)	160	2	8	23
Butter Sugar	1 (2 oz)	250	3	12	35
Carnival	1 med (1.3 oz)	170	2	7	25
Chocolate Chip	1 bite size (0.75 oz)	100	1	5	14
Chocolate Chip	1 med (1.3 oz)	170	2	8	24
Chocolate Chip	1 (2 oz)	250	3	11	36
Chocolate Chip Pecan	1 med (1.3 oz)	170	2	9	22
Chocolate Chip Walnut	1 med (1.3 oz)	180	2	9	22
Chocolate Chip Walnut	1 bite size (0.75 oz)	100	1	5	13
Chocolate Chip Walnut	1 (2 oz)	270	3	14	34
Double Chocolate Chip	1 med (1.3 oz)	180	2	9	23
Double Chocolate Chip	1 bite size (0.75 oz)	100	1	5	13
Oatmeal Raisin	1 med (1.3 oz)	160	2	7	23
Oatmeal Raisin	1 bite size (0.75 oz)	90	1	4	13
Otis Express Chocolate Chunk	1 (2 oz)	280	3	13	37
Otis Express Double Chocolate Chip	1 (2 oz)	270	3	14	35
Otis Express Oatmeal Raisin	1 (2 oz)	240	3	10	35
Otis Express Peanut Butter	1 (2 oz)	270	5	15	31
Peanut Butter	1 med (1.3 oz)	180	3	10	20
Pinnacle Checkpoint Chocolate Almond Coconut	1 (2.4 oz)	320	4	18	37
Pinnacle Mach One Mocha Chocolate Chunk	1 (2.4 oz)	300	3	13	43

FOOD	PORTION	CALS	PROT	FAT	CARB
Pinnacle Passport Peanut Butter Chocolate Chunk	1 (2.4 oz)	300	5	13	42
Pinnacle Ripcord Rocky Road	1 (2.4 oz)	310	3	15	41
Pinnacle Takeoff Triple Chocolate	1 (2.4 oz)	300	3	14	42
Pinnacle Transatlantic Turtle	1 (2.4 oz)	310	3	16	39
Travel Lite Low Fat Apple Cinnamon	1 (1.3 oz)	130	2	2	26
Travel Lite Low Fat Chocolate Chip	1 (1.3 oz)	130	2	2	27
Travel Lite Low Fat Ginger Spice	1 (1.3 oz)	130	2	2	26
Travel Lite Low Fat Oatmeal Rum Raisin	1 (1.3 oz)	130	2	2	26
White Chocolate Macadamia Nut	1 med (1.3 oz)	180	2	10	21
White Chocolate Macadamia Nut	1 (2 oz)	280	3	15	33
Pally					
Butter	5 (1 oz)	140	3	3	23
Carnival	5 (1 oz)	130	2	3	24
Cinnamon Biscuit	5 (1 oz)	130	2	3	23
Mariel Biscuit	6 (1 oz)	150	3	4	23
Tea Biscuits	5 (1 oz)	150	2	4	23
Parmalat					
Grisbi Lemon	1 (0.6 oz)	90	1	6	9
Peek Freans					
Arrowroot	4 (1.2 oz)	150	2	5	26
Assorted Creme	1 (1 oz)	130	1	6	19
Fruit Creme	2 (0.9 oz)	130	1	5	20
Ginger Crisp	4 (1.2 oz)	150	2	4	28
Nice	4 (1.2 oz)	160	2	6	25
Petit Beurre	4 (1 oz)	130	2	4	22
Rich Tea	4 (1.2 oz)	160	2	5	25
Shortcake	2 (0.9 oz)	140	1	7	18
Traditional Oatmeal	1 (0.7 oz)	90	1	3	15
Tropical Cremes Calypso Lime	2 (0.9 oz)	130	1	5	20
Pepperidge Farm					
Biscotti Almond	1 (0.7 oz)	90	2	4	12
Biscotti Chocolate Hazelnut	1 (0.7 oz)	90	2	5	11
Biscotti Cranberry Pistachio	1 (0.7 oz)	90	2	3	13

FOOD	PORTION	CALS	PROT	FAT	CARB
Bordeaux	4	130	2	5	19
Brussels	3	150	2	7	20
Chantilly Raspberry	2 (1 oz)	120	1	3	23
Chessman	3	120	2	8	18
Chocoate Chunk Soft Baked Double Chocolate	1 (0.9 oz)	130	2	7	15
Chocolate Chip	3	140	2	7	18
Chocolate Chunk Chesapeake	1 (0.7 oz)	140	2	8	15
Chocolate Chunk Minis Nantauket	4 (1 oz)	150	0	8	20
Chocolate Chunk Minis Sausalito	4 (1 oz)	160	1	9	18
Chocolate Chunk Montauk	1 (0.9 oz)	130	1	7	17
Chocolate Chunk Nantucket	1 (0.9 oz)	140	2	7	16
Chocolate Chunk Sausalito	1 (0.7 oz)	140	2	8	16
Chocolate Chunk Soft Baked	1	130	2	6	16
Chocolate Chunk Soft Baked Milk Chocolate Macadamia	1	130	2	7	16
Chocolate Chunk Soft Baked Reduced Fat	1	110	1	5	18
Chocolate Chunk Soft Baked White Chocolate Pecan	1	120	1	5	16
Chocolate Chunk Tahoe	1 (0.9 oz)	130	2	8	15
Fruitful Apricot Raspberry Cup	3	140	2	6	22
Fruitful Strawberry Cup	3	140	2	5	22
Geneva	3	160	2	9	19
Ginger Man	4 (1 oz)	130	2	4	21
Lemon Nut Crunch	3	170	2	9	18
Milano	3	180	2	10	21
Milano Endless Chocolate	3	180	2	10	21
Milano Milk Chocolate	3	170	2	9	21
Milano Double Chocolate	2 (0.7 oz)	140	2	8	17
Milano Mint	2	130	1	7	16
Milano Orange	2	130	1	7	16
Pirouettes Chocolate Laced	5 (1.1 oz)	180	2	10	20
Pirouettes Traditional	5 (1.2 oz)	170	2	9	20
Shortbread	2	140	2	7	16
Soft Baked Oatmeal Raisin	1 (0.9 oz)	130	2	7	16
Soft Baked Reduced Fat Oatmeal Raisin	1 (0.9 oz)	100	1	3	18
Spritzers Cool Key Lime	6 (1.1 oz)	140	1	7	21
Spritzers Ripe Red Raspberry	5 (1.1 oz)	140	1	7	21
Spritzers Zesty Lemon	5 (1.1 oz)	140	1	7	21

FOOD	PORTION	CALS	PROT	FAT	CARB
Sugar	3	140	2	6	20
Verona Strawberry	3 (1.1 oz)	140	2	5	22
Quaker					
Fruit & Oatmeal Bites Apple Crisp	1 pkg	140	2	3	27
Fruit & Oatmeal Bites Strawberry	1 pkg	140	2	3	27
Fruit & Oatmeal Bites Very Berry	1 pkg	140	2	3	27
Ralston					
Animal	12 (0.9 oz)	130	2	3	22
Chocolate Graham	2 (0.9 oz)	130	2	3	24
Cinnamon Grahams	2 (0.9 oz)	130	1	5	19
Cinnamon Grahams Low Fat	2 (0.9 oz)	110	2	2	22
Vanilla Wafers	7 (1.1 oz)	150	1	6	22
Real Torino					
Lady Fingers	3 (1 oz)	110	2	1	23
Reko					
Pizzelle Maple	5 (1 oz)	150	3	6	20
Pizzelle Vanilla	1 (6 g)	30	1	1	4
Royal					
Apple Bars	1 (1.1 oz)	100	1	2	21
Apple Cake	1 (1.1 oz)	110	1	3	19
Brownie Rounds	1 (1.1 oz)	130	1	6	19
Chocolate Chip	1 (1.1 oz)	140	1	6	20
Devilfood	1 (1 oz)	110	1	5	17
Fig Bars	1 (1.1 oz)	100	1	2	20
Oatmeal	1 (1.1 oz)	130	2	6	19
Raisin	1 (1 oz)	110	1	5	17
Strawberry Bars	1 (1.1 oz)	100	1	2	20
Salerno					
Mini Butter	25 (1 oz)	180	2	6	20
Mini Dinosaur Chocolate Graham	16 (1.1 oz)	140	2	5	22
Scotter Pie	1 (1.2 oz)	140	1	5	23
Santa Fe Farms					
Chocolate Chocolate Chip Fat Free	2 (1 oz)	60	2	0	16
Chocolate Mint Fat Free	2 (1 oz)	60	2	0	16
Ginger Fat Free	2 (1 oz)	70	2	0	17
Sargento					
MooTown Snackers Honey Graham Sticks & Vanilla Creme w/ Sprinkles	1 pkg (1 oz)	140	2	7	17

FOOD	PORTION	CALS	PROT	FAT	CARB
MooTown Snackers Vanilla Sticks & Chocolate Fudge Creme	1 pkg (1 oz)	130	1	6	18
Savion					
Chocolate Biscuits	5 (1 oz)	120	2	3	22
Tea Biscuits	5 (1 oz)	120	2	3	22
Tea Biscuits Vanilla	5 (1 oz)	120	2	3	22
Scotto's					
Biscotti Fat Free French Vanilla	4 (1 oz)	80	2	0	18
Season					
Hamantashen Poppy	1 (1 oz)	150	1	7	20
Hamantasken Apricot	1 (1 oz)	150	1	7	20
Simple Pleasures					
Almond	1 (0.3 oz)	37	1	2	5
Cinnamon Snaps	1 (0.2 oz)	31	1	1	6
Digestive	1 (0.3 oz)	46	1	2	6
Oatmeal	1 (0.5 oz)	74	1	3	5
Spice Snaps	1 (0.3 oz)	34	1	1	6
Sugar	1 (0.4 oz)	45	1	2	7
SnackWell's					
Bite Size Chocolate Chip	13 (1 oz)	130	2	4	22
Bite Size Double Chocolate Chip	13 (1 oz)	130	2	4	22
Bite Size Peanut Butter	13 (1 oz)	120	3	4	20
Caramel Delights	1 (0.6 oz)	70	1	2	13
Chocolate Sandwich	2 (0.8 oz)	110	1	3	20
Creme Sandwich	2 (0.9 oz)	110	1	3	20
Fat Free Devil's Food	1 (0.5 oz)	50	1	0	12
Golden Devil's Food	1 (0.5 oz)	50	1	1	11
Mint Creme	2 (0.9 oz)	110	1	4	19
Oatmeal Raisin	2 (0.9 oz)	110	2	3	20
Stella D'Oro					
Almond Toast Mandel	2 (1 oz)	110	2	3	21
Angel Wings	2 (0.9 oz)	140	2	9	13
Angelica	1 (0.8 oz)	100	2	4	15
Anginetti	4 (1.1 oz)	140	2	4	23
Anisette Sponge	2 (0.9 oz)	90	2	1	19
Anisette Toast	3 (1.2 oz)	130	2	1	27
Biscotti Almond	1 (0.8 oz)	100	2	3	15
Biscotti Chocolate Almond	1 (0.8 oz)	90	2	3	15
Biscotti Chocolate Chunk	1 (0.8 oz)	90	2	3	16
Biscotti Hazelnut	1 (0.8 oz)	100	2	4	15
Biscottini Cashews	1 (0.7 oz)	110	1	6	13
Breakfast Treats	1 (0.8 oz)	100	1	3	16
Breakfast Treats Chocolate	1 (0.8 oz)	100	2	4	15

FOOD	PORTION	CALS	PROT	FAT	CARB
Breakfast Treats Viennese Cinnamon	1 (0.8 oz)	100	1	3	17
Chinese Dessert Cookies	1 (1.2 oz)	170	2	9	21
Chocolate Castelets	2 (1 oz)	130	2	6	19
Egg Jumbo	2 (0.8 oz)	90	2	1	18
Fruit Slices Fat Free	1 (0.6 oz)	50	1	0	12
Kichel Low Sodium	21 (1 oz)	150	4	9	13
Lady Stella Assortment	3 (1 oz)	130	1	5	19
Margherite Chocolate	2 (1.1 oz)	140	2	6	22
Margherite Vanilla	2 (1.1 oz)	140	2	5	22
Roman Egg Biscuits	1 (1.2 oz)	140	2	5	21
Sesame Regina	3 (1.1 oz)	150	2	6	21
Swiss Fudge	2 (0.9 oz)	130	1	7	16
Stieffenhofer					
Choco Minis	4 (1 oz)	160	1	8	19
Snaky	3 (1 oz)	160	2	8	19
Streit's					
Wafers	3 (1 oz)	160	1	9	19
Suissette					
Swiss Chocolate Hearts	4 (1 oz)	170	2	10	17
Swiss Delight	4 (1 oz)	160	2	9	19
Swiss Praline	4 (1 oz)	150	1	9	17
Sunshine					
All American Butter	5 (1.1 oz)	140	2	6	21
All American Lemon Coolers	5 (1 oz)	140	1	6	21
All American Mini Chip-A-Roos	5 (1.1 oz)	160	1	8	21
Animal Crackers	14 (1.1 oz)	140	2	4	24
Ginger Snaps	7 (1 oz)	130	2	5	22
Golden Fruit Cranberry	1 (0.7 oz)	80	1	2	14
Golden Fruit Raisin	1 (0.7 oz)	80	1	2	15
Hydrox	3 (1.1 oz)	150	2	7	21
Hydrox Reduced Fat	3 (1.1 oz)	140	2	5	23
Oatmeal Country Style	2 (0.8 oz)	120	2	5	17
Sugar Wafers Peanut Butter Creme	4 (1.1 oz)	170	3	9	19
Sugar Wafers Vanilla Creme	3 (0.9 oz)	130	1	6	18
Vanilla Wafers	7 (1.1 oz)	150	2	7	21
Vienna Fingers	2 (1 oz)	140	2	6	21
Vienna Fingers Lemon	2 (1 oz)	140	2	6	21
Vienna Fingers Reduced Fat	2 (1 oz)	130	1	5	22
Sweet'N Low					
Sugar Free Amaretto Biscotti	4 (1 oz)	120	2	6	17
Sugar Free Chocolate Chip	4 (1 oz)	135	2	8	17
Sugar Free Cinnamon Graham	7 (1 oz)	120	2	6	19

FOOD	PORTION	CALS	PROT	FAT	CARB
Sugar Free Morning Crunch Bars	2 (1 oz)	120	2	6	19
Sugar Free Vanilla Wafers	7 (1 oz)	120	2	6	19
Sweetzels					
Chocolate Chip	7 (1 oz)	160	1	9	18
Ginger Snaps	4 (1.2 oz)	140	2	3	25
Vanilla Wafers	7 (1.1 oz)	137	2	5	22
Tastykake					
Chocolate Chip	1 (1.4 oz)	180	2	7	26
Chocolate Chip Bar	1 (2 oz)	270	2	12	39
Chocolate Fudge Iced	1 (1.4 oz)	170	4	7	25
Fudge Bar	1 (2 oz)	250	3	10	37
Lemon Bar	1 (2 oz)	260	2	10	41
Oatmeal Raisin Bar	1 (2 oz)	260	4	10	40
Oatmeal Raisin Boxed	3 (0.4 oz)	130	1	6	14
Oatmeal Raisin Iced	1 (1.4 oz)	170	3	6	27
Strawberry Bar	1 (2 oz)	260	2	10	41
Sugar Boxed	3 (0.4 oz)	120	1	6	18
The Source					
Barry's Raspberry Palmiers	1 (0.7 oz)	80	1	3	14
Tom's					
Animal Crackers	½ pkg (1 oz)	120	2	2	23
Big Cookie Chocolate Chip	1 pkg (2.75 oz)	340	4	16	49
Big Cookie Peanut Butter Chocolate Chip	1 pkg (2 oz)	280	3	15	37
Chocolate Chip	1 pkg (2 oz)	280	3	15	37
Confetti Chip	1 pkg (2 oz)	300	3	13	40
Fat Free Apple Bar	1 pkg (1.75 oz)	160	2	0	38
Fat Free Fig Bar	1 pkg (1.75 oz)	160	2	0	40
Vanilla Wafers	½ pkg (1 oz)	130	2	5	20
Tree Of Life					
Fat Free Almond Butter	1 (0.8 oz)	60	1	0	14
Fat Free Carrot Cake	1 (0.8 oz)	60	1	0	14
Fat Free Devil's Food Chocolate	1 (0.8 oz)	70	2	0	15
Fat Free Oatmeal Raisin	1 (0.8 oz)	70	2	0	16
Fruit Bars Fat Free Fig	1 (0.8 oz)	70	1	0	16
Fruit Bars Fat Free Peach Apricot	1 (0.8 oz)	70	1	0	17
Fruit Bars Fat Free Wildberry	1 (0.8 oz)	70	1	0	16
Monster Carob Chip	1 (4.7 oz)	700	10	35	95
Monster Granola	1 (4.7 oz)	700	10	30	95
Monster Macaroon	1 (4.7 oz)	750	5	45	85
Monster Peanut Butter	1 (4.7 oz)	700	15	35	85
Monster Fat Free Carrot Cake	1 cookie (3.8 oz)	240	4	0	60
Monster Fat Free Devil's Food Chocolate	1 cookie (3.8 oz)	320	8	0	80

FOOD	PORTION	CALS	PROT	FAT	CARB
Monster Fat Free Gingerbread	1 cookie (3.8 oz)	320	8	0	76
Monster Fat Free Maple Pecan	1 cookie (3.8 oz)	360	8	0	80
Oatmeal	1 (0.8 oz)	100	2	4	16
Sandwich Royal Vanilla	2 (0.9 oz)	120	1	5	17
Wheat Free Carob	1 (0.8 oz)	100	1	5	14
Wheat Free Maple Walnut	1 (0.8 oz)	100	2	6	13
Wheat Free Oatmeal	1 (0.8 oz)	90	1	5	11
Wheat Free Peanut Butter	1 (0.8 oz)	109	2	6	8
Twix					
Bars Chocolate Caramel	1 (0.9 oz)	140	1	7	18
Voortman					
Almonette	2 (1 oz)	150	1	8	17
Peanut Delight	1 (0.9 oz)	130	2	7	15
Turnovers Blueberry	1 (0.9 oz)	100	1	3	16
Turnovers Cherry	1 (0.9 oz)	100	1	3	16
Turnovers Strawberry	1 (0.9 oz)	100	1	3	16
Walkers					
Shortbread Triangles	2 (0.7 oz)	100	1	6	12
Weight Watchers					
Apple Raisin Bar	1 (0.75 oz)	70	1	2	14
Chocolate Chip	2 (1.06 oz)	140	2	5	22
Chocolate Sandwich	2 (1.06 oz)	140	2	4	23
Fruit Filled Fig	1 (0.7 oz)	70	1	0	16
Fruit Filled Raspberry	1 (0.7 oz)	70	1	0	16
Oatmeal Raisin	2 (1.06 oz)	120	2	2	22
Vanilla Sandwich	2 (1.06 oz)	140	1	3	25
White Eagle Bakery					
Chruscik	2 (1 oz)	140	2	8	16
Wortz					
Animal	9 (1.1 oz)	140	2	5	22
Chocolate Graham	2 (0.9 oz)	130	2	3	24
Cinnamon Grahams	2 (0.9 oz)	130	1	5	19
Vanilla Wafers	7 (1.1 oz)	150	1	6	22
refrigerated					
chocolate chip	1 (0.42 oz)	59	1	3	8
chocolate chip unbaked	1 oz	126	1	6	17
oatmeal	1 (0.4 oz)	56	1	3	8
oatmeal raisin	1 (0.4 oz)	56	1	3	8
peanut butter	1 (0.4 oz)	60	1	3	7
peanut butter dough	1 oz	130	2	7	15
sugar	1 (0.42 oz)	58	1	3	8
sugar dough	1 oz	124	1	6	17
Pillsbury					
Bunny	2	130	1	7	17
Chocolate Chip	1 (1 oz)	130	1	6	17

FOOD	PORTION	CALS	PROT	FAT	CARB
Chocolate Chip Reduced Fat	1 (1 oz)	110	1	3	19
Chocolate Chip w/ Walnuts	1 (1 oz)	140	1	7	17
Chocolate Chunk	1 (1 oz)	130	1	6	17
Christmas Tree	2	130	1	7	17
Double Chocolate	1 (1 oz)	130	1	6	17
Flag	2	130	1	7	17
Frosty	2	130	1	7	17
M&M's	1 (1 oz)	130	1	6	18
Oatmeal Chocolate Chip	1 (1 oz)	120	1	6	16
One Step Pan Chocolate Chip	⅛ pan (1 oz)	130	1	6	19
One Step Pan M&M's	⅛ pan (1 oz)	130	1	6	19
Peanut Butter	1 (1 oz)	120	2	6	15
Pumpkin	2	130	1	7	17
Reeses	1 (1 oz)	130	3	6	15
Shamrock	2	130	1	7	17
Sugar	2	130	1	3	19
Sugar Holiday Red & Green	2	130	1	6	19
Valentine	2	130	1	7	17
White Chocolate Chunk	1 (1 oz)	130	1	6	17
take-out					
biscotti w/ nuts chocolate dipped	1 (1.3 oz)	117	2	6	16
black & white	1 lg (3 oz)	302	4	9	52
finikia	1 (1.2 oz)	171	2	5	16
koulourakia butter cookie twist	1 (0.9 oz)	113	2	6	14

CORIANDER

Instant India

Tomato Coriander Paste	2 tbsp (1 oz)	90	1	6	8

CORN

(*see also* BRAN, CEREAL, CORNMEAL)

canned

cream style	½ cup	93	2	1	23
w/ red & green peppers	½ cup	86	3	1	21
white	½ cup	66	2	1	15
yellow	½ cup	66	2	1	15

Del Monte

Cream Style Golden	½ cup (4.4 oz)	90	2	1	20
Cream Style Golden No Salt Added	½ cup (4.4 oz)	60	1	1	14
Cream Style White	½ cup (4.4 oz)	100	2	1	21
Fiesta	½ cup (4.4 oz)	50	2	1	12
Gold & White Supersweet	½ cup (4.4 oz)	80	2	1	18
Whole Kernel Golden	½ cup (4.4 oz)	90	2	1	18

FOOD	PORTION	CALS	PROT	FAT	CARB
Whole Kernel Golden Supersweet No Salt Added	½ cup (4.4 oz)	60	2	1	11
Whole Kernel Golden Supersweet No Salt Added	½ cup (4.4 oz)	70	2	1	13
Whole Kernel Golden Supersweet No Sugar	½ cup (4.4 oz)	60	2	1	11
Whole Kernel Golden Supersweet Vacuum Packed	½ cup (3.7 oz)	70	2	1	13
Whole Kernel White Sweet	½ cup (4.4 oz)	60	2	1	11
Green Giant					
Cream Style	½ cup (4.5 oz)	100	2	1	22
Mexicorn	⅓ cup (2.7 oz)	60	2	0	14
Niblets	⅓ cup (2.7 oz)	70	2	0	15
Niblets 50% Less Sodium	⅓ cup (2.7 oz)	60	2	0	14
Niblets Extra Sweet	⅓ cup (2.6 oz)	50	2	1	10
Niblets No Added Sugar or Salt	⅓ cup (2.7 oz)	60	2	0	13
White Shoepeg	⅓ cup	80	2	1	16
Whole Sweet	½ cup (4.3 oz)	80	2	1	18
Whole Sweet 50% Less Sodium	½ cup (4.2 oz)	80	2	1	17
S&W					
Cream Style	½ cup (4.4 oz)	60	1	1	14
Whole Kernel	⅓ cup (3 oz)	70	2	2	12
fresh					
on-the-cob w/ butter cooked	1 ear	155	4	3	32
white cooked	½ cup	89	3	1	21
white raw	½ cup	66	2	1	15
yellow cooked	1 ear (2.7 oz)	83	3	1	19
yellow cooked	½ cup	89	3	1	21
yellow raw	1 ear (3 oz)	77	3	1	17
yellow raw	½ cup	66	2	1	15
frozen					
cooked	½ cup	67	2	tr	17
on-the-cob cooked	1 ear (2.2 oz)	59	2	tr	14
Birds Eye					
Gold & White Blend	½ cup (3.5 oz)	60	2	1	11
Green Giant					
Butter Sauce Niblets	⅔ cup (4.3 oz)	130	3	3	23
Butter Sauce Shoepeg White	¾ cup (4 oz)	120	3	3	21
Cream Corn	½ cup (4.1 oz)	110	2	1	23
Extra Sweet Niblets	⅔ cup (3.1 oz)	70	2	1	13

FOOD	PORTION	CALS	PROT	FAT	CARB
Harvest Fresh Niblets	⅔ cup (3.4 oz)	80	3	1	17
Harvest Fresh Shoepeg White	½ cup (2.6 oz)	70	2	1	14
Niblets	⅔ cup (2.9 oz)	80	2	1	17
On The Cob Extra Sweet	1 ear (4.4 oz)	120	4	2	22
On The Cob Nibblers	1 ear (2.1 oz)	70	2	1	14
On The Cob Niblets	1 ear (5 oz)	160	4	2	32
Select Extra Sweet White	⅔ cup (2.9 oz)	50	2	1	10
Select Shoepeg White	¾ cup (3.2 oz)	100	3	1	20
Stouffer's					
Souffle	½ cup (6 oz)	170	5	7	21
Tree Of Life					
Corn	⅔ cup (3.2 oz)	80	3	1	19
take-out					
fritters	1 (1 oz)	62	2	2	9
scalloped	½ cup	258	7	7	43
CORN CHIPS					
(*see* CHIPS)					
CORNISH HENS					
(*see* CHICKEN)					
CORNMEAL					
(*see also* POLENTA)					
corn grits cooked	1 cup	146	4	tr	31
corn grits uncooked	1 cup	579	14	2	124
white	1 cup (4.8 oz)	505	12	2	107
whole grain	1 cup (4.3 oz)	442	10	4	94
yellow	1 cup (4.8 oz)	505	12	2	107
yellow self-rising	1 cup (4.3 oz)	407	10	4	86
Albers					
White	3 tbsp	110	2	0	24
Yellow	3 tbsp	110	2	0	24
mix					
Hodgson Mill					
Cornbread Mix Jalapeno Mexican	¼ cup (1 oz)	100	4	1	21
Yellow Organic	¼ cup (1 oz)	100	3	1	22
Yellow Self Rising	¼ cup (1 oz)	90	3	1	21
Kentucky Kernal					
Sweet Cornbread Mix	¼ cup (1 oz)	120	2	2	24
take-out					
hush puppies	1 (0.75 oz)	74	3	3	10
CORNSTARCH					
Armour					
Cream Cornstarch	1 tbsp (0.4 oz)	40	0	0	9
COTTAGE CHEESE					
creamed	4 oz	117	14	5	3
creamed	1 cup (7.4 oz)	217	26	9	6
creamed w/ fruit	4 oz	140	11	4	15

FOOD	PORTION	CALS	PROT	FAT	CARB
dry curd	1 cup (5.1 oz)	123	25	1	3
dry curd	4 oz	96	20	tr	2
lowfat 1%	4 oz	82	14	1	3
lowfat 1%	1 cup (7.9 oz)	164	28	2	6
lowfat 2%	1 cup (7.9 oz)	203	31	4	8
lowfat 2%	4 oz	101	16	2	4
Breakstone's					
2% Fat Large Curd	½ cup (4.2 oz)	90	13	3	4
2% Fat Small Curd	½ cup (4.2 oz)	90	13	3	4
4% Fat Large Curd	½ cup (4.2 oz)	120	13	5	5
4% Fat Small Curd	½ cup (4.2 oz)	120	13	5	5
Cottage Doubles Peach	1 pkg (5.5 oz)	140	12	3	16
Dry Curd	¼ cup (1.9 oz)	45	8	0	3
Free	½ cup (4.4 oz)	80	13	0	6
Snack 2% Fat Small Curd	1 pkg (4 oz)	90	12	2	4
Snack 4% Fat Small Curd	1 pkg (4 oz)	110	12	5	4
Snack Free	1 pkg (4 oz)	70	12	0	6
Horizon Organic					
Cottage Cheese	½ cup (3.9 oz)	110	13	5	4
Knudsen					
1.5% Fat Small Curd Pineapple	½ cup (4.6 oz)	120	11	2	14
2% Fat Small Curd	½ cup (4.2 oz)	100	14	3	5
4% Fat Large Curd	½ cup (4.5 oz)	130	16	5	4
4% Fat Small Curd	½ cup (4.3 oz)	120	14	5	4
Free	½ cup (4.2 oz)	80	14	0	4
On The Go! 1.5% Fat Peach	1 pkg (4 oz)	110	10	2	13
On The Go! 1.5% Fat Pineapple	1 pkg (4 oz)	110	10	2	13
On The Go! 1.5% Fat Strawberry	1 pkg (4 oz)	110	10	2	13
On The Go! 1.5% Fat Tropical Fruit	1 pkg (4 oz)	110	10	2	13
On The Go! 2% Fat	1 pkg (4 oz)	90	13	2	5
On The Go! Fat Free	1 pkg (4 oz)	70	13	0	4
Light N'Lively					
1% Fat	½ cup (4 oz)	80	12	1	5
1% Fat Garden Salad	½ cup (4.2 oz)	80	12	2	5
1% Fat Peach & Pineapple	½ cup (4.3 oz)	110	11	1	15
Fat Free	½ cup (4.4 oz)	80	13	0	6
COTTONSEED					
kernels roasted	1 tbsp	51	3	4	2
COUSCOUS					
cooked	1 cup (5.5 oz)	176	6	tr	36
dry	1 cup (6.1 oz)	650	22	1	134
Melting Pot					
Calypso Cranberry	1 cup	200	7	0	42

FOOD	PORTION	CALS	PROT	FAT	CARB
Lentil Curry	1 cup	170	7	0	35
Lucky Seven	1 cup	190	7	1	38
Mango Salsa	1 cup	190	6	0	40
Roasted Garlic	1 cup	170	7	0	34
Sesame Ginger	1 cup	180	7	1	36
Sun-Dried Tomatoes	1 cup	190	8	1	36
Wild Mushroom	1 cup	190	8	0	38
COWPEAS					
catjang dried cooked	1 cup (2.9 oz)	200	14	1	35
common canned	1 cup	184	11	1	33
frozen cooked	½ cup	112	7	tr	20
leafy tips chopped cooked	1 cup	12	2	tr	1
leafy tips raw chopped	1 cup	10	1	tr	2
CRAB					
canned					
blue	3 oz	84	17	1	0
blue	1 cup	133	28	2	0
Bumble Bee					
Fancy Lump Meat	½ can (1.9 oz)	40	8	1	0
Fancy White Meat	½ can (1.9 oz)	28	6	0	1
fresh					
alaska king cooked	1 leg (4.7 oz)	129	26	2	0
alaska king cooked	3 oz	82	16	1	0
alaska king raw	3 oz	71	16	1	0
alaska king raw	1 leg (6 oz)	144	32	1	0
blue cooked	3 oz	87	17	2	0
blue cooked	1 cup	138	27	2	0
blue raw	1 crab (7 oz)	18	4	tr	tr
blue raw	3 oz	74	15	1	tr
dungeness raw	3 oz	73	15	1	1
dungeness raw	1 crab (5.7 oz)	140	28	2	1
queen steamed	3 oz	98	20	1	0
take-out					
baked	1 (3.8 oz)	160	29	2	4
cake	1 (2 oz)	160	11	10	5
kenagi korean crab cooked	1 serv (3 oz)	71	16	tr	0
soft-shell fried	1 (4.4 oz)	334	11	18	31
CRACKER CRUMBS					
cracker meal	1 cup (4 oz)	440	11	2	93
graham cracker crumbs	½ cup (4.4 oz)	540	9	13	97
Baker's Harvest					
Graham	⅛ cup (1 oz)	130	2	4	23
Kellogg's					
Corn Flake Crumbs	2 tbsp (0.4 oz)	40	1	0	9
CRACKERS					
(see also CRACKER CRUMBS)					
cheese	14 (½ oz)	71	1	4	8

FOOD	PORTION	CALS	PROT	FAT	CARB
cheese low sodium	14 (½ oz)	71	1	4	8
cheese w/ peanut butter filling	1 (0.24 oz)	34	1	2	4
crispbread	3	61	1	2	9
crispbread rye	1 (0.35 oz)	37	1	tr	8
crispbread rye	3	77	2	1	17
melba toast plain	1 (5 g)	19	1	tr	4
melba toast pumpernickel	1 (5 g)	19	1	tr	4
melba toast rye	1 (5 g)	19	1	tr	4
melba toast wheat	1 (5 g)	19	1	tr	4
milk	1 (0.42 oz)	55	1	2	8
peanut butter sandwich	1 (7 g)	34	1	2	4
rusk toast	1 (0.35 oz)	41	1	1	7
rye w/ cheese filling	1 (0.24 oz)	34	1	2	4
rye wafers plain	1 (0.9 oz)	84	2	tr	20
rye wafers seasoned	1 (0.8 oz)	84	2	2	16
saltines fat free low sodium	6 (1 oz)	118	3	tr	25
saltines fat free low sodium	3 (0.5 oz)	59	2	tr	12
snack cracker w/ cheese filling	1 (7 g)	33	1	2	4
water biscuits	3	92	2	3	16
wheat w/ cheese filling	1 (0.24 oz)	35	1	2	4
wheat w/ peanut butter filling	1 (0.24 oz)	35	1	2	4
wheat thins	7 (0.5 oz)	67	1	3	9
wheat thins low salt	7 (0.5 oz)	67	1	3	9
zwieback	1 oz	107	3	1	21
Ak-mak					
100% Whole Wheat	5 (1 oz)	116	5	2	19
Armenian Cracker Bread	1 sheet (1 oz)	100	4	2	19
Armenian Cracker Bread Whole Wheat	1 sheet (1 oz)	116	5	2	19
Round Cracker Bread No Seeds	1 (1 oz)	100	4	1	20
Round Cracker Bread Seeded	1 (1 oz)	100	4	2	19
Round Cracker Bread Whole Wheat	1 (1 oz)	116	5	2	19
Austin					
Cracker Sandwich Cheese On Cheese	6 (1.3 oz)	170	3	7	25
Cracker Sandwich Cheese Peanut Butter	6 (1.3 oz)	170	5	7	24
Cracker Sandwich Toasty Peanut Butter	6 (1.3 oz)	170	5	7	24

FOOD	PORTION	CALS	PROT	FAT	CARB
Cracker Sandwich Whole Wheat Cheese	6 (1.3 oz)	170	3	7	25
Baker's Harvest					
Cheese	23 (1 oz)	150	3	6	18
Cheese Reduced Fat	29 (1 oz)	130	3	4	21
Oyster	35 (0.5 oz)	70	1	2	11
Saltines Unsalted	5 (0.5 oz)	70	1	2	11
Saltines Deluxe	5 (0.5 oz)	60	1	2	10
Snackers	9 (1.1 oz)	160	2	8	19
Snackers Reduced Fat	10 (1.1 oz)	140	3	4	23
Snackers Unsalted	9 (1.1 oz)	160	2	8	19
Wheat Snacks	16 (1 oz)	140	3	6	20
Wheat Snacks Reduced Fat	16 (1.1 oz)	140	2	4	23
Woven Wheats	7 (1.1 oz)	140	3	5	21
Woven Wheats Reduced Fat	8 (1.1 oz)	130	3	3	24
Barbara's Bakery					
Cheese Bites	26 (1 oz)	120	3	2	24
Right Lite Rounds Original	5 (0.5 oz)	55	1	5	12
Rite Lite Rounds Tamari Sesame	5 (0.5 oz)	70	1	2	12
Wheatines All Flavors	1 lg sq (0.5 oz)	50	1	2	10
Blue Diamond					
Nut Thins Almond	16 (1 oz)	130	3	5	19
Nut Thins Hazelnut	16 (1 oz)	120	2	4	20
Nut Thins Pecan	16 (1 oz)	130	2	5	20
Cheetos					
Bacon Cheddar	1 pkg	190	3	9	25
Cheddar Cheese	1 pkg	210	3	11	23
Golden Toast	1 pkg	240	4	14	25
Cheez It					
Big	13 (1 oz)	150	4	8	16
Big Reduced Fat	15 (1 oz)	140	4	5	20
Heads & Tails	37 (1 oz)	140	1	6	18
Hot & Spicy	26 (1 oz)	150	4	8	17
Low Sodium	27 (1 oz)	160	4	8	16
Nacho	28 (1 oz)	150	3	7	16
Original	27 (1 oz)	160	4	8	16
Party Mix	½ cup (1 oz)	140	4	5	19
Party Mix Nacho	½ cup (1 oz)	130	3	5	20
Party Mix Reduced Fat	½ cup (1 oz)	130	4	3	21
Peanut Butter	1 pkg (1.3 oz)	190	4	10	22
Reduced Fat	29 (1 oz)	140	4	5	20
Snack Mix	½ cup (1 oz)	130	3	5	21
Snack Mix Big Crunch	¾ cup (1 oz)	110	3	6	20
Snack Mix Double Cheese	¾ cup (1 oz)	110	3	5	19
White Cheddar	26 (1 oz)	150	3	7	18

FOOD	PORTION	CALS	PROT	FAT	CARB
Courtney's					
Sun-Dried Tomato Organic	4 (0.5 oz)	60	1	1	10
Dare					
Breton	1 (5 g)	21	1	1	3
Breton Light	1 (5 g)	20	1	1	3
Breton Reduced Fat & Sodium	3 (0.5 oz)	60	2	2	9
Breton Minis	20 (0.6 oz)	89	2	4	11
Breton Minis Cheddar Cheese	20 (0.6 oz)	87	3	4	11
Breton Minis Garden Vegetable	20 (0.6 oz)	87	2	4	12
Vinta	1 (6 g)	30	1	1	4
Doritos					
Jalapeno Cheese	1 pkg	230	3	14	26
Nacho Cheddar	1 pkg	240	4	14	25
Eden					
Nori Nori Rice	15 (1 oz)	110	3	0	24
Estee					
Sugar Free Cracked Pepper	18	120	3	2	24
Sugar Free Golden	10	130	3	2	28
Sugar Free Wheat	17	100	3	2	18
Frito Lay					
Cheddar Snacks	1 pkg	200	5	10	27
Frookie					
Cheddar	17 (1 oz)	140	4	4	23
Cracked Pepper	8 (0.7 oz)	70	2	0	15
Garden Vegetable	13 (1 oz)	130	3	4	19
Garlic & Herb	8 (0.7 oz)	70	2	0	16
Pizza	17 (1 oz)	130	3	3	24
Snack & Party	10 (1 oz)	140	2	5	20
Water Crackers	8 (0.7 oz)	70	2	0	16
Wheat & Onion	12 (1 oz)	120	3	4	18
Wheat & Rye	13 (1 oz)	120	3	4	18
Gold'n Krackle					
Cheese	½ oz	65	2	2	9
Cheese & Oregano	½ oz	65	2	2	9
Hot & Spicy	½ oz	58	2	1	11
Onion & Garlic	½ oz	58	2	1	11
Plain	½ oz	58	2	1	11
Health Valley					
Healthy Pizza Garlic & Herb	6	50	2	0	11
Healthy Pizza Italiano	6	50	2	0	11
Healthy Pizza Zesty Cheese	6	50	2	0	11
Low Fat Mild Jalapeno	6	60	2	2	10
Low Fat Mild Ranch	6	60	2	2	10
Low Fat Roasted Garlic	6	60	2	2	10
Original Oat Bran	6	120	3	3	22

FOOD	PORTION	CALS	PROT	FAT	CARB
Original Rice Bran	6	110	3	3	19
Whole Wheat	5	50	2	0	11
Whole Wheat Cheese	5	50	2	0	11
Whole Wheat Herb	5	50	2	0	11
Whole Wheat No Salt Vegetable	5	50	2	0	11
Whole Wheat Onion	5	50	2	0	11
Whole Wheat Vegetable	5	50	3	0	11
Keebler					
Club 33% Reduced Fat	5 (0.6 oz)	70	1	2	12
Club 50% Reduced Sodium	4 (0.5 oz)	70	1	3	9
Club Original	4 (0.5 oz)	70	1	3	9
Elfin	23 (1 oz)	130	2	2	24
Export Soda	3 (0.5 oz)	60	1	2	10
Harvest Bakery Multigrain	2 (0.6 oz)	70	1	3	10
Munch'ems Cheddar	39 (1 oz)	140	3	5	20
Munch'ems Cheddar	30 (1 oz)	130	3	4	21
Munch'ems Chili Cheese	28 (1.1 oz)	130	2	4	23
Munch'ems Mexquite BBQ	40 (1 oz)	140	2	5	22
Munch'ems Ranch	40 (1 oz)	140	3	5	20
Munch'ems Ranch	33 (1 oz)	130	3	4	21
Munch'ems Salsa	28 (1.1 oz)	130	2	4	23
Munch'ems Seasoned Original	30 (1 oz)	130	3	5	20
Munch'ems Sour Cream & Onion	39 (1 oz)	140	3	5	20
Munch'ems Sour Cream & Onion 55% Reduced Fat	33 (1 oz)	130	2	4	22
Paks Cheese & Peanut Butter	1 pkg	190	6	9	22
Paks Club & Cheddar	1 pkg	190	3	11	20
Paks Toast & Peanut Butter	1 pkg	190	5	9	23
Paks Wheat & Cheddar	1 pkg (1.3 oz)	180	2	10	17
Toasteds Buttercrisp	5 (0.6 oz)	80	1	4	10
Toasteds Buttercrisp	9 (1 oz)	140	2	7	19
Toasteds Onion	9 (1 oz)	140	2	6	19
Toasteds Sesame	5 (0.6 oz)	80	1	4	10
Toasteds Sesame	9 (1 oz)	140	3	6	19
Toasteds Sesame Reduced Fat	10 (1 oz)	120	3	3	21
Toasteds Wheat	5 (0.6 oz)	80	1	4	10
Toasteds Wheat	9 (1 oz)	140	2	6	19
Toasteds Wheat Reduced Fat	5 (0.5 oz)	60	1	2	10
Toasteds Wheat Reduced Fat	10 (1 oz)	120	3	3	22

FOOD	PORTION	CALS	PROT	FAT	CARB
Town House	5 (0.6 oz)	80	1	5	9
Town House 50% Reduced Sodium	5 (0.6 oz)	80	1	5	10
Town House Reduced Fat	6 (0.6 oz)	70	1.	2	11
Town House Wheat	5 (0.6 oz)	80	1	4	10
Wheatables Honey Wheat	12 (1 oz)	140	2	6	20
Wheatables Original	12 (1 oz)	140	2	6	10
Wheatables Seven Grain	12 (1 oz)	140	2	6	20
Zesta Saltine 50% Reduced Sodium	5 (0.5 oz)	60	1	2	11
Zesta Saltine Fat Free	5 (0.5 oz)	50	1	0	11
Zesta Saltine Original	5 (0.5 oz)	60	1	2	10
Zesta Saltine Unsalted Top	5 (0.5 oz)	70	1	2	10
Zesta Soup & Oyster	42 (0.5 oz)	80	1	3	10
Lance					
Bonnie	6 (1⅛ oz)	160	3	7	23
Captain Wafers w/ Cream Cheese & Chives	1 pkg (1.3 oz)	190	4	9	22
Cheese-On-Wheat	1 pkg (1.3 oz)	190	4	10	21
Cranberry Bar Fat Free	1 (1.75 oz)	160	1	0	38
Lanchee	1 pkg (1¼ oz)	190	5	11	18
Malt	1 pkg (1¼ oz)	190	6	10	18
Nekot	1 pkg (1.5 oz)	210	6	10	25
Nip-Chee	1 pkg (1.3 oz)	190	4	10	21
Peanut Butter Wheat	1 pkg (1.3 oz)	190	5	11	20
Rye-Chee	1 pkg (1.4 oz)	210	4	11	22
Sour Dough w/ Cheddar & Sour Cream	1 pkg (1.6 oz)	240	4	15	23
Toastchee	1 pkg (1.4 oz)	200	7	12	19
Toasty	1 pkg (1¼ oz)	190	6	11	17
Wheat Italian	¾ cup (1.4 oz)	200	3	11	23
Wheat Pizza	¾ cup (1.4 oz)	200	3	10	23
Little Debbie					
Cheese Crackers w/ Peanut Butter	1 (0.9 oz)	140	3	8	16
Cheese On Cheese Crackers	1 (0.9 oz)	140	2	8	15
Cream Cheese & Chive	1 (0.9 oz)	140	2	7	17
Toasty Crackers w/ Peanut Butter	1 (0.9 oz)	140	3	7	16
Wheat Crackers w/ Cheddar Cheese	1 (0.9 oz)	140	3	8	15
Nabisco					
Zwieback	1 (8 g)	35	1	1	6
No-No					
Flatbreads Tortilla Corn Low Fat Sugar Free Everything	3 (1 oz)	95	3	1	18

FOOD	PORTION	CALS	PROT	FAT	CARB
Pepperidge Farm					
Butter Thins	4 (0.5 oz)	70	1	3	10
English Water Biscuits	4 (0.5 oz)	70	2	2	13
Goldfish Cheddar	55	140	4	6	19
Goldfish Cheddar 30% Less Sodium	60 (1.1 oz)	150	3	6	18
Goldfish Cheese Trio	58	140	4	6	19
Goldfish Original	55	140	3	6	19
Goldfish Parmesan Cheese	60	140	4	5	13
Goldfish Pizza Flavored	55 (1 oz)	140	3	6	19
Goldfish Pretzel	43 (1 oz)	120	3	3	22
Goldfish Toasted Wheat	41	150	4	7	19
Hearty Wheat	3 (0.6 oz)	80	2	4	10
Sesame	3 (0.5 oz)	70	1	3	9
Snack Mix Fat Free Goldfish	⅔ cup (0.9 oz)	90	3	0	20
Peter Pan					
Cheese Peanut Butter	1 pkg	210	5	10	23
Toast Peanut Butter	1 pkg	210	5	11	23
Premium					
Saltine Multigrain	5 (0.5 oz)	60	1	2	10
Ralston					
Cheese	23 (1 oz)	150	3	6	18
Cheese Reduced Fat	29 (1 oz)	130	3	4	21
Oyster	35 (0.5 oz)	70	1	2	11
Rich & Crisp	1 (0.5 oz)	70	1	3	9
Saltines Fat Free	5 (0.5 oz)	60	1	0	13
Saltines Deluxe	5 (0.5 oz)	60	1	2	10
Snackers	9 (1.1 oz)	160	2	8	19
Snackers Reduced Fat	10 (1.1 oz)	140	2	4	23
Snackers Unsalted	9 (1.1 oz)	160	2	8	19
Wheat Snacks	16 (1 oz)	140	3	6	20
Wheat Snacks Reduced Fat	16 (1.1 oz)	140	2	4	23
Woven Wheats	7 (1.1 oz)	140	3	5	21
Woven Wheats Reduced Fat	8 (1.1 oz)	130	3	3	24
RedOval Farms					
Stoned Wheat Thins Cracked Pepper	4 (0.6 oz)	70	1	3	10
Savory Thins					
Toasted Onion & Garlic	15 (1 oz)	110	3	1	23
Smucker's					
Snackers Grape	1 pkg (3.3 oz)	410	11	20	47
Snackers Strawberry	1 pkg (3.3 oz)	410	11	20	47
Sunshine					
Hi Ho	4 (0.5 oz)	70	1	4	8
Hi Ho Reduced Fat	5 (0.5 oz)	70	1	3	10
Krispy	5 (0.5 oz)	60	2	2	10
Krispy Fat Free	5 (0.5 oz)	50	1	0	11
Krispy Mild Cheddar	5 (0.5 oz)	60	2	2	10

FOOD	PORTION	CALS	PROT	FAT	CARB
Krispy Soup & Oyster	17 (0.5 oz)	60	2	2	11
Krispy Unsalted Tops	5 (0.5 oz)	60	2	2	10
Krispy Whole Wheat	5 (0.5 oz)	60	2	2	10
Tree Of Life					
Bite Size Fat Free Cracked Pepper	12 (0.5 oz)	55	1	0	12
Bite Size Fat Free Garden Vegetable	12 (0.5 oz)	55	2	0	12
Bite Size Fat Free Garlic & Herb	12 (0.5 oz)	55	2	0	12
Bite Size Fat Free Toasted Onion	12 (0.5 oz)	55	2	0	12
Oyster	40 (0.5 oz)	60	2	0	13
Saltine Cracked Pepper Fat Free	4 (0.5 oz)	60	2	0	13
Saltine Fat Free	4 (0.5 oz)	50	2	0	11
Venus					
Fat Free Cracked Pepper	11 (0.5 oz)	60	1	0	12
Fat Free Garden Vegetable	5 (0.5 oz)	60	2	0	12
Fat Free Garlic & Herb	11 (0.5 oz)	60	2	0	12
Fat Free Multi-Grain	5 (0.5 oz)	60	1	0	12
Fat Free Spicy Chili	10 (0.5 oz)	60	1	0	12
Fat Free Toasted Onion	5 (0.5 oz)	60	1	0	12
Fat Free Toasted Wheat	5 (0.5 oz)	60	2	0	12
Fat Free Tomato & Basil	10 (0.5 oz)	60	1	0	12
Fat Free Zesty Italian	10 (0.5 oz)	60	1	0	12
Garden Vegetable	6 (1 oz)	150	2	8	20
Honey Wheat	1 oz	140	2	5	21
Low Fat Cracker Bread	5 (0.5 oz)	60	1	2	10
Low Fat Water Crackers	4 (0.5 oz)	60	1	1	12
Sesame & Flaxseed	1 oz	130	3	3	23
Soup Original	0.5 oz	60	1	2	11
Toasted Wheat	6 (1 oz)	150	3	7	18
Wine Cheese Caviar Original	0.5 oz	60	1	2	11
Wine Cheese Caviar Pepper & Poppy	0.5 oz	60	1	2	11
Wasa					
Crispbread Hearty Rye	1 (0.5 oz)	45	1	0	9
Wisecrackers					
Low Fat Poblano Chili & Sweet Onion	4 (0.5 oz)	45	1	1	8
Wortz					
Cheese	23 (1 oz)	150	3	6	18
Oyster	35 (0.5 oz)	70	1	2	11
Rich & Crisp	1 (0.5 oz)	70	1	3	9
Saltines Fat Free	5 (0.5 oz)	60	1	0	13
Saltines Deluxe	5 (0.5 oz)	60	1	2	10

FOOD	PORTION	CALS	PROT	FAT	CARB
Wheat Snacks	16 (1 oz)	140	3	6	20
Wheat Snacks Reduced Fat	16 (1.1 oz)	140	2	4	23
Woven Wheats	7 (1.1 oz)	140	3	5	21
CRANBERRIES					
Ocean Spray					
Craisins	⅓ cup (1.4 oz)	130	0	0	33
Cran*Fruit Cranberry Orange	¼ cup	120	0	0	29
Cranberry Sauce Jellied	¼ cup	110	0	0	27
Fresh	2 oz	25	0	0	6
Whole Berry Sauce	¼ cup	110	0	0	28
CRANBERRY BEANS					
canned	1 cup	216	14	1	39
dried cooked	1 cup	240	17	1	43
CRANBERRY JUICE					
cranberry juice cocktail	6 oz	108	0	tr	27
cranberry juice cocktail low calorie	6 oz	33	0	0	9
cranberry juice cocktail frzn as prep	6 oz	102	0	0	26
Crystal Light					
Cranberry Breeze Drink	1 serv (8 oz)	5	0	0	0
Cranberry Breeze Drink Mix as prep	1 serv (8 oz)	5	0	0	0
Everfresh					
Cranberry Cocktail	1 can (8 oz)	140	0	0	36
Mott's					
Cocktail	8 fl oz	150	0	0	37
Nantucket Nectars					
Cocktail	8 oz	140	0	0	34
Ocean Spray					
Cocktail	8 oz	140	0	0	34
Cocktail Reduced Calorie	8 oz	50	0	0	13
Lightstyle Cranberry Juice Cocktail	8 oz	40	0	0	10
White Cranberry	1 cup (8 oz)	120	0	0	29
White Cranberry Peach	1 cup (8 oz)	120	0	0	30
White Cranberry Strawberry	1 cup (8 oz)	120	0	0	31
Veryfine					
Cocktail	1 bottle (10 oz)	180	0	0	45
Wellfleet Farms					
Cranberry	8 oz	130	0	0	33
CRAYFISH					
cooked	3 oz	97	20	1	0
CREAM					
(*see also* SOUR CREAM, SOUR CREAM SUBSTITUTES, WHIPPED TOPPINGS)					
creme fraiche	2 tbsp (1 oz)	100	1	11	1

FOOD	PORTION	CALS	PROT	FAT	CARB
half & half	1 cup (8.5 oz)	315	7	28	10
heavy whipping whipped	1 cup (4.1 oz)	411	5	44	7
light coffee	1 cup (8.4 oz)	496	6	46	9
light whipping cream whipped	1 cup (4.2 oz)	345	5	37	7
Land O Lakes					
Half & Half	2 tbsp (1 oz)	40	1	4	1
Heavy Whipping	1 tbsp (0.5 oz)	50	0	6	0
Organic Valley					
Half & Half	2 tbsp (1 oz)	40	1	3	1
CREAM CHEESE					
cream cheese	1 oz	99	2	10	1
cream cheese	1 pkg (3 oz)	297	6	30	2
Alpine Lace					
Reduced Fat Roasted Garlic & Herbs	1 tsp (1 oz)	60	4	4	2
Reduced Fat Sundried Tomato & Basil	2 tsp (1 oz)	70	4	5	2
Boar's Head					
Cream Cheese	2 tbsp (1 oz)	100	2	10	2
Breakstone's					
Temp-Tee Whipped	2 tbsp (0.8 oz)	80	2	8	tr
Galaxy					
Slices	1 slice (1 oz)	50	4	3	2
Horizon Organic					
Spreadable	2 tbsp	100	2	10	1
Organic Valley					
Cream Cheese	1 oz	100	2	9	1
Philadelphia					
Free	1 oz	30	4	0	2
Regular	1 oz	100	2	10	tr
Soft	2 tbsp (1 oz)	100	2	10	1
Soft Apple Cinnamon	2 tbsp (1.1 oz)	100	1	8	5
Soft Cheesecake	2 tbsp (1 oz)	110	2	9	4
Soft Chives & Onions	2 tbsp (1.1 oz)	110	1	10	2
Soft Garden Vegetable	2 tbsp (1.1 oz)	110	1	11	1
Soft Honey Nut	2 tbsp (1.1 oz)	110	2	10	4
Soft Pineapple	2 tbsp (1.1 oz)	100	1	9	4
Soft Salmon	3 tbsp (1.1 oz)	100	2	9	2
Soft Strawberry	2 tbsp (1.1 oz)	100	1	9	5
Soft Free	2 tbsp (1.2 oz)	30	5	0	2
Soft Free Garden Vegetable	2 tbsp (1.2 oz)	30	5	0	2
Soft Free Strawberries	2 tbsp (1.2 oz)	45	4	0	6
Soft Light	2 tbsp (1.1 oz)	70	3	5	2
Soft Light Jalapeno	2 tbsp (1.1 oz)	60	3	5	2
Soft Light Raspberry	2 tbsp (1.1 oz)	70	3	5	6
Soft Light Roasted Garlic	2 tbsp (1.1 oz)	70	3	5	2
Whipped	2 tbsp (0.7 oz)	70	1	7	tr

FOOD	PORTION	CALS	PROT	FAT	CARB
Whipped Chives	2 tbsp (0.7 oz)	70	1	6	tr
Whipped Smoked Salmon	2 tbsp (0.7 oz)	70	2	6	1
With Chives	1 oz	90	2	9	tr
CREAM OF TARTAR					
cream of tartar	1 tsp	8	0	0	2
CREPES					
Frieda's					
Ready-To-Use	2 (0.8 oz)	50	1	1	9
CRESS					
garden cooked	½ cup	16	1	tr	3
CROAKER					
atlantic breaded & fried	3 oz	188	15	11	6
atlantic raw	3 oz	89	15	3	0
CROCODILE					
cooked	3 oz	78	17	1	0
CROISSANT					
apple	1 (2 oz)	145	4	5	21
cheese	1 (2 oz)	236	5	12	27
plain	1 (2 oz)	232	5	12	26
plain	1 mini (1 oz)	115	2	6	13
Sara Lee					
Broccoli & Cheese	1 (3.7 oz)	280	11	13	30
French Style	1 (1.5 oz)	170	4	8	20
Ham & Swiss	1 (3.7 oz)	300	12	16	27
Petite	2 (2 oz)	230	6	11	26
take-out					
w/ egg & cheese	1 (4.5 oz)	368	13	25	24
w/ egg cheese & bacon	1 (4.5 oz)	413	16	28	24
w/ egg cheese & ham	1 (5.3 oz)	474	19	34	24
w/ egg cheese & sausage	1 (5.6 oz)	523	20	38	25
CROUTONS					
plain	1 cup (1 oz)	122	4	2	22
seasoned	1 cup (1.4 oz)	186	4	7	25
Pepperidge Farm					
Garlic	6 (0.2 oz)	30	1	1	5
Homestyle	6 (0.2 oz)	30	1	1	5
Sourdough	6 (0.2 oz)	35	1	2	4
Up Country Naturals					
Organic Whole Wheat Garlic & Herb	¼ cup (0.3 oz)	35	1	2	5
CUCUMBER					
fresh raw	1 (11 oz)	38	2	tr	8
fresh					
Chiquita					
Cucumber	⅓ med (3.5 oz)	15	1	0	3
take-out					
cucumber salad	3.5 oz	50	1	tr	11
tzatziki	½ cup (3.4 oz)	72	2	6	4

FOOD	PORTION	CALS	PROT	FAT	CARB
CURRANTS					
black fresh	½ cup	36	1	tr	9
zante dried	½ cup	204	3	tr	53
CUSK					
fillet baked	3 oz	106	23	1	0
CUSTARD					
home recipe					
baked	1 recipe 4 serv (19.8 oz)	549	29	26	60
flan	1 recipe 10 serv (53.7 oz)	2206	70	63	349
mix					
as prep w/ 2% milk	½ cup (4.7 oz)	148	7	4	24
as prep w/ 2% milk	1 recipe 4 serv (18.7 oz)	595	22	15	95
as prep w/ whole milk	½ cup (4.7 oz)	163	6	5	23
as prep w/ whole milk	1 recipe 4 serv (18.7 oz)	652	22	22	94
flan as prep w/ 2% milk	½ cup (4.7 oz)	135	4	2	26
flan as prep w/ 2% milk	1 recipe 4 serv (18.7 oz)	542	16	9	102
flan as prep w/ whole milk	½ cup (4.7 oz)	150	4	4	25
flan as prep w/ whole milk	1 recipe 4 serv (18.7 oz)	600	16	16	102
Betty Crocker					
Flan w/ Caramel Sauce as prep	1 serv	330	0	7	60
Jell-O					
Americana Custard Dessert as prep w/ 2% milk	½ cup (5 oz)	140	5	3	25
Flan as prep w/ 2% milk	½ cup (5.1 oz)	140	4	3	26
ready-to-eat					
Swiss Miss					
Egg Custard	1 pkg (4 oz)	153	5	5	22
take-out					
baked	½ cup (5 oz)	148	7	7	15
flan	½ cup (5.4 oz)	220	7	6	35
zabaione	½ cup (57.2 g)	135	3	5	13
CUTTLEFISH					
steamed	3 oz	134	28	1	1
DANDELION GREENS					
fresh cooked	½ cup	17	1	tr	3
DANISH PASTRY					
frozen					
Morton					
Honey Buns	1 (2.28 oz)	270	3	13	35
Honey Buns Mini	1 (1.3 oz)	160	2	8	19

FOOD	PORTION	CALS	PROT	FAT	CARB
ready-to-eat					
plain ring	1 (12 oz)	1305	21	71	152
Dolly Madison					
Danish Rollers	3 (2.8 oz)	290	3	10	46
Tastykake					
Cheese	1 (3 oz)	290	5	14	44
Lemon	1 (3 oz)	290	5	14	44
Raspberry	1 (3 oz)	290	5	14	44
take-out					
almond	1 (4¼ in) (2.3 oz)	280	5	16	30
apple	1 (4¼ in) (2.5 oz)	264	4	13	34
cheese	1 (3.2 oz)	353	6	25	29
cheese	1 (4¼ in) (2.5 oz)	266	6	16	26
cinnamon	1 (3.1 oz)	349	5	17	47
cinnamon	1 (4¼ in) (2.3 oz)	262	5	15	29
cinnimon nut	1 (4¼ in) (2.3 oz)	280	5	16	30
fruit	1 (3.3 oz)	335	5	16	45
lemon	1 (4¼ in) (2.5 oz)	264	4	13	34
raisin	1 (4¼ in) (2.5 oz)	264	4	13	34
raisin nut	1 (4¼ in) (2.3 oz)	280	5	16	30
raspberry	1 (4¼ in) (2.5 oz)	264	4	13	34
strawberry	1 (4¼ in) (2.5 oz)	264	4	13	34
DATES					
dried chopped	1 cup	489	4	1	131
dried whole	10	228	2	tr	61
jujube dried	1 oz	75	1	tr	19
Calavo					
Dried Pitted	5–6 (1.4 oz)	120	1	0	31
California Redi-Date					
Deglet Noor Dried	5–6 (1.4 oz)	120	1	0	31
Dromedary					
Chopped Dried	¼ cup	130	1	0	31
DEER					
(*see* VENISON)					
DELI MEATS/COLD CUTS					
(*see also* BEEF, CHICKEN, HAM, MEAT SUBSTITUTES, TURKEY)					
barbecue loaf pork & beef	1 oz	49	4	3	2
beerwurst beef	1 slice (2¾ in x ¹⁄₁₆ in)	20	1	2	tr
beerwurst beef	1 slice (4 in x ⅛ in)	75	3	7	tr
beerwurst pork	1 slice (2¾ in x ¹⁄₁₆ in)	14	1	1	tr
beerwurst pork	1 slice (4 in x ⅛ in)	55	4	4	tr
berliner pork & beef	1 oz	65	4	4	1
blood sausage	1 oz	95	4	9	tr
bologna beef	1 oz	88	4	8	tr
bologna beef & pork	1 oz	89	3	8	1

FOOD	PORTION	CALS	PROT	FAT	CARB
bologna pork	1 oz	70	4	6	tr
braunschweiger pork	1 slice (2½ in x ¼ in)	65	2	6	1
braunschweiger pork	1 oz	102	4	9	1
corned beef loaf	1 oz	43	7	2	0
dutch brand loaf pork & beef	1 oz	68	4	5	2
headcheese pork	1 oz	60	5	5	tr
honey loaf pork & beef	1 oz	36	4	1	2
honey roll sausage beef	1 oz	42	4	2	1
lebanon bologna beef	1 oz	60	6	4	1
liver cheese pork	1 oz	86	4	7	1
liverwurst pork	1 oz	92	4	8	1
luncheon meat beef	1 oz	87	4	7	1
luncheon meat pork & beef	1 oz	100	4	9	1
luncheon meat pork canned	1 oz	95	4	9	1
luncheon sausage pork & beef	1 oz	74	4	6	tr
luxury loaf pork	1 oz	40	5	1	1
mortadella beef & pork	1 oz	88	5	7	1
mother's loaf pork	1 oz	80	3	6	2
new england sausage pork & beef	1 oz	46	5	2	1
olive loaf pork	1 oz	67	3	5	3
peppered loaf pork & beef	1 oz	42	5	2	1
pepperoni pork & beef	1 slice (0.2 oz)	27	1	2	tr
pepperoni pork & beef	1 (9 oz)	1248	53	110	7
pickle & pimiento loaf pork	1 oz	74	3	6	2
picnic loaf pork & beef	1 oz	66	4	5	1
salami cooked beef & pork	1 oz	71	4	6	1
salami hard pork	1 slice (⅛ oz)	41	2	4	3
salami hard pork	1 pkg (4 oz)	460	26	38	2
salami hard pork & beef	1 slice (⅛ oz)	42	2	3	tr
salami hard pork & beef	1 pkg (4 oz)	472	26	39	3
sandwich spread pork & beef	1 oz	67	2	5	3
sandwich spread pork & beef	1 tbsp	35	1	3	2
summer sausage thuringer cervelat	1 oz	98	5	8	1
Boar's Head					
Bologna Beef	2 oz	150	7	13	0
Bologna Garlic	2 oz	150	7	13	1
Bologna Lowered Sodium	2 oz	150	8	13	0
Bologna Pork & Beef	2 oz	150	7	13	tr

FOOD	PORTION	CALS	PROT	FAT	CARB
Braunschweiger Lite	2 oz	120	9	8	1
Head Cheese	2 oz	90	10	5	tr
Liverwurst Strassburger	2 oz	170	8	15	1
Olive Loaf	2 oz	130	6	12	tr
Pastrami	2 oz	90	12	4	2
Prosciutto	1 oz	60	8	3	0
Red Pastrami	2 oz	90	12	4	2
Salami Beef	2 oz	120	10	9	0
Salami Cooked	2 oz	130	8	11	0
Salami Genoa	2 oz	180	12	14	1
Salami Hard	1 oz	110	6	9	tr
Spiced Ham	2 oz	120	7	10	1
Carl Buddig					
Beef	1 pkg (2.5 oz)	100	14	5	1
Corned Beef	1 pkg (2.5 oz)	100	14	5	tr
Pastrami	1 pkg (2.5 oz)	100	14	5	1
Hormel					
Liverwurst Spread	4 tbsp (2 oz)	130	8	10	2
Pepperoni Chunk	1 oz	140	5	13	0
Pepperoni Sliced	15 slices (1 oz)	140	5	13	0
Pepperoni Twin	1 oz	140	5	13	0
Pillow Pack Genoa Salami	2 oz	160	12	18	0
Pillow Pack Pepperoni	16 slices (1 oz)	140	5	13	0
Oscar Mayer					
Bologna	1 slice (1 oz)	90	3	8	1
Bologna Beef	1 slice (1 oz)	90	3	8	1
Bologna Garlic	1 slice (1.4 oz)	110	4	12	1
Bologna Wisconsin Made Ring	2 oz	180	6	16	2
Braunschweiger Spread	2 oz	190	8	17	2
Brunschweiger	1 slice (1 oz)	100	4	9	1
Free Bologna	1 slice (1 oz)	20	4	0	2
Light Bologna	1 slice (1 oz)	60	3	4	2
Light Bologna Beef	1 slice (1 oz)	60	3	4	2
Liver Cheese	1 slice (1.3 oz)	120	6	10	1
Luncheon Loaf Spiced	1 slice (1 oz)	70	4	5	2
Old Fashioned Loaf	1 slice (1 oz)	70	4	5	2
Olive Loaf	1 slice (1 oz)	70	3	6	2
Pepperoni	15 slices (1 oz)	140	6	13	0
Salami Cotto	1 slice (1 oz)	70	3	5	1
Salami Cotto Beef	1 slice (1 oz)	60	4	5	1
Salami For Beer	1 slices (1.6 oz)	110	6	9	1
Salami Hard	3 slices (1 oz)	100	6	9	0
Sandwich Spread	2 oz	130	4	10	8
Summer Sausage	2 slices (1.6 oz)	140	7	13	0
Summer Sausage Beef	2 slices (1.6 oz)	140	7	12	1
Spam					
Less Salt	2 oz	170	7	16	0

FOOD	PORTION	CALS	PROT	FAT	CARB
Lite	2 oz	110	9	8	0
Original	2 oz	170	7	16	0
Smoked	2 oz	170	7	16	0
take-out					
corned beef	2 oz	70	12	2	0
corned beef brisket	2 oz	90	11	5	0

DIETING AIDS

(*see* NUTRITION SUPPLEMENTS)

DINNER

(*see also* ASIAN FOOD, PASTA DISHES, POT PIES, SPANISH FOOD)

FOOD	PORTION	CALS	PROT	FAT	CARB
Amy's Organic					
Whole Meals Country Dinner	1 pkg (11 oz)	380	11	12	60
Banquet					
Beef Patty w/ Country Style Vegetables	1 meal (9.5 oz)	310	11	20	22
Boneless Pork Rib	1 meal (10 oz)	400	17	19	40
Boneless White Fried Chicken	1 meal (8.25 oz)	540	16	34	41
Chicken Parmigiana	1 meal (9.5 oz)	320	10	18	29
Chicken Fingers Meal	1 meal (7.1 oz)	740	22	43	67
Chicken Fried Beef Steak	1 pkg (10 oz)	420	15	23	39
Chicken Nuggets Meal	1 meal (6.75 oz)	430	14	23	42
Extra Helping Boneless Pork Riblet	1 meal (15.25 oz)	720	27	40	62
Extra Helping Fried Beef Steak	1 meal (16 oz)	820	29	50	63
Extra Helping Fried Chicken	1 meal (14.7 oz)	910	34	55	70
Extra Helping Meatloaf	1 meal (16 oz)	610	29	40	34
Extra Helping Salisbury Steak	1 meal (16.5 oz)	740	27	54	37
Extra Helping Turkey & Gravy w/ Dressing	1 meal (17 oz)	620	28	32	54
Extra Helping White Fried Chicken	1 meal (13 oz)	690	24	48	40
Extra Helping Yankee Pot Roast	1 meal (14.5 oz)	410	25	20	33
Family Size Brown Gravy & Salisbury Steak	1 serv	240	9	20	7
Family Size Brown Gravy & Sliced Beef	1 serv	140	13	8	5
Family Size Chicken & Broccoli Alfredo	1 serv	270	11	12	28
Family Size Country Style Chicken & Dumplings	1 serv	290	12	14	30
Family Size Creamy Broccoli Chicken Cheese & Rice	1 serv	280	14	14	25
Family Size Hearty Beef Stew	1 cup	170	10	7	18

FOOD	PORTION	CALS	PROT	FAT	CARB
Family Size Homestyle Gravy & Sliced Turkey	2 slices	140	7	10	5
Family Size Mushroom Gravy & Charbroiled Beef Patties	1 patty	250	11	20	6
Family Size Potato Ham & Broccoli Au Gratin	⅔ cup	210	7	13	16
Family Size Savory Gravy & Meatloaf	1 slice	120	10	13	7
Fish Sticks	1 meal (6.6 oz)	290	11	13	33
Grilled Chicken	1 meal (9.9 oz)	330	16	13	37
Honey Roast Turkey Breast	1 meal (9 oz)	270	11	12	29
Meatloaf	1 meal (9.5 oz)	280	12	16	23
Our Original Fried Chicken	1 meal (9 oz)	470	21	27	35
Pork Cutlet Meal	1 meal (10.25 oz)	420	11	25	36
Salisbury Steak	1 meal (9.5 oz)	380	12	24	28
Sliced Beef	1 meal (9 oz)	270	26	10	19
Turkey	1 meal (9.25 oz)	270	14	11	30
Veal Parmagiana	1 meal (8.75 oz)	330	13	14	37
Western Style Beef Patty	1 meal (9.5 oz)	360	14	21	28
White Meat Fried Chicken	1 meal (8.75 oz)	460	18	28	40
Yankee Pot Roast	1 meal (9.4 oz)	230	14	10	20
Birds Eye					
Chicken Viola! Zesty Garlic Chicken	2 cups (6.2 oz)	260	15	11	28
Chicken Voila! Alfredo	1 cup (6.1 oz)	230	15	8	26
Chicken Voila! Garden Herb	1 cup	310	16	15	28
Chicken Voila! Grilled Salsa	1 cup	240	14	5	35
Chicken Voila! Teriyaki	2 cups (6.4 oz)	240	13	9	26
Easy Recipe Creations Sweet & Sour w/ Pineapple Tidbits as prep	1⅔ cups (8.7 oz)	200	2	1	45
Steak Voila! Beef Sirloin Steak And Garlic Potatoes	1 cup	240	13	9	26
Turkey Voila! Homestyle w/ Roasted Potatoes	1 cup	200	12	6	24
Green Giant					
Create A Meal Broccoli Stir Fry as prep	1⅓ cups (9.9 oz)	290	27	13	16
Create A Meal Cheese & Herb Primavera as prep	1¼ cups (10 oz)	330	30	11	27
Create A Meal Garlic Herb as prep	1¼ cups (10 oz)	340	24	14	30
Create A Meal Hearty Vegetable Stew as prep	1¼ cups (10 oz)	280	23	9	25

FOOD	PORTION	CALS	PROT	FAT	CARB
Create A Meal Lemon Herb as prep	1½ cups (10 oz)	360	28	11	37
Create A Meal Mushroom & Wine as prep	1¼ cups (10 oz)	390	28	16	31
Create A Meal Vegetable Almond Stir Fry as prep	1⅓ cups (10 oz)	320	32	11	22
Healthy Choice					
Beef Pepper Steak Oriental	1 meal (9.5 oz)	260	19	5	34
Beef Pot Roast	1 meal (11 oz)	300	20	6	41
Beef Stroganoff	1 meal (11 oz)	320	22	8	40
Beef Tips Francais	1 meal (9.5 oz)	300	20	7	40
Beef Tips Portabello	1 meal (11.25 oz)	270	23	5	34
Bowls Chicken Teriyaki w/ Rice	1 meal (9.5 oz)	270	17	4	41
Bowls Country Chicken Bake	1 meal (9.5 oz)	230	18	8	22
Bowls Fiesta Chicken	1 meal (9.5 oz)	220	15	2	34
Bowls Garlic Lemon Chicken w/ Rice	1 meal (9.5 oz)	300	18	4	48
Bowls Roasted Potatoes w/ Ham	1 meal (8.5 oz)	210	17	4	26
Bowls Southwestern Chicken & Pasta	1 meal (9.5 oz)	320	31	4	39
Bowls Turkey Divan	1 meal (9.5 oz)	250	18	6	31
Charbroiled Beef Patty	1 meal (11 oz)	310	16	9	40
Chicken Cantonese	1 meal (10.75 oz)	280	22	6	34
Chicken Parmigiana	1 meal (11.5 oz)	330	19	8	46
Chicken & Vegetables Marsala	1 meal (11.5 oz)	240	20	4	32
Chicken Broccoli Alfredo	1 meal (11.5 oz)	300	25	7	34
Chicken Dijon	1 meal (11 oz)	270	23	5	33
Chicken Teriyaki	1 meal (11 oz)	270	17	6	37
Country Breaded Chicken	1 meal (10.25 oz)	350	16	9	51
Country Glazed Chicken Breast	1 meal (8.5 oz)	250	19	5	31
Country Herb Chicken	1 meal (12.15 oz)	320	16	8	44
Country Inn Roast Turkey	1 meal (10 oz)	250	20	6	28
Garlic Chicken Milano	1 meal (9.5 oz)	260	18	6	34
Grilled Chicken Sonoma	1 meal (9 oz)	230	16	4	30
Grilled Chicken w/ Mashed Potatoes	1 meal (8 oz)	180	16	4	18
Herb Baked Fish	1 meal (10.9 oz)	340	16	7	54
Herb Breaded Pork Patty	1 meal (8 oz)	280	18	6	38
Homestyle Chicken & Pasta	1 meal (9 oz)	270	21	6	32
Honey Glazed Chicken	1 meal (10 oz)	270	21	7	32
Honey Mustard Chicken	1 meal (9.5 oz)	290	21	6	38
Lemon Pepper Fish	1 meal (10.7 oz)	320	14	7	50
Mandarin Chicken	1 meal (10 oz)	280	20	3	44

FOOD	PORTION	CALS	PROT	FAT	CARB
Mesquite Beef w/ Barbecue Sauce	1 meal (11 oz)	320	21	9	36
Mesquite Chicken Barbecue	1 meal (10.5 oz)	310	18	5	48
Oriental Style Chicken & Vegetable Stir Fry	1 meal (11.9 oz)	360	19	6	57
Oven Roasted Beef	1 meal (10.15 oz)	280	18	8	35
Roast Turkey Breast	1 meal (8.5 oz)	220	18	5	28
Roasted Chicken	1 meal (11 oz)	230	20	5	23
Sesame Chicken	1 meal (10.8 oz)	360	19	7	54
Shrimp & Vegetables	1 meal (11.8 oz)	270	15	6	39
Sweet & Sour Chicken	1 meal (11 oz)	360	20	7	53
Traditional Meatloaf	1 meal (12 oz)	330	15	7	52
Traditional Breast Of Turkey	1 meal (10.5 oz)	290	22	5	40
Tradtional Salisbury Steak	1 meal (11.5 oz)	330	18	7	48
Tuna Casserole	1 meal (8 oz)	240	16	5	33
Kid Cuisine					
Circus Show Corn Dog	1 meal (8.8 oz)	490	8	20	70
Cosmic Chicken Nuggets	1 meal (9.1 oz)	500	18	25	50
Futuristic Fish Sticks	1 meal (8.25 oz)	410	9	16	57
Game Time Taco Roll Up	1 meal (7.35 oz)	420	9	18	55
High Flying Fried Chicken	1 meal (10.1 oz)	440	18	20	48
Parachuting Pork Ribettes	1 meal (7.55 oz)	390	16	19	39
Lean Cuisine					
Cafe Classics Baked Chicken	1 pkg (8.6 oz)	240	17	5	33
Cafe Classics Baked Fish	1 pkg (9 oz)	290	20	6	40
Cafe Classics Beef Peppercorn	1 pkg (8.75 oz)	260	16	7	32
Cafe Classics Beef Portobello	1 pkg (9 oz)	220	14	7	24
Cafe Classics Beef Pot Roast	1 pkg (9 oz)	210	13	6	25
Cafe Classics Chicken Carbonara	1 pkg (9 oz)	280	17	7	36
Cafe Classics Chicken Medallions w/ Creamy Cheese Sauce	1 pkg (9.37 oz)	300	19	7	40
Cafe Classics Chicken Mediterranean	1 pkg (10.5 oz)	260	17	4	38
Cafe Classics Chicken & Vegetables	1 pkg (10.5 oz)	240	19	5	30
Cafe Classics Chicken In Peanut Sauce	1 pkg (9 oz)	260	20	6	32
Cafe Classics Chicken In Wine Sauce	1 pkg (8.1 oz)	220	20	5	23
Cafe Classics Chicken L'Orange	1 pkg (9 oz)	230	20	2	33

FOOD	PORTION	CALS	PROT	FAT	CARB
Cafe Classics Chicken Parmesan	1 pkg (10.9 oz)	300	21	6	41
Cafe Classics Chicken Piccata	1 pkg (9 oz)	300	14	9	41
Cafe Classics Chicken w/ Basil Cream Sauce	1 pkg (8.5 oz)	260	17	7	33
Cafe Classics Country Vegetables & Beef	1 pkg (9 oz)	210	11	4	33
Cafe Classics Fiesta Chicken	1 pkg (9.25 oz)	270	17	5	40
Cafe Classics Glazed Chicken	1 pkg (8.5 oz)	240	22	6	25
Cafe Classics Glazed Turkey Tenderloins	1 pkg (9 oz)	260	14	5	41
Cafe Classics Grilled Chicken	1 pkg (9.4 oz)	250	22	5	29
Cafe Classics Grilled Chicken Salsa	1 pkg (8.9 oz)	270	15	7	36
Cafe Classics Herb Roasted Chicken	1 pkg (8 oz)	190	17	4	22
Cafe Classics Honey Mustard Chicken	1 pkg (8 oz)	270	19	4	40
Cafe Classics Honey Roasted Chicken	1 pkg (8.5 oz)	270	13	6	41
Cafe Classics Honey Roasted Pork	1 serv (9.5 oz)	250	17	6	32
Cafe Classics Meatloaf w/ Whipped Potatoes	1 pkg (9.4 oz)	260	20	7	28
Cafe Classics Oriental Beef	1 pkg (9.25 oz)	210	14	4	30
Cafe Classics Oven Roasted Beef	1 pkg (9.25 oz)	260	18	8	28
Cafe Classics Roasted Turkey Breast	1 pkg (9.75 oz)	270	13	2	49
Cafe Classics Salisbury Steak	1 pkg (9.5 oz)	280	24	8	29
Cafe Classics Sirloin Beef Peppercorn	1 pkg (8.75 oz)	220	15	7	23
Cafe Classics Southern Beef Tips	1 pkg (8.75 oz)	270	16	6	37
Everday Favorites Vegetable Lasagna	1 pkg (10.5 oz)	260	15	7	36
Everyday Favorite Chicken Florentine	1 pkg (8 oz)	220	13	5	32
Everyday Favorite Chicken Chow Mein	1 pkg (9 oz)	240	14	4	37
Everyday Favorites Homestyle Turkey	1 pkg (9.4 oz)	240	22	5	27

FOOD	PORTION	CALS	PROT	FAT	CARB
Everyday Favorites Hunan Beef & Broccoli	1 pkg (8.5 oz)	240	11	4	40
Everyday Favorites Mandarin Chicken	1 pkg (9 oz)	260	15	5	38
Everyday Favorites Roasted Chicken	1 pkg (8.1 oz)	260	14	7	34
Everyday Favorites Stuffed Cabbage	1 pkg (9.5 oz)	210	9	8	25
Everyday Favorites Swedish Meatballs	1 pkg (9.1 oz)	290	22	7	35
Hearty Portions Cheese & Spinach Manicotti	1 serv	370	25	8	50
Hearty Portions Chicken & Barbecue Sauce	1 serv	370	20	6	60
Hearty Portions Homestyle Beef Stroganoff	1 serv	350	23	9	44
Hearty Portions Jumbo Rigatoni w/ Meatballs	1 serv	440	25	9	64
Hearty Portions Oriental Glazed Chicken	1 serv	370	21	2	66
Hearty Portions Roasted Chicken w/ Mushrooms	1 serv	330	23	4	49
Skillet Sensations Beef Teriyaki & Rice	1 serv	280	14	3	48
Skillet Sensations Chicken Primavera	1 serv	320	20	5	50
Skillet Sensations Chicken Oriental	1 serv	280	17	3	46
Skillet Sensations Fiesta Beef & Rice	1 serv	300	19	4	48
Skillet Sensations Garlic Chicken	1 serv	340	20	5	56
Skillet Sensations Herb Chicken & Roasted Potatoes	1 serv	270	18	5	39
Skillet Sensations Roasted Turkey	1 serv	220	14	2	37
Skillet Sensations Savory Beef & Vegetables	1 serv	290	18	7	38
Skillet Sensations Three Cheese Chicken	1 serv	370	26	10	45
Luzianne					
Cajun Creole Dirty Rice	1 serv	160	4	1	35
Cajun Creole Etouffee	1 serv	200	5	1	42
Cajun Creole Gumbo	1 serv	160	4	1	33
Cajun Creole Jambalaya	1 serv	200	5	1	43

FOOD	PORTION	CALS	PROT	FAT	CARB
Marie Callender's					
Beef Stroganoff w/ Noodles	1 meal (13 oz)	600	20	27	59
Beef Tips In Mushroom Sauce	1 meal (13 oz)	430	25	19	39
Breaded Chicken Parmigiana	1 meal (16 oz)	860	30	32	63
Cheesy Rice w/ Chicken & Broccoli	1 meal (12 oz)	390	24	13	44
Chicken & Dumplings	1 meal (14 oz)	390	17	20	34
Chicken & Noodles	1 meal (13 oz)	520	21	30	42
Chicken Cordon Bleu	1 meal (13 oz)	610	23	28	58
Chicken Fried Beef Steak & Gravy	1 meal (15 oz)	650	20	37	50
Chicken Teriyaki	1 meal (13 oz)	510	24	12	71
Country Fried Chicken & Gravy	1 meal (16 oz)	620	24	30	63
Country Fried Pork Chop	1 meal (15 oz)	540	23	28	50
Escalloped Noodles & Chicken	1 meal (13 oz)	740	21	46	60
Glazed Chicken	1 meal (13 oz)	490	25	25	40
Grilled Southwestern Style Chicken	1 meal (14 oz)	410	24	11	43
Grilled Chicken & Mashed Potatoes	1 meal (10 oz)	340	24	16	20
Grilled Chicken Breast & Rice Pilaf	1 meal (11.75 oz)	360	20	14	36
Grilled Chicken In Mushroom Sauce	1 meal (14 oz)	480	32	15	54
Grilled Turkey Breast & Rice Pilaf	1 meal (11.75 oz)	310	22	10	34
Herb Roasted Chicken & Mashed Potatoes	1 meal (14 oz)	580	42	34	26
Honey Roasted Chicken	1 meal (14 oz)	440	45	17	27
Honey Smoked Ham Steak w/ Macroni & Cheese	1 meal (14 oz)	490	29	13	63
Meatloaf & Gravy w/ Mashed Potatoes	1 meal (14 oz)	540	23	30	42
Old Fashioned Beef Pot Roast & Gravy	1 meal (15 oz)	500	23	17	55
Roast Beef	1 meal (14.5 oz)	390	24	19	30
Sirloin Salisbury Steak & Gravy	1 meal (14 oz)	550	30	25	51
Skillet Meal Au Gratin Potatoes	⅔ cup (5 oz)	190	7	10	19
Skillet Meal Beef Pot Roast	½ pkg	290	20	9	33
Skillet Meal Beef Stroganoff	½ pkg	310	21	11	31
Skillet Meal Chicken & Rice w/ Broccoli & Cheese	½ pkg	440	30	14	47

FOOD	PORTION	CALS	PROT	FAT	CARB
Skillet Meal Chicken Teriyaki	½ pkg	340	21	1	61
Skillet Meal Herb Chicken	½ pkg	290	22	4	42
Skillet Meal Roasted Chicken & Vegetables	½ pkg	260	21	6	30
Skillet Meal White & Wild Rice In Cheese Sauce	1 cup	300	11	13	35
Swedish Meatballs	1 meal (12.5 oz)	520	28	26	44
Sweet & Sour Chicken	1 meal (14 oz)	570	23	15	66
Turkey w/ Gravy & Dressing	1 meal (14 oz)	500	31	19	52
Morton					
Breaded Chicken Pattie	1 meal (6.75 oz)	290	10	17	24
Chicken Nuggets	1 meal (7 oz)	340	12	19	31
Chili Gravy w/ Beef Enchilada & Tamale	1 meal (10 oz)	270	7	9	40
Fried Chicken	1 meal (9 oz)	470	20	30	30
Gravy & Charbroiled Beef Patty	1 meal (9 oz)	310	10	18	26
Gravy & Salisbury Steak	1 meal (9 oz)	310	7	20	24
Gravy & Turkey w/ Stuffing	1 meal (9 oz)	240	10	10	27
Tomato Sauce w/ Meat Loaf	1 meal (9 oz)	250	9	13	24
Veal Parmagiana w/ Tomato Sauce	1 meal (8.75 oz)	290	8	15	30
Nature's Choice					
Broccoli Parmesan Alfredo	1 pkg (12 oz)	270	20	9	29
Nature's Entree					
Hearty Stew	1 pkg (12 oz)	290	18	9	34
Tuscany White Bean	1 pkg (12 oz)	330	21	8	42
Patio					
Ranchera	1 pkg (13 oz)	470	13	22	55
Stouffer's					
Baked Chicken Breast w/ Mashed Potatoes	1 serv (12.2 oz)	330	25	14	25
Beef Stroganoff	1 pkg (9.75 oz)	390	23	20	30
Chicken A La King	1 pkg (9.5 oz)	350	17	13	41
Creamed Chicken	1 pkg (6.5 oz)	260	15	19	8
Creamed Chipped Beef	½ cup (5.5 oz)	160	10	11	6
Creamy Chicken & Broccoli	1 pkg (8.9 oz)	320	19	15	26
Escalloped Chicken & Noodles	1 pkg (10 oz)	430	17	27	30
Fish w/ Macaroni & Cheese	1 serv (9.5 oz)	460	22	20	47
Glazed Chicken w/ Rice	1 serv (11.8 oz)	290	21	6	39
Green Pepper Steak	1 pkg (10.5 oz)	330	17	9	45
Homestyle Baked Chicken & Gravy & Whipped Potatoes	1 pkg (8.9 oz)	270	22	12	19

FOOD	PORTION	CALS	PROT	FAT	CARB
Homestyle Beef Pot Roast & Browned Potatoes	1 pkg (8.9 oz)	250	16	8	29
Homestyle Fish Filet w/ Macaroni & Cheese	1 pkg (9 oz)	430	24	21	37
Homestyle Fried Chicken & Whipped Potatoes	1 pkg (7.5 oz)	310	17	12	33
Homestyle Meatloaf & Whipped Potatoes	1 pkg (9.9 oz)	330	20	16	26
Homestyle Roast Turkey w/ Gravy Stuffing & Whipped Potatoes	1 pkg (9.6 oz)	320	19	13	31
Homestyle Salisbury Steak & Gravy & Macaroni & Cheese	1 pkg (9.6 oz)	350	24	16	27
Meatloaf	1 serv (5.5 oz)	210	16	12	9
Meatloaf w/ Whipped Potatoes	1 serv (11.5 oz)	380	22	18	33
Stuffed Pepper	1 pkg (10 oz)	200	11	5	27
Swedish Meatballs	1 pkg (10.25 oz)	480	24	24	43
Swanson					
Beef Pot Roast	1 pkg (14 oz)	320	19	8	44
Chicken Parmigiana w/ Spaghetti	1 pkg (11 oz)	380	17	17	41
Turkey Breast	1 pkg (11.7 oz)	330	18	6	50
Tamarind Tree					
Alu Chole	1 pkg (9.2 oz)	350	12	6	63
Channa Dal Masala	1 pkg (9.2 oz)	340	13	5	62
Dal Makhini	1 pkg (9.2 oz)	330	14	6	55
Dhingri Mutter	1 pkg (9.2 oz)	290	8	5	53
Navratan Korma	1 pkg (9.2 oz)	430	12	15	60
Palak Paneer	1 pkg (9.2 oz)	380	14	15	46
Saag Chole	1 pkg (9.2 oz)	370	14	10	55
Vegetable Jalfrazi	1 pkg (9.2 oz)	310	8	6	57
Tyson					
BBQ Chicken Potato & Vegetable Medley	1 pkg (14.7 oz)	560	19	21	73
Beef Stir Fry	1 pkg (14 oz)	430	26	5	70
Blackened Chicken Spanish Rice & Corn	1 pkg (8.8 oz)	260	17	5	36
Chicken Primavera	1 pkg (11.3 oz)	350	25	6	48
Chicken Divan Candied Carrots & Pasta	1 pkg (9.8 oz)	370	20	15	38
Chicken Francais Sliced Potatoes & Green Beans	1 pkg (8.8 oz)	260	19	10	23

FOOD	PORTION	CALS	PROT	FAT	CARB
Chicken Kiev Rice Pilaf & Broccoli Carrots	1 pkg (9.1 oz)	440	18	25	36
Chicken Marsala Carrots & Red Potatoes	1 pkg (8.8 oz)	180	15	5	19
Chicken Mesquite Corn & Pea Medley & Au Gratin Potatoes	1 pkg (8.8 oz)	320	18	8	44
Chicken Picatta	1 pkg (8.8 oz)	190	17	6	18
Chicken Stir Fry Kit	2¾ cups (14 oz)	430	24	5	73
Chicken w/ Broccoli & Cheese Carrots & Pasta	1 pkg (8.8 oz)	270	20	12	19
Chicken w/ Mushroom Sauce Rice Pilaf & Candied Carrots	1 pkg (8.8 oz)	220	15	6	27
Chicken w/ Tabasco BBQ Sauce	1 pkg (8.8 oz)	260	13	7	37
Fried Chicken & Gravy w/ Mashed Potatoes & Corn	1 pkg (10.8 oz)	360	16	15	39
Grilled Chicken Corn O'Brien & Ranch Beans	1 pkg (8.8 oz)	230	19	4	30
Grilled Italian Chicken Pasta & Vegetable Medley	1 pkg (8.8 oz)	190	21	4	19
Honey Dijon Chicken Pasta & Pea Medley	1 pkg (11.3 oz)	340	20	7	49
Roasted Chicken w/ Garlic Sauce Pasta & Vegetable Medley	1 pkg (8.8 oz)	210	17	7	20
Weight Watchers					
Smart One Grilled Salisbury Steak	1 pkg (8.5 oz)	250	18	9	24
Smart Ones Chicken Mirabella	1 pkg (9.2 oz)	180	11	2	30
Smart Ones Fiesta Chicken	1 pkg (8.5 oz)	210	13	2	35
Smart Ones Honey Mustard Chicken	1 pkg (8.5 oz)	200	11	2	35
Smart Ones Lemon Herb Chicken Piccata	1 pkg (8.5 oz)	190	11	2	33
Smart Ones Pepper Steak	1 pkg (10 oz)	240	18	5	32
Smart Ones Risotto w/ Cheese & Mushrooms	1 pkg (10 oz)	290	11	7	47
Smart Ones Roast Turkey Medallions & Mushrooms	1 pkg (8.5 oz)	180	11	2	30

FOOD	PORTION	CALS	PROT	FAT	CARB
Smart Ones Shrimp Marinara	1 pkg (9 oz)	180	9	2	31
Smart Ones Stuffed Turkey Breast	1 pkg (10 oz)	260	13	7	37
Smart Ones Swedish Meatballs	1 pkg (9 oz)	280	19	70	34
Yves					
Veggie Country Stew	1 pkg (10.5 oz)	170	17	0	24
DIP					
Breakstone's					
Bacon & Onion	2 tbsp (1.1 oz)	60	2	5	2
Chesapeake Clam	2 tbsp (1.1 oz)	50	1	4	1
Free Creamy Salsa	2 tbsp (1.1 oz)	20	1	0	3
Free French Onion	2 tbsp (1.1 oz)	25	2	0	4
Free Ranch	2 tbsp (1.1 oz)	25	2	0	4
French Onion	2 tbsp (1.1 oz)	50	1	5	2
Toasted Onion	2 tbsp (1.1 oz)	50	1	5	2
Cheez Whiz					
Medium Cheese & Salsa	2 tbsp (1.2 oz)	100	3	8	3
Mild Cheese & Salsa	2 tbsp (1.2 oz)	100	3	8	3
Chi-Chi's					
Fiesta Bean	2 tbsp (0.9 oz)	35	1	2	4
Fiesta Cheese	2 tbsp (0.9 oz)	40	1	3	3
Fritos					
Bean	2 tbsp (1.2 oz)	40	2	1	6
Chili Cheese	1.2 oz	45	1	3	3
French Onion	2 tbsp (1.1 oz)	60	1	5	4
Hot Bean	2 tbsp (1.2 oz)	40	2	1	5
Jalapeno & Cheddar Cheese	2 tbsp (1.2 oz)	50	1	4	4
Guiltless Gourmet					
Black Bean Mild	2 tbsp (1 oz)	30	2	0	5
Black Bean Spicy	2 tbsp (1 oz)	30	2	0	5
Knudsen					
Free Creamy Salsa	2 tbsp (1.1 oz)	20	1	0	3
Free French Onion	2 tbsp (1.1 oz)	25	2	0	4
Free Ranch	2 tbsp (1.1 oz)	25	2	0	4
Kraft					
Avocado	2 tbsp (1.1 oz)	60	1	4	4
Bacon & Horseradish	2 tbsp (1.1 oz)	60	1	5	3
Clam	2 tbsp (1.1 oz)	60	1	4	4
Free French Onion	2 tbsp (1.1 oz)	25	2	0	4
Free Ranch	2 tbsp (1.1 oz)	25	2	0	4
Free Salsa	2 tbsp (1.1 oz)	20	1	0	4
French Onion	2 tbsp (1.1 oz)	60	1	4	4
Green Onion	2 tbsp (1.1 oz)	60	1	4	4
Jalapeno Cheese	2 tbsp (1.1 oz)	60	1	4	3

FOOD	PORTION	CALS	PROT	FAT	CARB
Premium Sour Cream	2 tbsp (1.1 oz)	50	1	4	1
Premium Sour Cream Bacon & Horseradish	2 tbsp (1.1 oz)	60	2	5	2
Premium Sour Cream Bacon & Onion	2 tbsp (1.1 oz)	60	2	5	2
Premium Sour Cream Creamy Onion	2 tbsp (1.1 oz)	45	1	4	2
Ranch	2 tbsp (1.1 oz)	60	1	5	3
Ruffles					
French Onion	2 tbsp	70	1	5	4
Ranch	2 tbsp (1.2 oz)	70	1	6	4
Snyder's Of Hanover					
Microwavable Hot Nacho Cheese	2 tbsp	48	1	3	5
Microwavable Mild Cheese	2 tbsp	45	2	3	2
Mustard Pretzel	2 tbsp	60	1	2	12
Sour Cream & Onion	2 tbsp	60	1	5	2
Taco Bell					
Fat Free Black Bean	2 tbsp (1.2 oz)	30	2	0	6
Tyson					
Bleu Cheese For Dipping Wings	2 tbsp (1.4 oz)	140	1	14	3
Utz					
Fat Free Sour Cream & Onion	2 tbsp (1.1 oz)	30	1	0	7
Jalapeno & Cheddar	2 tbsp (1 oz)	30	0	3	2
Low Fat Desert Garden	2 tbsp (1.1 oz)	40	1	2	5
Low Fat Salsa Con Queso	2 tbsp (1 oz)	40	1	2	5
Mild Cheddar	2 tbsp (1 oz)	45	2	3	2
Sour Cream & Onion	2 tbsp (1 oz)	60	1	5	2
DOCK					
fresh cooked	3½ oz	20	1	1	3
DOLPHINFISH					
fresh baked	3 oz	93	20	1	0
fresh fillet baked	5.6 oz	174	38	1	0
DOUGHNUTS					
cake type unsugared	1 (1.6 oz)	198	2	11	23
chocolate glazed	1 (1.5 oz)	175	2	8	24
chocolate sugared	1 (1.5 oz)	175	2	8	24
chocolate coated	1 (1.5 oz)	204	2	13	21
creme filled	1 (3 oz)	307	6	21	26
french cruller glazed	1 (1.4 oz)	169	1	8	24
frosted	1 (1.5 oz)	204	2	13	21
honey bun	1 (2.1 oz)	242	4	14	27
jelly	1 (3 oz)	289	5	16	33
old fashioned	1 (1.6 oz)	198	2	11	23
sugared	1 (1.6 oz)	192	2	10	23

FOOD	PORTION	CALS	PROT	FAT	CARB
wheat glazed	1 (1.6 oz)	162	3	9	19
wheat sugared	1 (1.6 oz)	162	3	9	19
yeast glazed	1 (2.1 oz)	242	4	14	27
Dolly Madison					
Chocolate Frosted	1 (1.1 oz)	140	1	8	15
Donut Gems Chocolate	4 (2 oz)	260	3	15	28
Donut Gems Crunch	3 (2 oz)	220	3	10	31
Donut Gems Powdered	4 (2 oz)	230	3	11	30
English Cruller	1 (2 oz)	250	2	14	31
Glazed Whirl	1 (1.6 oz)	210	2	11	25
Glazed Yeast	1 (1.5 oz)	190	2	9	23
Old Fashioned	1 (2.1 oz)	280	4	16	28
Plain	1 (1.2 oz)	140	2	7	15
Powdered	1 (1 oz)	120	1	6	14
Dutch Mill					
Cider	1 (2.1 oz)	240	3	10	35
Cinnamon	1 (1.8 oz)	210	3	11	26
Donut Holes Double-Dipped Chocolate	3 (1.4 oz)	220	2	16	19
Donut Holes Shootin' Stars	3 (1.4 oz)	190	2	10	23
Double-Dipped Chocolate	1 (2.1 oz)	280	3	17	31
Glazed	1 (2.1 oz)	250	3	12	34
Glazed Chocolate	1 (2.4 oz)	270	3	11	40
Plain	1 (1.8 oz)	210	3	12	25
Sugared	1 (1.8 oz)	220	3	11	27
Hostess					
Blueberry	1 (1.7 oz)	210	2	13	21
Donettes Crumb	3 (1.5 oz)	170	2	8	23
Donettes Frosted	3 (1.5 oz)	200	2	12	21
Donettes Powdered	3 (1.5 oz)	180	2	9	23
Frosted	1 (1.4 oz)	180	2	11	19
O's Raspberry Filled	1 (2.2 oz)	230	3	10	34
Old Fashioned Glazed	1 (2.1 oz)	260	2	13	33
Plain	1 (1.1 oz)	140	2	7	15
Powdered	1 (1.3 oz)	150	2	8	19
Little Debbie					
Donut Sticks	1 (1.6 oz)	210	2	12	24
Mini Powdered	1 pkg (2.5 oz)	290	3	14	38
Tastykake					
Mini Plain Glaze	1 pkg (2.5 oz)	260	3	11	40
Mini Powdered Sugar	1 pkg (2.5 oz)	260	3	12	38
Mini Rich Frosted	1 pkg (3 oz)	370	5	22	43
Tom's					
Chocolate Gem	1 pkg (2.5 oz)	320	4	18	37
Dunkin' Sticks	1 pkg (2.5 oz)	370	2	22	43
Powdered Gems	1 pkg (2.5 oz)	320	3	18	41

FOOD	PORTION	CALS	PROT	FAT	CARB
DRESSING					
(see STUFFING/DRESSING)					
DRINK MIXERS					
(see also SODA, WATER)					
whiskey sour mix	2 oz	55	0	0	14
Daily's					
Bloody Mary Original	1 serv (6 oz)	50	0	0	14
Margarita Daiquiri Strawberry	1 serv (4 oz)	180	0	0	47
Margarita Green Demon	1 serv (3 oz)	80	0	0	19
Pina Colada	1 serv (3 oz)	160	0	2	37
Tabasco					
Bloody Mary Mix	1 serv (8.4 oz)	56	2	tr	11
Bloody Mary Mix Extra Spicy	1 serv (8.4 oz)	58	3	tr	11
DRUM					
freshwater fillet baked	5.4 oz	236	35	10	0
freshwater baked	3 oz	130	19	5	0
DUCK					
w/ skin roasted	1 cup (4.9 oz)	472	27	40	0
w/ skin w/ bone leg roasted	3 oz	184	23	10	0
w/ skin w/o bone breast roasted	3 oz	172	21	9	0
w/o skin roasted	1 cup (4.9 oz)	281	33	16	0
w/o skin w/ bone leg braised	1 cup (6.1 oz)	310	51	10	0
w/o skin w/o bone breast broiled	1 cup (6.1 oz)	244	48	4	0
wild w/ skin raw	½ duck (9.5 oz)	571	47	41	0
wild w/o skin breast raw	½ breast (2.9 oz)	102	16	4	0
Grimaud Farms					
Muscovy Duck Confit	1 serv (3 oz)	170	20	10	tr
DUMPLING					
Health Is Wealth					
Potstickers Chicken Free	2 (1.6 oz)	80	4	4	11
Potstickers Pork Free	2 (1.6 oz)	80	4	4	11
Potstickers Vegetable	2 (1.6 oz)	90	7	3	11
Steamed Dumpling	2 (1.6 oz)	50	7	2	12
Pepperidge Farm					
Apple	1 (3 oz)	230	3	11	30
Peach	1 (3 oz)	320	3	11	50
DURIAN					
fresh	3.5 oz	141	3	2	29
EDAMAME					
(see SOYBEANS)					
EEL					
fresh cooked	3 oz	200	20	13	0
fresh cooked	1 fillet (5.6 oz)	375	38	24	0

FOOD	PORTION	CALS	PROT	FAT	CARB
raw	3 oz	156	16	10	0
smoked	3.5 oz	330	19	28	0

EGG
(see also EGG DISHES, EGG SUBSTITUTES)

chicken

FOOD	PORTION	CALS	PROT	FAT	CARB
fresh	1	75	6	5	1
frozen	1	75	6	5	1
frozen	1 cup	363	30	24	3
hard cooked	1	77	6	5	1
hard cooked chopped	1 cup	210	17	14	2
poached	1	74	6	5	1
white only	1	17	4	0	tr
white only	1 cup	121	26	0	2
Horizon Organic					
Medium	1 (1.5 oz)	70	6	4	1
Organic Valley					
Brown Extra Large	1 (2.2 oz)	90	8	6	tr
Brown Large	1 (2 oz)	80	7	6	tr
Brown Medium	1 (1.8 oz)	70	6	5	tr

other poultry

FOOD	PORTION	CALS	PROT	FAT	CARB
duck	1 (2.5 oz)	130	9	10	1
duck 100 year old	1 (1 oz)	49	4	3	1
duck preserved hard core	1 (1.8 oz)	80	6	6	1
duck preserved soft core	1 (1.8 oz)	80	7	6	1
duck salted	1 (1 oz)	54	4	4	2
goose	1 (5 oz)	267	20	19	2
quail	1 (9 g)	14	1	1	tr
turkey	1 (2.7 oz)	135	9	9	1

EGG DISHES

frozen

FOOD	PORTION	CALS	PROT	FAT	CARB
Weight Watchers					
Handy Ham & Cheese Omelet	1 (4 oz)	220	13	5	30

take-out

FOOD	PORTION	CALS	PROT	FAT	CARB
deviled	2 halves	145	6	13	1
omelette plain	1 serv (3.5 oz)	172	15	13	tr
salad	½ cup	307	13	28	2
scotch egg	1 (4.2 oz)	301	14	21	16
scrambled plain	2 (3.3 oz)	199	13	15	2
scrambled w/ whole milk & margarine	1 serv	365	24	27	5
sunny side up	1	91	6	7	1

EGG ROLLS
(see also ASIAN FOODS)

FOOD	PORTION	CALS	PROT	FAT	CARB
egg roll wrapper fresh	1	83	3	tr	16
Chun King					
Chicken Mini	6	210	6	9	25
Chicken Restaurant Style	1 (3 oz)	190	6	9	22

FOOD	PORTION	CALS	PROT	FAT	CARB
Pork & Shrimp Mini	6	210	6	9	27
Shrimp Mini	6	190	5	6	28
Shrimp Restaurant Style	1 (3 oz)	180	5	7	25
Health Is Wealth					
Broccoli	1 (3 oz)	150	4	5	23
Oriental Vegetable	1 (3 oz)	160	4	4	23
Oriental Chicken Free	1 (3 oz)	120	8	4	21
Pizza	1 (3 oz)	200	7	9	23
Spinach	1 (3 oz)	180	7	8	20
Spring Rolls	1 (1.6 oz)	70	2	2	10
Veggie	1 (3 oz)	130	4	4	21
La Choy					
Chicken Mini	6	210	6	9	25
Chicken Restaurant Style	1 (3 oz)	210	6	9	25
Pork Restaurant Style	1 (3 oz)	220	5	11	24
Pork & Shrimp Bite Size	12	210	6	10	25
Pork & Shrimp Mini	6	210	6	9	27
Shrimp Mini	6	190	5	6	28
Shrimp Restaurant Style	1 (3 oz)	180	5	7	25
Sweet & Sour Chicken Restaurant Style	1 (3 oz)	220	6	9	29
Vegetable w/ Lobster Mini	6	190	5	7	27
Worthington					
Vegetarian Egg Rolls	1 (3 oz)	180	6	8	20
take-out					
lobster	1 (4.8 oz)	270	8	7	43
lumpia vegetable & shrimp	2 (3 oz)	120	4	0	26
meat & shrimp	1 (4.8 oz)	320	10	12	41
pork & shrimp	1 (5 oz)	300	13	10	41
shrimp	1 (3 oz)	170	6	5	24
spicy pork	1 (3 oz)	200	6	9	23
vegetable	1 (3 oz)	170	5	4	28
EGG SUBSTITUTES					
frozen	¼ cup	96	7	7	2
frozen	1 cup	384	27	27	8
liquid	1 cup (8.8 oz)	211	30	8	2
liquid	1½ oz	40	6	2	tr
powder	0.35 oz	44	5	1	2
powder	0.7 oz	88	11	3	4
Better'n Eggs					
Fat Free Cholesterol Free	¼ cup (2 oz)	30	6	0	1
Egg Beaters					
Eggs Substitute	¼ cup	30	5	0	1
Morningstar Farms					
Breakfast Sandwich Bagel Scramblers Pattie Cheese	1 (5.9 oz)	320	28	5	40

FOOD	PORTION	CALS	PROT	FAT	CARB
Breakfast Sandwich English Muffin Scramblers Pattie	1 (5.1 oz)	240	22	3	32
Breakfast Sandwich English Muffin Scramblers Pattie Cheese	1 (6 oz)	280	28	3	35
Scramblers	¼ cup (2 oz)	35	6	0	2
EGGNOG					
eggnog	1 cup	342	10	19	34
eggnog	1 qt	1368	39	76	138
eggnog flavor mix as prep w/ milk	9 oz	260	8	8	39
Oberweis					
Egg Nog	½ cup	240	3	15	25
EGGNOG SUBSTITUTES					
Silk					
Nog	½ cup	90	3	2	15
EGGPLANT					
slices grilled	4 (7 oz)	38	2	0	0
whole peeled raw	1 (1 lb)	117	5	1	28
Progresso					
Caponata	2 tbsp (1 oz)	25	0	2	2
TastyBite					
Punjab Eggplant	½ pkg (5 oz)	130	5	8	9
take-out					
baba ghannouj	¼ cup	55	2	4	5
caponata	2 tbsp (1 oz)	30	1	2	3
iman bayildi eggplant w/ onion & tomato	1 serv (15.6 oz)	345	3	28	25
indian eggplant runi	1 serv	180	2	14	13
papoutsakis little shoes	1 serv (15.5 oz)	245	12	16	15
ELDERBERRIES					
fresh	1 cup	105	1	1	27
ELDERBERRY JUICE					
elderberry	7 oz	76	4	0	16
ELK					
roasted	3 oz	124	26	2	0
ENDIVE					
fresh	3.5 oz	9	2	tr	tr
ENERGY BARS					
(*see also* CEREAL BARS, ENERGY DRINKS, NUTRITION SUPPLEMENTS)					
AllGoode Organics					
Amazin' Peanut Raisin	1 bar	210	7	11	25
Banana Nut Nirvana	1 bar	190	5	8	30
Cashew Almond Passion	1 bar	210	7	9	25
Chocolate Peanut Pleasure	1 bar	200	5	9	29
Honey Nut Harvest	1 bar	210	7	9	29

FOOD	PORTION	CALS	PROT	FAT	CARB
Nutty Chocolate Apricot	1 bar	200	6	10	26
Balance					
Oasis Strawberry Cheesecake	1 bar (1.69 oz)	180	8	3	28
Benecol					
Chocolate Crisp	1 bar (1.2 oz)	130	3	3	23
Chocolate Crisp	1 bar (1.2 oz)	130	3	3	23
Peanut Crisp	1 bar (1.2 oz)	140	3	4	23
Better Bar					
Chocolate Coated Caramel Pecan	1 bar (1.8 oz)	180	18	4	15
Chocolate Coated Peanut	1 bar (1.8 oz)	180	18	4	15
Yogurt Coated Raspberry	1 bar (1.8 oz)	180	18	3	15
Breakthru					
Organic Chocolate Fudge	1 bar (2.1 oz)	230	10	3	39
Organic Cinnamon Crunch	1 bar (2.1 oz)	220	12	3	37
Organic Honey Graham	1 bar (2.1 oz)	220	12	3	37
Organic Mocha Fudge	1 bar (2.1 oz)	230	10	3	39
Centrum					
Energy Chocolate Nougat	1 (1.98 oz)	220	8	5	34
Energy Chocolate Peanut Butter	1 (1.98 oz)	220	8	5	34
Clif Bar					
Apricot	1 bar (2.4 oz)	220	8	3	43
Carrot Cake	1 bar (2.4 oz)	240	10	4	43
Chocolate Brownie	1 bar (2.4 oz)	240	10	4	41
Chocolate Almond Fudge	1 bar (2.4 oz)	230	10	5	36
Chocolate Chip	1 bar (2.4 oz)	240	10	4	41
Chocolate Chip Peanut Crunch	1 bar (2.4 oz)	240	12	5	39
Cookies'N Cream	1 bar (2.4 oz)	230	10	4	39
Cranberry Apple Cherry	1 bar (2.4 oz)	220	8	2	44
Crunchy Peanut Butter	1 bar (2.4 oz)	240	12	5	39
GingerSnap	1 bar (2.4 oz)	230	10	4	42
Ensure					
All Flavors	1 bar (2.1 oz)	230	9	6	35
Extend					
Chocolate Chip Crunch	1 bar (1.4 oz)	160	3	3	31
Peanut Butter Crunch	1 bar (1.4 oz)	160	4	3	30
Glucerna					
All Flavors	1 bar (1.3 oz)	140	6	4	24
HeartBar					
Cranberry	1 bar (1.8 oz)	190	13	3	27
Original	1 bar (1.76 oz)	180	14	3	26
Jenny Craig					
Meal Bar Chocolate Peanut	1 bar (2 oz)	220	10	5	33
Meal Bar Lemon Meringue	1 bar (2 oz)	210	10	5	31
Meal Bar Milk Chocolate	1 bar (2 oz)	210	10	5	33

FOOD	PORTION	CALS	PROT	FAT	CARB
Meal Bar Oatmeal Raisin	1 bar (1.97 oz)	210	10	3	35
Meal Bar Yogurt Peanut	1 bar (2 oz)	220	10	5	33
Kashi					
GoLean Chocolate Peanut Butter	1 (2.7 oz)	280	13	6	50
GoLean Honey Vanilla Yogurt	1 (2.7 oz)	280	11	4	53
GoLean Strawberry Vanilla Yogurt	1 (2.7 oz)	280	11	4	53
Lean Body For Her					
Chocolate Honey Peanut	1 bar (1.76 oz)	190	16	7	10
Luna					
Chai Tea	1 bar (1.7 oz)	180	10	4	27
Chocolate Pecan Pie	1 bar (1.7 oz)	180	10	5	24
LemonZest	1 bar (1.7 oz)	180	10	4	24
Nutz Over Chocolate	1 bar (1.7 oz)	180	10	5	24
S'Mores	1 bar (1.7 oz)	180	10	4	26
Sesame Raisin Crunch	1 bar (1.7 oz)	170	10	3	26
Toasted Nuts 'n Cranberry	1 bar (1.7 oz)	170	10	3	26
Tropical Crisp	1 bar (1.7 oz)	180	10	5	24
Met-Rx					
Big 100 Gram Bar Peanut Butter	1 bar (3.5 oz)	340	26	4	52
Source/One Chocolate Cheesecake	1 bar (2.1 oz)	160	15	5	21
Nutiva					
Flaxseed & Raisin Organic	1 bar (1.4 oz)	280	14	19	12
Hempseed Bar Organic	1 bar (1.4 oz)	210	9	14	11
Nutribar					
Chocolate Covered Belgian Chocolate	1 bar (2.3 oz)	252	13	8	33
Chocolate Covered Chocolate Fudge	1 bar (2.3 oz)	267	14	8	35
Chocolate Covered Hazelnut	1 bar (2.3 oz)	261	13	8	34
Chocolate Covered Mocha Almond	1 bar (2.3 oz)	261	13	8	34
Chocolate Covered Peanut	1 bar (2.3 oz)	262	13	9	34
Yogurt Covered Peach Apricot	1 bar (2.3 oz)	261	13	8	34
Yogurt Covered Raspberry	1 bar (2.3 oz)	261	13	8	34
Yogurt Covered Wildberry	1 bar (2.3 oz)	261	13	8	34
Odwalla Bar!					
Peanut Crunch	1 bar (2.2 oz)	260	8	7	40
PermaLean					
Protein Crunch Chocoholic Chocolate	1 bar (1.8 oz)	170	21	3	10

FOOD	PORTION	CALS	PROT	FAT	CARB
Protein Crunch Chocolate Raspberry	1 bar (1.8 oz)	180	21	2	9
Protein Crunch Stark Raving Peanutz	1 bar (1.8 oz)	180	21	4	9
PowerBar					
Apple Cinnamon	1 bar (2.3 oz)	230	10	3	45
Banana	1 bar (2.3 oz)	230	9	2	45
Chocolate	1 bar (2.3 oz)	230	10	2	45
Essentials Chocolate	1 bar (1.9 oz)	180	10	4	28
Harvest Blueberry	1 bar (2.3 oz)	240	7	4	45
Harvest Strawberry	1 bar (2.3 oz)	240	7	4	45
Malt-Nut	1 bar (2.3 oz)	230	10	3	45
Mocha	1 bar (2.3 oz)	230	10	3	45
Oatmeal Raisin	1 bar (2.3 oz)	230	10	3	45
Peanut Butter	1 bar (2.3 oz)	230	10	3	45
Power Gel Strawberry Banana	1 pkg	110	0	0	28
Vanilla Crisp	1 bar (2.3 oz)	230	9	3	45
Wild Berry	1 bar (2.3 oz)	230	10	3	45
Revival					
Marshmallow Krunch	1 bar (2.1 oz)	220	17	3	30
Protein Bars Chocolate Temptation	1 bar (2.1 oz)	220	15	4	31
Protein Bars Peanut Butter Chocolate Pal	1 bar (2.1 oz)	240	16	6	30
Protein Bars Peanut Butter Pal	1 bar (2.1 oz)	240	17	5	29
Slim-Fast					
Crispy Peanut Caramel	1 bar	120	1	4	21
Dutch Chocolate	1 bar	140	5	5	20
Meal On-The-Go Apple Cobbler	1 bar	220	8	5	33
Meal On-The-Go Chocolate Cookie Dough	1 bar	220	8	5	35
Meal On-The-Go Honey Peanut	1 bar	220	8	5	34
Meal On-The-Go Milk Chocolate Peanut	1 bar	220	8	5	36
Meal On-The-Go Oatmeal Raisin	1 bar	220	8	5	36
Meal On-The-Go Rich Chocolate Brownie	1 bar	220	8	5	34
Meal On-The-Go Toasted Oat & Spice	1 bar	220	8	5	35
Peanut Butter	1 bar	150	6	5	19
Peanut Butter Crunch	1 bar	130	1	4	21
Sweet Success					
Chewy Chocolate Brownie	1 bar (1.2 oz)	120	2	4	23

FOOD	PORTION	CALS	PROT	FAT	CARB
Think!					
Apple Spice	1 bar (2 oz)	205	5	3	40
Chocolate Almond Coconut Raisin	1 bar (2 oz)	243	6	7	39
Chocolate Fruit Harvest	1 bar (2 oz)	217	5	3	43
ZonePerfect					
Honey Peanut	1 bar (1.8 oz)	200	14	7	22
ENERGY DRINKS					
(*see also* ENERGY BARS, NUTRITION SUPPLEMENTS)					
California Joe					
All Natural Protein Drink Mix as prep	1 serv (8 oz)	165	12	4	21
Fat Burner					
Diet Fruit Punch	8 fl oz	0	8	0	0
Hansen's					
D-Stress	1 can (8.2 oz)	110	0	0	31
Energy	1 can (8.3 oz)	120	0	0	32
Healthy Pleasures					
Chocolate Irish Cream	1 bottle (10.5 oz)	260	12	2	45
Kashi					
GoLean Shake Man	1 pkg (2.5 oz)	260	30	1	34
GoLean Shake Woman	1 pkg (2.5 oz)	250	30	2	32
Nantucket Nectars					
Super Nectars Ginkgo Mango	8 oz	150	0	0	38
Super Nectars Protein Smoothie	8 oz	170	2	1	38
Super Nectars Red Guarana Tea	8 oz	110	0	0	26
NutraShake					
Citrus	1 pkg (4 oz)	200	6	0	44
Citrus Free	1 serv (4 oz)	200	6	0	44
Vanilla	1 serv (8 oz)	400	12	12	62
Vanilla No Added Sugar	1 serv (4 oz)	200	7	8	25
Pounds Off					
Dark Chocolate Ectasy	1 can (11 oz)	200	11	3	39
French Vanilla	1 can (11 oz)	220	12	3	41
Powerade					
Fruit Punch	8 fl oz	70	0	0	19
Lemon Lime	8 fl oz	70	0	0	19
Mountain Blast	8 fl oz	70	0	0	19
Red Bull					
Energy Drink	1 can (8.3 oz)	113	0	0	28
Slim-Fast					
Chocolate as prep w/ fat free milk	1 serv	190	14	1	32
Chocolate Malt as prep w/ fat free milk	1 serv	190	14	1	32

FOOD	PORTION	CALS	PROT	FAT	CARB
JumpStart Chocolate as prep w/ fat free milk	1 serv	240	18	2	39
JumpStart Vanilla as prep w/ fat free milk	1 serv	240	18	2	39
Strawberry as prep w/ fat free milk	1 serv	190	14	1	32
Vanilla as prep w/ fat free milk	1 serv	190	14	1	32
SoBe					
Adrenaline Rush	1 can (8.3 oz)	140	1	0	36
Drive	8 oz	120	0	0	32
Edge	8 fl oz	110	0	0	30
Elixir 3C Strawberry Carrot	8 fl oz	90	0	0	25
Jing Essentials	1 bottle (14 oz)	140	0	0	36
Jing Essentials Citrus Soy Blend	1 bottle (14 oz)	170	1	1	44
Karma	8 oz	120	0	0	33
Lean Sugar Free Metabolic Enhancer Diet Green Tea	8 fl oz	5	0	0	1
Lean Sugar Free Metabolic Enhancer Diet Orange Carrot	8 fl oz	10	0	0	2
Lizard Lightning Orange Mango	8 fl oz	130	0	0	33
Qi Essential Berry Soy Blend	1 bottle (14 oz)	170	1	1	44
Qi Essentials	1 bottle (14 oz)	140	0	0	36
Shen Essentials	1 bottle (14 oz)	140	0	0	36
Shen Essentials Peach Soy Blend	1 bottle (14 oz)	170	1	1	44
Tsunami Orange Cream	8 fl oz	110	0	0	29
Sweet Success					
Creamy Milk Chocolate	1 can	200	10	3	36
Creamy Milk Chocolate as prep w/ skim milk	1 serv	180	11	1	36
TwinLab					
Hydra Fuel	16 fl oz	132	0	0	33
Nitro Fuel	16 oz	460	15	0	100
Ultra Fuel	1 bottle (16 oz)	400	0	0	100
Ultra Slim-Fast					
Cafe Mocha as prep w/ fat free milk	1 serv	200	14	2	36
Chocolate Fudge as prep w/ fat free milk	1 serv	200	14	3	36
Chocolate Malt as prep w/ fat free milk	1 serv	200	14	2	36
Chocolate Royale as prep w/ fat free milk	1 serv	200	14	2	36

FOOD	PORTION	CALS	PROT	FAT	CARB
Fruit Juice Mixable as prep w/ juice	1 serv	200	12	1	44
Milk Chocolate as prep w/ fat free milk	1 serv	210	14	2	34
Ready-To-Drink Apple Cranberry Raspberry	1 serv	220	7	2	46
Ready-To-Drink Cappuccino Delight	1 serv	220	10	2	42
Ready-To-Drink Chocolate Royale	1 serv	220	10	3	38
Ready-To-Drink Creamy Milk Chocolate	1 serv	220	10	3	42
Ready-To-Drink Dark Chocolate Fudge	1 serv	220	10	3	42
Ready-To-Drink Orange Strawberry Banana	1 serv	220	7	2	46
Ready-To-Drink Orange Pineapple	1 serv	220	7	2	46
Ready-To-Drink Strawberries N' Cream	1 serv	220	10	3	40
Strawberry as prep w/ fat free milk	1 serv	200	14	1	37
Vanilla as prep w/ fat free milk	1 serv	200	14	1	37
ENGLISH MUFFIN					
frozen					
Weight Watchers					
Sandwich	1 (4 oz)	210	13	5	28
ready-to-eat					
apple cinnamon	1	138	4	2	28
crumpets	1 (1.5 oz)	80	3	0	16
granola	1	155	6	1	31
mixed grain	1	155	6	1	31
plain	1	134	4	1	26
plain toasted	1	133	4	1	26
raisin cinnamon	1	138	4	2	28
sourdough	1	134	4	1	26
wheat	1	127	5	1	26
whole wheat	1	134	6	1	27
Milton's					
Multi-Grain	1 (2 oz)	150	4	1	33
Wonder					
Cinnamon Raisin	1 (2.1 oz)	140	5	2	26
Original	1 (2 oz)	130	4	1	25
Sourdough	1 (2 oz)	130	4	1	25
take-out					
w/ butter	1 (2.2 oz)	189	5	6	30
w/ cheese & sausage	1 (4 oz)	393	15	24	29

FOOD	PORTION	CALS	PROT	FAT	CARB
w/ egg cheese & canadian bacon	1 (4.8 oz)	289	17	13	28
w/ egg cheese & sausage	1 (5.8 oz)	487	22	31	31
EPAZOTE					
fresh	1 tbsp (1 g)	tr	0	0	tr
FALAFEL					
take-out					
falafel	1 (1.2 oz)	57	2	3	5
FAT					
(see also BUTTER, BUTTER BLENDS, BUTTER SUBSTITUTES, MARGARINE, OIL)					
beef cooked	1 oz	193	3	20	0
beef tallow	1 tbsp (13 g)	115	0	13	0
chicken	1 cup	1846	0	205	0
chicken	1 tbsp	115	0	13	0
cocoa butter	1 tbsp	120	0	14	0
duck	1 tbsp (13 g)	115	0	13	0
goose	1 tbsp	115	0	13	0
goose	1 oz	257	0	29	0
lamb new zealand	1 oz	182	2	19	0
lard	1 tbsp (13 g)	115	0	13	0
lard	1 cup (205 g)	1849	0	205	0
nutmeg butter	1 tbsp	120	0	14	0
pork backfat	1 oz	230	1	25	0
pork cooked	1 oz	178	3	18	0
salt pork	1 oz	212	23	23	0
shortening	1 cup	1812	0	205	0
shortening	1 tbsp	113	0	13	0
turkey	1 tbsp	115	0	13	0
ucuhuba butter	1 tbsp	120	0	14	0
FAT SUBSTITUTES					
Smucker's					
Baking Healthy 100% Fat Free	1 tbsp	30	0	0	7
FAVA BEANS					
Progresso					
Fava Beans	½ cup (4.6 oz)	110	6	1	20
FEIJOA					
fresh	1 (1.75 oz)	25	1	tr	5
puree	1 cup	119	3	2	26
FENNEL					
fresh bulb	1 (8.2 oz)	72	3	tr	17
fresh sliced	1 cup	27	1	tr	6
FENUGREEK					
seed	1 tsp	12	1	tr	2
FIBER					
Benefiber					
Supplement	1 pkg (4 g)	20	0	0	4

FOOD	PORTION	CALS	PROT	FAT	CARB
Metamucil					
Fiber Wafers Apple Crisp	2	120	2	5	17
ND Labs					
Pure Apple Fiber	1 tbsp (7 g)	16	0	0	7
FIDDLEHEAD FERNS					
fresh	3.5 oz	34	5	tr	6
FIGS					
calimyrna	3 (5.4 oz)	120	1	0	28
dried cooked	½ cup	140	2	1	16
dried whole	10	477	6	2	122
FIREWEED					
leaves chopped	1 cup (0.8 oz)	24	1	1	4
FISH					
(*see also individual names,* FISH SUBSTITUTES, SUSHI)					
frozen					
breaded fillet	1 (2 oz)	155	9	7	14
sticks	1 stick (1 oz)	76	4	3	7
Gorton's					
Baked Au Gratin	1 piece (4.6 oz)	130	14	5	7
Baked Broccoli Cheddar	1 piece (4.6 oz)	130	14	5	7
Baked Primavera	1 piece (4.6 oz)	120	15	5	4
Batter Dipped Portions	1 piece (2.5 oz)	170	6	11	12
Crunchy Golden Fillets Breaded	2 (3.8 oz)	250	10	14	21
Crunchy Golden Sticks	6 (3.8 oz)	250	12	13	21
Garlic & Herb	2 pieces (3.6 oz)	220	10	11	21
Garlic Butter Crumb	1 piece (4.6 oz)	170	17	9	5
Grilled Cajun Blackened	1 piece (3.8 oz)	120	16	6	1
Grilled Garlic Butter	1 piece (3.8 oz)	120	16	6	1
Grilled Italian Herb	1 piece (3.8 oz)	130	17	6	2
Grilled Lemon Butter	1 piece (3.8 oz)	120	16	6	1
Grilled Lemon Pepper	1 piece (3.8 oz)	120	16	6	1
Parmesan	2 pieces (3.6 oz)	260	10	15	20
Ranch	1 piece (3.6 oz)	240	9	13	22
Southern Fried Country Style	2 pieces (3.6 oz)	230	10	14	16
Tenders	3.5 pieces (4 oz)	250	11	14	20
Tenders Extra Crunchy	3.5 pieces (4 oz)	270	11	12	29
Mrs. Paul's					
Buttered Fillet Microwave	1 fillet	80	10	4	10
Fillet Sandwich Microwave	1	280	10	15	27
Fillets Microwave	1 fillet	280	12	19	16
Fish Sticks 40 Crunchy	4 (2.75 oz)	200	10	10	18
Fish Sticks Microwave	5	290	10	20	18
Seafood Platter Combination	9 oz	600	19	33	55
take-out					
fish cake	1 (4.7 oz)	166	18	7	6

FOOD	PORTION	CALS	PROT	FAT	CARB
jamaican brown fish stew	1 serv	426	48	22	9
kedgeree	5.6 oz	242	21	11	15
mousse	1 serv (3.5 oz)	185	13	14	3
stew	1 cup (7.9 oz)	157	19	4	10
taramasalata	2 tbsp	124	1	14	1
FISH OIL					
cod liver	1 tbsp	123	0	14	0
herring	1 tbsp	123	0	14	0
menhaden	1 tbsp	123	0	14	0
salmon	1 tbsp	123	0	14	0
sardine	1 tbsp	123	0	14	0
shark	1 oz	270	0	29	0
whale	1 oz	270	0	29	0
FISH PASTE					
fish paste	2 tsp	15	1	1	tr
FISH SUBSTITUTES					
Loma Linda					
Ocean Platter not prep	⅓ cup (0.9 oz)	90	14	1	8
Worthington					
Fillets	2 (3 oz)	180	16	10	8
Tuno	½ cup (1.9 oz)	80	6	6	2
FLAXSEED					
Bite Me					
Flax Bar	1 bar (1.8 oz)	242	7	11	30
FLOUNDER					
fresh					
cooked	3 oz	99	21	1	0
cooked	1 fillet (4.5 oz)	148	31	2	0
take-out					
battered & fried	3.2 oz	211	13	11	15
breaded & fried	3.2 oz	211	13	11	15
FLOUR					
buckwheat whole groat	1 cup (4.2 oz)	402	15	4	85
corn masa	1 cup (4 oz)	416	11	4	87
cottonseed lowfat	1 oz	94	14	tr	10
peanut defatted	1 cup	196	31	tr	21
peanut defatted	1 oz	92	15	tr	10
peanut lowfat	1 cup	257	20	13	19
potato	1 cup (6.3 oz)	628	14	1	143
rice brown	1 cup (5.5 oz)	574	11	4	121
rice white	1 cup (5.5 oz)	578	9	2	127
rye dark	1 cup (4.5 oz)	415	18	3	88
rye light	1 cup (3.6 oz)	374	9	1	82
rye medium	1 cup (3.6 oz)	361	10	2	79
sesame lowfat	1 oz	95	14	tr	10
triticale whole grain	1 cup (4.6 oz)	439	17	2	95
white all-purpose	1 cup (4.4 oz)	455	13	1	95
white bread	1 cup (4.8 oz)	495	16	2	99

FOOD	PORTION	CALS	PROT	FAT	CARB
white cake unsifted	1 cup (4.8 oz)	496	11	1	107
white self-rising	1 cup (4.4 oz)	443	12	1	93
white unbleached	1 cup (4.4 oz)	455	13	1	95
whole wheat	1 cup (4.2 oz)	407	16	2	87
All Trump					
Flour	¼ cup (1 oz)	100	4	0	22
Betty Crocker					
Softasilk Velvet Cake Flour	¼ cup (1 oz)	100	2	0	23
Gold Medal					
All Purpose	¼ cup (1 oz)	100	3	0	22
Better For Bread	¼ cup (1 oz)	100	4	0	22
Organic All Purpose	¼ cup (1 oz)	100	3	0	22
Self Rising	¼ cup (1 oz)	100	3	0	22
Unbleached	¼ cup (1 oz)	100	3	0	22
Wondra	¼ cup	100	3	0	23
Hodgson Mill					
White Unbleached Organic	¼ cup (1 oz)	100	3	0	23
Whole Wheat Graham Organic	¼ cup (1 oz)	100	3	1	22
La Pina					
Flour	¼ cup (1 oz)	100	2	0	23
Red Band					
All Purpose	¼ cup (1 oz)	100	2	0	23
Self-Rising	¼ cup (1 oz)	100	2	0	22
Robin Hood					
All Purpose	¼ cup (1 oz)	100	3	0	22
Self-Rising	¼ cup (1 oz)	100	3	0	22
Unbleached	¼ cup (1 oz)	100	3	0	22
Whole Wheat	¼ cup (1 oz)	90	4	1	21
FRANKFURTER					
(*see* HOT DOG)					
FRENCH BEANS					
dried cooked	1 cup	228	12	1	43
FRENCH FRIES					
(*see* POTATOES)					
FRENCH TOAST					
frozen					
french toast	1 slice (2 oz)	126	4	4	19
home recipe					
as prep w/ 2% milk	1 slice	149	7	7	16
as prep w/ whole milk	1 slice	151	7	7	16
take-out					
sticks	5 (4.9 oz)	513	8	29	58
w/ butter	2 slices (4.7 oz)	356	10	19	36

FOOD	PORTION	CALS	PROT	FAT	CARB
FROG'S LEGS					
as prep w/ seasoned flour & fried	1 (0.8)	70	4	5	15
FROSTING					
(*see* CAKE ICING)					
FRUCTOSE					
Estee					
Fructose	1 tsp	15	0	0	4
Packet	1 pkg	10	0	0	3
FRUIT DRINKS					
(*see also individual names,* LEMONADE)					
frozen					
citrus juice drink as prep	1 cup	114	1	0	28
citrus juice drink not prep	1 can (12 fl oz)	684	5	tr	171
fruit punch not prep	1 can (12 fl oz)	678	1	tr	173
Tree Of Life					
Organic Smoothie Banana Raspberry Strawberry	⅔ cup (5 oz)	90	1	0	23
Organic Smoothie Mango Strawberry Raspberry	⅔ cup (5 oz)	70	1	0	18
Organic Smoothie Strawberry Banana	⅔ cup (5 oz)	90	7	0	23
Organic Smoothie Strawberry Blueberry Banana	⅔ cup (5 oz)	90	1	0	22
mix					
Crystal Light					
Fruit Punch as prep	1 serv (8 oz)	5	0	0	0
Lemon-Lime Drink as prep	1 serv (8 oz)	5	0	0	0
Passion Fruit Pineapple Drink as prep	1 serv (8 oz)	5	0	0	tr
Pineapple Orange Drink as prep	1 serv (8 oz)	5	0	0	0
Strawberry Orange Banana as prep	1 serv (8 oz)	5	0	0	0
Strawberry Kiwi as prep	1 serv (8 oz)	5	0	0	0
Watermelon Strawberry as prep	1 serv (8 oz)	5	0	0	0
Kool-Aid					
Cherry as prep	1 serv (8 oz)	60	0	0	16
Grape Berry Splash Drink as prep	1 serv (8 oz)	70	0	0	17
Grape Berry Splash Drink as prep w/ sugar	1 serv (8 oz)	100	0	0	25

FOOD	PORTION	CALS	PROT	FAT	CARB
Kickin' Kiwi Lime Drink as prep	1 serv (8 oz)	60	0	0	16
Kickin' Kiwi Lime Drink as prep w/ sugar	1 serv (8 oz)	100	0	0	25
Lemon-Lime Drink as prep w/ sugar	1 serv (8 oz)	100	0	0	25
Man-O-Mango Berry Drink as prep	1 serv (8 oz)	60	0	0	16
Man-O-Mango Berry Drink as prep w/ sugar	1 serv (8 oz)	100	0	0	25
Oh Yeah Orange Pineapple Drink as prep	1 serv (8 oz)	60	0	0	16
Oh Yeah Orange Pineapple Drink as prep w/ sugar	1 serv (8 oz)	100	0	0	25
Pina-Pineapple Drink as prep	1 serv (8 oz)	60	0	0	17
Pina-Pineapple Drink as prep w/ sugar	1 serv (8 oz)	100	0	0	25
Roarin' Raspberry Cranberry Drink as prep	1 serv (8 oz)	70	0	0	17
Roarin' Raspberry Cranberry Drink as prep w/ sugar	1 serv (8 oz)	100	0	0	25
Slammin' Strawberry Kiwi Drink as prep	1 serv (8 oz)	70	0	0	17
Slammin' Strawberry Kiwi Drink as prep w/ sugar	1 serv (8 oz)	100	0	0	25
Strawberry Raspberry Drink as prep	1 serv (8 oz)	60	0	0	16
Strawberry Raspberry Drink as prep w/ sugar	1 serv (8 oz)	100	0	0	25
Sugar Free Tropical Punch as prep	1 serv (8 oz)	5	0	0	0
Tropical Punch as prep	1 serv (8 oz)	60	0	0	16
Tropical Punch as prep w/ sugar	1 serv (8 oz)	100	0	0	25
Watermelon Cherry Drink as prep	1 serv (8 oz)	60	0	0	16
Watermelon Cherry Drink as prep w/ sugar	1 serv (8 oz)	100	0	0	25
Tang					
Orange Pineapple as prep	1 serv (8 oz)	100	0	0	24
ready-to-drink					
cranberry apricot drink	6 fl oz	118	0	0	30
orange grapefruit juice	8 fl oz	107	1	tr	25
orange & apricot	8 fl oz	128	1	tr	32
pineapple & grapefruit	8 fl oz	117	1	tr	29
pineapple & orange drink	8 fl oz	125	3	0	29

FOOD	PORTION	CALS	PROT	FAT	CARB
Apple & Eve					
Apple Cranberry	8 oz	120	1	0	30
Capri Sun					
Fruit Punch	1 pkg (7 oz)	100	0	0	26
Maui Punch	1 pkg (7 oz)	100	0	0	27
Mountain Cooler	1 pkg (7 oz)	90	0	0	24
Pacific Cooler	1 pkg (7 oz)	100	0	0	26
Red Berry	1 pkg (7 oz)	100	0	0	26
Safari Punch	1 pkg (7 oz)	100	0	0	25
Strawberry Kiwi Drink	1 pkg (7 oz)	100	0	0	26
Surfer Cooler Drink	1 pkg (7 oz)	100	0	0	27
Citrus Squeeze					
California Punch	8 oz	130	0	0	33
Florida Punch	8 oz	120	0	0	30
Coco Lopez					
Mango Kiwi	8 fl oz	130	0	0	33
Crystal Light					
Fruit Punch	1 serv (8 oz)	5	0	0	0
Kiwi Strawberry	1 serv (8 oz)	5	0	0	0
Orange Strawberry Banana Drink	1 serv (8 oz)	5	0	0	0
Del Monte					
Peach Raspberry	5.5 fl oz	160	1	0	40
Pineapple Banana Orange	5.5 fl oz	170	1	0	44
Strawberry Peach Banana	5.5 fl oz	150	1	0	39
Dole					
Apple Berry Burst	8 fl oz	120	0	0	31
Cranberry Apple	8 fl oz	120	0	0	30
Fruit Fiesta	8 fl oz	140	0	—	34
Fruit Punch	1 carton (10 oz)	160	0	0	39
Mountain Cherry	8 fl oz	150	0	0	30
Orange Peach Mango	8 oz	120	1	0	28
Orange Strawberry Banana	8 oz	120	1	0	28
Orchard Peach	8 oz	140	1	0	34
Pineapple Orange	8 oz	120	2	0	27
Pineapple Orange Strawberry	8 oz	130	0	0	32
Tropical Fruit	8 oz	160	0	0	38
Eden					
Organic Apple Cherry Juice	8 oz	120	0	0	30
Everfresh					
Cranberry-Apple Drink	1 can (8 oz)	120	0	0	31
Grape-Strawberry	1 can (8 oz)	120	0	0	31
Kiwi-Strawberry	1 can (8 oz)	120	0	0	30
Mandarin Orange Mango Drink	1 can (8 oz)	120	0	0	29

FOOD	PORTION	CALS	PROT	FAT	CARB
Orange Banana Strawberry Drink	1 can (8 oz)	120	0	0	30
Tropical Fruit Punch	1 can (8 oz)	120	0	0	30
Wild Blackberry Lime Drink	1 can (8 oz)	120	0	0	29
Fresh Samantha					
Banana Strawberry	1 cup (8 oz)	130	4	0	11
Carrot Orange	1 cup (8 oz)	100	4	0	8
Desperately Seeking C	1 cup (8 oz)	110	4	0	9
Protein Blast	1 cup (8 oz)	160	9	1	10
Super Juice	1 cup (8 oz)	140	4	1	11
The Big Bang	1 cup (8 oz)	100	2	0	8
Fruitopia					
Fruit Integration	8 fl oz	110	0	0	29
Guzzler					
Island Punch	8 fl oz	140	0	0	29
Juicy Juice					
Apple Grape	1 box (8.45 oz)	140	0	0	34
Berry	1 box (8.45 oz)	130	0	0	37
Punch	1 box (4.23 oz)	70	0	0	17
Punch	1 box (8.45 oz)	140	0	0	34
Tropical	1 box (8.45 oz)	140	0	0	34
Kool-Aid					
Bursts Great Bluedini	1 (7 oz)	100	0	0	24
Bursts Kickin' Kiwi Lime	1 (7 oz)	100	0	0	24
Bursts Oh Yeah Orange Pineapple	1 (7 oz)	100	0	0	24
Bursts Slammin' Strawberry Kiwi	1 (7 oz)	100	0	0	24
Bursts Tropical Punch	1 (7 oz)	100	0	0	24
Splash Grape Berry Punch	1 serv (8 oz)	120	0	0	31
Splash Kiwi Strawberry Drink	1 serv (8 oz)	110	0	0	29
Splash Tropical Punch	1 serv (8 oz)	120	0	0	31
Mauna La'i					
Island Guava	8 oz	130	0	0	32
Paradise Passion	8 oz	130	0	0	32
Mott's					
Berry	1 box (8 oz)	100	0	0	26
Fruit Punch	1 box (8 oz)	110	0	0	27
Fruit Punch	8 fl oz	130	0	0	32
Nantucket Nectars					
Apple Raspberry	8 oz	140	0	0	34
California Melonberry	8 oz	110	0	0	28
Cranberry Apple	8 oz	140	0	0	36
Fruit Punch	8 oz	130	0	0	32

FOOD	PORTION	CALS	PROT	FAT	CARB
Kiwi Berry	8 oz	120	0	0	30
Orange Passionfruit	8 oz	120	0	0	29
Orange Mango	8 oz	130	0	0	32
Pineapple Orange Guava	8 oz	120	0	0	31
Watermelon Strawberry	8 oz	120	0	0	30
Oberweis					
Fruit Punch	8 oz	120	0	0	30
Ocean Spray					
Cran*Blueberry	8 oz	160	0	0	41
Cran*Cherry	8 oz	160	0	0	39
Cran*Currant	8 oz	140	0	0	33
Cran*Grape	8 oz	170	0	0	41
Cran*Mango	8 oz	130	0	0	33
Cran*Raspberry	8 oz	140	0	0	36
Cran*Raspberry Reduced Calorie	8 oz	50	0	0	13
Cran*Strawberry	8 oz	140	0	0	36
Cran*Tangerine	8 oz	130	0	0	33
Cranapple	8 oz	160	0	0	41
Cranapple Reduced Calorie	8 oz	50	0	0	13
Cranicot	8 oz	160	0	0	40
Crazy Kiwi Passion	8 oz	130	0	0	32
Fruit Punch	8 oz	130	0	0	32
Kiwi Strawberry	8 oz	120	0	0	31
Lightstyle Cran*Grape	8 oz	40	0	0	9
Lightstyle Cran*Mango	8 oz	40	0	0	10
Lightstyle Cran*Raspberry	8 oz	40	0	0	10
Mandarin Magic	8 oz	120	0	0	31
Ruby Red & Tangerine Grapefruit	8 oz	130	0	0	32
Ruby Red & Mango	8 oz	130	0	0	33
Shasta Plus					
Apple-Strawberry	1 can (11.5 oz)	160	0	0	41
Fruit Punch	1 can (11.5 oz)	160	0	0	39
Pineapple-Cherry	1 can (11.5 oz)	160	0	0	40
Snapple					
Cranberry Raspberry	8 fl oz	120	0	0	29
Diet Cranberry Raspberry	8 fl oz	10	0	0	2
Fruit Punch	8 fl oz	110	0	0	29
Kiwi Strawberry	8 fl oz	110	0	0	28
Snapricot Orange	8 fl oz	120	0	0	30
Squeezit					
Berry B. Wild	1 bottle (7 oz)	110	0	0	28
Blue Raspberry	1 bottle (7 oz)	110	0	0	28
Cherry Cola	1 bottle (7 oz)	110	0	0	27
Chucklin' Cherry	1 bottle (7 oz)	110	0	0	28

FOOD	PORTION	CALS	PROT	FAT	CARB
Green Apple	1 bottle (7 oz)	110	0	0	27
Grumpy Grape	1 bottle (7 oz)	110	0	0	28
Lemon Lime	1 bottle (7 oz)	110	0	0	28
Rockin' Red Puncher	1 bottle (7 oz)	110	0	0	24
Smarty Arty Orange	1 bottle (7 oz)	110	0	0	27
Strawberry	1 bottle (7 oz)	110	0	0	29
Tropical Punch	1 bottle (7 oz)	110	0	0	28
Watermelon	1 bottle (7 oz)	110	0	0	28
Tropicana					
Berry Punch	8 fl oz	130	0	0	32
Citrus Punch	8 fl oz	140	0	0	36
Fruit Punch	8 oz	130	0	0	32
Tangerine Orange Juice	8 fl oz	110	2	0	25
Twister Apple Raspberry Blackberry	1 bottle (10 fl oz)	160	0	1	38
Twister Citrus Punch	1 bottle (10 oz)	180	0	0	45
Twister Cranberry Punch	1 bottle (10 oz)	170	0	0	43
Twister Fruit Punch	1 bottle (10 oz)	170	0	0	43
Twister Ruby Red Tangerine	1 bottle (10 oz)	160	0	0	40
Twister Strawberry Kiwi	1 bottle (10 oz)	160	0	0	42
V8					
Splash Berry Blend	8 oz	110	0	0	28
Veryfine					
Apple Cranberry	1 bottle (10 oz)	190	0	0	48
Apple Quenchers Black Cherry White Grape	8 fl oz	120	0	0	30
Apple Quenchers Cranberry Tangerine	8 fl oz	120	0	0	31
Apple Quenchers Peach Kiwi	8 fl oz	130	0	0	33
Apple Quenchers Peach Plum	8 fl oz	130	0	0	32
Apple Quenchers Pear Passionfruit	8 fl oz	120	0	0	31
Apple Quenchers Raspberry Cherry	8 fl oz	120	0	0	31
Apple Quenchers Raspberry Lime	8 fl oz	120	0	0	30
Apple Quenchers Strawberry Banana	8 fl oz	120	0	0	30
Chillers Artic Mango Tangerine	8 fl oz	110	0	0	27
Chillers Freezing Fruit Punch	8 fl oz	130	0	0	33
Chillers Lemon Lime Blizzard	8 fl oz	120	0	0	29

FOOD	PORTION	CALS	PROT	FAT	CARB
Chillers Shivering Strawberry Melon	1 can (11.5 oz)	160	0	0	41
Chillers Tropical Freeze	8 fl oz	120	0	0	30
Cranberry Raspberry	8 fl oz	160	0	0	41
Fruit Punch	1 bottle (10 oz)	170	0	0	42
Juice-Ups Berry	8 fl oz	140	0	0	34
Juice-Ups Fruit Punch	8 fl oz	140	0	0	34
Juice-Ups Orange Punch	8 fl oz	140	0	0	35
Orange Strawberry	8 fl oz	120	0	0	31
Papaya Punch	1 bottle (10 oz)	160	0	0	39
Pineapple Orange	1 bottle (10 oz)	160	0	0	39
Strawberry Banana	1 can (11.5 oz)	160	0	0	40
Strawberry Banana Punch	1 can (11.5 oz)	190	0	0	48
Wellfleet Farms					
Cranberry & Georgia Peach	8 oz	140	0	0	35
Cranberry & Granny Smith Apple	8 oz	130	0	0	33
Cranberry & Key Lime	8 oz	140	0	0	35
FRUIT MIXED					
(see also individual names)					
canned					
fruit cocktail in heavy syrup	½ cup	93	1	tr	24
fruit cocktail juice pack	½ cup	56	1	tr	15
fruit cocktail water pack	½ cup	40	1	tr	10
fruit salad juice pack	½ cup	62	1	tr	16
tropical fruit salad in heavy syrup	½ cup	110	1	tr	29
Del Monte					
Cherry Mixed Light Syrup	½ cup (4.4 oz)	90	1	0	22
Chunk Mixed In Heavy Syrup	½ cup (4.5 oz)	100	0	0	24
Chunky Mixed Fruit Naturals	½ cup (4.4 oz)	60	0	0	15
Chunky Mixed In Extra Light Syrup	½ cup (4.4 oz)	60	0	0	15
Citrus Salad	½ cup (4.4 oz)	80	0	0	20
Fruit Cocktail Fruit Naturals	½ cup (4.4 oz)	60	0	0	15
Fruit Cocktail In Extra Light Syrup	½ cup (4.4 oz)	60	0	0	15
Fruit Cocktail In Heavy Syrup	½ cup (4.5 oz)	100	0	0	24
Fruit Cup Fruit Naturals Mixed	1 pkg (4 oz)	50	0	0	13
Fruit Cup Mixed In Extra Light Syrup	1 pkg (4 oz)	50	0	0	13
Fruit Salad In Extra Light Syrup	½ cup (4.5 oz)	70	1	0	22
Fruit To Go Fruity Combo	1 pkg (4 oz)	70	1	0	18
Fruit To Go Wild Berry Jumble	1 pkg (4 oz)	80	1	0	20

FOOD	PORTION	CALS	PROT	FAT	CARB
Fruitrageous Crazy Cherry Mixed	1 pkg (4 oz)	90	1	0	22
Orchard Select California Mixed	½ cup (4.5 oz)	80	1	0	19
Snack Cups Mixed Fruit In Heavy Syrup	1 serv (4 oz)	80	0	0	20
SunFresh Ambrosia Salad	½ cup	70	0	0	16
Tropical Fruit Salad	½ cup (4.3 oz)	60	0	0	16
Tropical Fruit Salad In Light Syrup	½ cup (4.4 oz)	80	0	0	21
Very Cherry Mixed Fruit	½ cup (4.4 oz)	90	1	0	22
Mott's					
Fruitsations Banana	1 pkg (4 oz)	90	0	0	23
Fruitsations Cherry	1 pkg (4 oz)	70	0	0	19
Fruitsations Mango Peach	1 pkg (4 oz)	70	0	0	22
Fruitsations Mixed Berry	1 pkg (4 oz)	90	0	0	22
Fruitsations Pear	1 pkg (4 oz)	90	0	0	23
Fruitsations Strawberry	1 pkg (4 oz)	80	0	0	19
Fruitsations Tropical Fruit	1 pkg (4 oz)	70	0	0	19
Healthy Harvest Peach Medley	1 pkg (3.9 oz)	50	0	0	13
Ocean Spray					
Cran*Fruit Cranberry Raspberry	¼ cup	120	0	0	29
Cran*Fruit Cranberry Strawberry	¼ cup	120	0	0	29
Sunfresh					
Ambrosia Salad	½ cup (4.5 oz)	70	0	0	16
Mixed Fruit In Light Syrup	½ cup (4.6 oz)	90	1	0	20
Tropical Salad In Extra Light Syrup	½ cup (4.5 oz)	80	1	0	20
White House					
Apple Banana Sauce	1 pkg (4 oz)	100	0	0	23
Apple Mixed Berry Sauce	1 pkg (4 oz)	110	0	0	23
Apple Peach Sauce	1 pkg (4 oz)	100	0	0	23
dried					
mixed	11 oz pkg	712	7	1	188
Paradise					
Old English Fruit & Peel Mix	1 tbsp (0.8 oz)	70	6	0	18
Sun-Maid					
Tropical Medley	¼ cup (1.4 oz)	130	1	0	32
frozen					
mixed fruit sweetened	1 cup	245	4	tr	61
Birds Eye					
Mixed Fruit	½ cup (4.4 oz)	90	1	0	23
Tree Of Life					
Organic Mixed Berries	¾ cup (5 oz)	60	0	0	16

FOOD	PORTION	CALS	PROT	FAT	CARB
FRUIT SNACKS					
Betty Crocker					
Fruit Gushers All Flavors	1 pkg (0.9 oz)	90	0	1	20
Fruit String Thing All Flavors	1 pkg (0.7 oz)	80	0	1	17
Favorite Brands					
Cherry Fruit Snack	1 pkg (0.9 oz)	80	1	0	19
Creepy Crawler Fruit Snacks	1 pkg (0.9 oz)	80	1	0	19
Dinosaur Fruit Snack	1 pkg (0.9 oz)	80	1	0	19
Grape Fruit Snack	1 pkg (0.9 oz)	80	1	0	19
Space Alien Fruit Snack	1 pkg (0.9 oz)	80	1	0	19
Sports Fruit Snacks	1 pkg (0.9 oz)	80	1	0	19
Strawberry Fruit Snack	1 pkg (0.9 oz)	80	1	0	19
Teenage Mutant Ninja Turtle Fruit Snacks	1 pkg (0.9 oz)	80	1	0	19
The Mega Roll Strawberry	1 pkg (1 oz)	110	0	3	22
The Roll Cherry	1 pkg (0.75 oz)	80	0	2	16
The Roll Strawberry	1 pkg (0.75 oz)	80	0	2	16
Troll Fruit Snacks	1 pkg (0.9 oz)	80	1	0	19
Zoo Animal Fruit Snacks	1 pkg (0.9 oz)	80	1	0	19
General Mills					
Fruit Snacks All Flavors	1 pkg (0.9 oz)	80	0	0	21
Health Valley					
Bakes Apple	1 bar	70	2	0	19
Bakes Date	1 bar	70	2	0	19
Bakes Raisin	1 bar	70	2	0	19
Fruit Bars Apple	1	140	3	0	35
Fruit Bars Apricot	1	140	3	0	35
Fruit Bars Date	1	140	3	0	34
Fruit Bars Raisin	1	140	2	0	35
Sensible Foods					
Crackin' Fruit Cherry Berry	1 pkg (0.6 oz)	51	1	0	13
Sunbelt					
Fruit Jammers	1 pkg (1 oz)	100	0	1	23
Sunkist					
100% Fruit Roll All Flavors	1 (0.5 oz)	50	0	0	12
Weight Watchers					
Apple & Cinnamon	1 pkg (0.5 oz)	50	0	0	13
Apple Chips	1 pkg (0.75 oz)	70	0	0	18
Peach & Strawberry	1 pkg (0.5 oz)	50	0	0	13
GARLIC					
Dorot					
Frozen Crushed Cubes	1 cube (4 g)	5	0	0	1
GEFILTE FISH					
sweet	1 piece (1.5 oz)	35	4	1	3
GELATIN					
mix					
low calorie	½ cup	8	2	0	0

FOOD	PORTION	CALS	PROT	FAT	CARB
mix artificially sweetened as prep	½ cup (4.1 oz)	8	1	0	1
mix artificially sweetened as prep	1 pkg 4 serv (16.5 oz)	33	5	0	3
mix as prep	½ cup (4.7 oz)	80	2	0	19
mix as prep	1 pkg 4 serv (19 oz)	319	7	0	76
mix not prep	1 pkg (3 oz)	324	7	0	77
mix w/ fruit as prep	½ cup (3.7 oz)	73	1	tr	18
mix w/ fruit as prep	1 pkg 8 serv (19 oz)	588	10	2	144
powder unsweetened	1 pkg (7 g)	23	6	0	0
powder unsweetened	1 oz	94	24	0	0
Jell-O					
1-2-3-Brand Strawberry as prep	⅔ cup (5.2 oz)	130	2	2	26
Apricot as prep	½ cup (5 oz)	80	2	0	19
Berry Black as prep	½ cup (5 oz)	80	2	0	19
Berry Blue as prep	½ cup (5 oz)	80	2	0	19
Black Cherry as prep	½ cup (5 oz)	80	2	0	19
Cherry as prep	½ cup (5 oz)	80	2	0	19
Cranberry Raspberry as prep	½ cup (5 oz)	80	2	0	19
Cranberry Strawberry as prep	½ cup (5 oz)	80	2	0	19
Cranberry as prep	½ cup (5 oz)	80	0	0	19
Grape as prep	½ cup (5 oz)	80	2	0	19
Lemon as prep	½ cup (5 oz)	80	2	0	19
Lime as prep	½ cup (5 oz)	80	2	0	19
Mango as prep	½ cup (5 oz)	80	2	0	19
Mixed Fruit as prep	½ cup (5 oz)	80	2	0	19
Orange as prep	½ cup (5 oz)	80	2	0	19
Peach as prep	½ cup (5 oz)	80	2	0	19
Peach Passion Fruit as prep	½ cup (5 oz)	80	2	0	19
Pineapple as prep	½ cup (5 oz)	80	2	0	19
Raspberry as prep	½ cup (5 oz)	80	2	0	19
Sparkling White Grape as prep	½ cup (5 oz)	80	2	0	19
Strawberry Banana as prep	½ cup (5 oz)	80	2	0	19
Strawberry Kiwi as prep	½ cup (5 oz)	80	2	0	19
Strawberry as prep	½ cup (5 oz)	80	2	0	19
Sugar Free Cherry as prep	½ cup (4.2 oz)	10	1	0	0
Sugar Free Cranberry as prep	½ cup (4.2 oz)	10	1	0	0
Sugar Free Lemon as prep	½ cup (4.2 oz)	10	1	0	0
Sugar Free Lime as prep	½ cup (4.2 oz)	10	1	0	0

FOOD	PORTION	CALS	PROT	FAT	CARB
Sugar Free Mixed Fruit as prep	½ cup (4.2 oz)	10	1	0	0
Sugar Free Orange as prep	½ cup (4.2 oz)	10	1	0	0
Sugar Free Raspberry as prep	½ cup (4.2 oz)	10	1	0	0
Sugar Free Strawberry Banana as prep	½ cup (4.2 oz)	10	1	0	0
Sugar Free Strawberry as prep	½ cup (4.2 oz)	10	1	0	0
Sugar Free Strawberry Kiwi as prep	½ cup (4.2 oz)	10	1	0	0
Sugar Free Watermelon as prep	½ cup (4.2 oz)	10	1	0	0
Watermelon as prep	½ cup (5 oz)	80	2	0	19
Wild Strawberry as prep	½ cup (5 oz)	80	2	0	19
ready-to-eat					
Handi-Snacks					
Gels Blue Raspberry	1 serv (4 oz)	80	0	0	20
Gels Cherry	1 serv (4 oz)	80	0	0	20
Gels Orange	1 serv (3.5 oz)	80	0	0	20
Gels Strawberry	1 serv (3.5 oz)	80	0	0	20
Hunt's					
Snack Pack Gels Cherry	1 serv (3.5 oz)	100	0	0	25
Snack Pack Gels Raspberry Berry	1 serv (3.5 oz)	100	0	0	25
Snack Pack Gels Strawberry	1 serv (3.5 oz)	100	0	0	25
Snack Pack Gels Strawberry Orange	1 serv (3.5 oz)	100	0	0	25
Jell-O					
Berry Black	1 serv (3.5 oz)	70	1	0	17
Berry Blue	1 serv (3.5 oz)	70	1	0	17
Cherry	1 serv (3.5 oz)	70	1	0	17
Orange	1 serv (3.5 oz)	70	1	0	17
Orange Strawberry Banana	1 serv (3.5 oz)	70	1	0	17
Raspberry	1 serv (3.5 oz)	70	1	0	17
Rhymin' Lymon	1 serv (3.5 oz)	70	1	0	17
Strawberry	1 serv (3.5 oz)	70	1	0	17
Strawberry Kiwi	1 serv (3.5 oz)	10	1	0	0
Sugar Free Orange	1 serv (3.2 oz)	10	1	0	0
Sugar Free Raspberry	1 serv (3.2 oz)	10	1	0	0
Sugar Free Strawberry	1 serv (3.2 oz)	10	1	0	0
Tropical Berry	1 serv (3.5 oz)	10	1	0	0
Tropical Fruit Punch	1 serv (3.5 oz)	70	1	0	17
Wild Watermelon	1 serv (3.5 oz)	70	1	0	17
Swiss Miss					
Gels Berry Strawberry	1 pkg (3.5 oz)	79	1	0	18

FOOD	PORTION	CALS	PROT	FAT	CARB
Gels Berry Lemon	1 pkg (3.5 oz)	79	1	0	18
Gels Raspberry Orange	1 pkg (3.5 oz)	79	1	0	18
Gels Strawberry Raspberry	1 pkg (3.5 oz)	79	1	0	18
GIBLETS					
capon simmered	1 cup (5 oz)	238	38	8	0
chicken floured & fried	1 cup (5 oz)	402	47	19	6
chicken simmered	1 cup (5 oz)	228	37	7	1
turkey simmered	1 cup (5 oz)	243	39	7	3
GINGER					
Eden					
Pickled w/ Shiso Leaves	1 tbsp	15	0	0	3
GINKGO NUTS					
canned	1 oz	32	1	tr	6
dried	1 oz	99	3	tr	21
GINSENG					
dried	1 oz	90	5	tr	20
fresh	1 oz	28	1	tr	6
GIZZARDS					
chicken simmered	1 cup (5 oz)	222	5	5	2
turkey simmered	1 cup (5 oz)	236	43	6	1
GOAT					
roasted	3 oz	122	23	3	0
GOOSE					
w/ skin roasted	½ goose (1.7 lbs)	2362	195	170	0
w/ skin roasted	6.6 oz	574	47	41	0
w/o skin roasted	5 oz	340	41	18	0
w/o skin roasted	½ goose (1.3 lbs)	1406	171	75	0
GOOSEBERRIES					
canned in light syrup	½ cup	93	1	tr	24
fresh	1 cup	67	1	1	15
GRANOLA					
(*see* CEREAL, CEREAL BARS)					
GRAPE JUICE					
bottled	1 cup	155	1	tr	38
frzn sweetened not prep	6 oz	386	1	1	96
grape drink	6 oz	84	0	0	22
Capri Sun					
Drink	1 pkg (7 oz)	100	0	0	25
Daily					
Drink	8 oz	110	0	0	27
Everfresh					
Juice	1 can (8 oz)	150	0	0	38
Juicy Juice					
Drink	1 box (8.45 oz)	140	0	0	34
Drink	1 box (4.23 oz)	70	0	0	17
Kool-Aid					
Bursts Grape Drink	1 (7 oz)	100	0	0	25
Drink as prep w/ sugar	1 serv (8 oz)	100	0	0	25

FOOD	PORTION	CALS	PROT	FAT	CARB
Drink Mix as prep	1 serv (8 oz)	60	0	0	16
Sugar Free Drink Mix as prep	1 serv (8 oz)	5	0	0	0
Mott's					
100% Juice	1 box (8 oz)	130	0	0	33
Grape Juice	8 fl oz	130	0	0	31
Nantucket Nectars					
100% Juice	8 oz	160	0	0	39
Grapeade	8 oz	130	0	0	33
Shasta Plus					
Grape Drink	1 can (11.5 oz)	160	0	0	39
Veryfine					
100% Juice	1 bottle (10 oz)	200	0	0	47
Chillers Glacial Grape	1 can (11.5 oz)	160	0	0	41
Grape Drink	1 bottle (10 oz)	160	0	0	41
Juice-Ups	8 fl oz	130	0	0	32
Welch's					
100% White	8 oz	160	0	0	39
GRAPE LEAVES					
take-out					
dolmas	5 (4.2 oz)	200	2	11	23
GRAPEFRUIT					
canned					
juice pack	½ cup	46	1	tr	11
unsweetened	1 cup	93	1	tr	22
water pack	½ cup	44	1	tr	11
Sunfresh					
Red & White	½ cup (4.4 oz)	45	1	0	9
fresh					
pink	½	37	1	tr	9
pink sections	1 cup	69	1	tr	18
red	½	37	1	tr	9
red sections	1 cup	69	1	tr	18
white	½	39	1	tr	10
white sections	1 cup	76	2	tr	19
Ocean Spray					
Fresh	2 oz	50	1	0	14
GRAPEFRUIT JUICE					
fresh	1 cup	96	1	tr	23
frzn as prep	1 cup	102	1	tr	24
frzn not prep	6 oz	302	4	1	72
sweetened	1 cup	116	1	tr	28
Apple & Eve					
Made In The Shade Ruby Red	8 fl oz	130	0	0	32
Everfresh					
Juice	1 can (8 oz)	90	0	0	22
Ruby Red Cocktail	1 can (8 oz)	130	0	0	32

FOOD	PORTION	CALS	PROT	FAT	CARB
Fresh Samantha					
Juice	1 cup (8 oz)	90	1	0	7
Mott's					
100% Juice	8 fl oz	110	2	0	27
Nantucket Nectars					
100% Juice	8 oz	100	1	0	23
100% Ruby Red	8 oz	100	0	0	25
Ocean Spray					
100% Juice	8 oz	100	1	0	24
100% Juice Pink	8 oz	110	0	0	28
Ruby Red Drink	8 oz	130	0	0	33
Tropicana					
Golden	8 oz	90	1	0	22
Ruby Red	8 oz	90	1	0	22
Twister Pink	1 bottle (10 oz)	140	0	0	34
W/ Double Vitamin C	8 fl oz	110	1	0	27
Veryfine					
100% Juice	1 bottle (10 oz)	110	0	0	25
Pink	1 bottle (10 oz)	150	0	0	38
Ruby Red	8 fl oz	120	0	0	29
GRAPES					
thompson seedless in heavy syrup	½ cup	94	1	tr	25
thompson seedless water pack	½ cup	48	1	tr	13
Chiquita					
Grapes	1½ cups (4.8 oz)	90	1	1	24
GRAVY					
canned					
au jus	1 cup	38	3	tr	6
beef	1 cup	124	9	6	11
beef	1 can (10 oz)	155	11	7	14
chicken	1 cup	189	5	14	13
mushroom	1 cup	120	3	6	13
turkey	1 cup	122	6	5	12
Campbell					
Beef	¼ cup	29	1	1	4
Brown	¼ cup	46	1	3	4
Chicken	¼ cup	42	1	2	4
Turkey	¼ cup	29	1	1	3
mix					
au jus as prep w/ water	1 cup	32	1	1	4
brown as prep w/ water	1 cup	75	2	2	13
chicken as prep	1 cup	83	3	2	14
mushroom as prep	1 cup	70	2	1	14
onion as prep w/ water	1 cup	77	2	1	16
pork as prep	1 cup	76	2	2	13
turkey as prep	1 cup	87	3	2	15

FOOD	PORTION	CALS	PROT	FAT	CARB
Bournvita					
Extract	2 heaping tsp	34	1	1	7
Bovril					
Extract	1 heaping tsp	9	2	0	tr
Durkee					
Au Jus as prep	¼ cup	5	0	0	1
Brown as prep	¼ cup	10	0	1	3
Brown Mushroom as prep	¼ cup	15	1	0	3
Brown Onion as prep	¼ cup	15	1	0	4
Chicken as prep	¼ cup	20	1	1	4
Country as prep	¼ cup	35	1	2	5
Homestyle as prep	¼ cup	15	1	1	3
Onion as prep	¼ cup	10	1	0	3
Pork as prep	¼ cup	10	1	0	3
Sausage as prep	¼ cup	35	1	2	5
Swiss Steak as prep	¼ cup	15	0	0	4
Turkey as prep	¼ cup	20	1	0	4
French's					
Au Jus as prep	¼ cup	5	0	0	1
Brown as prep	¼ cup	10	0	1	3
Chicken as prep	¼ cup	25	1	1	4
Country as prep	¼ cup	35	1	2	5
Herb Brown as prep	¼ cup	15	1	1	3
Homestyle as prep	¼ cup	10	0	1	3
Mushroom as prep	¼ cup	10	0	1	3
Onion as prep	¼ cup	15	0	1	4
Pork as prep	¼ cup	10	0	1	3
Turkey as prep	¼ cup	20	1	0	4
Loma Linda					
Gravy Quik Chicken	1 tbsp (5 g)	20	1	0	3
Marmite					
Extract	1 heaping tsp	9	2	0	tr
McCormick					
Au Jus Natural as prep	¼ cup	5	0	0	1
Beef & Herb as prep	¼ cup	30	1	1	3
Chicken as prep	¼ cup	20	0	0	4
Turkey as prep	¼ cup	20	0	0	3
GREAT NORTHERN BEANS					
canned					
great northern	1 cup	300	19	1	55
Eden					
Organic	½ cup (4.6 oz)	110	5	1	20
Green Giant					
Great Northern	½ cup (4.4 oz)	100	6	1	18
dried					
cooked	1 cup	210	15	1	37
Hurst					
HamBeens w/ Ham	3 tbsp (1.2 oz)	120	7	1	22

FOOD	PORTION	CALS	PROT	FAT	CARB
GREEN BEANS					
canned					
green beans	½ cup	13	1	tr	3
italian	½ cup	13	1	tr	3
italian low sodium	½ cup	13	1	tr	3
low sodium	½ cup	13	1	tr	3
Del Monte					
Cut	½ cup (4.2 oz)	20	1	0	4
Cut Italian	½ cup (4.2 oz)	30	1	0	6
Cut No Salt Added	½ cup (4.2 oz)	20	1	0	4
French Style	½ cup (4.2 oz)	20	1	0	4
French Style No Salt Added	½ cup (4.2 oz)	20	1	0	4
French Style Seasoned	½ cup (4.2 oz)	20	1	0	4
Whole	½ cup (4.2 oz)	20	1	0	4
S&W					
Blue Lake Cut	½ cup (4.2 oz)	20	1	0	4
French Style	½ cup (4.2 oz)	20	1	0	4
Whole Small	½ cup (4.2 oz)	20	1	0	4
fresh					
cooked	½ cup	22	1	tr	5
raw	½ cup	17	1	tr	4
frozen					
cooked	½ cup	18	1	tr	4
italian cooked	½ cup	18	1	tr	4
Green Giant					
Cut	¾ cup (2.8 oz)	25	1	0	5
Harvest Fresh & Almonds	⅔ cup (2.8 oz)	60	2	3	5
Stouffer's					
Green Bean Mushroom Casserole	1 serv (4 oz)	130	3	8	12
Tree Of Life					
Cut	⅔ cup (2.8 oz)	25	1	0	4
GROUNDCHERRIES					
fresh	½ cup	37	1	tr	8
GROUPER					
cooked	3 oz	100	21	1	0
cooked	1 fillet (7.1 oz)	238	50	3	0
GUAVA					
fresh	1	45	1	1	11
GUAVA JUICE					
Nantucket Nectars					
Cocktail	8 oz	130	0	0	33
GUINEA HEN					
w/ skin raw	½ hen (12.1 oz)	545	81	22	0
w/o skin raw	½ hen (9.3 oz)	292	55	7	0
HADDOCK					
fresh cooked	1 fillet (5.3 oz)	168	36	1	0
fresh cooked	3 oz	95	21	1	0

FOOD	PORTION	CALS	PROT	FAT	CARB
fresh raw	3 oz	74	16	1	0
roe raw	1 oz	37	7	tr	tr
smoked	3 oz	99	21	1	0
smoked	1 oz	33	7	tr	0
take-out					
breaded & fried	1 piece (3.5 oz)	187	23	9	3
HALIBUT					
atlantic & pacific cooked	3 oz	119	23	2	0
atlantic & pacific cooked	½ fillet (5.6 oz)	223	42	5	0
atlantic & pacific raw	3 oz	93	18	2	0
greenland baked	3 oz	203	16	15	0
fresh					
greenland baked	5.6 oz	380	29	28	0
HALVA					
(see SESAME)					
HAM					
(see also HAM DISHES, PORK, TURKEY)					
boneless 11% fat roasted	3 oz	151	19	8	0
canned extra lean roasted	3 oz	116	18	4	tr
canned extra lean roasted	1 cup	190	30	7	1
canned extra lean 4% fat	3 oz	116	18	4	tr
center slice country style lean roasted	4 oz	220	31	9	tr
chopped	1 oz	65	5	5	0
chopped canned	1 oz	68	5	5	tr
ham & cheese loaf	1 oz	73	9	6	1
ham & cheese spread	1 oz	69	5	5	1
ham & cheese spread	1 tbsp	37	2	3	tr
ham salad spread	1 oz	61	2	4	3
ham salad spread	1 tbsp	32	1	2	2
minced	1 oz	75	5	6	1
patty cooked	1 patty (2 oz)	203	8	18	1
prosciutto	1 oz	55	8	2	tr
sliced extra lean 5% fat	1 oz	37	5	1	tr
sliced regular 11% fat	1 oz	52	5	3	1
steak boneless extra lean	1 (2 oz)	69	11	2	0
westphalian smoked	1 oz	105	5	10	0
Alpine Lace					
Boneless Cooked 98% Fat Free	2 slices (2 oz)	60	9	1	2
Honey Ham 98% Fat Free	2 slices (2 oz)	60	9	1	2
Smoked Virginia 98% Fat Free	2 slices (2 oz)	60	9	1	2
Armour					
Chopped Ham canned	2 oz	130	8	11	1
Deviled Ham Spread	1 pkg (3 oz)	210	13	18	0
Lean Slices Brown Sugar	1 pkg (2.5 oz)	90	13	2	4

FOOD	PORTION	CALS	PROT	FAT	CARB
Boar's Head					
Black Forest Smoked	2 oz	60	10	1	2
Cappy	2 oz	60	10	2	3
Deluxe	2 oz	60	9	1	2
Deluxe Lowered Sodium	2 oz	50	10	1	tr
Maple Glazed Honey	2 oz	60	10	1	3
Pepper	2 oz	60	10	1	2
Rosemary & Sundried Tomato	2 oz	70	10	3	2
Sweet Slice Smoked	3 oz	100	15	3	1
Virgina	2 oz	60	9	1	3
Virginia Smoked	2 oz	60	9	1	2
Carl Buddig					
Ham Sliced w/ Natural Juices	1 pkg (2.5 oz)	120	12	7	1
Honey Ham Sliced w/ Natural Juice	1 pkg (2.5 oz)	120	12	7	3
Lean Slices Oven Roasted Honey Ham	1 pkg (2.5 oz)	90	13	2	4
Lean Slices Smoked	1 pkg (2.5 oz)	80	14	2	1
Hillshire					
Deli Select Honey Ham	6 slices (2 oz)	60	10	2	2
Hormel					
Black Label Canned (refrigerated)	3 oz	100	14	5	1
Black Label Canned (self stable)	3 oz	110	14	5	0
Cure 81 Half Ham	3 oz	100	16	5	0
Curemaster	3 oz	80	14	3	0
Deviled Ham	4 tbsp (2 oz)	150	9	12	2
Ham & Cheese Patties	1 patty (2 oz)	190	7	17	0
Ham Patties	1 (2 oz)	180	7	17	1
Light & Lean 97 Sliced	1 slice (1 oz)	25	4	1	0
Primissimo Proscuitti	2 oz	120	15	7	0
Spiral Cure 81	3 oz	150	15	9	1
Louis Rich					
Carving Board Baked	2 slices (1.6 oz)	50	8	2	1
Carving Board Honey Glazed Thin	6 slices (2.1 oz)	70	11	2	2
Carving Board Honey Glazed Traditional	2 slices (1.6 oz)	50	8	2	1
Carving Board Smoked	1 slice (1.6 oz)	45	8	2	0
Dinner Slices Baked	1 slice (3.3 oz)	80	16	2	1
Oscar Mayer					
Baked	3 slices (2.2 oz)	70	11	3	2
Boiled	3 slices (2.2 oz)	60	10	3	0
Chopped	1 slice (1 oz)	50	4	3	1
Dinner Slice	3 oz	80	14	3	0

FOOD	PORTION	CALS	PROT	FAT	CARB
Dinner Steaks	1 (2 oz)	60	10	2	0
Free Baked	3 slices (1.6 oz)	35	7	0	1
Free Honey	3 slices (1.6 oz)	35	7	0	2
Free Smoked	3 slices (1.6 oz)	35	7	0	1
Honey	3 slices (2.2 oz)	70	10	3	2
Lower Sodium	3 slices (2.2 oz)	70	10	3	2
Smoked	3 slices (2.2 oz)	60	11	3	0
Spam					
Spread	4 tbsp (2 oz)	140	8	12	1
Wampler					
Black Forest	2 oz	60	10	2	2
HAM DISHES					
take-out					
croquettes	1 (3.1 oz)	217	12	14	11
salad	½ cup	287	16	23	5
HAM SUBSTITUTES					
Yves					
Veggie Ham Deli Slices	1 serv (2.2 oz)	80	14	0	6
HAMBURGER					
Kid Cuisine					
Buckaroo Beef Patty Sandwich w/ Cheese	1 meal (8.5 oz)	410	12	15	58
take-out					
double patty w/ bun	1 reg	544	30	28	43
double patty w/ cheese & bun	1 reg	457	28	28	22
double patty w/ cheese & double bun	1 reg	461	22	22	44
double patty w/ cheese ketchup mayonnaise onion pickle tomato & bun	1 reg	416	21	21	35
double patty w/ ketchup mayonnaise onion pickle tomato & bun	1 reg	649	30	35	53
double patty w/ ketchup cheese mayonnaise mustard pickle tomato & bun	1 lg	706	38	44	40
double patty w/ ketchup mustard mayonnaise onion pickle tomato & bun	1 lg	540	34	27	40

FOOD	PORTION	CALS	PROT	FAT	CARB
double patty w/ ketchup mustard onion pickle & bun	1 reg	576	32	32	39
single patty w/ bacon ketchup cheese mustard onion pickle & bun	1 lg	609	32	37	37
single patty w/ bun	1 reg	275	12	12	31
single patty w/ bun	1 lg	400	23	23	25
single patty w/ cheese & bun	1 reg	320	15	15	32
single patty w/ cheese & bun	1 lg	608	30	33	47
single patty w/ ketchup cheese ham mayonnaise pickle tomato & bun	1 lg	745	40	48	38
single patty w/ ketchup mustard mayonnaise onion pickle tomato & bun	1 reg	279	13	13	27
triple patty w/ cheese & bun	1 lg	769	56	51	27
triple patty w/ ketchup mustard pickle & bun	1 lg	693	50	41	29

HAMBURGER SUBSTITUTES
(see also MEAT SUBSTITUTES)

FOOD	PORTION	CALS	PROT	FAT	CARB
Amy's Organic					
Veggie Burger California	1 (2.5 oz)	100	4	3	17
Veggie Burger Chicago	1 (2.5 oz)	100	6	4	9
Veggie Burger Texas	1 (2.5 oz)	130	12	3	15
Boca Burgers					
Hint of Garlic	1 patty (2.5 oz)	110	14	2	9
Vegan Original	1 patty (2.5 oz)	84	12	0	9
Franklin Farms					
Veggiburger Portabella	1 (3 oz)	120	15	2	11
GardenVegan					
Fat-Free Patty	1 patty (2.5 oz)	140	11	0	23
Gardenburger					
Classic Greek	1 (2.5 oz)	120	6	3	17
Fire Roasted Vegetable	1 (2.5 oz)	120	7	3	17
Hamburger Style	1 (2.5 oz)	90	16	0	7
Hamburger Style w/ Cheese	1 (2.5 oz)	110	16	3	7
Savory Mushroom	1 (2.5 oz)	120	6	3	18
Green Giant					
Southwestern Style	1 patty (3.2 oz)	140	18	4	9

FOOD	PORTION	CALS	PROT	FAT	CARB
Harmony Farms					
Soy Burgers Onion	1 (2.5 oz)	90	10	3	7
Soy Burgers Garlic	1 (2.5 oz)	110	12	3	10
Soy Burgers Mushroom	1 (2.5 oz)	110	11	3	9
Lightlife					
Barbecue Grilles	1 patty (2.7 oz)	120	10	4	11
Lemon Grilles	1 patty (2.7 oz)	140	11	6	11
Light Burgers	1 (3 oz)	130	16	1	12
Tamari Grilles	1 patty (2.7 oz)	120	11	5	9
Loma Linda					
Patty Mix not prep	⅓ cup (0.9 oz)	90	14	1	7
Redi-Burger	⅝ in slice (3 oz)	120	18	3	7
Vege-Burger	¼ cup (1.9 oz)	70	11	2	2
Morningstar Farms					
Better'n Burger	1 (2.7 oz)	80	13	0	8
Garden Grille	1 patty (2.5 oz)	120	6	3	18
Garden Veggie Patties	1 patty (2.4 oz)	100	10	3	9
Hard Rock Cafe Veggie Burger	1 (3 oz)	170	6	8	18
Harvest Burger Italian Style	1 patty (3.2 oz)	140	17	5	8
Harvest Burger Original	1 (3.2 oz)	140	18	4	8
Harvest Burger Southwestern	1 (3.2 oz)	140	16	4	9
Spicy Black Bean Burger	1 (2.7 oz)	110	11	1	16
Natural Touch					
Garden Veggie Pattie	1 (2.4 oz)	110	10	3	8
Okara Pattie	1 (2.2 oz)	110	11	5	4
Original Veggie Burger Kit not prep	¼ pkg (0.8 oz)	80	14	0	6
Southwestern Veggie Burger Kit not prep	¼ pkg (0.9 oz)	90	12	0	9
Spicy Black Bean Burger	1 (2.7 oz)	100	11	1	15
Vegan Burger	1 (2.7 oz)	70	11	0	6
Superburgers					
Vegan Organic Original	1 (3 oz)	98	10	2	14
Vegan Organic Smoked	1 (3 oz)	98	10	2	14
Vegan Organic TexMex	1 (3 oz)	110	10	1	14
V'dora					
Vegetable BurgerLites	1 (3.3 oz)	58	4	0	4
Worthington					
Granburger not prep	3 tbsp (0.6 oz)	60	10	1	3
Prosage Patties	1 (1.3 oz)	80	9	3	3
Vegetarian Burger	¼ cup (1.9 oz)	60	9	2	2
Yves					
Black Bean & Mushroom Burgers	1 (3 oz)	100	12	0	13

FOOD	PORTION	CALS	PROT	FAT	CARB
Garden Vegetable Patties	1 (3 oz)	90	11	0	11
Veggie Burger	1 (3 oz)	119	16	2	9
HAZELNUTS					
dried blanched	1 oz	191	4	19	5
dried unblanched	1 oz	179	4	18	4
dry roasted unblanched	1 oz	188	3	19	5
oil roasted unblanched	1 oz	187	4	18	5
HEART					
beef simmered	3 oz	148	24	5	tr
chicken simmered	1 cup (5 oz)	268	11	11	tr
lamb braised	3 oz	158	21	7	2
pork braised	1	191	30	7	1
pork braised	1 cup	215	34	7	1
turkey simmered	1 cup (5 oz)	257	39	9	3
veal braised	3 oz	158	25	6	tr
HEARTS OF PALM					
canned	1 cup (5.1 oz)	41	4	1	7
canned	1 (1.2 oz)	9	1	tr	2
HEMP					
HempNut					
Shelled Hempseed	1 oz	162	9	13	3
Nutiva					
Hempseed	1½ tbsp (0.5 oz)	70	4	5	3
HERBAL TEA					
(*see* TEA/HERBAL TEA)					
HERBS/SPICES					
(*see also individual names*)					
chinese five spice	1 tsp	7	0	tr	2
Chi-Chi's					
Seasoning Mix	1 tsp (3 g)	10	0	0	1
Eden					
Furikake Seasoning	½ tsp	5	0	0	1
Instant India					
Curry Paste Cilantro Garlic	2 tbsp (1 oz)	110	2	3	4
Curry Paste Ginger Garlic	2 tbsp (1 oz)	90	1	3	8
McCormick					
Big'n Season	1 tbsp (8 g)	30	0	0	5
Buffalo Wings					
Meat Loaf Seasoning	1 tsp (4 g)	15	0	0	2
HERRING					
atlantic cooked	3 oz	172	20	10	0
atlantic cooked	1 fillet (5 oz)	290	33	17	0
atlantic raw	3 oz	134	15	8	0
pacific baked	3 oz	213	18	15	0
pacific fillet baked	5.1 oz	360	30	26	0
roe canned	1 oz	34	6	1	tr
roe raw	1 oz	37	7	tr	tr
smoked	3.5 oz	210	22	14	0

FOOD	PORTION	CALS	PROT	FAT	CARB
take-out					
atlantic kippered	1 fillet (1.4 oz)	87	10	5	0
atlantic pickled	½ oz	39	2	3	1
fried	1 serv (3.5 oz)	233	23	15	2
HICKORY NUTS					
dried	1 oz	187	4	18	5
HOMINY					
canned					
white	1 cup (5.6 oz)	482	2	1	23
Van Camp					
Golden	½ cup (4.3 oz)	80	4	1	17
White	½ cup (4.3 oz)	80	1	1	16
HONEY					
honey	1 cup (11.9 oz)	1031	1	0	279
wild honey	1 tbsp	60	0	0	17
HONEYDEW					
fresh					
cubed	1 cup	60	1	tr	16
wedge	⅒	46	1	tr	12
Chiquita					
Wedge	⅒ melon (4.7 oz)	50	1	0	13
HORSE					
roasted	3 oz	149	24	5	0
HORSERADISH					
wasabi root raw	1 (5.9 oz)	184	8	1	40
wasabi root raw sliced	1 cup (4.6 oz)	142	6	1	31
Boar's Head					
Horseradish	1 tsp (5 g)	5	0	0	0
Eden					
Wasabi Powder	1 tsp	10	0	0	1
Kraft					
Cream Style	1 tsp (5 g)	0	0	0	0
Horseradish Sauce	1 tsp (5 g)	20	0	2	tr
Prepared	1 tsp (5 g)	0	0	0	0
HOT COCOA					
(*see* COCOA)					
HOT DOG					
beef	1 (2 oz)	180	7	16	1
beef	1 (1.5)	142	5	13	1
beef & pork	1 (2 oz)	183	6	17	1
beef & pork	1 (1.5 oz)	144	5	13	1
chicken	1 (1.5 oz)	116	6	9	3
pork cheesefurter smokie	1 (1.5 oz)	141	6	12	1
turkey	1 (1.5 oz)	102	6	8	1
Applegate Farms					
Chicken Natural Uncured	1 (1.5 oz)	120	14	5	1
Natural Turkey	1 (1.5 oz)	120	14	5	1

FOOD	PORTION	CALS	PROT	FAT	CARB
Boar's Head					
Beef	1 (2 oz)	160	7	14	1
Beef Lite	1 (1.6 oz)	90	7	6	0
Pork & Beef	1 (2 oz)	150	7	14	0
Health Is Wealth					
Uncured Beef	1 (1.5 oz)	80	6	6	1
Uncured Chicken	1 (1.5 oz)	100	8	8	1
Healthy Choice					
Beef Low Fat	1 (1.8 oz)	70	6	3	7
Low Fat Turkey Pork Beef	1 (1.4 oz)	60	5	2	5
Hormel					
Fat Free	1 (1.8 oz)	45	5	0	5
Fat Free Beef	1 (1.8 oz)	45	6	0	5
Kid Cuisine					
Mystical Mini Corn Dogs	4 pieces	230	8	14	18
Louis Rich					
Bun Length	1 (2 oz)	110	6	8	3
Cheese	1 (1.6 oz)	90	6	6	2
Franks	1 (1.6 oz)	80	5	6	2
Organic Vallely					
All-Natural Beef	1 (1.6 oz)	90	7	6	1
Oscar Mayer					
Beef	1 (1.6 oz)	140	5	13	1
Big & Juicy Franks Deli Style	1 (2.7 oz)	230	9	22	1
Big & Juicy Franks Original	1 (2.7 oz)	240	9	22	1
Big & Juicy Franks Quarter Pound	1 (4 oz)	350	13	32	2
Big & Juicy Weiners Hot 'N Spicy	1 (2.7 oz)	220	10	20	1
Big & Juicy Weiners Smokie Links	1 (2.7 oz)	220	10	19	1
Big & Juicy Wieners Original	1 (2.7 oz)	240	9	22	1
Bun-Length Beef	1 (2 oz)	180	6	17	2
Cheese	1 (1.6 oz)	140	5	13	1
Fat Free Beef	1 (1.8 oz)	40	7	0	3
Fat Free Turkey & Beef	1 (1.8 oz)	40	6	0	3
Jumbo Beef	1 (2 oz)	180	6	17	2
Light Beef	1 (2 oz)	110	6	8	2
Wieners	1 (1.6 oz)	150	5	13	1
Wieners Bun-Length	1 (2 oz)	190	6	17	2
Wieners Jumbo	1 (2 oz)	180	6	17	2
Wieners Light	1 (2 oz)	110	7	8	2
Wieners Little	6 (2 oz)	180	6	17	2
Wampler					
Chicken	1 (2 oz)	120	7	11	0
take-out					
corndog	1	460	17	19	56

FOOD	PORTION	CALS	PROT	FAT	CARB
w/ bun chili	1	297	14	13	31
w/ bun plain	1	242	10	15	18
HOT DOG SUBSTITUTES					
Lightlife					
Smart Deli Jumbo's	1 link (2.7 oz)	80	16	0	4
Smart Dogs	1 (1.5 oz)	45	9	0	2
Tofu Pups	1 (1.4 oz)	60	8	3	2
Wonder Dogs	1 (1.5 oz)	60	9	2	2
Loma Linda					
Big Franks	1 (1.8 oz)	110	10	7	2
Big Franks Low Fat	1 (1.8 oz)	80	11	3	3
Corn Dogs	1 (2.5 oz)	150	7	4	22
Morningstar Farms					
America's Original Veggie Dog	1 (2 oz)	80	11	1	6
Meatfree Corn Dog	1 (2.5 oz)	150	7	4	22
Meatfree Mini Corn Dog	4 (2.7 oz)	170	11	5	21
Natural Touch					
Vege Frank	1 (1.6 oz)	100	10	6	2
Worthington					
Veja Links Low Fat	1 (1.1 oz)	40	5	2	1
Yves					
Good Dog	1 (1.8 oz)	70	13	2	2
Tofu Dogs	1 (1.3 oz)	45	9	1	2
Veggie Dogs	1 (1.6 oz)	60	11	0	1
Veggie Dogs Chili	1 (1.6 oz)	50	10	0	3
Veggie Dogs Jumbo	1 (2.7 oz)	100	16	2	7
Veggie Dogs Jumbo Hot N' Spicy	1 (2.7 oz)	106	19	2	4
HUMMUS					
hummus	1 cup	420	12	21	50
take-out					
hummus	⅓ cup	140	4	7	17
HYACINTH BEANS					
dried cooked	1 cup	228	16	1	40
ICE CREAM AND FROZEN DESSERTS					
(*see also* ICES AND ICE POPS, PUDDING POPS, SHERBET, YOGURT FROZEN)					
chocolate	½ cup (4 fl oz)	143	3	7	19
dixie cup chocolate	1 (3.5 fl oz)	125	2	6	16
dixie cup strawberry	1 (3.5 fl oz)	112	2	5	16
dixie cup vanilla	1 (3.5 fl oz)	116	2	6	14
french vanilla soft serve	½ gal	3014	56	180	306
french vanilla soft serve	½ cup (4 fl oz)	185	4	11	19
strawberry	½ cup (4 fl oz)	127	2	6	18
vanilla	½ cup (4 fl oz)	132	2	7	16
vanilla light	½ cup (2.3 oz)	92	3	3	15
vanilla rich	½ cup (2.6 oz)	178	3	12	17
vanilla soft serve	½ cup	111	4	2	19

FOOD	PORTION	CALS	PROT	FAT	CARB
vanilla 10% fat	½ gal	2153	38	115	254
vanilla 16% fat	½ gal	2805	33	190	256
vanilla light	½ gal	1469	41	45	232
vanilla light	1 cup	184	5	6	29
vanilla light soft serve	1 cup	223	8	5	38
vanilla light soft serve	½ gal	1787	64	37	307
Ben & Jerry's					
Bovinity Divinity	½ cup	290	4	18	30
Butter Pecan	½ cup	330	6	25	22
Cherry Garcia	½ cup	260	5	16	26
Chocolate Chip Cookie Dough	½ cup	300	5	16	34
Chocolate Fudge Brownie	½ cup	280	5	15	32
Chubby Hubby	½ cup	350	6	21	33
Chunky Monkey	½ cup	310	5	19	32
Coconut Almond Fudge Chip	½ cup	310	5	22	24
Coffee Heath Bar Crunch	½ cup	310	4	18	32
Dilbert's World Totally Nuts	½ cup	310	5	21	27
Low Fat Blackberry Cobbler	½ cup	180	3	3	34
Low Fat Coconut Cream Pie	½ cup	160	4	3	29
Low Fat Mocha Latte	½ cup	150	5	2	28
Low Fat S'mores	½ cup	190	5	2	35
Mint Chocolate Cookie	½ cup	280	4	17	28
New York Super Fudge Chunk	½ cup	320	5	21	28
No Fat Chocolate Comfort	½ cup	150	4	2	29
Orange & Cream	½ cup	230	3	14	23
Peanut Butter Cup	½ cup	380	7	25	32
Phish Food	½ cup	300	4	14	41
Phish Stick	1	330	4	20	38
Pistachio Pistachio	½ cup	240	5	15	20
Pop Cookie Dough	1	420	5	25	44
Pop Totally Nuts	1	370	6	29	24
Pop Vanilla	1	330	4	23	29
Pop Vanilla Heath Bar Crunch	1	330	4	22	33
S'mores Bar	1	350	5	18	43
Triple Caramel Chunk	½ cup	290	4	17	32
Vanilla World's Best	½ cup	250	4	16	22
Vanilla Caramel Fudge	½ cup	300	4	17	33
Vanilla Heath Bar Crunch	½ cup	310	4	19	30
Wavy Gravy	½ cup	340	7	20	32
Better Than Ice Creme					
Soy Vanilla as prep	½ cup	110	1	3	21
Bon Bons					
Dark Chocolate	5 pieces	190	2	13	16
Milk Chocolate	5 pieces	200	2	14	17

FOOD	PORTION	CALS	PROT	FAT	CARB
Breyers					
Butter Pecan	½ cup (2.4 oz)	180	3	12	14
Caramel Praline Crunch	½ cup (2.6 oz)	180	3	9	22
Cherry Vanilla	½ cup (2.4 oz)	150	3	8	17
Chocolate	½ cup (2.4 oz)	160	2	9	18
Chocolate Chip	½ cup (2.4 oz)	170	3	10	17
Chocolate Chip Cookie Dough	½ cup (2.5 oz)	180	3	10	20
Chocolate Rainbow	½ cup (2.4 oz)	120	3	10	16
Coffee	½ cup (2.4 oz)	150	3	9	15
Cookies N Cream	½ cup (2.4 oz)	170	3	9	19
Creamsicle	½ cup (2.8 oz)	130	2	4	22
Double Chocolate Fudge	½ cup (2.6 oz)	150	2	9	23
Fat Free Caramel Praline	½ cup (2.5 oz)	120	3	0	25
Fat Free Chocolate	½ cup (2.4 oz)	90	3	0	19
Fat Free Mint Cookies N Cream	½ cup (2.4 oz)	100	3	0	21
Fat Free Strawberry	½ cup (2.4 oz)	90	3	0	19
Fat Free Take Two Vanilla Strawberry	½ cup (2.4 oz)	80	3	0	19
Fat Free Vanilla	½ cup (2.4 oz)	90	3	0	19
Fat Free Vanilla Chocolate Strawberry	½ cup (2.4 oz)	90	3	0	19
Fat Free Vanilla Fudge Twirl	½ cup (2.5 oz)	100	3	0	22
French Vanilla	½ cup (2.4 oz)	160	4	10	15
Fruit Rainbow	½ cup (2.4 oz)	140	2	8	16
Hershey w/ Almonds	½ cup (2.7 oz)	190	3	8	23
Light Butter Pecan	½ cup (2.3 oz)	120	4	4	19
Light Caramel Praline Pecan	½ cup (3 oz)	180	4	5	30
Light French Chocolate	½ cup (2.4 oz)	150	4	5	22
Light Mint Chocolate Chip	½ cup (2.4 oz)	140	3	5	21
Light Vanilla	½ cup (2.4 oz)	130	3	5	18
Light Vanilla Chocolate Strawberry	½ cup (2.4 oz)	120	4	3	19
Light Low Fat Brown Marble Fudge	½ cup (2.6 oz)	130	4	2	26
Light Low Fat French Vanilla	½ cup (2.3 oz)	110	3	2	20
Light Low Fat Swiss Almond Fudge	½ cup (2.5 oz)	130	4	3	24
Low Fat Butter Pecan	½ cup (2.6 oz)	150	3	7	21
Low Fat Vanilla	½ cup (2.6 oz)	120	3	3	22
Low Fat Vanilla Chocolate Strawberry	½ cup (2.6 oz)	120	3	3	22
Mint Chocolate Chip	½ cup (2.4 oz)	170	3	10	17
No Sugar Added Fudge Twirl	½ cup (2.6 oz)	100	3	5	14

FOOD	PORTION	CALS	PROT	FAT	CARB
No Sugar Added Mint Chocolate Chip	½ cup (2.4 oz)	100	3	5	12
No Sugar Added Vanilla	½ cup (2.4 oz)	90	3	5	11
No Sugar Added Vanilla Chocolate Strawberry	½ cup (2.4 oz)	90	3	5	11
Peach	½ cup (2.4 oz)	130	2	6	17
Peanut Butter Cup	½ cup (2.7 oz)	210	4	12	24
Rocky Road	½ cup (2.5 oz)	180	2	9	24
Soft'N Creamy Vanilla	½ cup (2.3 oz)	150	2	7	19
Soft'N Creamy Vanilla Chocolate Strawberry	½ cup (2.3 oz)	150	2	7	19
Strawberry	½ cup (2.4 oz)	130	2	7	15
Take Two Vanilla Chocolate	½ cup (2.5 oz)	160	3	9	17
Take Two Vanilla Orange Sherbet	½ cup (2.7 oz)	130	2	5	21
Vanilla	½ cup (2.4 oz)	150	3	9	15
Vanilla Chocolate Strawberry	½ cup (2.4 oz)	150	2	8	16
Vanilla Fudge Twirl	½ cup (2.6 oz)	160	3	8	19
Viennetta Cappuccino	½ cup (2.4 oz)	190	3	11	19
Viennetta Chocolate	½ cup (2.4 oz)	190	3	12	18
Viennetta Vanilla	½ cup (2.4 oz)	190	3	11	19
Butterfinger					
Bar	1 (2.5 oz)	190	2	13	16
California Joe					
Soft Serve Chocolate	½ cup (2.5 oz)	72	5	0	11
Soft Serve Vanilla	½ cup (2.5 oz)	70	5	0	11
Carnation					
Cup Chocolate	1 (3 oz)	140	2	8	16
Cup Chocolate Malt	1 (12 oz)	270	7	6	48
Cup Strawberry	1 (3 oz)	100	1	5	12
Cup Vanilla	1 (5 oz)	170	2	10	19
Cup Vanilla	1 (3 oz)	100	1	6	11
Cup Vanilla Malt	1 (12 oz)	260	6	6	48
Sundae Cup Strawberry	1 (5 oz)	200	2	8	29
Sunday Cup Chocolate	1 (5 oz)	210	2	9	30
Cool Creations					
Cookies & Cream Sandwich	1 (3.5 oz)	240	2	11	34
Mickey Mouse Bar	1 (2.5 oz)	120	2	8	10
Mini Sandwich	1 (2.3 oz)	110	1	5	16
Dippin' Dots					
Dipping Dots Chocolate	⅝ cup (3 oz)	190	4	9	22
Drumstick					
Cone Chocolate	1 (4.6 oz)	320	6	17	36
Cone Chocolate Dipped	1 (4.6 oz)	320	5	16	40
Cone Vanilla	1 (4.6 oz)	340	6	19	35

FOOD	PORTION	CALS	PROT	FAT	CARB
Cone Vanilla Caramel	1 (4.6 oz)	360	6	20	38
Cone Vanilla Fudge	1 (4.6 oz)	360	5	20	39
Edy's					
3 Musketeers	½ cup	160	3	7	22
Dreamery Banana Split	½ cup	240	3	11	31
Dreamery Black Raspberry Avalanche	½ cup	270	4	16	27
Dreamery Caramel Toffee Bar Heaven	½ cup	290	4	16	32
Dreamery Cashew Praline Parfait	½ cup	280	4	16	30
Dreamery Chocolate Truffle Explosion	½ cup	280	5	15	31
Dreamery Chocolate Peanut Butter Chunk	½ cup	310	7	18	29
Dreamery Coney Island Waffle Cone	½ cup	310	4	18	32
Dreamery Cool Mint	½ cup	300	4	17	32
Dreamery Deep Dish Apple Pie	½ cup	280	3	15	34
Dreamery Dulce De Leche	½ cup	270	4	14	32
Dreamery Grandma's Cookie Dough	½ cup	300	4	17	32
Dreamery Harvest Peach	½ cup	230	3	13	25
Dreamery New York Strawberry Cheesecake	½ cup	260	4	15	27
Dreamery Nothing But Chocolate	½ cup	280	5	14	34
Dreamery Nuts About Malt	½ cup	290	5	17	29
Dreamery Raspberry Brownie A La Mode	½ cup	130	3	14	34
Dreamery Raspberry Brownie A La Mode	½ cup	270	3	14	34
Dreamery Strawberry Fields	½ cup	220	3	12	26
Dreamery Tiramisu	½ cup	260	4	13	31
Dreamery Vanilla	½ cup	260	5	15	25
Grand Black Cherry Vanilla	½ cup	140	2	7	17
Grand Blue Ribbon Chocolate Cake	½ cup	180	3	10	20
Grand Butter Pecan	½ cup	170	3	10	16
Grand Cherry Chocolate Chip	½ cup	160	2	8	19
Grand Chocolate	½ cup	150	3	8	16
Grand Chocolate Caramel Swirl	½ cup	170	2	9	19

FOOD	PORTION	CALS	PROT	FAT	CARB
Grand Chocolate Chips	½ cup	170	3	9	18
Grand Chocolate Fudge Mousse	½ cup	160	2	8	19
Grand Chocolate Fudge Sundae	½ cup	170	3	9	20
Grand Coffee	½ cup	140	2	8	15
Grand Cookie Dough	½ cup	180	3	9	21
Grand Cookies'N Cream	½ cup	160	3	8	19
Grand Double Fudge Brownie	½ cup	170	2	9	19
Grand Espresso Chip	½ cup	150	2	8	17
Grand French Vanilla	½ cup	160	2	9	17
Grand French Vanilla Fudge Pie	½ cup	160	2	8	20
Grand Mint Chocolate Chips	½ cup	170	3	9	18
Grand Neapolitan	½ cup	140	2	7	16
Grand Nutty Cone Crunch	½ cup	180	3	10	19
Grand Real Strawberry	½ cup	130	2	6	16
Grand Rocky Road	½ cup	170	3	10	17
Grand Spumoni	½ cup	150	3	8	16
Grand Strawberry Cupcake	½ cup	140	2	6	19
Grand Tin Roof Sundae	½ cup	170	3	9	18
Grand Utimate Caramel Cup	½ cup	170	2	8	22
Grand Vanilla	½ cup	140	2	8	15
Grand Vanillaberry Bar	½ cup	130	2	5	19
Grand Light Butter Pecan	½ cup	120	3	5	16
Grand Light Chocolate Raspberry Escape	½ cup	130	3	5	19
Grand Light Chocolate Fudge Mousse	½ cup	120	3	4	17
Grand Light Cookie Dough	½ cup	130	3	5	19
Grand Light Cookies'N Cream	½ cup	120	3	4	18
Grand Light Crazy For Caramel	½ cup	120	3	4	19
Grand Light French Silk	½ cup	130	3	5	19
Grand Light Mint Chocolate Chips	½ cup	120	3	5	17
Grand Light Peanut Butter Cups	½ cup	120	3	5	17
Grand Light Rocky Road	½ cup	120	3	4	17
Grand Light S'Mores & More	½ cup	130	3	4	22
Grand Light Strawberry Shortcake	½ cup	110	2	4	18
Grand Light Vanilla	½ cup	100	3	3	15

FOOD	PORTION	CALS	PROT	FAT	CARB
Homemade All Natural Vanilla	½ cup	130	3	7	14
Homemade Brownies A La Mode	½ cup	150	3	7	18
Homemade Chocolate Chip Cookie Jar	½ cup	180	3	10	19
Homemade Chocolate Chip Mousse	½ cup	170	3	9	19
Homemade Double Chocolate Chunk	½ cup	170	3	9	19
Homemade Mint Chocolate Chunk	½ cup	170	3	9	18
Homemade Strawberries & Cream	½ cup	120	2	6	15
Homemade Vanilla Custard	½ cup	150	4	8	15
M&M's Almond	½ cup	180	3	10	21
M&M's Mint	½ cup	200	3	11	21
M&M's Vanilla	½ cup	180	3	9	22
Milky Way	½ cup	160	3	7	21
Snickers	½ cup	180	3	9	21
Snickers Cruncher	½ cup	190	3	10	21
Twix	½ cup	190	3	9	23
Twix Peanut Butter	½ cup	190	3	11	20
Flintstones					
Cool Cream	1 (2.75 oz)	90	1	2	18
Push-Up Pebbles Treats	1 (2.75 oz)	120	1	6	15
Haagen-Dazs					
Bars Chocolate & Almonds	1 (3.7 oz)	380	6	27	27
Bars Chocolate & Dark Chocolate	1 (3.6 oz)	350	5	24	28
Bars Chocolate Peanut Butter Swirl	1 (3 oz)	320	6	23	21
Bars Coffee & Almond Crunch	1 (3.7 oz)	370	5	27	27
Bars Cookies & Cream Crunch	1 (3.6 oz)	370	5	26	30
Bars Dulce De Leche Caramel	1 (3.7 oz)	370	4	24	34
Bars Tropical Coconut	1 (3.5 oz)	340	5	24	25
Bars Vanilla & Almonds	1 (3.7 oz)	380	6	28	26
Bars Vanilla & Dark Chocolate	1 (3.6 oz)	350	5	24	27
Bars Vanilla & Milk Chocolate	1 (3.5 oz)	340	5	24	25
Butter Pecan	½ cup	310	5	23	21
Cappuccino Commotion	½ cup	310	5	21	25
Cherry Vanilla	½ cup	240	4	15	23

FOOD	PORTION	CALS	PROT	FAT	CARB
Chocolate	½ cup	270	5	18	22
Chocolate Chocolate Fudge	½ cup	290	5	18	27
Chocolate Chocolate Chip	½ cup	300	5	20	26
Chocolate Swiss Almond	½ cup	300	4	20	24
Cinnamon	½ cup	250	4	17	20
Coffee	½ cup	270	5	18	21
Coffee Mocha Chip	½ cup	290	5	19	25
Cookie Dough Chip	½ cup	310	4	20	29
Cookies & Cream	½ cup	270	5	17	23
Creme Caramel Pecan	½ cup	320	5	20	29
Dulce De Leche Caramel	½ cup	290	5	17	28
Low Fat Chocolate	½ cup	170	7	3	29
Low Fat Coffee Fudge	½ cup	170	5	3	32
Low Fat Strawberry	½ cup	150	5	2	28
Low Fat Vanilla	½ cup	170	7	3	29
Macadamia Brittle	½ cup	300	4	20	25
Mango	½ cup	250	4	14	28
Mint Chip	½ cup	300	5	19	26
Pineapple Coconut	½ cup	230	4	12	25
Pistachio	½ cup	290	5	20	22
Rum Raisin	½ cup	270	4	17	22
Strawberry	½ cup	250	4	16	23
Vanilla	½ cup	270	5	18	21
Vanilla Chocolate Chip	½ cup	310	5	20	26
Vanilla Fudge	½ cup	290	5	18	25
Vanilla Swiss Almond	½ cup	300	5	20	24
Healthy Choice					
Butter Pecan Crunch	½ cup	120	3	2	22
Cappuccino Chocolate Chunk	½ cup	120	3	2	22
Cappuccino Mocha Crunch	½ cup	120	3	2	22
Cherry Chocolate Chunk	½ cup	110	3	2	19
Chocolate Chocolate Chunk	½ cup	120	3	2	21
Coconut Cream Pie	½ cup	120	3	2	23
Cookies 'N Cream	½ cup	120	3	2	21
Cookies Creme De Mint	½ cup	130	3	2	24
Fudge Brownie	½ cup	120	3	2	22
Mint Chocolate Chip	½ cup	120	3	2	21
Old Fashioned Blueberry Hill	½ cup	120	2	2	23
Old Fashioned Butterscotch Blonde	½ cup	140	3	2	26
Old Fashioned Cherry Vanilla	½ cup	120	2	2	22

FOOD	PORTION	CALS	PROT	FAT	CARB
Old Fashioned Strawberry	½ cup	110	2	2	20
Peanut Butter Cup	½ cup	110	3	2	19
Praline & Caramel	½ cup	130	3	2	25
Praline Caramel Cluster	½ cup	130	3	2	25
Rocky Road	½ cup	140	3	2	28
Turtle Fudge Cake	½ cup	130	3	2	25
Vanilla	½ cup	100	3	2	18
Vanilla Bean	½ cup	110	3	2	19
Wild Raspberry Truffle	½ cup	120	3	2	22
Klondike					
Choco Taco Fudge Grande	1 bar (3.2 oz)	310	41	17	36
Oreo Ice Cream Cookie Sandwich	1 (2.6 oz)	240	4	10	35
Original	1 (3.3 oz)	290	4	19	25
Nestle Crunch					
Chocolate	1 bar (3 oz)	200	2	14	17
Crunch King	1 (4 oz)	270	3	19	21
Nuggets	8 pieces	310	4	21	25
Reduced Fat	1 (2.5 oz)	130	3	7	14
Vanilla	1 bar (3 oz)	200	2	14	16
NutraShake					
High Calorie High Protein All Flavors	1 serv (4 oz)	200	6	10	24
Perry's					
No Fat No Sugar Added Caramel	½ cup (2.8 oz)	90	4	0	25
No Fat No Sugar Added Chocolate	½ cup (2.6 oz)	80	5	0	21
No Fat No Sugar Added Peach	½ cup (2.9 oz)	90	3	0	24
No Fat No Sugar Added Strawberry	½ cup (2.8 oz)	90	4	0	23
No Fat No Sugar Added Vanilla	½ cup (2.6 oz)	80	4	0	21
Rice Dream					
Carob	½ cup (3.2 oz)	150	1	6	24
Carob Almong	½ cup (3.2 oz)	170	1	8	24
Cocoa Marble Fudge	½ cup (3.2 oz)	150	1	6	25
Cookies N' Dream	½ cup (3.2 oz)	170	1	7	26
Mint Chocolate Chip	½ cup (3.2 oz)	170	1	8	26
Neapolitan	½ cup (3.2 oz)	150	1	6	24
Vanilla Swiss Almond	½ cup (3.2 oz)	180	1	8	25
Rice Dream Supreme					
Cappuccino Almond Fudge	½ cup (3.2 oz)	170	1	8	24
Cherry Chocolate Chunk	½ cup (3.2 oz)	170	1	7	27
Chocolate Almond Chunk	½ cup (3.2 oz)	170	2	8	25
Chocolate Fudge Brownie	½ cup (3.2 oz)	170	1	7	28

FOOD	PORTION	CALS	PROT	FAT	CARB
Double Espresso Bean	½ cup (3.2 oz)	160	1	7	24
Mint Chocolate Cookie	½ cup (3.2 oz)	170	1	8	26
Peanut Butter Cup	½ cup (3.2 oz)	180	3	8	25
Pralines N' Dream	½ cup (3.2 oz)	180	1	9	25
Silhouette					
The Skinny Cow Low Fat Ice Cream Sandwich Vanilla	1	130	5	2	23
Starbucks					
Biscotti Bliss	½ cup	240	4	12	30
Caffe Almond Fudge	½ cup	260	5	13	30
Caffe Almond Roast	1 bar	280	4	18	26
Dark Roast Expresso Swirl	½ cup	220	4	10	29
Italian Roast Coffee	½ cup	230	5	12	26
Javachip	½ cup	250	4	13	29
Low Fat Latte	½ cup	170	5	3	31
Low Fat Mocha Mambo	½ cup	170	5	3	32
Vanilla Mochachip	½ cup	270	4	16	27
Tofutti					
Cuties Chocolate	1 (1.4 oz)	130	2	5	16
Cuties Vanilla	1 (1.4 oz)	121	2	5	17
Monkey Bars Peanut Butter	1 bar (2.5 oz)	220	3	13	22
Turkey Hill					
Black Cherry	½ cup	140	2	7	18
Butter Pecan	½ cup	170	2	11	16
Cookies 'N Cream	½ cup	160	2	9	19
Light Butter Pecan	½ cup	130	3	6	17
Light Choco Mint Chip	½ cup	140	3	5	19
Light Vanilla & Chocolate	½ cup	110	3	3	18
Light Vanilla Bean	½ cup	110	3	3	18
Neapolitan	½ cup	150	2	8	18
Rocky Road	½ cup	170	3	8	23
Tin Roof Sundae	½ cup	160	2	9	19
Vanilla & Chocolate	½ cup	150	2	8	17
Vanilla Bean	½ cup	140	2	8	16
Weight Watchers					
Chocolate Chip Cookie Dough Sundae	1 (2.64 oz)	190	3	5	35
Chocolate Mousse	1 bar	40	2	1	9
Chocolate Treat	1 bar	100	3	1	20
English Toffee Crunch	1 bar	110	2	6	12
Orange Vanilla Treat	1 bar	40	2	1	10
Vanilla Sandwich	1 bar	150	3	3	28
take-out					
cone vanilla light soft serve	1 (4.6 oz)	164	4	6	24
gelato chocolate hazelnut	½ cup (5.3 oz)	370	9	29	26
gelato vanilla	½ cup (3 oz)	211	3	15	18
sundae caramel	1 (5.4 oz)	303	7	9	49

FOOD	PORTION	CALS	PROT	FAT	CARB
sundae hot fudge	1 (5.4 oz)	284	6	9	48
sundae strawberry	1 (5.4 oz)	269	6	8	45

ICE CREAM CONES AND CUPS

sugar cone	1	40	1	tr	8

Dutch Mill

Chocolate Covered Wafer Cups	1 (0.5 oz)	80	1	5	8

Frookie

Chocolate Crunch	1 (0.4 oz)	50	1	1	10
Honey Crunch	1 (0.4 oz)	45	1	1	9

Keebler

Fudge Dipped Cup	1 (0.3 oz)	35	0	2	6
Ice Creme Cup	1 (0.2 oz)	15	0	0	4

ICE CREAM TOPPINGS

butterscotch	2 tbsp (1.4 oz)	103	1	tr	27
caramel	2 tbsp (1.4 oz)	103	1	tr	27
marshmallow cream	1 oz	88	1	tr	23
marshmallow cream	1 jar (7 oz)	615	3	tr	157
strawberry	1 cup (11.5 oz)	863	1	1	225
walnuts in syrup	2 tbsp (1.4 oz)	167	2	9	22

Hershey

Chocolate Shop Double Chocolate	1 tbsp (0.7 oz)	50	0	0	13
Chocolate Shoppe Apple Pie A La Mode	2 tbsp (1.3 oz)	100	0	0	25
Chocolate Shoppe Chocolate Mini	1 tbsp (0.7 oz)	50	0	0	13
Chocolate Shoppe Hot Fudge Fat Free	2 tbsp (1.4 oz)	100	1	0	23
Chocolate Shoppe Sprinkles Reeses	1 tbsp (0.5 oz)	70	1	4	10

Kraft

Caramel	2 tbsp (1.4 oz)	120	2	0	28
Chocolate	2 tbsp (1.4 oz)	110	2	0	26
Hot Fudge	2 tbsp (1.4 oz)	140	1	5	24
Pineapple	2 tbsp (1.4 oz)	110	0	0	28
Strawberry	2 tbsp (1.4 oz)	110	0	0	29

Smucker's

Plate Scapers Caramel	2 tbsp	100	1	0	25

ICED TEA

mix

Crystal Light

Decaffeinated as prep	1 serv (8 oz)	5	0	0	tr
Iced Tea as prep	1 serv (8 oz)	5	0	0	0
Peach Tea as prep	1 serv (8 oz)	5	0	0	0
Raspberry Tea as prep	1 serv (8 oz)	5	0	0	0

FOOD	PORTION	CALS	PROT	FAT	CARB
Lipton					
100% Tea Decaffeinated as prep	1 serv	0	0	0	0
100% Tea Unsweetened as prep	1 serv	0	0	0	0
100% Tea as prep	1 serv	0	0	0	0
Calorie Free as prep	1 serv	0	0	0	0
Decaffeinated Ice Tea Brew as prep	1 serv (8 oz)	0	0	0	0
Decaffeinated Lemon as prep	1 serv	90	0	0	22
Diet Decaffeinated Lemon as prep	1 serv	5	0	0	1
Diet Lemon as prep	1 serv	5	0	0	1
Diet Peach as prep	1 serv	5	0	0	1
Diet Raspberry as prep	1 serv	5	0	0	1
Diet Tea & Lemondage as prep	1 serv	10	0	0	2
Herbal Iced Collection	1 tea bag	0	0	0	tr
Ice Tea Brew as prep	1 serv (8 oz)	0	0	0	0
Lemon as prep	1 serv	90	0	0	22
Lemon as prep	1 pkg (0.5 oz)	50	0	0	13
Natural Brew 100% Tea Decaffeinated as prep	1 serv	0	0	0	0
Natural Brew 100% Tea as prep	1 serv	0	0	0	0
Natural Brew Diet Lemon as prep	1 serv	5	0	0	1
Natural Brew Diet Peach as prep	1 serv	5	0	0	1
Natural Brew Diet Tropical as prep	1 serv	5	0	0	1
Natural Brew Tropical as prep	1 serv	90	0	0	22
Natural Brew Unsweetened Lemon as prep	1 serv	0	0	0	tr
Peach as prep	1 serv	90	0	0	22
Rasberry as prep	1 serv	90	0	0	22
Tea & Lemonade as prep	1 serv	90	0	0	22
Nestea					
100% Tea	2 tsp (1 g)	0	0	0	tr
100% Tea Decafe	2 tsp (1 g)	0	0	0	tr
Ice Teasers Lemon	1 serv (0.5 oz)	5	0	0	1
Ice Teasers Orange	1 serv (0.5 oz)	5	0	0	1
Ice Teasers Wild Cherry	1 serv (0.5 oz)	5	0	0	1
Lemon	2 tsp (1 g)	5	0	0	1
Lemon & Sugar	2 tbsp (0.7 oz)	80	0	0	19
Lemonade Tea	2 tbsp (0.7 oz)	80	0	0	19

FOOD	PORTION	CALS	PROT	FAT	CARB
Sugar Free	2 tbsp (0.7 oz)	5	0	0	1
Sugar Free Decafe	1 tbsp (0.7 oz)	5	0	0	1
Sun Tea	1 tsp (1 g)	0	0	0	tr
ready-to-drink					
Crystal Light					
Lemon	1 serv (8 oz)	5	0	0	0
Peach Tea	1 serv (8 oz)	5	0	0	0
Raspberry Tea	1 serv (8 oz)	5	0	0	0
Honest Tea					
Gold Rush Herbal Cinnamon	8 fl oz	9	0	0	3
Lipton					
Carribean Cooler	1 can (12 oz)	130	0	0	34
Diet Lemon	8 oz	0	0	0	0
Diet Lemon	1 bottle (16 oz)	10	0	0	0
Green Tea & Passion Fruit	1 bottle (16 oz)	160	0	0	38
Lemon	8 oz	80	0	0	20
Lemon	1 can (12 oz)	120	0	0	33
Lemon	1 bottle (16 oz)	180	0	0	42
Natural Lemon	1 box (8 oz)	100	0	0	25
Peach	8 oz	80	0	0	20
Peach	1 bottle (16 oz)	220	0	0	52
Raspberry	8 oz	80	0	0	20
Raspberry	1 bottle (16 oz)	220	0	0	52
Raspberry Blast	1 can (12 oz)	130	0	0	35
Southern Style Extra Sweet No Lemon	1 bottle (16 oz)	240	0	0	58
Southern Style Lemon	1 bottle (16 oz)	200	0	0	50
Southern Style Sweetened No Lemon	1 bottle (16 oz)	200	0	0	48
Sweet	8 oz	80	0	0	20
Sweetened No Lemon	1 bottle (16 oz)	140	0	0	36
Sweetened Lemon	8 oz	80	0	0	20
Tangerine Twist	1 can (12 oz)	120	0	0	33
Tea & Lemonade	1 bottle (16 oz)	220	0	0	52
Unsweetened No Lemon	1 bottle (16 oz)	0	0	0	0
Mad River					
Red Tea w/ Guarana	8 oz	90	0	0	24
Nantucket Nectars					
Diet	8 oz	5	0	0	1
Diet Green Tea	8 oz	5	0	0	1
Half & Half	8 oz	90	0	0	23
Iced Tea	8 oz	80	0	0	20
Matt Fee	8 oz	80	0	0	20
Raspberry	8 oz	90	0	0	23
Savannah	8 oz	80	0	0	20
Snapple					
Diet Lemon	8 fl oz	0	0	0	1
Diet Peach	8 fl oz	0	0	0	1

FOOD	PORTION	CALS	PROT	FAT	CARB
Diet Raspberry	8 fl oz	0	0	0	1
Ginseng Tea	8 fl oz	80	0	0	20
Green Tea w/ Lemon	8 fl oz	100	0	0	25
Lemon	8 fl oz	100	0	0	25
Peach	8 fl oz	100	0	0	26
Raspberry	8 fl oz	100	0	0	26
Turkey Hill					
Diet	1 cup	0	0	0	0
Diet Decaffeinated	1 cup	0	0	0	0
Green Tea w/ Ginseng & Honey	1 cup	70	17	0	17
Raspberry Tea	1 cup	110	0	0	28
Regular	1 cup	90	0	0	22
ICES AND ICE POPS					
(*see also* ICE CREAM AND FROZEN DESSERTS, PUDDING POPS, SHERBET, YOGURT FROZEN)					
fruit & juice bar	1 (3 fl oz)	75	1	tr	19
gelatin pop	1 (1.5 oz)	31	1	0	7
ice coconut pineapple	½ cup (4 fl oz)	109	0	3	23
ice pop	1 (2 fl oz)	42	0	0	11
Ben & Jerry's					
Sorbet Devil's Food Chocolate	½ cup	170	2	3	36
Sorbet Doonesberry	½ cup	140	0	0	33
Sorbet Lemon Swirl	½ cup	120	0	0	30
Sorbet Purple Passion Fruit	½ cup	140	0	0	29
Carnation					
Cup Orange Sherbet	1 (5 oz)	150	1	2	32
Cup Orange Sherbet	1 (3 oz)	90	1	1	19
Cold Fusion					
Protein Juice Bar All Flavors	1 bar (3.8 oz)	130	11	0	23
Cool Creations					
Ice Pop	1 pop (2 oz)	50	0	0	13
Mickey Mouse Bar	1 (4 oz)	170	2	11	17
Surprise Pops	1 (2 oz)	60	0	0	14
Dole					
Fruit'n Juice Coconut	1 bar (4 oz)	210	3	7	33
Fruit'n Juice Lemonade	1 bar (4 oz)	120	1	0	28
Fruit'n Juice Lime	1 bar (4 oz)	110	0	0	28
Fruit'n Juice Peach Passion	1 bar (2.5 oz)	70	0	0	17
Fruit'n Juice Pineapple Coconut	1 bar (4 oz)	150	1	4	27
Fruit'n Juice Pineapple Orange Banana	1 bar (2.5 oz)	70	0	0	16
Fruit'n Juice Pineapple Orange Banana	1 bar (4 oz)	110	0	0	26
Fruit'n Juice Raspberry	1 bar (2.5 oz)	70	0	0	16

FOOD	PORTION	CALS	PROT	FAT	CARB
Fruit'n Juice Strawberry	1 bar (2.5 oz)	70	0	0	17
Fruit'n Juice Strawberry	1 bar (4 oz)	110	0	0	26
Grape No Sugar Added	1 bar (1.75 oz)	25	0	0	6
Raspberry	1 bar (1.75 oz)	45	0	0	11
Raspberry No Sugar Added	1 bar (1.75 oz)	25	0	0	6
Strawberry	1 bar (1.75 oz)	45	0	0	11
Strawberry No Sugar Added	1 bar (1.75 oz)	25	0	0	6
Edy's					
Fruit Bars Strawberry	1 (3 oz)	80	0	0	21
Sherbet Berry Rainbow	½ cup	130	1	1	29
Sherbet Lime	½ cup	130	1	2	28
Sherbet Orange Cream	½ cup	120	2	2	23
Sherbet Raspberry	½ cup	130	1	1	28
Sherbet Starburst Orange & Cherry	½ cup	150	1	2	33
Sherbet Starburst Strawberry	½ cup	160	1	3	33
Sherbet Swiss Orange	½ cup	150	1	3	30
Sherbet Tropical Rainbow	½ cup	130	1	1	29
Sorbet Coconut	½ cup	140	1	3	28
Sorbet Lemon	½ cup	140	0	0	35
Sorbet Mandarin Orange	½ cup	130	0	0	32
Sorbet Peach	½ cup	130	0	0	32
Sorbet Raspberry	½ cup	130	0	0	33
Sorbet Strawberry	½ cup	120	0	0	31
Whole Fruit Bars Creamy Coconut	1 bar	120	3	3	21
Whole Fruit Bars Lemonade	1 bar	80	0	0	20
Whole Fruit Bars Lime	1 bar	80	0	0	20
Whole Fruit Bars Tangerine	1 bar	80	0	0	20
Whole Fruit Bars Wild Berry	1 bar	80	0	0	21
Flinstones					
Push-Up Sherbet Treats	1 (2.75 oz)	100	1	2	20
Frozfruit					
Banana Cream	1 bar (4 oz)	150	1	7	20
Cantaloupe	1 bar (4 oz)	60	0	0	35
Cappuccino Cream	1 bar (3 oz)	140	1	6	18
Cherry	1 bar (4 oz)	70	1	0	18
Coconut Cream	1 bar (4 oz)	170	2	11	17
Kiwi Strawberry	1 bar (4 oz)	90	0	0	23
Lemon	1 bar (4 oz)	90	0	0	22
Lemon Iced Tea	1 bar (4 oz)	80	0	0	19
Lime	1 bar (4 oz)	90	0	0	21
Orange	1 bar (4 oz)	90	0	0	21
Pina Colada Cream	1 bar (4 oz)	170	2	8	23
Pineapple	1 bar (4 oz)	80	0	0	19

FOOD	PORTION	CALS	PROT	FAT	CARB
Raspberry	1 bar (4 oz)	80	0	0	20
Strawberry	1 bar (4 oz)	80	0	0	20
Strawberry Banana Cream	1 bar (4 oz)	140	1	6	22
Strawberry Cream	1 bar (4 oz)	130	1	5	21
Tropical	1 bar (4 oz)	90	0	0	23
Watermelon	1 bar (4 oz)	50	0	0	13
Haagen-Dazs					
Sorbet Chocolate	½ cup	120	2	0	28
Sorbet Manago	½ cup	120	0	0	31
Sorbet Orange	½ cup	120	0	0	30
Sorbet Orchard Peach	½ cup	130	0	0	33
Sorbet Raspberry	½ cup	120	0	0	30
Sorbet Strawberry	½ cup	120	0	0	30
Sorbet Zesty Lemon	½ cup	120	0	0	31
Sorbet Bar Chocolate	1 (2.7 oz)	80	1	0	20
Sorbet Bars Raspberry & Vanilla Yogurt	1 (2.5 oz)	90	2	0	21
Sorbet Bars Strawberry & Vanilla Ice Cream	1 (2.5 oz)	110	1	5	15
Mr. Freeze					
Assorted	2 bars (3 oz)	45	0	0	11
Tropical	2 bars (3 oz)	45	0	0	11
Natural Choice					
Organic Banana	½ cup (3.6 oz)	110	0	0	28
Organic Blueberry	½ cup (3.6 oz)	100	0	0	27
Organic Kiwi	½ cup (3.6 oz)	110	0	0	28
Organic Lemon	½ cup (3.6 oz)	110	0	0	28
Organic Mango	½ cup (3.6 oz)	110	0	0	28
Organic Strawberry	½ cup (3.6 oz)	110	0	0	28
Organic Strawberry Kiwi	½ cup (3.6 oz)	110	0	0	28
INSTANT BREAKFAST					
(see BREAKFAST DRINKS)					
JACKFRUIT					
fresh	3.5 oz	70	1	tr	4
JALAPENO					
(see PEPPERS)					
JAM/JELLY/PRESERVES					
apple butter	1 tbsp (0.6 oz)	33	0	0	9
orange marmalade	1 pkg (0.5 oz)	34	0	0	9
quince jam	0.5 oz	43	0	0	8
raspberry jelly	0.5 oz	37	0	0	9
red currant jam	0.5 oz	34	1	0	8
red currant jelly	0.5 oz	38	0	0	9
Eden					
Cherry Butter	1 tbsp	35	0	0	9
Organic Apple Butter	1 tbsp	20	0	0	5

FOOD	PORTION	CALS	PROT	FAT	CARB
Estee					
Fruit Spread Apple Spice	1 tbsp	16	0	0	4
Fruit Spread Apricot	1 tbsp	16	0	0	4
Fruit Spread Grape	1 tbsp	16	0	0	4
Fruit Spread Peach	1 tbsp	16	0	0	4
Fruit Spread Red Raspberry	1 tbsp	16	0	0	4
Fruit Spread Strawberry	1 tbsp	16	0	0	4
Polaner					
All Fruit Peach	1 tbsp	40	0	0	8
All Fruit Raspberry	1 tbsp	40	0	0	10
Smucker's					
Concord Grape Jelly	1 tbsp	50	0	0	13
Peach Preserves	1 tbsp	50	0	0	13
Simply Fruit Red Raspberry	1 tbsp	40	0	0	10
Tabasco					
Spicy Pepper Jelly	1 tbsp (0.6 oz)	50	0	0	12
White House					
Apple Butter	1 tbsp (0.6 oz)	35	0	0	9
JAPANESE FOOD					
(*see* ASIAN FOOD, SUSHI)					
JAVA PLUM					
fresh	1 cup	82	1	tr	21
KALE					
fresh					
chopped cooked	½ cup	21	1	tr	4
scotch chopped cooked	½ cup	18	1	tr	4
frozen					
chopped cooked	½ cup	20	2	tr	4
KEFIR					
kefir	7 oz	132	6	8	10
KETCHUP					
Del Monte					
Ketchup	1 tbsp (0.5 oz)	15	0	0	4
Estee					
Ketchup	1 tbsp	15	0	0	5
Heinz					
Ketchup	1 tbsp (0.6 oz)	15	0	0	4
McIlhenny					
Spicy	1 tbsp (0.6 oz)	20	0	0	5
Muir Glen					
Organic	1 tbsp (0.6 oz)	15	0	0	3
Smucker's					
Tomato	1 tbsp	25	0	0	7
Tree Of Life					
Ketchup	1 tbsp (0.5 oz)	10	0	0	3
KIDNEY					
beef simmered	3 oz	122	22	3	0
lamb braised	3 oz	117	20	3	1

FOOD	PORTION	CALS	PROT	FAT	CARB
pork cooked	1 cup	211	36	7	0
pork cooked	3 oz	128	22	4	0
veal braised	3 oz	139	22	5	0
KIDNEY BEANS					
canned					
kidney beans	1 cup	208	13	1	38
red	1 cup	216	13	1	40
Eden					
Organic Cannellini	½ cup (4.6 oz)	100	6	1	17
Green Giant					
Dark Red	½ cup (4.5 oz)	110	6	0	18
Light Red	½ cup (4.5 oz)	110	8	0	20
Hunt's					
Kidney	½ cup (4.5 oz)	94	6	1	20
Progresso					
Dark Red	½ cup (4.5 oz)	110	8	0	20
Red	½ cup (4.6 oz)	110	7	1	20
S&W					
Dark Red Premium	½ cup (4.6 oz)	100	7	1	23
Van Camp					
Dark Red	½ cup (4.6 oz)	90	6	0	20
Light Red	½ cup (4.6 oz)	90	6	0	20
dried					
california red cooked	1 cup	219	16	tr	40
cooked	1 cup	225	15	1	40
red cooked	1 cup	225	15	1	40
royal red cooked	1 cup	218	17	tr	39
KIWIS					
fresh	1 med	46	1	tr	11
Chiquita					
Fresh	2 med (5.2 oz)	100	2	1	24
KNISH					
take-out					
cheese & blueberry	1 (7 oz)	378	24	13	40
cheese & cherry	1 (7 oz)	378	24	13	40
everything	1 (7 oz)	221	7	8	34
kashe	1 (7 oz)	270	7	8	45
potato	1 lg (7 oz)	332	8	12	49
potato	1 med (3.5 oz)	166	4	6	25
potato w/ broccoli & cheese	1 (7 oz)	312	12	15	33
potato w/ spinach & mushroom	1 (7 oz)	214	6	8	32
KOHLRABI					
raw sliced	½ cup	19	1	tr	4
sliced cooked	½ cup	24	1	tr	5
KRILL					
fresh	1 oz	22	3	1	tr

FOOD	PORTION	CALS	PROT	FAT	CARB
LAMB					
(see also LAMB DISHES)					
cubed lean only braised	3 oz	190	29	7	0
cubed lean only broiled	3 oz	158	24	6	0
ground broiled	3 oz	240	21	17	0
leg lean & fat Choice roasted	3 oz	219	22	14	14
loin chop w/ bone lean & fat Choice broiled	1 chop (2.3 oz)	201	16	15	0
loin chop w/ bone lean only Choice broiled	1 chop (1.6 oz)	100	14	5	0
new zealand lean & fat cooked	3 oz	259	21	19	0
new zealand lean only cooked	3 oz	175	25	8	0
rib chop lean & fat Choice broiled	3 oz	307	19	25	0
rib chop lean only Choice broiled	3 oz	200	24	11	0
shank lean & fat Choice braised	3 oz	206	24	11	0
shank lean & fat Choice roasted	3 oz	191	22	11	0
shoulder chop w/ bone lean & fat Choice braised	1 chop (2.5 oz)	244	21	17	0
shoulder chop w/ bone lean only Choice braised	1 chop (1.9 oz)	152	19	8	0
sirloin lean & fat Choice roasted	3 oz	248	21	21	0
LAMB DISHES					
take-out					
curry	¾ cup	345	26	17	22
moussaka	5.6 oz	312	15	21	16
stew	¾ cup	124	10	5	11
LAMBSQUARTERS					
chopped cooked	½ cup	29	3	1	5
LEEKS					
cooked	1 (4.4 oz)	38	1	tr	9
raw	1 (4.4 oz)	76	2	tr	18
LEMON GRASS					
fresh	1 cup (2.4 oz)	66	1	tr	17
LEMON JUICE					
Canarino					
Italian Hot Lemon Beverage	1 cup	0	0	0	0
Realemon					
Juice	1 tsp (5 ml)	0	0	0	0

FOOD	PORTION	CALS	PROT	FAT	CARB
LEMONADE					
frozen					
not prep	1 can (6 oz)	397	1	tr	103
mix					
powder as prep w/ water	9 fl oz	113	0	tr	29
Country Time					
Lem'n Berry Sippers Cranberry Raspberry Lemonade as prep	1 serv (8 oz)	90	0	0	21
Lem'n Berry Sippers Raspberry Lemonade as prep	1 serv (8 oz)	90	0	0	21
Lem'n Berry Sippers Strawberry Lemonade as prep	1 serv (8 oz)	90	0	0	21
Lem'n Berry Sippers Wildberry Lemonade as prep	1 serv (8 oz)	90	0	0	21
Lem'n Berry Sippers Sugar Free Strawberry Lemonade as prep	1 serv (8 oz)	5	0	0	0
Lemonade as prep	1 serv (8 oz)	70	0	0	17
Pink as prep	1 serv (8 oz)	70	0	0	17
Sugar Free Pink as prep	1 serv (8 oz)	5	0	0	0
Sugar Free as prep	1 serv (8 oz)	5	0	0	0
Crystal Light					
Lemonade as prep	1 serv (8 oz)	5	0	0	0
Pink as prep	1 serv (8 oz)	5	0	0	0
Kool-Aid					
Lemonade as prep	1 serv (8 oz)	70	0	0	17
Mix as prep w/ sugar	1 serv (8 oz)	100	0	0	25
Pink as prep w/ sugar	1 serv (8 oz)	100	0	0	25
Soarin' Strawberry Lemonade as prep	1 serv (8 oz)	70	0	0	17
Soarin' Strawberry Lemonade as prep w/ sugar	1 serv (8 oz)	100	0	0	25
Sugar Free Soarin' Strawberry Lemonade as prep	1 serv (8 oz)	5	0	0	0
Sugar Free Mix as prep	1 serv (8 oz)	5	0	0	0
ready-to-drink					
Crystal Light					
Lemonade	1 serv (8 oz)	5	0	0	0
Pink	1 serv (8 oz)	5	0	0	0
Everfresh					
Lemonade	1 can (8 oz)	120	0	0	29
Ruby Red	1 can (8 oz)	110	0	0	27

FOOD	PORTION	CALS	PROT	FAT	CARB
Nantucket Nectars					
Authentic	8 oz	120	0	0	30
Pink	8 oz	120	0	0	30
Newman's Own					
Lemonade	1 bottle (10 oz)	140	0	0	34
Roadside Virginia	8 fl oz	110	0	0	27
Shasta Plus					
Lemonade	1 can (11.5 oz)	160	0	0	40
Snapple					
Diet Pink	8 fl oz	20	0	0	4
Lemonade	8 fl oz	120	0	0	30
Pink	8 fl oz	120	0	0	29
Turkey Hill					
Lemonade	1 cup	120	0	0	29
Veryfine					
Chillers	1 can (11.5 oz)	190	0	0	48
Chillers Cherry	8 fl oz	120	0	0	29
Chillers Peach	8 fl oz	120	0	0	31
Chillers Pink	1 can (11.5 oz)	180	0	0	45
Chillers Strawberry	1 can (11.5 oz)	170	0	0	43
LENTILS					
dried cooked	1 cup	231	18	1	40
Natural Touch					
Lentil Rice Loaf	1 in slice (3.2 oz)	170	8	9	14
Shiloh Farms					
Organic Green not prep	¼ cup (1.6 oz)	150	11	0	27
TastyBite					
Bengal Lentils	½ pkg (5 oz)	190	7	5	30
Jodhpur Lentils	½ pkg (5 oz)	190	6	9	22
take-out					
indian sambar	1 serv	236	15	5	37
yemiser selatta eithopian lentil salad	1 serv (3 oz)	115	4	7	11
LETTUCE					
(see also SALAD)					
bibb	1 head (6 oz)	21	2	tr	4
boston	1 head (6 oz)	21	2	tr	4
cornsalad field salad	1 cup (1.9 oz)	7	1	tr	1
iceberg	1 head (19 oz)	70	5	1	11
Dole					
Iceberg	1 cup (3 oz)	15	1	0	3
Romaine	1½ cups (3 oz)	15	1	0	2
Shredded	1½ cup (3 oz)	15	1	0	3
Earthbound Farm					
Romaine Salad Organic	1½ cups (2.9 oz)	15	3	0	3
LILY ROOT					
dried	1 oz	89	2	1	21
fresh	1 oz	32	1	tr	8

FOOD	PORTION	CALS	PROT	FAT	CARB
LIMA BEANS					
canned					
large	1 cup	191	12	tr	36
lima beans	½ cup	93	6	tr	17
Del Monte					
Green	½ cup (4.4 oz)	80	4	0	15
Eden					
Organic Baby	½ cup (4.6 oz)	100	6	1	17
S&W					
Small Green	½ cup (4.4 oz)	80	4	0	15
dried					
baby cooked	1 cup	229	15	1	42
cooked	½ cup	104	6	tr	20
large cooked	1 cup	217	15	1	39
Hurst					
HamBeans Baby Limas w/ Ham	1 serv	120	7	1	22
HamBeans Large Limas w/ Ham	1 serv	120	7	1	22
frozen					
cooked	½ cup	94	6	tr	18
fordhook cooked	½ cup	85	5	tr	16
Birds Eye					
Baby	½ cup	130	7	0	24
Fordhook	½ cup	100	6	0	19
Green Giant					
Butter Sauce	⅔ cup (3.6 oz)	120	6	3	18
Harvest Fresh Baby	½ cup (2.7 oz)	80	4	0	15
LIME JUICE					
Realime					
Juice	1 tsp (5 ml)	0	0	0	0
LING					
blue raw	3.5 oz	83	17	1	0
fresh baked	3 oz	95	21	1	0
fresh fillet baked	5.3 oz	168	37	1	0
LINGCOD					
baked	3 oz	93	19	1	0
fillet baked	5.3 oz	164	34	2	0
LIQUOR/LIQUEUR					
(*see also* BEER AND ALE, CHAMPAGNE, DRINK MIXERS, MALT, WINE, WINE COOLERS)					
aquavit	1 oz	65	0	0	0
bloody mary	5 oz	116	1	tr	5
bourbon & soda	4 oz	105	0	0	0
coffee liqueur	1½ oz	174	0	tr	24
coffee w/ cream liqueur	1½ oz	154	1	7	10
cognac	1 oz	67	0	0	tr
creme de menthe	1½ oz	186	0	tr	21
daiquiri	2 oz	111	0	0	4

FOOD	PORTION	CALS	PROT	FAT	CARB
gin	1½ oz	110	0	0	0
gin & tonic	7.5 oz	171	0	0	16
manhattan	2 oz	128	0	0	2
martini	2½ oz	156	0	0	tr
pina colada	4½ oz	262	1	3	40
rum	1½ oz	97	0	0	0
screwdriver	7 oz	174	1	tr	18
sloe gin fizz	2½ oz	132	0	0	4
tequila sunrise	5½ oz	189	1	tr	15
vodka	1½ oz	97	0	0	0
whiskey	1½ oz	105	0	0	tr
LIVER					
beef braised	3 oz	137	21	4	3
beef pan-fried	3 oz	184	23	7	7
chicken stewed	1 cup (5 oz)	219	34	8	1
duck raw	1 (1.5 oz)	60	8	2	2
goose raw	1 (3.3 oz)	125	15	4	6
lamb braised	3 oz	187	26	7	2
lamb fried	3 oz	202	22	11	3
pork braised	3 oz	140	22	4	3
sheep raw	3.5 oz	131	21	4	0
turkey simmered	1 cup (5 oz)	237	34	8	5
veal braised	3 oz	140	18	6	2
veal fried	3 oz	208	25	10	3
LOBSTER					
northern cooked	1 cup	142	30	1	2
northern cooked	3 oz	83	17	1	1
northern raw	3 oz	77	77	1	tr
northern raw	1 lobster (5.3 oz)	136	28	1	1
spiny steamed	3 oz	122	22	2	3
spiny steamed	1 (5.7 oz)	233	43	3	5
Progresso					
Lobster Sauce	½ cup (4.3 oz)	100	3	7	6
take-out					
newburg	1 cup	485	46	27	13
LOGANBERRIES					
frzn	1 cup	80	2	tr	19
LOTUS					
root raw sliced	10 slices	45	2	tr	14
root sliced cooked	10 slices	59	1	tr	14
seeds dried	1 oz	94	4	1	18
Eden					
Root	1 serv (0.3 oz)	35	1	0	8
LOX					
(*see* SALMON)					
LUPINES					
dried cooked	1 cup	197	26	5	16

FOOD	PORTION	CALS	PROT	FAT	CARB
MACADAMIA NUTS					
dry roasted w/ salt	10–12 nuts (1 oz)	200	2	22	4
oil roasted	1 oz	204	2	22	4
Hawaiian Host					
Chocolate Covered	1 piece (0.5 oz)	53	1	6	8
MacFarms of Hawaii					
Chocolate Covered	¼ cup (1.3 oz)	210	3	16	18
Dry Roasted Salted	¼ cup (1.3 oz)	220	3	23	4
Kona Coffee Dark Chocolate Covered	¼ cup (1.3 oz)	210	3	16	18
MACKEREL					
canned					
jack	1 can (12.7 oz)	563	84	23	0
jack	1 cup	296	44	12	0
dried					
Eden					
Bonito Flakes	2 tbsp	4	1	0	0
fresh					
atlantic cooked	3 oz	223	20	15	0
atlantic raw	3 oz	174	16	12	0
jack baked	3 oz	171	22	9	0
jack fillet baked	6.2 oz	354	45	18	0
king baked	3 oz	114	22	2	0
king fillet baked	5.4 oz	207	40	4	0
pacific baked	3 oz	171	22	9	0
pacific fillet baked	6.2 oz	354	45	18	0
spanish cooked	3 oz	134	20	5	0
spanish cooked	1 fillet (5.1 oz)	230	34	9	0
spanish raw	3 oz	118	16	5	0
smoked					
atlantic	3.5 oz	296	19	24	0
MALANGA					
fresh	½ cup	137	2	tr	32
MALT					
nonalcoholic	12 fl oz	32	1	0	5
MALTED MILK					
chocolate as prep w/ milk	1 cup	229	9	9	30
chocolate flavor powder	3 heaping tsp (¾ oz)	79	1	1	18
natural flavor as prep w/ milk	1 cup	237	10	10	27
natural flavor powder	3 heaping tsp (¾ oz)	87	2	2	19
Carnation					
Chocolate	3 tbsp (0.7 oz)	90	1	1	18
Original	3 tbsp (0.7 oz)	90	3	2	15
MAMMY-APPLE					
fresh	1	431	4	4	106

FOOD	PORTION	CALS	PROT	FAT	CARB
MANGO					
fresh	1	135	1	1	35
Del Monte					
In Extra Light Syrup	½ cup (4.4 oz)	100	0	1	25
Rainforest Farms					
Slices Dried	6 slices (1.3 oz)	140	1	1	33
MANGO JUICE					
Fresh Samantha					
Mango Mama	1 cup (8 oz)	120	2	0	10
Guzzler					
Mango Passion	8 fl oz	140	0	0	22
Ocean Spray					
Mango Mango	8 oz	130	0	0	33
Snapple					
Mango Madness	8 fl oz	110	0	0	29
Tang					
Drink Mix as prep	1 serv (8 oz)	100	0	0	25
MARGARINE					
stick corn	1 stick (4 oz)	815	1	91	1
stick corn	1 tsp	34	0	4	0
tub corn	1 tsp	34	0	4	0
tub diet	1 tsp	17	0	2	0
Take Control					
Spread	1 tbsp (0.5 oz)	50	0	6	0
Weight Watchers					
Light	1 tbsp	45	0	4	2
Light Sodium Free	1 tbsp	45	0	4	2
MARINADE					
(*see* SAUCE)					
MARSHMALLOW					
marshmallow	1 cup (1.6 oz)	146	1	tr	37
Just Born					
Peeps	5 (1.5 oz)	160	1	0	40
MATZO					
egg	1 (1 oz)	111	4	1	22
egg & onion	1 (1 oz)	111	3	1	22
plain	1 (1 oz)	112	3	tr	24
whole wheat	1 (1 oz)	99	4	tr	22
Manischewitz					
Matzo Meal	¼ cup (1 oz)	130	3	0	23
MAYONNAISE					
mayonnaise	1 cup	1577	2	175	6
reduced calorie	1 tbsp	34	0	3	2
reduced calorie	1 cup	556	1	46	38
Blue Plate					
Squeeze	1 tbsp	100	0	11	0
Hellman's					
Mayonnaise	1 tbsp	100	0	11	0

FOOD	PORTION	CALS	PROT	FAT	CARB
Kraft					
Fat Free	1 tbsp (0.6 oz)	10	0	0	2
Light	1 tbsp (0.5 oz)	50	0	5	2
Real	1 tbsp (0.5 oz)	100	0	11	0
Weight Watchers					
Fat Free	1 tbsp	10	0	0	3
Light	1 tbsp	25	0	2	1
Light Low Sodium	1 tbsp	25	0	2	1
MAYONNAISE TYPE SALAD DRESSING					
home recipe	1 tbsp	25	1	2	2
home recipe	1 cup	400	11	24	38
mayonnaise type salad dressing	1 cup	916	2	78	56
reduced calorie w/o cholesterol	1 tbsp	68	7	7	2
Miracle Whip					
Free	1 tbsp (0.5 oz)	15	0	0	2
Light	1 tbsp (0.5 oz)	35	0	3	2
Salad Dressing	1 tbsp (0.6 oz)	70	0	7	2
Nasoya					
Nayonaise	1 tbsp	35	0	4	1
Nayonaise Dijon	1 tbsp	30	0	3	1
Weight Watchers					
Fat Free Whipped Dressing	1 tbsp	15	0	0	3
MEAT STICKS					
jerky beef	1 lg piece (0.7 oz)	67	8	3	3
jerky beef	1 oz	96	11	4	4
smoked	1 oz	156	6	14	2
smoked	1 (0.7 oz)	109	4	10	1
Big Ones					
BBQ	1 (1 oz)	130	5	12	1
Hot n'Spicy	1 (1 oz)	130	6	12	1
Original	1 (1 oz)	130	5	12	1
Teriyaki	1 (1 oz)	130	6	12	2
Jack Link's					
Kippered Beefsteak Teriyaki	1 oz	80	13	1	5
Lance					
Beef & Cheese	1 pkg (1.5 oz)	150	9	11	3
Beef Jerky	1 piece (0.25 oz)	30	2	2	tr
Beef Snack	1 piece (0.63 oz)	100	4	8	1
Hot Sausage	1 piece (0.9 oz)	60	4	5	1
Lowrey's					
Smokehouse Tender Hickory Smoked	1 pkg (1 oz)	80	10	2	5
Smokehouse Tender Original	1 pkg (1 oz)	60	11	1	2

FOOD	PORTION	CALS	PROT	FAT	CARB
Smokehouse Tender Peppered	1 pkg (1 oz)	60	11	1	2
Oberto					
Beef Jerky	1 pkg (1.3 oz)	100	15	1	8
Pemmican					
Original Tender Kippered Beef Steak	1	110	12	5	3
Peppered Tender Kippered Beef Steak	1	110	12	5	3
Rough Cut					
Beef Steak Hot	1 pkg (1 oz)	70	10	1	2
Beef Steak Original	1 pkg (1 oz)	60	10	1	2
Beef Steak Peppered	1 pkg (1 oz)	60	10	1	2
Rustlers Roundup					
Beef Jerky	1 serv (5 g)	20	2	2	tr
Flamin' Hot	1 serv (8 g)	40	2	3	1
Smoky Steak	1 serv (0.8 oz)	60	8	2	1
Spicy	1 serv (0.5 oz)	70	3	6	1
Slim Jim					
Spicy	1 (4½ in) (0.3 oz)	50	2	4	0
Spicy Big	1 (.44 oz)	70	1	6	1
Spicy Giant	1 (0.97 oz)	150	6	14	2
Spicy Super	1 (0.64 oz)	100	4	9	1

MEAT SUBSTITUTES

(*see also* BACON SUBSTITUTES, CANADIAN BACON SUBSTITUTES, CHICKEN SUBSTITUTES, HAMBURGER SUBSTITUTES, SAUSAGE SUBSTITUTES, AND TURKEY SUBSTITUTES)

FOOD	PORTION	CALS	PROT	FAT	CARB
simulated meat product	1 oz	88	11	1	11
Amy's Organic					
Whole Meals Veggie Loaf	1 pkg (10 oz)	260	8	5	47
Boca Burgers					
Chef Max's Original	1 patty (2.5 oz)	110	14	2	9
Frieda's					
SoyTaco	1 oz	50	4	3	3
Soyrizo	4 tbsp (1.9 oz)	120	7	9	5
Ken & Robert's					
Veggie Pockets	1 (4.5 oz)	250	8	8	40
Veggie Pockets Bar B Que	1 (4.5 oz)	290	10	8	45
Veggie Pockets Broccoli & Cheddar	1 (4.5 oz)	250	9	8	38
Veggie Pockets Greek	1 (4.5 oz)	250	10	8	37
Veggie Pockets Indian	1 (4.5 oz)	260	8	8	40
Veggie Pockets Pizza	1 (4.5 oz)	270	9	8	41
Veggie Pockets Pot Pie	1 (4.5 oz)	250	8	9	38
Veggie Pockets Potato & Cheddar	1 (4.5 oz)	260	6	8	42
Veggie Pockets Santa Fe	1 (4.5 oz)	250	8	8	39
Veggie Pockets Tex Mex	1 (4.5 oz)	260	9	8	46

FOOD	PORTION	CALS	PROT	FAT	CARB
Lightlife					
Foney Baloney	3 slices (1.5 oz)	60	8	3	2
Gimme Lean Beef	2 oz	70	9	0	8
Smart Deli Bologna	3 slices (1.5 oz)	50	10	0	2
Smart Deli Ham	3 slices (1.5 oz)	50	10	0	2
Smart Deli Peppercorn	3 slices (1.5 oz)	45	10	0	1
Smart Deli Stickes Soylami	1 oz	40	9	0	1
Smart Deli Sticks Pepperoni	1 oz	45	9	0	2
Smart Ground Original	⅓ cup (1.9 oz)	70	12	0	5
Smart Ground Taco	⅓ cup (2 oz)	60	10	0	6
Loma Linda					
Dinner Cuts	2 slices (3.2 oz)	90	17	2	3
Nuteena	⅜ in slice (1.9 oz)	160	6	13	6
Sandwich Spread	¼ cup (1.9 oz)	80	4	5	7
Savory Dinner Loaf Mix not prep	⅓ cup (0.9 oz)	90	14	2	7
Swiss Stake	1 piece (3.2 oz)	120	9	6	8
Tender Bits	6 pieces (3 oz)	110	11	5	7
Tender Rounds	6 pieces (2.8 oz)	120	14	5	5
Vita Burger Chunks not prep	¼ cup (0.7 oz)	70	10	1	6
Vita Burger Granules	3 tbsp (0.7 oz)	70	10	1	6
Morningstar Farms					
Burger Style Recipe Crumbles	⅔ cup (1.9 oz)	80	10	3	4
Ground Meatless	½ cup (1.9 oz)	60	10	0	4
Harvest Burger Recipe Crumbles	½ cup (2 oz)	70	12	0	5
Quarter Prime	1 patty (3.4 oz)	140	24	2	6
Natural Touch					
Dinner Entree	1 patty (3 oz)	220	19	15	2
Loaf Mix not prep	4 tbsp (1 oz)	100	14	1	10
Stroganoff Mix not prep	4 tbsp (0.8 oz)	90	5	4	10
Taco Mix not prep	3 tbsp (0.6 oz)	60	8	1	4
Vegan Burger Crumbles	½ cup (1.9 oz)	60	10	0	4
Quorn					
Grounds	⅔ cup (3 oz)	80	13	3	5
Worthington					
Beef Style Meatless	⅜ in slice (1.9 oz)	110	9	7	4
Bolono	3 slices (2 oz)	80	10	4	2
Choplets	2 slices (3.2 oz)	90	17	2	3
Corned Beef Meatless	4 slices (2 oz)	140	10	9	5
Country Stew	1 cup (8.4 oz)	210	13	9	20
Dinner Roast	¾ in slice (3 oz)	180	12	12	5
FriPats	1 patty (2.2 oz)	130	14	6	4
Multigrain Cutlets	2 slices (3.2 oz)	100	15	2	5
Numete	⅜ in slice (1.9 oz)	130	6	10	5
Prime Stakes	1 piece (3.2 oz)	120	10	7	4

FOOD	PORTION	CALS	PROT	FAT	CARB
Prosage Roll	⅝ in slice (1.9 oz)	140	10	10	2
Protose	⅜ in slice (1.9 oz)	130	13	7	5
Salami Meatless	3 slices (2 oz)	130	12	8	2
Savory Slices	3 slices (2.9 oz)	150	10	9	6
Smoked Beef Meatless	6 slices (2 oz)	120	11	6	6
Stakelets	1 piece (2.5 oz)	140	12	8	6
Veelets	1 patty (2.5 oz)	180	14	9	10
Vegetable Skallops	½ cup (3 oz)	90	15	2	3
Vegetable Steaks	2 pieces (2.5 oz)	80	15	2	3
Wham	2 slices (1.6 oz)	80	7	5	1
Yves					
Veggie Bologna	4 slices (2.2 oz)	70	15	0	2
Veggie Ground Italian	⅓ cup (2 oz)	60	10	0	4
Veggie Ground Round Italian	⅓ cup (1.9 oz)	60	10	0	4
Veggie Ground Round Original	2 oz	60	10	0	4
Veggie Pizza Pepperoni Slices	1 serv (1.7 oz)	70	14	0	4
Veggie Salami Deli Slices	1 serv (2.2 oz)	90	17	0	5
MELON					
melon balls frzn	1 cup	55	1	tr	14
Sunfresh					
Melon Salad In Extra Light Syrup	½ cup (4.5 oz)	45	0	0	10
MELON JUICE					
Ocean Spray					
Mega Melon	8 oz	130	0	0	33
MEXICAN FOOD					
(*see* SALSA, SAUCE, SPANISH FOODS, TORTILLA)					
MILK					
canned					
condensed sweetened	1 oz	123	3	3	21
condensed sweetened	1 cup	982	24	27	166
evaporated	½ cup	169	9	10	13
evaporated skim	½ cup	99	10	tr	14
Carnation					
Evaporated	½ cup	150	2	8	3
Evaporated Fat Free	½ cup (4 fl oz)	100	9	0	4
Evaporated Lowfat	½ cup	110	2	2	3
Sweetened Condensed	⅓ cup	330	3	8	22
dried					
buttermilk	1 tbsp	25	2	tr	3
nonfat instantized	1 pkg (3.2 oz)	244	32	tr	47
Carnation					
Nonfat	⅓ cup	80	8	0	12
Saco					
Cultured Buttermilk	4 tbsp (0.8 oz)	80	5	tr	13

FOOD	PORTION	CALS	PROT	FAT	CARB
Sanalac					
Powder	¼ cup (0.8 oz)	85	8	tr	13
refrigerated					
1%	1 cup	102	8	3	12
1%	1 qt	409	32	10	47
1% protein fortified	1 qt	477	39	12	54
1% protein fortified	1 cup	119	10	3	14
2%	1 cup	121	8	5	12
2%	1 qt	485	33	19	47
buffalo	7 oz	224	8	16	10
buttermilk	1 cup	99	8	2	12
buttermilk	1 qt	396	32	9	47
camel	7 oz	160	10	8	10
donkey	7 oz	86	4	2	12
goat	1 cup	168	9	10	11
goat	1 qt	672	35	40	43
human	1 cup	171	3	11	17
indian buffalo	1 cup	236	9	17	13
low sodium	1 cup	149	8	8	11
mare	7 oz	98	4	4	12
nonfat	1 cup	86	8	tr	12
nonfat	1 qt	342	33	2	48
nonfat protein fortified	1 qt	400	39	2	55
nonfat protein fortified	1 cup	100	10	1	14
sheep	1 cup	264	15	17	13
whole	1 cup	150	8	8	11
Cool Cow					
Low Fat	1 cup (8 oz)	110	9	3	12
Farmland					
Skim Plus	1 cup (8 oz)	110	11	0	17
Horizon Organic					
Fat Free	1 cup (8 oz)	80	8	0	12
Land O Lakes					
1% Lowfat	1 carton (10 oz)	120	10	3	13
Fat Free	1 carton (10 oz)	100	10	5	13
Whole	1 carton (10 oz)	180	10	10	13
NutraBalance					
LactaCare	1 pkg (8 oz)	500	18	18	64
Organic Valley					
Low Fat	1 cup	100	8	3	12
Nonfat	1 cup	80	8	0	13
Reduced Fat	1 cup	130	8	5	12
Whole	1 cup	150	8	8	12
Stonyfield Farm					
Organic Whole Milk	1 cup (8 oz)	180	9	10	12
Organic Whole Milk Vanilla	1 cup (8 oz)	230	8	8	30

FOOD	PORTION	CALS	PROT	FAT	CARB
Turkey Hill					
Cool Moos 2% Reduced Fat	1 cup	130	8	5	12
Cool Moos Whole Milk	1 cup	160	8	8	12
MILK DRINKS					
chocolate milk	1 cup	208	8	8	26
chocolate milk	1 qt	833	32	34	103
chocolate milk 1%	1 cup	158	8	3	26
chocolate milk 1%	1 qt	630	32	10	104
chocolate milk 2%	1 cup	179	8	5	26
strawberry flavor mix as prep w/ whole milk	9 oz	234	8	8	33
Horizon Organic					
Lowfat Chocolate Milk	1 cup (8 oz)	160	9	3	26
Land O Lakes					
Chocolate	1 cup (8.4 oz)	200	8	7	27
Organic Valley					
Chocolate Milk Reduced Fat	1 cup	180	8	5	26
Quik					
Banana Lowfat	1 cup (8.4 oz)	200	7	5	31
Banana Powder	2 tbsp (0.8 oz)	90	0	0	27
Chocolate	1 cup (8.4 oz)	230	7	8	33
Chocolate Lowfat	1 carton (8.4 oz)	200	8	5	30
Cookies n Cream Powder	2 tbsp (0.8 oz)	100	1	1	21
Strawberry	1 cup (8.4 oz)	230	7	8	33
Strawberry Lowfat	1 carton (8.4 oz)	210	8	5	35
Strawberry Powder	2 tbsp (0.8 oz)	90	0	0	22
Turkey Hill					
Cool Moos Chocolate 1% Lowfat	1 cup	180	8	3	32
Cool Moos Orange Cream 1% Lowfat	1 cup	190	8	3	33
Cool Moos Strawberry 1% Lowfat	1 cup	160	8	3	27
Cool Moos Vanilla 1% Lowfat	1 cup	160	8	3	26
MILK SUBSTITUTES					
imitation milk	1 cup	150	4	8	15
imitation milk	1 qt	600	17	33	60
8th Continent					
Soymilk Low Fat Chocolate	1 bottle (8 oz)	140	7	3	23
Soymilk Low Fat Original	1 bottle (8 oz)	80	7	3	8
Soymilk Low Fat Vanilla	1 bottle (8 oz)	90	7	3	11
Better Than Milk					
Rice Original	2 tbsp (0.66 oz)	78	0	2	15
Rice Original Light	2 tbsp (0.66 oz)	66	0	0	17
Rice Vanilla	2 tbsp (0.66 oz)	78	0	2	15
Rice Vanilla Light	2 tbsp (0.66 oz)	66	0	0	17

FOOD	PORTION	CALS	PROT	FAT	CARB
Soy Carob	2 tbsp (1 oz)	90	3	2	18
Soy Chocolate	2 tbsp (1.1 oz)	112	3	2	21
Soy Light	2 tbsp (0.66 oz)	73	6	2	8
Soy Original	2 tbsp (0.8 oz)	100	2	3	16
Soy Vanilla	2 tbsp (0.7 oz)	77	6	2	8
Blue Diamond					
Almond Breeze Chocolate	8 oz	120	1	3	21
Almond Breeze Original	8 oz	60	1	2	8
Almond Breeze Vanilla	8 oz	90	1	3	15
EdenBlend					
Organic	8 oz	120	7	3	18
Edensoy					
Organic Light	8 oz	93	5	2	14
Organic Light Vanilla	8 oz	120	4	2	21
Galaxy					
Veggi Milk Chocolate	1 cup (8 oz)	150	9	2	26
Veggie Milk Original	1 cup (8 oz)	110	9	3	13
Harmony Farms					
Original Rice Beverage	1 cup (8 oz)	90	13	0	21
Harmony House					
Enriched Rice Beverage	1 cup (8 oz)	90	1	0	21
Enriched Soy Beverage	1 cup (8 oz)	90	13	0	21
Original Soy Beverage	1 cup (8 oz)	90	13	0	21
Health Valley					
Soo Moo	1 cup	110	6	0	22
NutraBalance					
NuTaste	1 pkg (8 oz)	80	8	2	7
Rice Dream					
Carob	1 box (8 oz)	150	1	3	32
Chocolate	1 box (8 oz)	170	1	3	36
Chocolate Enriched	1 box (8 oz)	170	1	3	36
Organic Original	1 box (8 oz)	120	1	2	25
Organic Original Enriched	1 box (8 oz)	120	1	2	25
Vanilla	1 box (8 oz)	130	1	2	28
Vanilla Enriched	1 box (8 oz)	130	1	2	28
Silk					
Chocolate	1 cup	140	5	4	23
Organic Plain	1 cup	100	7	4	8
Vanilla	1 bottle (11 oz)	140	8	5	14
Soy Dream					
Carob	8 oz	210	7	5	36
Chocolate Enriched	8 oz	210	7	5	35
Original	8 oz	140	8	5	14
Original Enriched	8 oz	140	8	5	14
Vanilla	8 oz	170	8	5	23
Vanilla Enriched	8 oz	140	8	5	23
Tree Of Life					
Original Rice Beverage	1 cup (2.9 oz)	90	13	0	21

FOOD	PORTION	CALS	PROT	FAT	CARB
Vitasoy					
1% Low Fat Vanilla Delight	8 oz	90	4	2	13
Carob Supreme	8 fl oz	150	8	5	20
Creamy Unsweetened	8 oz	80	6	4	5
Creamy Original	8 fl oz	110	9	5	9
Enriched Light Original	8 fl oz	60	4	2	7
Enriched Light Vanilla	8 fl oz	90	4	2	13
Green Tea Soymilk	8 oz	130	7	4	16
Original Creamy	8 fl oz	110	7	4	12
Original Light	8 fl oz	60	4	2	7
Rich Chocolate	8 fl oz	160	7	4	24
Rich Cocoa	8 fl oz	150	8	5	21
Vanilla Light	8 fl oz	90	4	2	14
Vanilla Delite	8 fl oz	120	7	4	14
White Wave					
Mocha	1 cup	140	6	4	20
MILKFISH					
baked	3 oz	162	22	7	0
MILKSHAKE					
chocolate	10 oz	360	10	11	58
strawberry	10 oz	319	10	8	53
thick shake chocolate	10.6 oz	356	9	8	63
thick shake vanilla	11 oz	350	12	10	56
vanilla	10 oz	314	10	8	51
MILLET					
cooked	1 cup (6.1 oz)	207	6	2	41
MINERAL WATER					
(*see* WATER)					
MISO					
dried	1 oz	86	7	3	10
miso	½ cup	284	16	8	39
Eden					
Organic Genmai	1 tbsp	25	2	1	3
MOLASSES					
blackstrap	1 tbsp (0.7 oz)	47	0	0	12
blackstrap	1 cup (11.5 oz)	771	0	tr	199
molasses	1 tbsp (0.7 oz)	53	0	0	14
molasses	1 cup (11.5 oz)	873	0	1	226
Brer Rabbit					
Dark	1 tbsp	60	0	0	16
Mott's					
Sulphured	1 tbsp	50	0	0	12
Unsulphured	1 tbsp	50	0	0	14
MONKFISH					
baked	3 oz	82	16	2	0
MOOSE					
roasted	3 oz	114	25	1	0

FOOD	PORTION	CALS	PROT	FAT	CARB
MOTH BEANS					
dried cooked	1 cup	207	14	1	37
MOUSSE					
frozen					
Sara Lee					
Chocolate	⅛ pkg (4.3 oz)	400	5	25	37
Weight Watchers					
Chocolate Mousse	1 (2.75 oz)	190	6	5	31
take-out					
chocolate	½ cup (7.1 oz)	447	9	33	33
orange	½ cup	87	3	5	19
MUFFIN					
frozen					
Pepperidge Farm					
Blueberry	1 (2 oz)	180	2	7	28
Bran w/ Raisins	1 (2 oz)	180	4	6	30
Corn	1 (2 oz)	190	3	7	28
Orange Cranberry	1 (2 oz)	180	2	6	29
Sara Lee					
Blueberry	1 (2.2 oz)	220	3	11	27
Corn	1 (2.2 oz)	260	3	14	30
Weight Watchers					
Chocolate Chocolate Chip	1 (2.5 oz)	190	3	2	39
Fat Free Banana	1 (2.5 oz)	170	3	0	41
Fat Free Blueberry	1 (2.5 oz)	160	3	0	38
home recipe					
blueberry as prep w/ 2% milk	1 (2 oz)	163	4	6	23
blueberry as prep w/ whole milk	1 (2 oz)	165	6	6	23
corn as prep w/ 2% milk	1 (2 oz)	180	4	7	25
corn as prep w/ whole milk	1 (2 oz)	183	4	7	25
plain as prep w/ 2% milk	1 (2 oz)	169	4	7	24
plain as prep w/ whole milk	1 (2 oz)	172	4	7	24
wheat bran as prep w/ 2% milk	1 (2 oz)	161	4	7	24
wheat bran as prep w/ whole milk	1 (2 oz)	164	4	7	24
mix					
blueberry	1 (1¾ oz)	149	3	4	24
corn	1 (1.75 oz)	160	4	5	25
wheat bran as prep	1 (1¾ oz)	138	5	5	23
Betty Crocker					
Apple Cinnamon as prep	1	170	1	7	23
Apple Streusel as prep	1	210	2	8	33
Banana Nut as prep	1	170	2	6	27
Cranberry Orange as prep	1	150	2	5	25

FOOD	PORTION	CALS	PROT	FAT	CARB
Double Chocolate as prep	1	220	2	11	30
Golden Corn as prep	1	160	2	5	24
Lemon Poppyseed as prep	1	180	1	8	24
Sunkist Lemon Poppyseed as prep	1	190	2	7	29
Twice The Blueberries as prep	1	140	2	3	25
Wild Blueberry as prep	1	170	2	5	28
Gold Medal					
Corn	1	160	3	6	25
Hodgson Mill					
Bran	¼ cup (1.3 oz)	130	4	1	27
Cornbread	¼ cup (1.3 oz)	130	4	1	28
Whole Wheat	¼ cup (1.3 oz)	130	4	1	27
Robin Hood					
Apple Cinnamon	1	170	3	8	23
Banana Nut	1	170	3	8	21
Blueberry	1	160	3	6	24
Caramel Nut	1	170	3	7	24
Sweet Rewards					
Low Fat Apple Cinnamon as prep	1	140	2	2	26
ready-to-eat					
blueberry	1 (2 oz)	158	3	4	27
corn	1 (2 oz)	174	3	5	29
oat bran wheat free	1 (2 oz)	154	4	4	28
toaster type blueberry	1	103	2	3	18
toaster type corn	1	114	2	4	19
toaster type wheat bran w/ raisins	1 (1.3 oz)	106	2	3	19
Dolly Madison					
Blueberry	1 (1.75 oz)	170	2	7	26
Mega Banana Nut	1 (5.9 oz)	620	8	31	78
Mega Blueberry	1 (5.9 oz)	590	8	28	78
Mega Chocolate Chip	1 (5.9 oz)	620	8	29	78
Mega Cranberry Orange	1 (5.9 oz)	590	6	28	79
Mega Cream Cheese	1 (5.9 oz)	620	7	33	73
Dutch Mill					
Apple Oat Bran	1 (2 oz)	180	3	5	31
Banana Walnut	1 (2 oz)	220	3	6	33
Carrot	1 (2 oz)	190	3	7	31
Corn	1 (2 oz)	190	4	6	31
Cranberry Orange	1 (2 oz)	170	3	6	26
Raisin Bran	1 (2 oz)	230	2	5	37
Hostess					
Banana Bran Low Fat	1 (2.7 oz)	240	4	3	47
Blueberry Low Fat	1 (2.7 oz)	230	4	3	47
Hearty Banana Nut	1 (5.9 oz)	620	8	31	78

FOOD	PORTION	CALS	PROT	FAT	CARB
Hearty Blueberry	1 (5.9 oz)	590	8	28	78
Hearty Chocolate Chip	1 (5.9 oz)	620	8	29	78
Hearty Cranberry Orange	1 (5.9 oz)	590	6	28	79
Hearty Cream Cheese	1 (5.9 oz)	620	7	33	73
Mini Banana Walnut	3 (1.2 oz)	160	2	9	16
Mini Blueberry	3 (1.2 oz)	150	1	8	18
Mini Chocolate Chip	3 (1.2 oz)	160	2	9	17
Mini Cinnamon Apple	3 (1.2 oz)	160	1	9	16
Mini Cinnamon Bites	3 (1.1 oz)	130	1	6	18
Mini Rocky Road	3 (1.2 oz)	160	2	9	17
Muffin Loaf Apple Spice	1 (3.7 oz)	430	3	18	61
Muffin Loaf Banana Nut	1 (3.8 oz)	460	4	20	63
Muffin Loaf Blueberry	1 (3.8 oz)	440	5	19	62
Muffin Loaf Chocolate Chocolate Chip	1 (3.8 oz)	400	5	17	58
Muffin Loaf Raspberry	1 (3.8 oz)	440	5	19	62
Oat Bran	1 (1.5 oz)	160	2	8	21
Otis Spunkmeyer					
Apple Cinnamon	1 (2 oz)	220	3	11	27
Low Fat Wild Blueberry	1 (2.25 oz)	200	3	4	38
Mayport Almond Poppy Seed	½ muffin (2 oz)	210	3	12	23
Mayport Banana Nut	1 (2.25 oz)	270	3	14	33
Mayport Cheese Streusel	½ muffin (2 oz)	220	3	10	30
Mayport Chocolate Chocolate Chip	1 (2.25 oz)	260	4	13	33
Mayport Chocolate Chip	½ muffin (2 oz)	240	3	13	28
Mayport Cinnamon Spice	½ muffin (2 oz)	230	3	13	26
Mayport Corn	½ muffin (2 oz)	230	3	13	26
Mayport Harvest Bran	1 (2.25 oz)	240	4	10	34
Mayport Lemon	½ muffin (2 oz)	230	3	13	27
Mayport Orange	½ muffin (2 oz)	230	3	13	27
Mayport Pineapple	½ muffin (2 oz)	210	3	12	25
Mayport Wild Blueberry	1 (2.25 oz)	230	3	13	27
Mayport Low Fat Apple Cinnamon	1 (4 oz)	380	5	6	75
Mayport Low Fat Banana Nut	1 (4 oz)	350	6	6	70
Mayport Low Fat Chocolate Chocolate Chip	1 (4 oz)	370	7	6	73
Uncle Wally's					
Fat Free Apple Cinnamon Delight	1 (1.9 oz)	110	3	0	28
Weight Watchers					
Fat Free Apple Crisp	1 (2.5 oz)	160	3	0	37
Fat Free Cranberry Orange	1 (2.5 oz)	160	3	0	38
Fat Free Double Chocolate	1 (2.5 oz)	180	3	0	40
Fat Free Wild Blueberry	1 (2.5 oz)	160	3	0	36

FOOD	PORTION	CALS	PROT	FAT	CARB
Low Fat Apple Cinnamon	1 (2.5 oz)	170	4	3	35
Low Fat Blueberry	1 (2.5 oz)	180	4	3	37
Low Fat Carrot	1 (2.5 oz)	160	4	3	34
Low Fat Chocolate Chip	1 (2.5 oz)	180	4	3	38
Low Fat Cranberry Orange	1 (2.5 oz)	180	4	3	38
Low Fat Lemon Poppy	1 (2.5 oz)	190	4	3	38
take-out					
raisin bran lowfat	1 (4 oz)	270	5	1	61
MULBERRIES					
fresh	1 cup	61	2	1	14
MULLET					
striped cooked	3 oz	127	21	4	0
striped raw	3 oz	99	16	3	0
MUNG BEANS					
dried cooked	1 cup	213	14	1	39
MUNGO BEANS					
dried cooked	1 cup	190	14	1	33
MUSHROOMS					
canned					
chanterelle	3.5 oz	12	1	1	tr
pieces	½ cup	19	1	tr	4
straw	1 cup (6.4 oz)	58	7	1	8
BinB					
Pieces & Stems	1 can (4.2 oz)	30	3	0	4
Sliced	1 can (4.2 oz)	30	3	0	4
Sliced w/ Garlic	1 can (4.2 oz)	35	3	1	4
Whole	1 can (4.2 oz)	30	3	0	4
Green Giant					
Pieces & Stems	½ cup (4.2 oz)	30	3	0	4
Sliced	½ cup (4.2 oz)	30	2	0	3
Whole	½ cup (4.2 oz)	30	3	0	4
dried					
chanterelle	1 oz	25	5	tr	tr
cloud ears	1 cup (1 oz)	80	3	tr	20
shiitake	4 (½ oz)	44	1	tr	11
tree ear	½ cup (0.4 oz)	36	1	tr	10
wood ear mok yee	½ cup (0.4 oz)	25	2	tr	8
Eden					
Shiitake	6 (0.4 oz)	35	2	0	7
fresh					
chanterelle	3.5 oz	11	2	tr	tr
morel	3.5 oz	9	2	tr	0
oyster raw	1 sm (0.5 oz)	6	1	tr	1
oyster raw	1 lg (5.2 oz)	55	6	1	9
portabella	1 serv (2 oz)	14	1	tr	3
raw sliced	½ cup	9	1	tr	2
shitake cooked	4 (2.5 oz)	40	1	tr	10
sliced cooked	½ cup	21	2	tr	4

FOOD	PORTION	CALS	PROT	FAT	CARB
MUSKRAT					
roasted	3 oz	199	26	10	0
MUSSELS					
blue raw	3 oz	73	10	2	3
blue raw	1 cup	129	18	3	6
fresh blue cooked	3 oz	147	20	4	6
MUSTARD					
dry mustard	1 tsp	15	1	1	1
Boar's Head					
Delicatessen Style	1 tsp (5 g)	0	0	0	0
Honey	1 tsp (5 g)	10	0	0	2
Eden					
Organic Stone Ground	1 tsp	0	0	0	1
Kraft					
Horseradish Mustard	1 tsp (5 g)	0	0	0	0
Mustard	1 tsp (5 g)	0	0	0	0
Luzianne					
Creole Mustard	1 tbsp	10	1	0	2
Tree Of Life					
Dijon	1 tsp (5 g)	0	0	0	0
Stone Ground	1 tsp (5 g)	0	0	0	0
Yellow	1 tsp (5 g)	0	0	0	0
MUSTARD GREENS					
fresh chopped cooked	½ cup	11	2	tr	1
fresh raw chopped	½ cup	7	1	tr	1
frozen chopped cooked	½ cup	14	2	tr	2
Birds Eye					
Chopped	1 cup (3 oz)	30	2	0	2
NATTO					
natto	½ cup	187	16	10	13
NAVY BEANS					
canned					
navy	1 cup	296	20	1	54
dried					
cooked	1 cup	259	16	1	48
Hurst					
HamBeens w/ Ham	3 tbsp (1.2 oz)	120	8	1	20
NECTARINE					
fresh	1	67	1	1	16
Chiquita					
Fresh	1 med (4.9 oz)	70	1	1	16
NEUFCHATEL					
neufchatel	1 oz	74	3	7	1
neufchatel	1 pkg (3 oz)	221	8	20	3
Horizon Organic					
Neufchatel	2 tbsp	70	3	6	tr
Organic Valley					
Neufchatel	1 oz	70	2	6	1

FOOD	PORTION	CALS	PROT	FAT	CARB
Philadelphia					
Neufchatel	1 oz	70	3	6	tr
NOODLE DISHES					
Hormel					
Microcup Meals Noodles & Chicken	1 cup (7.5 oz)	200	8	9	20
Hunt's					
Noodles & Chicken	1 cup (8.7 oz)	176	12	6	21
Noodles & Beef	1 cup (8.7 oz)	151	10	4	22
Kraft					
Noodle Classics Cheddar Cheese as prep	1 cup (7.4 oz)	400	13	19	47
Noodle Classics Savory Chicken as prep	1 cup (8.5 oz)	340	10	13	46
Lipton					
Noodles & Sauce Alfredo Broccoli as prep	1 cup (2.2 oz)	340	12	14	43
Noodles & Sauce Alfredo as prep	1 cup (2.2 oz)	330	15	14	42
Noodles & Sauce Beef as prep	1 cup (2.1 oz)	280	8	10	43
Noodles & Sauce Butter as prep	1 cup (2.2 oz)	310	8	14	41
Noodles & Sauce Butter & Herb as prep	1 cup (2.2 oz)	300	9	13	42
Noodles & Sauce Chicken Broccoli as prep	1 cup (2.1 oz)	310	11	11	44
Noodles & Sauce Chicken Tetrazzini as prep	1 cup (2 oz)	300	10	12	41
Noodles & Sauce Chicken as prep	1 cup (2.1 oz)	290	8	11	42
Noodles & Sauce Creamy Chicken as prep	1 cup (2.1 oz)	320	11	13	42
Noodles & Sauce Parmesan as prep	1 cup (2.1 oz)	330	14	15	40
Noodles & Sauce Sour Cream & Chives as prep	1 cup (2.2 oz)	310	10	14	41
Noodles & Sauce Stroganoff as prep	1 cup (2 oz)	300	11	11	40
take-out					
noodle pudding	½ cup	132	6	7	11
NOODLES					
chow mein	1 cup (1.6 oz)	237	4	14	25
egg	1 cup (38 g)	145	5	2	27
egg cooked	1 cup (5.6 oz)	213	8	2	40
japanese soba cooked	1 cup (4 oz)	113	6	tr	24
japanese somen cooked	1 cup (6.2 oz)	231	7	tr	48

FOOD	PORTION	CALS	PROT	FAT	CARB
korean acorn noodles not prep	2 oz	195	7	tr	41
rice cooked	1 cup (6.2 oz)	192	2	tr	44
spinach/egg cooked	1 cup (5.6 oz)	211	8	3	39
Azumaya					
Spinach	1 cup	210	8	1	42
Thin Cut	1 cup	210	8	1	43
Wide Cut	1 cup	210	8	1	43
Chun King					
Chow Mein	½ cup (1 oz)	137	3	6	19
Eden					
Kudzu	2 oz	200	0	0	48
Hodgson Mill					
Four Color Veggie Egg	2 oz	200	9	2	37
Whole Wheat Egg	2 oz	190	10	2	34
La Choy					
Chow Mein	½ cup (1 oz)	137	3	6	19
Chow Mein Crispy Wide	½ cup (1 oz)	148	3	8	16
Rice	½ cup (1 oz)	121	2	3	21
Manischewitz					
Fine Yolk Free	1½ cups	210	8	1	40
Nasoya					
Chinese	1 cup	210	8	1	43
Japanese	1 cup	210	8	1	43
Spinach	1 cup	210	8	1	42
NOPALES					
cooked	1 cup (5.2 oz)	23	2	tr	5
raw sliced	1 cup (3 oz)	14	1	tr	3
NUTRITION SUPPLEMENTS					
(*see also* BREAKFAST DRINKS, CEREAL BARS, ENERGY BARS, ENERGY DRINKS, SPORTS DRINKS)					
Enlive!					
Drink All Flavors	1 box (8.1 oz)	300	10	0	65
Ensure					
Supplement All Flavors	1 can (8 fl oz)	250	9	6	40
Essential					
Protein Powder	1 serv (0.6 oz)	70	16	tr	6
Glucerna					
Shakes All Flavors	1 can (8 oz)	220	10	9	29
Met-Rx					
Lite	1 pkg (1.6 oz)	170	25	1	16
Original	1 pkg (2.5 oz)	250	37	2	22
Protein Shake	1 can	200	25	3	20
Ultra	1 pkg (2.6 oz)	250	40	2	19
Nestle					
Additions	2⅓ tsp (0.7 oz)	100	6	5	9
NutraBalance					
EggPro	1 tbsp (7.5 g)	30	6	0	1

FOOD	PORTION	CALS	PROT	FAT	CARB
Nutribar					
Shake Chocolate Supreme as prep w/ 2% milk	1 serv (10 oz) (4.6 oz)	262	14	8	34
Shake Vanilla as prep w/ 2% milk	1 (10 oz)	259	14	7	35
PermaLean					
Protein Powder Bodacious Berry	1 scoop (1 oz)	104	20	tr	1
Protein Powder Chocoholic Chocolate	1 scoop (1 oz)	104	20	tr	5
Pounds Off					
All Flavors	1 bar (2.1 oz)	210	11	5	32
NUTS MIXED					
(see also individual names)					
dry roasted w/ peanuts	1 oz	169	5	15	7
dry roasted w/ peanuts salted	1 oz	169	5	15	7
mixed nuts chocolate covered	¼ cup (1.5 oz)	240	4	17	20
oil roasted w/ peanuts	1 oz	175	5	16	6
oil roasted w/ peanuts salted	1 oz	175	5	16	6
oil roasted w/o peanuts	1 oz	175	4	16	6
oil roasted w/o peanuts salted	1 oz	175	4	16	6
Estee					
Fruit & Nut Mix	¼ cup	210	6	12	19
OCTOPUS					
fresh steamed	3 oz	140	25	2	4
OHELOBERRIES					
fresh	1 cup	39	1	tr	10
OIL					
(see also FAT)					
almond	1 cup	1927	0	218	0
almond	1 tbsp	120	0	14	0
apricot kernel	1 cup	1927	0	218	0
apricot kernel	1 tbsp	120	0	14	0
avocado	1 cup	1927	0	218	0
avocado	1 tbsp	124	0	14	0
babassu palm	1 tbsp	120	0	14	0
butter oil	1 cup	1795	1	204	0
canola	1 cup	1927	0	218	0
canola	1 tbsp	124	0	14	0
coconut	1 tbsp	117	0	14	0
corn	1 tbsp	120	0	14	0
corn	1 cup	1927	0	218	0
cottonseed	1 cup	1927	0	218	0
cottonseed	1 tbsp	120	0	14	0

FOOD	PORTION	CALS	PROT	FAT	CARB
cupu assu	1 tbsp	120	0	14	0
grapeseed	1 tbsp	120	0	14	0
hazelnut	1 cup	1927	0	218	0
hazelnut	1 tbsp	120	0	14	0
mustard	1 tbsp	124	0	14	0
mustard	1 cup	1927	0	218	0
oat	1 tbsp	120	0	14	0
olive	1 tbsp	119	0	14	0
olive	1 cup	1909	0	216	0
palm	1 cup	1927	0	218	0
palm	1 tbsp	120	0	14	0
palm kernel	1 cup	1879	0	218	0
palm kernel	1 tbsp	117	0	14	0
peanut	1 tbsp	119	0	14	0
peanut	1 cup	1909	0	216	0
poppyseed	1 tbsp	120	0	14	0
pumpkin seed	1 oz	217	0	29	0
rice bran	1 tbsp	120	0	14	0
safflower	1 tbsp	120	0	14	0
safflower	1 cup	1927	0	218	0
sesame	1 tbsp	120	0	14	0
sheanut	1 tbsp	120	0	14	0
soybean	1 tbsp	120	0	14	0
soybean	1 cup	1927	0	218	0
sunflower	1 tbsp	120	0	14	0
sunflower	1 cup	1927	0	218	0
teaseed	1 tbsp	120	0	14	0
tomatoseed	1 tbsp	120	0	14	0
vegetable soybean & cottonseed	1 tbsp	120	0	14	0
vegetable soybean & cottonseed	1 cup	1927	0	218	0
walnut	1 cup	1927	0	218	0
walnut	1 tbsp	120	0	14	0
wheat germ	1 tbsp	120	0	14	0
Eden					
Olive Spanish Extra Virgin	1 tbsp	120	0	14	0
Safflower	1 tbsp (0.5 oz)	120	0	14	0
House Of Tsang					
Hot Chili Sesame	1 tsp (5 g)	45	0	5	0
Mongolian Fire	1 tsp (5 g)	45	0	5	0
Pure Sesame	1 tsp (5 g)	45	0	5	0
Singapore Curry	1 tsp (5 g)	45	0	5	0
Wok Oil	1 tbsp (0.5 oz)	130	0	14	0
Italica					
Olive Oil	1 tbsp	120	0	9	0
Orville Redenbacher's					
Popping	1 tbsp (0.5 oz)	120	0	14	0

FOOD	PORTION	CALS	PROT	FAT	CARB
Pam					
Butter	⅓ sec spray	0	0	0	0
Cooking Spray	⅓ sec spray	0	0	0	0
Olive Oil	⅓ sec spray	0	0	0	0
Progresso					
Olive Extra Mild	1 tbsp (0.5 oz)	120	0	14	0
Olive Extra Virgin	1 tbsp (0.5 oz)	120	0	14	0
Olive Riviera Blend	1 tbsp (0.5 oz)	120	0	14	0
Tree Of Life					
Olive Extra Virgin Organic	1 tbsp (0.5 g)	130	0	14	0
Weight Watchers					
Butter Spray	⅓ sec spray	0	0	0	0
Cooking Spray	⅓ sec spray	0	0	0	0
OKRA					
fresh					
sliced cooked	½ cup	25	1	tr	6
sliced cooked	8 pods	27	2	tr	6
frozen					
sliced cooked	1 pkg (10 oz)	94	5	1	21
sliced cooked	½ cup	34	2	tr	8
Birds Eye					
Cut	¾ cup (2.9 oz)	25	1	0	5
Whole	9 pods (3 oz)	25	1	0	5
OLIVES					
green olive tapenade	1 tbsp	25	0	3	1
spanish stuffed	5 (0.5 oz)	15	0	1	1
Italia In Tavola					
Black Olives Paste	1 tbsp (0.5 oz)	20	0	2	tr
Progresso					
Olive Salad (drained)	2 tbsp (0.8 oz)	25	0	3	1
Tee Pee					
Spanish Green	2 oz	98	1	10	1
Vlasic					
Ripe Colossal Pitted	2 (0.6 oz)	20	0	2	1
Ripe Jumbo Pitted	3 (0.6 oz)	25	0	2	1
Ripe Large Pitted	4 (0.5 oz)	25	0	3	1
Ripe Medium Pitted	5 (0.5 oz)	25	0	3	1
Ripe Sliced	¼ cup (0.5 oz)	25	0	3	1
Ripe Small Pitted	6 (0.5 oz)	25	0	3	1
ONION					
canned					
chopped	½ cup	21	1	tr	5
whole	1 (2.2 oz)	12	1	tr	3
Boar's Head					
Sweet Vidalia In Sauce	1 tbsp	10	0	0	2
fresh					
chopped cooked	½ cup	47	1	tr	11
raw chopped	½ cup	30	1	tr	7

FOOD	PORTION	CALS	PROT	FAT	CARB
scallions raw sliced	½ cup	16	1	tr	4
welsh raw	3½ oz	34	2	tr	7
Antioch Farms					
Vidalia	1 med	60	1	0	14
frozen					
rings	7 (2.5 oz)	285	4	19	27
rings cooked	2 (0.7 oz)	81	1	5	8
Birds Eye					
Pearl Onions In Cream Sauce	½ cup (4.4 oz)	60	2	2	8
take-out					
fried	½ cup (7.5 oz)	176	3	11	17
rings breaded & fried	8 to 9	275	4	16	31
OPOSSUM					
roasted	3 oz	188	26	9	0
ORANGE					
canned					
Del Monte					
Mandarin In Light Syrup	½ cup (4.5 oz)	80	0	0	19
Dole					
FruitBowls Mandarin Oranges	1 pkg (4 oz)	70	0	0	18
fresh					
california navel	1	65	1	tr	16
california valencia	1	59	1	tr	14
florida	1	69	1	tr	17
sections	1 cup	85	2	tr	21
ORANGE JUICE					
canned	1 cup	104	1	tr	25
chilled	1 cup	110	2	1	25
fresh	1 cup	111	2	tr	26
frzn as prep	1 cup	112	2	tr	27
frzn not prep	6 oz	339	5	tr	81
mandarin orange	7 oz	94	2	tr	20
orange drink	6 oz	94	0	0	24
Big Juicy					
Drink	8 oz	110	0	0	28
Capri Sun					
Drink	1 pkg (7 oz)	100	0	0	25
Everfresh					
Juice	1 can (8 oz)	100	0	0	24
Ruby Red Orange Drink	1 can (8 oz)	130	0	0	33
Fresh Samantha					
Juice	1 cup (8 oz)	100	1	0	8
Horizon Organic					
Juice Pulp Free	8 fl oz	110	2	0	26

FOOD	PORTION	CALS	PROT	FAT	CARB
Juicy Juice					
Punch	1 box (8.45 oz)	130	0	0	33
Punch	1 box (4.23 oz)	60	0	0	15
Kool-Aid					
Drink Mix Orange as prep	1 serv (8 oz)	60	0	0	16
Orange Drink as prep w/ sugar	1 serv (8 oz)	100	0	0	25
Minute Maid					
Simply Orange 100%	8 fl oz	110	2	0	26
Simply Orange Calcium Fortified	8 fl oz	110	2	0	26
Simply Orange Grove Made	8 fl oz	110	2	0	26
Mott's					
100% Juice	1 box (8 oz)	130	2	0	31
100% Juice	8 fl oz	130	2	0	31
Nantucket Nectars					
100% Juice	8 oz	120	0	0	28
NutraShake					
Fourtified	1 pkg (4 oz)	50	0	0	12
Ocean Spray					
100% Juice	8 oz	120	0	0	31
Shasta Plus					
Orange Drink	1 can (11.5 oz)	160	0	0	40
Snapple					
Orangeade	8 fl oz	120	0	0	29
Tang					
Orange Drink as prep	1 serv (8 oz)	90	0	0	23
Sugar Free Orange as prep	1 serv (8 oz)	5	0	0	0
Tropicana					
Double Vitamin C	8 fl oz	110	2	0	26
Juice	8 oz	110	2	0	26
Ruby Red	8 oz	110	2	0	26
Season's Best	8 oz	110	1	0	27
Season's Best Homestyle	8 fl oz	110	1	0	27
Tropical	8 oz	110	2	0	25
With Calcium	8 fl oz	110	2	0	26
Veryfine					
100% Juice	1 bottle (10 oz)	150	0	0	37
Chillers Arctic Orange	8 fl oz	130	0	0	33
Juice Blend	1 can (11.5 oz)	160	0	0	39
Orange Drink	1 bottle (10 oz)	160	0	0	41

ORGAN MEATS

(*see* BRAINS, GIBLETS, GIZZARD, HEART, KIDNEY, LIVER, SWEETBREADS)

ORIENTAL FOOD

(*see* ASAIN FOOD, EGG ROLLS, DINNER, NOODLES, RICE, SUSHI)

OYSTERS

FOOD	PORTION	CALS	PROT	FAT	CARB
canned eastern	1 cup	170	18	6	10
canned eastern	3 oz	58	6	2	3

FOOD	PORTION	CALS	PROT	FAT	CARB
eastern cooked	6 med	58	6	2	3
eastern cooked	3 oz	117	12	4	7
eastern raw	6 med	58	6	2	3
eastern raw	1 cup	170	18	6	10
pacific raw	1 med	41	5	1	2
pacific raw	3 oz	69	8	2	4
steamed	1 med	41	5	1	2
steamed	3 oz	138	16	4	8
Bumble Bee					
Fancy Whole	2 oz	70	7	3	3
Smoked	½ can (1.9 oz)	120	10	7	6
take-out					
breaded & fried	6 (4.9 oz)	368	13	18	40
oysters rockefeller	3 oysters	66	7	2	5
stew	1 cup	278	15	18	15
PANCAKE/WAFFLE SYRUP					
low calorie	1 tbsp	12	0	0	3
maple	1 tbsp (0.8 oz)	52	0	0	13
pancake syrup	1 tbsp (0.7 oz)	57	0	0	15
pancake syrup	1 cup (11 oz)	903	0	0	238
pancake syrup light	1 oz	46	0	0	13
pancake syrup w/ butter	1 tbsp (0.7 oz)	59	0	tr	15
Estee					
Maple	¼ cup	80	0	0	20
Mrs. Butter-worth's					
Original	¼ cup (2 oz)	230	0	0	56
Smucker's					
Breakfast Syrup Sugar Free	¼ cup (2 oz)	30	0	0	8
PANCAKES					
frozen					
buttermilk	1 4 in diam (1.3 oz)	83	2	1	16
plain	1 4 in diam (1.3 oz)	83	2	1	16
Eggo					
Buttermilk	3 (4.1 oz)	270	7	8	44
home recipe					
plain	1 (4 in diam)	86	2	4	11
mix					
buckwheat	1 (4 in diam)	62	2	2	9
buttermilk	1 4 in diam (1.3 oz)	74	2	1	14
plain	1 4 in diam (1.3 oz)	74	2	1	14
sugar free low sodium	1 (3 in diam)	44	1	tr	9
whole wheat	1 (4 in diam)	92	4	3	13
Betty Crocker					
Buttermilk as prep	3	200	5	3	20
Original as prep	3	200	6	3	39
Bisquick					
Shake 'N Pour Blueberry as prep	3	210	6	4	40

FOOD	PORTION	CALS	PROT	FAT	CARB
Bruce					
Sweet Potato Pancakes	2	210	6	3	39
Estee					
Pancake Mix as prep	4 (4 in diam)	180	4	0	40
Hodgson Mill					
Buckwheat	⅓ cup (1.8 oz)	160	5	1	36
Hungry Jack					
Potato as prep	3 (3 in diam)	90	3	2	16
Robin Hood					
Buttermilk as prep	3	230	8	6	35
take-out					
blueberry	1 (4 in diam)	84	2	4	11
buckwheat	1 (4 in diam)	55	2	2	6
potato	1 (4 in diam)	78	2	6	4
w/ butter & syrup	2 (8.1 oz)	520	8	14	91
PAPAYA					
fresh	1	117	2	tr	30
fresh cubed	1 cup	54	1	tr	14
Sunfresh					
In Extra Light Syrup	½ cup (4.5 oz)	70	1	0	17
PAPAYA JUICE					
Everfresh					
Premium Drink	1 can (8 oz)	140	0	0	35
Nantucket Nectars					
Cocktail	8 oz	120	0	0	30
PARSLEY					
fresh chopped	½ cup	11	1	tr	2
PARSNIPS					
fresh cooked	1 (5.6 oz)	130	2	tr	31
fresh sliced cooked	½ cup	63	1	tr	15
PASSION FRUIT JUICE					
purple	1 cup	126	1	tr	34
yellow	1 cup	149	2	tr	36
PASTA					
(*see also* NOODLES, PASTA DINNERS, PASTA SALAD)					
dry					
corn cooked	1 cup (4.9 oz)	176	4	1	39
corn spaghetti	2 oz	180	4	2	35
elbows	1 cup	389	13	2	78
elbows cooked	1 cup (4.9 oz)	197	7	1	40
shells small cooked	1 cup (4 oz)	162	5	1	33
shells small protein fortified cooked	1 cup (4 oz)	189	9	tr	36
spaghetti cooked	1 cup (4.9 oz)	197	7	1	40
spaghetti protein fortified cooked	1 cup (4.9 oz)	230	11	tr	44
spinach spaghetti cooked	1 cup (4.9 oz)	182	6	1	37
spirals cooked	1 cup (4.7 oz)	189	6	tr	38

FOOD	PORTION	CALS	PROT	FAT	CARB
vegetable cooked	1 cup (4.7 oz)	172	6	tr	36
whole wheat cooked	1 cup (4.9 oz)	174	7	tr	37
whole wheat spaghetti cooked	1 cup (4.9 oz)	174	7	1	37
Annie Chun's					
Soba Noodles	2 oz	200	8	1	39
Barilla					
Conchiglie Rigate	1 cup (2 oz)	200	6	1	40
Gemelli as prep	1 cup (2 oz)	200	7	1	42
Tortelloni Ricotta & Asparagus	¾ cup	240	7	8	32
Tortelloni Ricotta & Spinach	¾ cup	220	8	8	28
Cuore					
Capellini cooked	1⅓ cup (2 oz)	190	7	1	39
Fusilli cooked	1⅓ cup (2 oz)	190	7	1	39
Tortiglioni cooked	1⅓ cup (2 oz)	190	7	1	39
DeCecco					
Whole Wheat Linguine cooked	2 oz	180	8	2	33
Duc Amici					
Pasta Lite Low Carb Fusilli	2 oz	160	28	1	10
Eden					
Organic Extra Fine	2 oz	210	9	2	40
Organic Gemelli	2 oz	210	8	2	40
Organic Pesto Gemelli	2 oz	210	8	1	41
Organic Ribbons Saffron	2 oz	210	9	2	40
Organic Spaghetti Semolina	2 oz	200	8	1	40
Organic Spaghetti 50% Whole Grain	2 oz	210	8	1	41
Organic Spirals Kamut Vegetable	2 oz	210	8	2	40
Organic Spirals Sesame Rice	2 oz	200	8	2	37
Organic Spirals Mixed Grain	2 oz	210	8	2	41
Organic Spirals Spinach	2 oz	210	8	1	41
Organic Vegetable Alphabets	2 oz	200	8	1	40
Spirals Rye	2 oz	200	6	0	44
Goya					
Coditos not prep	½ cup	230	8	1	47
Hodgson Mill					
Four Color Veggie Bows	2 oz	200	8	1	41
Four Color Veggie Rotini Spirals	2 oz	200	8	1	41
Four Color Veggie Wagon Wheels	2 oz	200	8	1	41
Pastamania! Durum Wheat Fettuccine	2 oz	200	8	2	38

FOOD	PORTION	CALS	PROT	FAT	CARB
Pastamania! Fettuccine Garlic & Parsley	2 oz	200	8	2	38
Pastamania! Fettuccine w/ Jerusalem Artichoke	2 oz	210	8	2	41
Pastamania! Fettucinne w/ Mushroom	2 oz	210	8	2	41
Pastamania! Fusilli Tre Colore w/ Tomato & Spinach	2 oz	200	7	1	40
Pastamania! Pesto Fettuccine	2 oz	200	8	2	38
Pastamania! Sea Shell Mix	2 oz	200	8	1	40
Pastamania! Spinach Fettuccine	2 oz	200	8	2	37
Pastamania! Thin Linguine	2 oz	200	8	2	38
Pastamania! Tomato Spinach & Durum Wheat	2 oz	210	8	2	40
Spaghetti Whole Wheat	2 oz	190	9	1	34
Lundberg					
Spaghetti Organic Brown Rice	2 oz	210	4	2	44
Ronzoni					
Lasagne	2½ pieces (2 oz)	210	7	1	42
fresh					
cooked	2 oz	75	3	1	14
spinach cooked	2 oz	74	3	1	14
Di Giorno					
Angel's Hair	1 cup	160	6	2	31
Beef & Roasted Garlic Tortellini	1 cup	340	14	11	46
Fettuccine	1 cup	200	8	2	38
Four Cheese Raviolo	1 cup	350	14	15	40
Herb Linguine	1 cup	200	8	2	38
Italian Sausage Ravioli In Green Bell Pepper Pasta	1¼ cup	350	14	12	45
Lemon Chicken Tortellini In Cracked Black Pepper Pasta	1 cup	270	13	5	42
Light Cheese Ravioli	1 cup	280	15	7	40
Linguine	1 cup	200	8	2	38
Mozzarella Garlic Tortelloni	1 cup	300	15	8	42
Pesto Tortelloni	1 cup	320	16	8	46
Portabello Mushroom Tortelloni	1 cup	310	13	7	48
Red Bell Pepper Fettuccine	1 cup	200	8	2	38

FOOD	PORTION	CALS	PROT	FAT	CARB
Spinach Fettuccine	1 cup	190	8	2	38
Sun-Dried Tomato Ravioli	1⅓ cup	380	17	14	48
Three Cheese Tortellini	¾ cup	250	11	7	37
home recipe					
made w/o egg cooked	2 oz	71	2	1	14
plain made w/ egg cooked	2 oz	74	3	1	13
PASTA DINNERS					
canned					
Chef Boyardee					
99% Fat Free Beef Ravioli	1 cup (8.6 oz)	210	9	1	41
99% Fat Free Cheese Ravioli	1 cup (8.8 oz)	210	7	1	44
Beef Ravioli	1 cup (8.6 oz)	230	9	5	37
Beefaroni	1 cup (8.7 oz)	260	10	7	37
Macaroni & Cheese	½ can (7.5 oz)	180	8	2	35
Mini Ravioli	1 cup (8.8 oz)	252	8	6	37
Spaghetti & Meat Balls	1 cup (8.4 oz)	240	9	10	32
Tortellini Cheese	½ can (7 oz)	230	9	1	48
Tortellini Meat	½ can (7 oz)	260	10	4	48
Franco-American					
Beef Raviolios	1 can (7.7 oz)	250	9	5	39
Beefy Mac	1 can (7.5 oz)	228	9	8	30
Elbow Macaroni & Cheese	1 can (7.5 oz)	187	6	6	25
Spaghetti 'N Beef	1 can (7.5 oz)	226	10	8	30
Spaghetti w/ Meatballs	1 can (7.2 oz)	249	10	9	33
Kid's Kitchen					
Microwave Meals Cheezy Mac & Beef	1 cup (7.5 oz)	260	15	7	33
Microwave Meals Noodle Rings & Chicken	1 cup (7.5 oz)	150	10	4	17
Microwave Meals Spaghetti Rings & Franks	1 cup (7.5 oz)	240	9	9	32
Progresso					
Beef Ravioli	1 cup (9.1 oz)	260	9	5	45
Cheese Ravioli	1 cup (9.1 oz)	220	7	2	43
frozen					
Amy's Organic					
Macaroni & Cheese	1 pkg (9 oz)	390	17	14	50
Macaroni & Soy Cheese	1 pkg (9 oz)	360	16	14	42
Pasta Primavera	1 pkg (9.5 oz)	320	15	12	39
Ravioli w/ Sauce	1 pkg (9.5 oz)	340	15	12	44
Tofu Vegetable Lasagna	1 pkg (9.5 oz)	300	18	10	41
Vegetable Lasagna	1 pkg (9.5 oz)	300	15	10	39
Whole Meals Cannelloni	1 pkg (9 oz)	260	11	11	32
Banquet					
Chicken Pasta Primavera	1 meal (9.5 oz)	320	11	12	40

FOOD	PORTION	CALS	PROT	FAT	CARB
Family Size Egg Noodles w/ Beef & Brown Gravy	1 serv	150	11	5	16
Family Size Lasagna w/ Meat Sauce	1 cup	270	14	10	33
Family Size Macaroni & Cheese	1 cup	230	8	7	32
Fettuccine Alfredo	1 meal (9.5 oz)	350	11	16	40
Homestyle Noodles & Chicken	1 meal (12 oz)	390	12	19	44
Lasagna w/ Meat Sauce	1 meal (9.5 oz)	260	10	8	38
Macaroni & Cheese	1 meal (12 oz)	420	15	14	57
Birds Eye					
Easy Recipe Creations Chicken Primavera as prep	2¼ cups (8.7 oz)	260	9	11	31
Pasta Secrets Italian Pesto	2⅓ cups (6.4 oz)	240	9	9	32
Pasta Secrets Primavera	2⅓ cups (6.6 oz)	230	9	10	26
Pasta Secrets Ranch	2⅓ cups (6.6 oz)	300	7	15	29
Pasta Secrets Three Cheese	2 cups (6.1 oz)	230	9	8	31
Pasta Secrets White Cheddar	2 cups (6.3 oz)	240	7	10	30
Pasta Secrets Zesty Garlic	2 cups (5.9 oz)	240	7	10	31
Green Giant					
Create A Meal Creamy Alfredo as prep	1¼ cups (10 oz)	380	34	12	33
Create A Meal Creamy Cheddar as prep	1½ cups (10 oz)	290	20	10	29
Create A Meal Creamy Chicken Noodle as prep	1¼ cups (10 oz)	350	28	11	34
Pasta Accents Alfredo	2 cups (5.6 oz)	210	9	5	25
Pasta Accents Creamy Cheddar	2⅓ cups (6.7 oz)	250	9	8	36
Pasta Accents Florentine	2 cups (7.3 oz)	310	13	9	44
Pasta Accents Garden Herb Seasoning	2 cups (6.8 oz)	230	9	7	32
Pasta Accents Garlic Seasoning	2 cups (6.6 oz)	260	7	10	36
Pasta Accents Primavera	2¼ cups (7 oz)	320	13	12	40
Pasta Accents White Cheddar Sauce	1¾ cups (5.6 oz)	300	10	12	38
Healthy Choice					
Beef Macaroni	1 meal (8.5 oz)	220	12	4	34
Bowls Cheese & Chicken Tortellini	1 meal (8.7 oz)	250	11	5	40
Breaded Chicken Breast Strips w/ Macaroni & Cheese	1 meal (8 oz)	270	22	5	34
Cheese Ravioli Parmigiana	1 meal (9 oz)	260	11	5	44
Chicken Fettuccine Alfredo	1 meal (8.5 oz)	280	21	7	30

FOOD	PORTION	CALS	PROT	FAT	CARB
Fettuccine Alfredo	1 meal (8 oz)	240	11	5	37
Lasagna Roma	1 meal (13.5 oz)	420	26	9	59
Macaroni & Cheese	1 meal (9 oz)	240	12	5	36
Manicotti w/ Three Cheeses	1 meal (11 oz)	300	15	9	40
Spaghetti & Sauce w/ Seasoned Beef	1 meal (10 oz)	260	14	8	43
Stuffed Pasta Shells	1 meal (10.35 oz)	370	18	6	60
Kid Cuisine					
Magical Macaroni & Cheese	1 meal (10.6 oz)	440	10	13	72
Lean Cuisine					
Cafe Classics Bow Tie Pasta & Chicken	1 pkg (9.5 oz)	220	15	4	32
Cafe Classics Cheese Lasagna w/ Chicken Scaloppini	1 pkg (10 oz)	270	22	8	27
Cafe Classics Shrimp & Angel Hair Pasta	1 pkg (10 oz)	240	15	5	35
Everyday Favorites	1 pkg (10 oz)	270	13	6	40
Everyday Favorites Alfredo Pasta Primavera	1 pkg (10 oz)	290	11	7	46
Everyday Favorites Angel Hair Pasta	1 pkg (10 oz)	240	9	4	43
Everyday Favorites Cheese Cannelloni	1 pkg (9.1 oz)	230	21	4	28
Everyday Favorites Cheese Ravioli	1 pkg (8.5 oz)	260	12	7	38
Everyday Favorites Chicken Lasagna	1 pkg (10 oz)	280	20	7	34
Everyday Favorites Classic Cheese Lasagna	1 pkg (11.5 oz)	290	20	6	38
Everyday Favorites Fettucini Alfredo	1 pkg (9.25 oz)	280	13	7	42
Everyday Favorites Fettucini Primavera	1 pkg (10 oz)	270	13	7	38
Everyday Favorites Lasagna w/ Meat Sauce	1 pkg (10.5 oz)	300	23	8	35
Everyday Favorites Macaroni & Cheese	1 pkg (10 oz)	290	15	7	42
Everyday Favorites Macaroni & Beef	1 pkg (10 oz)	270	15	4	43
Everyday Favorites Penne Pasta	1 pkg (10 oz)	260	9	4	47
Everyday Favorites Spaghetti w/ Meat Sauce	1 pkg (11.5 oz)	290	11	5	50
Everyday Favorites Spaghetti w/ Meatballs	1 pkg (9.5 oz)	270	16	6	37

FOOD	PORTION	CALS	PROT	FAT	CARB
Everyday Favorites	1 pkg (9.25 oz)	270	21	6	33
Family Style Favorites Five Cheese Lasagna	1 serv (8 oz)	210	14	5	27
Skillet Sensations Chicken Alfredo	1 serv	280	20	6	36
Marie Callender's					
Cheese Ravioli In Marinara Sauce w/ Spirals & Garlic Bread	1 meal (16 oz)	750	25	29	96
Extra Cheese Lasagna	1 meal (15 oz)	590	27	27	61
Fettuccine Alfredo & Garlic Bread	1 meal (14 oz)	920	23	55	62
Fettuccine Alfredo Supreme	1 meal (13 oz)	450	15	27	35
Fettuccine Primavera w/ Tortellini	1 meal (14 oz)	750	19	49	57
Fettuccine w/ Broccoli & Chicken	1 meal (13 oz)	710	26	43	53
Lasagna w/ Meat Sauce	1 meal (15 oz)	630	29	31	59
Macaroni & Cheese	1 meal (12 oz)	540	25	24	55
Skillet Meal Chicken Alfredo	½ pkg	490	28	29	32
Skillet Meal Penne Pasta & Meatballs	½ pkg	600	26	31	53
Skillet Meal Rigatoni Vegetables In Cheese Sauce	1 cup	290	12	12	32
Spaghetti w/ Meat Sauce & Garlic Bread	1 meal (17 oz)	670	27	25	65
Stuffed Pasta Trio	1 meal (10.5 oz)	380	15	16	40
Morton					
Macaroni & Cheese	1 serv (8 oz)	240	9	8	34
Spaghetti w/ Meat Sauce	1 meal (8.5 oz)	200	5	6	30
Mrs. Paul's					
Seafood Rotini	9 oz	240	12	6	34
Quorn					
Fettuccine Alfredo	1 pkg (10.5 oz)	360	17	16	40
Lasagna	1 pkg (10.5 oz)	360	23	12	43
Stouffer's					
Cheddar Pasta w/ Beef & Tomatoes	1 pkg (11 oz)	450	25	19	45
Cheese Manicotti	1 pkg (9 oz)	380	18	17	38
Cheese Ravioli	1 pkg (10.6 oz)	380	15	13	51
Chicken Lasagna	1 serv (7.8 oz)	320	13	17	29
Fettucini Alfredo	1 pkg (10 oz)	520	16	28	17
Fettucini Primavera	1 pkg (10 oz)	430	13	20	49
Five Cheese Lasagna	1 pkg (10.75 oz)	360	21	13	40
Grilled Chicken & Angel Hair Pasta	1 pkg (10.9 oz)	380	25	13	40

FOOD	PORTION	CALS	PROT	FAT	CARB
Homestyle Chicken Fettucini	1 pkg (10.5 oz)	390	31	15	32
Homestyle Chicken Parmigiana w/ Spaghetti	1 pkg (12 oz)	460	24	16	54
Homestyle Veal Parmigiana w/ Spaghetti	1 pkg (11.9 oz)	430	21	17	49
Lasagna Bake	1 pkg (10.25 oz)	370	18	12	47
Lasagna w/ Meat Sauce	1 pkg (10.5 oz)	370	23	14	39
Macaroni & Cheese	1 cup (6 oz)	320	13	16	31
Macaroni & Cheese w/ Broccoli	1 pkg (10.5 oz)	360	15	17	37
Macaroni & Beef	1 pkg (11.5 oz)	420	20	20	40
Noodles Romanoff	1 pkg (12 oz)	490	18	25	48
Pasta Shells w/ American Cheese	1 cup (6 oz)	260	11	10	31
Salisbury Steak w/ Macaroni & Cheese	1 serv (11.3 oz)	410	26	19	34
Spaghetti w/ Meat Sauce	1 pkg (10 oz)	350	15	12	46
Spaghetti w/ Meatballs	1 pkg (12.6 oz)	440	19	15	56
Tuna Noodle Casserole	1 pkg (10 oz)	320	20	10	37
Turkey Tettrazini	1 pkg (10 oz)	360	19	17	33
Vegetable Lasagna	1 pkg (10.5 oz)	440	21	20	43
Weight Watchers					
Garden Lasagna	1 pkg (11 oz)	270	14	7	36
Homestyle Macaroni & Cheese	1 pkg (9 oz)	290	12	7	45
Smart Ones Angel Hair Pasta	1 pkg (9 oz)	180	9	2	32
Smart Ones Bowtie Pasta & Mushrooms Marsala	1 pkg (9.65 oz)	270	11	7	40
Smart Ones Chicken Fettucini	1 pkg (10 oz)	300	21	7	39
Smart Ones Creamy Rigatoni w/ Broccoli & Chicken	1 pkg (9 oz)	230	14	2	40
Smart Ones Fettucini Alfredo w/ Broccoli	1 pkg (8.5 oz)	230	13	6	32
Smart Ones Lasagna Florentine	1 pkg (10 oz)	200	11	2	33
Smart Ones Lasagna Alfredo	1 pkg (9 oz)	300	14	7	46
Smart Ones Lasagna w/ Meat Sauce	1 pkg (10.25 oz)	270	18	6	36
Smart Ones Lasagna w/ Meat Sauce	1 pkg (9 oz)	240	13	2	43
Smart Ones Macaroni & Cheese	1 pkg (9 oz)	220	9	2	42

FOOD	PORTION	CALS	PROT	FAT	CARB
Smart Ones Pasta & Spinach Romano	1 pkg (10.4 oz)	260	12	8	35
Smart Ones Pasta w/ Tomato Basil Sauce	1 pkg (9.6 oz)	260	10	7	40
Smart Ones Penne Pasta w/ Sun-Dried Tomatoes	1 pkg (10 oz)	280	11	8	40
Smart Ones Penne Pollo	1 pkg (10 oz)	290	22	6	38
Smart Ones Ravioli Florentine	1 pkg (8.5 oz)	220	9	2	43
Smart Ones Spaghetti Marinara	1 pkg (9 oz)	280	9	7	46
Smart Ones Spaghetti w/ Meat Sauce	1 pkg (10 oz)	280	15	6	41
Smart Ones Spicy Penne & Ricotta	1 pkg (10.2 oz)	280	11	6	45
Smart Ones Tuna Noodle Casserole	1 pkg (9.5 oz)	270	13	7	38
Smart Ones Zita Mozzarella	1 pkg (9 oz)	290	11	7	47
Yves					
Veggie Lasagna	1 pkg (10.5 oz)	300	17	3	51
Veggie Macaroni	1 pkg (10.5 oz)	230	14	2	38
Veggie Penne	1 pkg (10.5 oz)	220	12	2	36
home recipe					
macaroni & cheese	1 cup	430	17	22	40
spaghetti w/ meatballs & tomato sauce	1 cup	330	19	12	39
mix					
Hamburger Helper					
Ravioli as prep	1 cup	280	20	10	30
Ravioli w/ White Cheese Topping as prep	1 cup	310	20	10	34
Hodgson Mill					
Macaroni & Cheese Whole Wheat	1 serv	250	11	2	45
Kraft					
Deluxe Macaroni & Cheese Four Cheese Blend as prep	1 cup (6.2 oz)	320	14	10	44
Deluxe Macaroni & Cheese Original as prep	1 cup (6.1 oz)	320	14	10	44
Light Deluxe Macaroni & Cheese as prep	1 cup (6.5 oz)	290	14	5	48
Macaroni & Cheese All Shapes as prep	1 cup (6.9 oz)	410	12	18	49
Macaroni & Cheese Original as prep	1 cup (6.9 oz)	410	12	18	49
Macaroni & Cheese Original as prep light recipe	1 cup (6.4 oz)	290	12	6	48

FOOD	PORTION	CALS	PROT	FAT	CARB
Premium Macaroni & Cheese Cheesy Alfredo as prep	1 cup (6.9 oz)	410	11	19	49
Premium Macaroni & Cheese Mild White Cheddar as prep	1 cup (6.8 oz)	410	12	19	49
Premium Macaroni & Cheese Thick 'N Creamy as prep	1 cup (7.6 oz)	420	13	19	50
Premium Macaroni & Cheese Three Cheese as prep	1 cup (6.9 oz)	410	12	18	49
Spaghetti Classics Mild Italian as prep	1 cup (9.1 oz)	240	11	3	46
Spaghetti Classics Tangy Italian as prep	1 cup (8.9 oz)	240	11	2	46
Spaghetti Classics Zesty Cheese as prep	1 cup (8.6 oz)	240	11	2	46
Spaghetti Classics w/ Meat Sauce as prep	1 cup (8.2 oz)	330	11	10	47
Lipton					
Pasta & Sauce Angel Hair Chicken Broccoli as prep	1 cup	260	8	8	43
Pasta & Sauce Angel Hair Parmesan as prep	1 cup	280	8	11	41
Pasta & Sauce Bow Tie Chicken Primavera as prep	1 cup	290	9	10	43
Pasta & Sauce Bow Tie Italian Cheese as prep	1 cup	300	10	12	41
Pasta & Sauce Butter & Herbs as prep	1 cup	270	7	10	40
Pasta & Sauce Cheddar Broccoli as prep	1 cup	340	11	11	49
Pasta & Sauce Chicken Herb Parmesan as prep	1 cup	80	8	9	43
Pasta & Sauce Chicken Stir-Fry as prep	1 cup	270	8	8	43
Pasta & Sauce Creamy Garlic as prep	1 cup	350	10	13	50
Pasta & Sauce Creamy Mushroom as prep	1 cup	320	10	11	46
Pasta & Sauce Garlic & Butter Linguine as prep	1 cup	260	7	9	40
Pasta & Sauce Mild Cheddar Cheese as prep	1 cup	290	10	10	41
Pasta & Sauce Roasted Garlic Chicken as prep	1 cup	290	9	10	43

FOOD	PORTION	CALS	PROT	FAT	CARB
Pasta & Sauce Roasted Garlic & Olive Oil w/ Tomato as prep	1 cup	270	8	9	42
Pasta & Sauce Rotini Primavera as prep	1 cup	320	10	12	45
Pasta & Sauce Savory Herb w/ Garlic as prep	1 cup	280	8	9	52
Pasta & Sauce Three Cheese Rotini as prep	1 cup	320	11	12	44
Melting Pot					
Terrazza Black Beans & Penne	1 cup	180	8	1	36
Terrazza Florentine Red Beans & Fusilli	1 cup	220	10	1	43
Terrazza Red Lentils & Bow Ties	1 cup	240	13	2	42
Terrazza Tuscan White Beans & Gemell	1 cup	220	10	1	44
Velveeta					
Rotini & Cheese w/ Broccoli as prep	1 cup (7.2 oz)	400	18	16	47
Shells & Cheese Bacon as prep	1 cup (6.8 oz)	360	17	14	43
Shells & Cheese Original as prep	1 cup (6.6 oz)	360	16	13	44
Shells & Cheese Salsa as prep	1 cup (7.5 oz)	380	17	14	47
ready-to-eat					
Tyson					
Rosemary Penne	1 pkg (12.5 oz)	330	25	5	45
shelf-stable					
Hormel					
Microcup Meals Lasagna	1 cup (7.5 oz)	250	8	14	24
Microcup Meals Macaroni & Cheese	1 cup (7.5 oz)	260	11	11	30
Microcup Meals Ravioli w/ Tomato Sauce	1 cup (7.5 oz)	220	8	6	34
Microcup Meals Spaghetti & Meatballs	1 cup (7.5 oz)	220	11	7	28
Kid's Kitchen					
Microwave Meals Beefy Macaroni	1 cup (7.5 oz)	190	11	6	23
Microwave Meals Macaroni & Cheese	1 cup (7.5 oz)	260	11	11	30
Microwave Meals Mini Ravioli	1 cup (7.5 oz)	240	10	7	34
Microwave Meals Spaghetti & Meatballs	1 cup (7.5 oz)	220	11	7	28

FOOD	PORTION	CALS	PROT	FAT	CARB
Microwave Meals Spaghetti Ring & Meatballs	1 cup (7.5 oz)	250	11	7	35
Lunch Bucket					
Beef Ravioli In Tomato Sauce	1 pkg (7.5 oz)	180	5	4	32
Italian Pasta w/ Chicken	1 pkg (7.5 oz)	130	5	2	24
Lasagna 'n Meatsauce	1 pkg (7.5 oz)	160	5	3	29
Macaroni 'n Beef in Meatsauce	1 pkg (7.5 oz)	180	0	5	10
Macaroni 'n Cheese	1 pkg (7.5 oz)	190	7	7	24
Pasta 'n Chicken	1 pkg (7.5 oz)	150	5	5	22
Spaghetti 'n Meatsauce	1 pkg (7.5 oz)	160	5	3	29
take-out					
lasagna	1 piece (2.5 in x 2.5 in)	374	22	21	25
macaroni & cheese	1 cup	230	9	10	26
manicotti	¾ cup (6.4 oz)	273	14	12	28
rigatoni w/ sausage sauce	¾ cup	260	10	12	28
spaghetti w/ meatballs & cheese	1 cup	407	21	19	38
PASTA SALAD					
mix					
Kraft					
Herb & Garlic as prep	¾ cup (4.9 oz)	280	6	14	34
Pasta Salad Classic Ranch w/ Bacon as prep	¾ cup (4.7 oz)	350	7	22	32
Pasta Salad Creamy Ceasar as prep	¾ cup (4.8 oz)	340	7	21	31
Pasta Salad Garden Primavera as prep	¾ cup (5 oz)	240	8	8	35
Pasta Salad Italian 97% Fat Free as prep	¾ cup (4.9 oz)	190	8	2	34
Pasta Salad Parmesan Peppercorn as prep	¾ cup (4.9 oz)	360	7	23	29
Suddenly Salad					
Classic Pasta	¾ cup	250	7	8	38
Classic Pasta Reduced Fat Recipe	¾ cup	210	7	4	38
Garden Italian 98% Fat Free	¾ cup	140	5	1	28
take-out					
elbow macaroni salad	3.5 oz	160	3	5	26
italian style pasta salad	3.5 oz	140	3	7	15
mustard macaroni salad	3.5 oz	190	4	10	23
pasta salad w/ vegetables	3.5 oz	140	4	4	21
PATE					
antipasto pate	1 can (2.25 oz)	110	3	9	3
chicken liver canned	1 oz	238	4	4	2

FOOD	PORTION	CALS	PROT	FAT	CARB
chicken liver canned	1 tbsp (13 g)	109	2	2	1
duck pate	1 oz	96	4	8	1
fish pate	1 oz	76	3	7	1
goose liver smoked canned	1 tbsp (13 g)	60	1	6	1
goose liver smoked canned	1 oz	131	3	12	1
liver canned	1 oz	90	4	8	tr
liver canned	1 tbsp (13 g)	41	5	4	tr
mushroom anchovy pate	1 can (2.25 oz)	130	2	11	7
pate foie gras	1 oz	127	3	13	1
pork pate	1 oz	107	3	10	1
pork pate en croute	1 oz	91	3	7	3
rabbit pate	1 oz	66	5	5	1
salmon pate	1 can (2.25 oz)	140	6	10	6
shrimp	1 can (2.25 oz)	140	6	10	7
smoked turkey	1 can (2.25 oz)	170	6	13	7
PEACH					
canned					
spiced in heavy syrup	1 cup	180	1	tr	49
Del Monte					
Fruit Cup Diced Extra Light Syrup	1 pkg (4 oz)	50	0	0	13
Fruit Cup Diced In Heavy Syrup	1 serv (4 oz)	80	0	0	20
Fruit Cup Fruit Naturals Diced	1 pkg (4 oz)	50	0	0	13
Fruit Pleasures Raspberry Flavor	½ cup (4.5 oz)	80	1	0	20
Fruit To Go Banana Berry Peaches	1 pkg (4 oz)	70	1	0	17
Fruitrageous Peachy Pie	1 pkg (4 oz)	80	1	0	21
Fruitrageous Wild Raspberry Flavor	1 pkg (4 oz)	80	1	0	20
Halves Ginger Flavor	½ cup (4.5 oz)	90	0	0	22
Halves In Extra Light Syrup	½ cup (4.4 oz)	60	0	0	15
Halves In Heavy Syrup	½ cup (4.5 oz)	100	0	0	24
Halves Melba In Heavy Syrup	½ cup (4.5 oz)	100	0	0	24
Slice Fruit Natural	½ cup (4.4 oz)	60	0	0	15
Sliced In Extra Light Syrup	½ cup (4.4 oz)	60	0	0	14
Sliced In Heavy Syrup	½ cup (4.5 oz)	100	0	0	24
Sliced Natural Raspberry Flavor	½ cup (4.4 oz)	80	0	0	20
Sliced Natural Harvest Spice Flavor	½ cup (4.5 oz)	80	1	0	21
Whole Spiced In Heavy Syrup	½ cup (4.2 oz)	100	0	0	24

FOOD	PORTION	CALS	PROT	FAT	CARB
dried					
halves	1 cup	383	6	1	98
halves	10	311	5	1	80
halves cooked w/ sugar	½ cup	139	1	tr	36
halves cooked w/o sugar	½ cup	99	1	tr	25
fresh					
peach	1	37	1	tr	10
sliced	1 cup	73	1	tr	19
Chiquita					
Peach	1 med (3.4 oz)	40	14	0	10
frozen					
slices sweetened	1 cup	235	2	tr	60
PEACH JUICE					
nectar	1 cup	134	1	tr	35
Nantucket Nectars					
The Original	8 oz	120	0	0	30
PEANUT BUTTER					
chunky	2 tbsp	188	8	16	7
chunky	1 cup	1520	62	129	56
chunky w/o salt	1 cup	1520	62	129	56
chunky w/o salt	2 tbsp	188	8	16	7
smooth	1 cup	1517	63	128	53
smooth	2 tbsp	188	8	16	7
smooth w/o salt	2 tbsp	188	8	16	7
smooth w/o salt	1 cup	1517	63	129	53
Estee					
Creamy Low Sodium	2 tbsp (1 oz)	190	7	15	7
Jif					
Apple Cinnamon	2 tbsp (1.3 oz)	200	6	16	11
Berry Blend	2 tbsp (1.2 oz)	200	6	17	10
Chocolate Silk	2 tbsp (1.3 oz)	190	5	15	14
Creamy	2 tbsp (1.1 oz)	190	8	16	7
Extra Crunchy	2 tbsp (1.1 oz)	190	8	16	7
Reduced Fat Creamy	2 tbsp (1.3 oz)	190	8	12	15
Reduced Fat Crunchy	2 tbsp (1.3 oz)	190	8	12	15
Simply	2 tbsp (1.1 oz)	190	8	16	6
Peanut Wonder					
Low Sodium	2 tbsp	100	4	3	13
Regular	2 tbsp	100	4	3	13
Reese's					
Peanut Butter Chips	1 tbsp (0.5 oz)	80	3	4	7
PEANUTS					
chocolate coated	10 (1.4 oz)	208	5	13	20
chocolate coated	1 cup (5.2 oz)	773	19	50	74
cooked	½ cup	102	4	7	14
dry roasted	1 cup	855	35	73	31
dry roasted w/ salt	30 nuts (1 oz)	170	7	14	6
oil roasted	1 oz	163	7	14	5

FOOD	PORTION	CALS	PROT	FAT	CARB
oil roasted	1 cup	837	38	71	27
oil roasted w/o salt	1 cup	837	38	71	27
oil roasted w/o salt	1 oz	163	7	14	5
spanish oil roasted	1 oz	162	8	14	5
spanish oil roasted w/o salt	1 oz	162	8	14	5
unroasted	1 oz	159	7	14	5
valencia oil roasted	1 cup	848	39	74	23
valencia oil roasted	1 oz	165	8	14	5
valencia oil roasted w/o salt	1 oz	165	8	14	5
valencia oil roasted w/o salt	1 cup	848	40	74	23
virginia oil roasted	1 oz	161	8	14	5
virginia oil roasted	1 cup	826	37	70	28
Estee					
Candy Coated	¼ cup	200	5	9	23
Frito Lay					
Honey Roasted	1 serv (1.5 oz)	270	10	21	10
Hot	1 serv (1.1 oz)	190	7	16	6
Salted	1 oz	200	7	16	5
Lance					
Honey Toasted	1 pkg (1⅜ oz)	220	9	15	13
Roasted	1 pkg (1¾ oz)	190	9	14	6
Salted	1 pkg (1⅛ oz)	200	9	15	6
Salted Long Tube	¼ cup (1 oz)	180	8	14	5
Little Debbie					
Salted	¼ cup (1 oz)	160	7	14	5
Tom's					
Double Coated	1 pkg (1.35 oz)	220	8	15	15
Toasted	1 pkg (1.4 oz)	240	11	19	7
Weight Watchers					
Honey Roasted	1 pkg (0.7 oz)	100	7	5	7
PEAR					
canned					
halves in heavy syrup	1 cup	188	1	tr	49
halves juice pack	1 cup	123	1	tr	32
Del Monte					
Fruit Cup Diced In Heavy Syrup	1 pkg (4 oz)	80	0	0	20
Fruit Cup Diced Extra Light Syrup	1 pkg (4 oz)	50	0	0	13
Fruit To Go Peachy Peaches	1 pkg (4 oz)	70	1	0	17
Halves Fruit Naturals	½ cup (4.4 oz)	60	0	0	15
Halves In Extra Light Syrup	½ cup (4.4 oz)	60	0	0	15
Halves In Heavy Syrup	½ cup (4.5 oz)	100	0	0	24
Orchard Select Sliced Bartlett	½ cup (4.4 oz)	80	1	0	20
Sliced In Extra Light Syrup	½ cup (4.5 oz)	60	0	0	15

FOOD	PORTION	CALS	PROT	FAT	CARB
dried					
halves	10	459	3	1	122
halves	1 cup	472	3	1	125
halves cooked w/ sugar	½ cup	196	1	tr	52
fresh					
asian	1 (4.3 oz)	51	1	tr	13
pear	1	98	1	1	25
sliced w/ skin	1 cup	97	1	1	25
Chiquita					
Pear	1 med (5.8 oz)	100	18	1	25
PEAS					
canned					
green	½ cup	59	4	tr	11
green low sodium	½ cup	59	4	tr	11
Del Monte					
Sweet	½ cup (4.4 oz)	60	3	0	13
Sweet No Salt Added	½ cup (4.4 oz)	60	3	0	11
Sweet Very Young Small	½ cup (4.4 oz)	60	3	0	10
Green Giant					
Sweet	½ cup (4.3 oz)	60	4	0	11
Sweet 50% Less Sodium	½ cup (4.3 oz)	60	4	0	11
LeSueur					
Early Peas	½ cup (4.2 oz)	60	4	0	12
Early Peas 50% Less Sodium	½ cup (4.2 oz)	60	4	0	11
Sweet	½ cup (4.2 oz)	60	4	0	12
Sweet 50% Less Sodium	½ cup (4.2 oz)	60	4	0	11
S&W					
Petite	½ cup (4.4 oz)	70	4	0	12
Small	½ cup (4.4 oz)	70	4	0	12
dried					
split cooked	1 cup	231	16	1	41
Hurst					
HamBeens Green Split Peas w/ Ham	1 serv	120	8	1	21
fresh					
green cooked	½ cup	67	4	tr	13
green raw	½ cup	58	4	tr	11
snap peas cooked	½ cup	34	3	tr	6
snap peas raw	½ cup	30	2	tr	5
frozen					
green cooked	½ cup	63	4	tr	11
snap peas cooked	½ cup	42	3	tr	7
snap peas cooked	1 pkg (10 oz)	132	9	1	23
Birds Eye					
Butter Peas	½ cup (2.7 oz)	110	7	1	20
Crowder	½ cup (3 oz)	120	8	1	22
Field Peas w/ Snaps	⅔ cup (3.4 oz)	130	9	1	24
Purple Hull Peas	½ cup (2.8 oz)	110	7	1	21

FOOD	PORTION	CALS	PROT	FAT	CARB
Green Giant					
Butter Sauce	¾ cup (4 oz)	100	4	2	16
Butter Sauce LeSueur Baby Peas	¾ cup (4 oz)	100	5	2	16
Harvest Fresh LeSueur Baby	⅔ cup (3.2 oz)	70	4	0	13
Harvest Fresh Sugar Snap	⅔ cup (3.2 oz)	50	3	0	10
Harvest Fresh Sweet	⅔ cup (3.3 oz)	60	4	0	12
LeSueur Baby Sweet	⅔ cup (2.8 oz)	60	5	0	11
LeSueur Early June	⅔ cup (2.8 oz)	80	5	0	11
LeSueur Early June w/ Mushrooms	¾ cup (3 oz)	60	4	0	10
Select Sugar Snap	¾ cup (2.8 oz)	35	2	0	7
Sweet	⅔ cup (3.1 oz)	70	4	0	13
La Choy					
Snow Pea Pods	½ pkg (3 oz)	35	2	2	4
Tree Of Life					
Peas	⅔ cup (3.1 oz)	70	5	0	12
shelf-stable					
TastyBite					
Agra Peas & Greens	½ pkg (5 oz)	260	8	14	26
take-out					
pea & potato curry	1 serv (7 oz)	284	5	22	19
pea curry	1 serv (4.4 oz)	438	5	42	11
PECANS					
dry roasted	1 oz	187	2	18	6
dry roasted salted	1 oz	187	2	18	6
halves dry roasted w/ salt	20 (1 oz)	200	3	21	4
halves dried	1 cup	721	8	73	20
oil roasted	1 oz	195	2	20	5
oil roasted salted	1 oz	195	2	20	5
PECTIN					
powder	¼ pkg (0.4 oz)	39	0	0	11
Slim Set					
Packet	1 pkg	208	0	0	44
Powder	1 tbsp	3	0	0	1
Sure Jell					
For Lower Sugar Recipes	1 tsp (2.8 g)	20	0	0	4
Fruit Pectin	1 tsp (3.6 g)	20	0	0	4
PEPEAO					
dried	½ cup	36	1	tr	10
PEPPERS					
canned					
chili green	1 cup (5.5 oz)	29	1	tr	6
chili green hot chopped	½ cup	17	1	tr	4
chili red hot	1 (2.6 oz)	18	1	tr	4
chili red hot chopped	½ cup	17	1	tr	4
green halves	½ cup	13	1	tr	3

FOOD	PORTION	CALS	PROT	FAT	CARB
jalapeno chopped	½ cup	17	1	tr	3
red halves	½ cup	13	1	tr	3
Chi-Chi's					
Chilies Diced Green	2 tbsp (1.2 oz)	10	0	0	1
Chilies Green Whole	¾ pepper (1 oz)	10	0	0	1
Progresso					
Cherry Sliced & So Hot	2 tbsp (1 oz)	25	0	2	2
Hot Cherry	1 (1 oz)	10	0	0	2
Pepper Salad (drained)	2 tbsp (1 oz)	15	0	1	1
Roasted	1 piece (1 oz)	10	0	0	3
Sweet Fried w/ Onions	2 tbsp (0.9 oz)	20	0	2	2
Tuscan	3 (1 oz)	10	0	0	2
Rosarita					
Jalapeno Whole w/ Escabeche	¼ cup (1.2 oz)	8	1	tr	1
Vlasic					
Hot Sliced Cherry	1 oz	5	0	0	1
Jalapeno Sliced	1 oz	10	0	0	2
Mild Cherry	1 oz	5	0	0	1
Pepper Rings Hot	1 oz	5	0	0	1
Pepper Rings Mild	1 oz	5	0	0	1
dried					
ancho	1 (0.6 oz)	48	2	1	9
pasilla	1 (7 g)	24	1	1	4
fresh					
banana fresh	1 (4 in) (1.2 oz)	9	1	tr	2
banana fresh	1 cup (4.4 oz)	33	2	1	7
chili green hot fresh	1	18	1	tr	4
chili green hot fresh chopped	½ cup	30	2	tr	7
chili red fresh chopped	½ cup	30	2	tr	7
chili red hot fresh	1 (1.6 oz)	18	1	tr	4
green chopped cooked	½ cup	19	1	tr	5
green cooked	1 (2.6 oz)	20	1	tr	5
green fresh	1 (2.6 oz)	20	1	tr	5
habanero chile	1 tsp	9	1	tr	2
jalapeno fresh sliced	1 cup (3.2 oz)	27	1	1	5
red chopped cooked	½ cup	19	1	tr	5
red cooked	1 (2.6 oz)	20	1	tr	5
red fresh	1 (2.6 oz)	20	1	tr	5
serrano fresh chopped	1 cup (3.7 oz)	34	2	tr	7
yellow fresh	10 strips	14	1	tr	3
yellow fresh	1 (6.5 oz)	50	2	tr	12
Chiquita					
Pepper	1 med (5.2 oz)	30	1	0	7
frozen					
Birds Eye					
Diced Green	¾ cup (2.9 oz)	20	1	0	4

FOOD	PORTION	CALS	PROT	FAT	CARB
PERCH					
fresh					
cooked	3 oz	99	21	1	0
cooked	1 fillet (1.6 oz)	54	11	1	0
ocean perch atlantic cooked	3 oz	103	20	2	0
ocean perch atlantic cooked	1 fillet (1.8 oz)	60	12	1	0
ocean perch atlantic raw	3 oz	80	16	1	0
PERSIMMONS					
fresh japanese	1	118	1	tr	31
PHEASANT					
breast w/o skin raw	½ breast (6.4 oz)	243	44	6	0
leg w/o skin raw	1 (3.6 oz)	143	24	5	0
roasted	3.5 oz	215	33	9	0
w/ skin raw	½ pheasant (14 oz)	723	91	37	0
w/o skin raw	½ pheasant (12.4 oz)	470	83	13	0
PHYLLO DOUGH					
phyllo dough	1 oz	85	2	2	15
sheet	1	57	1	1	10
PICANTE					
(*see* SALSA)					
PICKLES					
Claussen					
Bread 'N Butter Chips	4 slices (1 oz)	20	0	0	4
Deli Style Hearty Garlic Whole	½ (1 oz)	5	0	0	1
Kosher Dill Spears	1 spear (1.2 oz)	5	0	0	1
Kosher Dills Halves	1 half (1 oz)	5	0	0	1
Kosher Dills Mini	1 (0.8 oz)	5	0	0	1
Kosher Dills Whole	½ (1 oz)	5	0	0	1
New York Deli Style Half Sours Whole	½ (1 oz)	5	0	0	1
Sandwich Slices Bread 'N Butter	2 (1.2 oz)	25	0	0	5
Sandwich Slices Deli Style Hearty Garlic	2 (1.2 oz)	5	0	0	1
Sandwich Slices Kosher Dills	2 (1.2 oz)	5	0	0	1
Super Slices For Burgers	1 (0.8 oz)	5	0	0	1
Vlasic					
Hamburger Dill Chips	1 oz	5	0	0	1
Kosher Cross Cuts	1 oz	5	0	0	1
Kosher Spears	1 oz	5	0	0	1
Kosher Whole	1 oz	5	0	0	1
Sweet Butter Chips	1 oz	30	0	0	7
Sweet Gerkins	1 oz	35	0	0	9
Whole Dills	1 oz	5	0	0	1

FOOD	PORTION	CALS	PROT	FAT	CARB
PIE					
frozen					
apple	⅛ of 9 in pie (4.4 oz)	297	2	14	43
blueberry	⅛ of 9 in pie (4.4 oz)	289	2	13	44
cherry	⅛ of 9 in pie (4.4 oz)	325	3	14	50
chocolate creme	⅙ of 8 in pie (4 oz)	344	3	22	38
coconut creme	⅙ of 7 in pie (2.2 oz)	191	1	11	24
lemon meringue	⅙ of 8 in pie (4.5 oz)	303	2	10	53
peach	⅙ of 8 in pie (4.1 oz)	261	2	12	39
Amy's Organic					
Apple	1 serv (8 oz)	280	4	12	42
Mrs. Smith's					
Apple	1 slice (4.3 oz)	350	3	19	41
Blueberry	1 slice (4.6 oz)	330	3	17	43
Cappuccino	1 slice (4.2 oz)	300	4	13	45
Cherry	1 slice (4.3 oz)	320	3	17	41
Cherry Crumb	1 slice (4.2 oz)	320	3	12	52
Chocolate Cream	1 slice (4.6 oz)	340	3	18	43
Chocolate Mint Cream	1 slice (4.3 oz)	360	3	15	53
Coconut Custard	1 slice (4.4 oz)	260	6	14	28
Cookies 'N Cream	1 slice (4.3 oz)	360	4	16	52
Dutch Apple	1 slice (4.4 oz)	330	3	13	50
French Silk	1 slice (4.4 oz)	560	4	40	48
Key West Lime	1 slice (4.3 oz)	430	5	18	62
Lemon Cream	1 slice (5 oz)	440	3	26	49
Lemonade	1 slice (4.3 oz)	340	3	15	51
Mince	1 slice (4.6 oz)	380	3	17	53
Mixed Berry	1 slice (4.2 oz)	300	2	13	44
Peach	1 slice (4.6 oz)	320	3	17	40
Peach Lattice	1 slice (4.2 oz)	290	2	13	42
Peanut Butter Silk	1 slice (4.6 oz)	600	8	41	51
Pecan	1 slice (4.8 oz)	560	6	27	75
Pumpkin Custard	1 slice (4.6 oz)	270	5	13	35
Raspberry	1 slice (4.6 oz)	330	3	17	44
S'Mores Cream	1 slice (4.3 oz)	360	3	16	53
Strawberry Banana	1 slice (4.3 oz)	330	3	15	48
Sweet Potato Custard	1 slice (4.6 oz)	340	4	17	44
Sara Lee					
Apple 45% Reduced Fat	⅛ pie (4.5 oz)	290	4	8	51
Chocolate Silk	⅕ pie (4.8 oz)	500	4	32	49
Coconut Cream	⅕ pie (4.8 oz)	480	4	31	47

FOOD	PORTION	CALS	PROT	FAT	CARB
Homestyle Apple	⅛ pie (4.6 oz)	340	3	16	46
Homestyle Blueberry	⅛ pie (4.6 oz)	360	3	15	54
Homestyle Cherry	⅛ pie (4.6 oz)	320	3	16	42
Homestyle Dutch Apple	⅛ pie (4.6 oz)	350	3	15	53
Homestyle Mince	⅛ pie (4.6 oz)	390	3	17	56
Homestyle Peach	⅛ pie (4.6 oz)	320	3	14	46
Homestyle Pecan	⅛ pie (4.2 oz)	520	5	24	70
Homestyle Pumpkin	⅛ pie (4.6 oz)	260	4	11	37
Homestyle Raspberry	⅛ pie (4.6 oz)	380	3	19	48
Lemon Meringue	⅙ pie (5 oz)	350	2	11	59
Weight Watchers					
Mississippi Mud	1 piece (2.45 oz)	160	4	5	26
home recipe					
pecan	⅛ of 9 in pie (4.3 oz)	502	6	27	64
pumpkin	⅛ of 9 in pie (5.4 oz)	316	7	14	41
mix					
banana cream no-bake	⅛ of 9 in pie (3.2 oz)	231	3	12	29
chocolate mousse no-bake	⅛ of 9 in pie (3.3 oz)	247	3	15	28
coconut creme no-bake	⅛ of 9 in pie (3.3 oz)	259	3	17	27
Jell-O					
No Bake Chocolate Silk as prep	⅙ pie (4.4 oz)	320	5	16	37
snack					
apple	1 (3 oz)	266	2	14	33
apple fried	1 (6.4 oz)	404	4	21	55
blueberry fried	1 (6.4 oz)	404	4	21	55
cherry	1 (3 oz)	266	2	14	33
cherry fried	1 (6.4 oz)	404	4	21	55
lemon	1 (3 oz)	266	2	14	33
lemon fried	1 (6.4 oz)	404	4	21	55
peach fried	1 (6.4 oz)	404	4	21	55
strawberry fried	1 (6.4 oz)	404	4	21	55
Dolly Madison					
Apple	1 (4.5 oz)	480	3	22	67
Blueberry	1 (4.5 oz)	480	3	21	70
Cherry	1 (4.5 oz)	470	3	22	65
Chocolate Pudding	1 (4.5 oz)	530	4	25	71
Lemon	1 (4.5 oz)	500	3	24	66
Peach	1 (4.5 oz)	480	3	21	66
Pecan	1 (3 oz)	360	3	19	44
Pecan Fried	1 (4.5 oz)	530	4	21	80
Pineapple	1 (4.5 oz)	460	4	21	62

FOOD	PORTION	CALS	PROT	FAT	CARB
Hostess					
Apple	1 (4.5 oz)	480	3	22	67
Blackberry	1 (4.5 oz)	520	3	21	79
Blueberry	1 (4.5 oz)	480	3	21	70
Cherry	1 (4.5 oz)	470	3	22	65
French Apple	1 (4.5 oz)	480	3	22	67
Lemon	1 (4.5 oz)	500	3	24	66
Peach	1 (4.5 oz)	480	3	21	68
Pineapple	1 (4.5 oz)	460	4	21	62
Strawberry	1 (4.5 oz)	510	3	23	71
Lance					
Pecan	1 (3 oz)	350	4	17	46
Tastykake					
Apple	1 (4 oz)	270	3	11	41
Blueberry	1 (4 oz)	300	3	11	49
Cherry	1 (4 oz)	290	3	11	46
Coconut Creme	1 (4 oz)	370	5	21	42
French Apple	1 (4.2 oz)	310	3	11	52
Lemon	1 (4 oz)	300	3	13	44
Peach	1 (4 oz)	280	3	11	43
Pineapple	1 (4 oz)	290	3	12	45
Pineapple Cheese	1 (4 oz)	320	5	12	50
Pumpkin	1 (4 oz)	340	4	14	47
Strawberry	1 (3.5 oz)	320	3	12	51
Tastyklair	1 (4 oz)	400	5	20	50
Tom's					
Apple	1 pkg (3 oz)	330	2	17	42
Banana Marshmallow	1 pkg (2.75 oz)	320	3	11	54
Cherry	1 pkg (3 oz)	320	2	18	37
Chocolate Marshmallow	1 pkg (2.75 oz)	320	3	11	53
take-out					
apple	⅛ of 9 in pie (5.4 oz)	411	4	19	58
banana cream	⅛ of 9 in pie (5.2 oz)	398	7	20	49
blueberry	⅛ of 9 in pie (5.2 oz)	360	4	18	49
butterscotch	⅛ of 9 in pie (4.5 oz)	355	6	18	42
cherry	⅛ of 9 in pie (6.3 oz)	486	5	22	69
coconut creme	⅛ of 9 in pie (4.7 oz)	396	6	21	46
coconut custard	⅛ of 8 in pie (3.6 oz)	271	6	14	32
custard	⅛ of 9 in pie (4.5 oz)	262	7	11	34

FOOD	PORTION	CALS	PROT	FAT	CARB
lemon meringue	⅛ of 9 in pie (4.5 oz)	362	5	16	50
mince	⅛ of 9 in pie (5.8 oz)	477	18	18	79
pecan	⅙ of 8 in pie (4 oz)	452	5	21	65
pumpkin	⅙ of 8 in pie (3.8 oz)	229	4	10	30
vanilla cream	⅛ of 9 in pie (4.4 oz)	350	6	18	41
PIE CRUST					
frozen					
baked	⅛ of 9 in pie (0.6 oz)	82	1	5	8
baked	9 in shell (4.4 oz)	647	6	41	63
puff pastry baked	1 shell (1.4 oz)	223	3	15	18
Pepperidge Farm					
Puff Pastry Sheets	⅙ sheet (1.4 oz)	170	3	11	14
Puff Pastry Shell	1 (1.6 oz)	190	4	13	16
Puff Pastry Squares	1 sq (2 oz)	240	4	16	19
Pet-Ritz					
Deep Dish	⅛ pie (0.7 oz)	90	1	5	11
Tart Shells	1 (1 oz)	130	1	8	13
home recipe					
9-inch crust	1	900	11	60	79
baked	9 in shell (6.3 oz)	949	12	62	86
baked	⅛ of 9 in crust (0.8 oz)	119	1	8	11
mix					
as prep	9 in crust (5.6 oz)	801	11	49	81
as prep	⅛ of 9 in pie (0.7 oz)	100	1	6	10
Betty Crocker					
Pie Crust as prep	⅛ crust	110	1	8	9
ready-to-eat					
chocolate cookie crumb baked	⅛ of 9 in pie (1 oz)	139	1	9	15
chocolate cookie crumb baked	9 in crust (7.7 oz)	1130	12	69	122
chocolate cookie crumb chilled	9 in crust (7.8 oz)	1127	12	69	121
chocolate cookie crumb chilled	⅛ of 9 in pie (1 oz)	142	1	9	15
graham cracker baked	⅛ of 9 in pie (1 oz)	148	1	8	20
graham cracker baked	9 in crust (8.4 oz)	1181	10	60	156
graham cracker chilled	⅛ of 9 in pie (1 oz)	150	1	8	20
graham cracker chilled	9 in crust (8.6 oz)	1182	10	60	155

FOOD	PORTION	CALS	PROT	FAT	CARB
vanilla wafer cracker crumbs baked	9 in crust (6.1 oz)	937	7	64	89
vanilla wafer cracker crumbs baked	⅛ of 9 in pie (0.8 oz)	119	1	8	11
vanilla wafer cracker crumbs chilled	⅛ of 9 in pie (0.8 oz)	117	1	8	11
vanilla wafer cracker crumbs chilled	9 in crust (6.2 oz)	934	7	64	88
Keebler					
Graham Single Serve	1 (0.8 oz)	120	1	6	15
Reduced Fat Graham	⅛ pie (0.7 oz)	90	1	4	14
PIE FILLING					
apple	1 can (21 oz)	599	1	1	156
cherry	1 can (21 oz)	683	3	1	175
pumpkin pie mix	1 cup	282	3	tr	71
Comstock					
MoreFruit Light Cherry	⅓ cup (2.9 oz)	60	0	0	13
Red Ruby Cherry	⅓ cup (3.1 oz)	90	0	0	23
Smucker's					
Pie Glaze Strawberry	2 oz	80	0	0	21
PIEROGI					
pierogi	¾ cup (4.4 oz)	307	11	19	24
Health Is Wealth					
Potato & Cheddar	2 (2.8 oz)	140	5	2	27
Potato & Onion	2 (2.8 oz)	140	4	2	27
Mrs. T's					
Jalapeno & Cheddar	3 (4.2 oz)	190	7	3	35
Potato & Cheddar	3 (4.2 oz)	180	7	3	34
Potato & Onion	3 (4.2 oz)	180	6	2	34
Sweet Potato	3 (4.2 oz)	300	5	0	35
PIGNOLIA					
(*see* PINE NUTS)					
PIG'S EARS AND FEET					
ear simmered	1	184	18	12	tr
feet pickled	1 oz	58	4	5	tr
feet pickled	1 lb	921	61	73	tr
feet simmered	3 oz	165	16	11	0
Hormel					
Pickled Feet	2 oz	80	7	6	0
Pickled Hocks	2 oz	110	9	8	0
PIGEON					
w/ skin & bone	3.5 oz	169	21	10	0
PIGEON PEAS					
dried cooked	½ cup	102	6	tr	20
dried cooked	1 cup	204	11	1	39
PIKE					
northern cooked	½ fillet (5.4 oz)	176	38	1	0
northern cooked	3 oz	96	21	1	0

FOOD	PORTION	CALS	PROT	FAT	CARB
northern raw	3 oz	75	16	1	0
roe raw	1 oz	37	7	tr	tr
walleye baked	3 oz	101	21	1	0
walleye fillet baked	4.4 oz	147	30	2	0
PILLNUTS					
canarytree dried	1 oz	204	3	23	1
PIMIENTOS					
Dromedary					
Peeled	½ tsp (4 g)	0	0	0	0
Unpeeled	½ tsp (4 g)	0	0	0	0
PINE NUTS					
pignolia dried	1 tbsp	51	2	5	1
pignolia dried	1 oz	146	7	14	4
pinyon dried	1 oz	161	3	17	5
Progresso					
Pignoli	1 jar (1 oz)	170	10	13	2
PINEAPPLE					
canned					
chunks in heavy syrup	1 cup	199	1	tr	52
chunks juice pack	1 cup	150	1	tr	39
crushed in heavy syrup	1 cup	199	1	tr	52
tidbits in heavy syrup	1 cup	199	1	tr	52
tidbits in juice	1 cup	150	1	tr	19
tidbits in water	1 cup	79	1	tr	20
Del Monte					
Chunks In Heavy Syrup	½ cup (4.3 oz)	90	0	0	24
Chunks In Its Own Juice	½ cup (4.3 oz)	70	0	0	17
Crushed In Heavy Syrup	½ cup (4.3 oz)	90	0	0	24
Crushed In Its Own Juice	½ cup (4.3 oz)	70	0	0	17
Fruit Cup Tidbits	1 pkg (4 oz)	50	1	0	15
Sliced In Heavy Syrup	2 slices (4.1 oz)	90	0	0	23
Sliced In Its Own Juice	½ cup (4 oz)	60	0	0	16
Spears In Its Own Juice	½ cup (4.3 oz)	70	0	0	17
Tidbits In Its Own Juice	½ cup (4.3 oz)	70	0	0	17
Wedges In Its Own Juice	½ cup (4.3 oz)	70	0	0	17
Dole					
Chunks Juice Pack	½ cup	60	0	0	15
Sunfresh					
In Extra Light Syrup	½ cup (4.6 oz)	80	0	0	17
fresh					
diced	1 cup	77	1	tr	19
Bonita Hill					
Golden Extra Sweet	2 slices (3.9 oz)	60	1	0	16
PINEAPPLE JUICE					
canned	1 cup	139	1	tr	34
frzn as prep	1 cup	129	1	tr	32
frzn not prep	6 oz	387	3	tr	96

FOOD	PORTION	CALS	PROT	FAT	CARB
Del Monte					
Juice From	6 fl oz	80	1	0	20
Dole					
Chilled	8 oz	130	0	0	30
PINK BEANS					
dried					
cooked	1 cup	252	15	1	47
PINTO BEANS					
canned					
pinto	1 cup	186	11	1	35
Chi-Chi's					
Pinto Beans	½ cup (4.3 oz)	100	6	1	18
Eden					
Organic Spicy	½ cup (4.6 oz)	125	6	0	24
Green Giant					
Pinto Beans	½ cup (4.4 oz)	110	6	1	20
Progresso					
Pinto Beans	½ cup (4.6 oz)	110	7	1	18
dried					
cooked	1 cup	235	14	1	44
Hurst					
HamBeens w/ Ham	3 tbsp (1.2 oz)	120	7	1	20
frozen					
cooked	3 oz	152	9	tr	29
PISTACHIOS					
dried	1 cup	739	26	62	32
dry roasted	1 oz	172	4	15	8
dry roasted salted	1 cup	776	19	68	35
dry roasted salted	1 oz	172	4	15	8
dry roasted w/ salt	47 nuts (1 oz)	160	6	13	8
Lance					
Pistachios	1 pkg (1⅛ oz)	90	4	7	4
PITANGA					
fresh	1 cup	57	1	1	13
PIZZA					
Amy's Organic					
Cheese	1 (13 oz)	310	13	11	39
Pocket Sandwich Cheese Pizza	1 (4.5 oz)	290	14	9	38
Pocket Sandwich Veggie Pepperoni Pizza	1 (4.5 oz)	220	12	7	28
Roasted Vegetable	1 (12 oz)	270	6	8	43
Spinach	1 (14 oz)	320	13	11	40
Appian Way					
Pizza Mix Thick Crust	⅓ pie (4.2 oz)	290	10	5	51
Pizza Mix Thin Crust	⅓ pie (4.1 oz)	250	7	3	48
Banquet					
Pepperoni	1 pie (6.75 oz)	490	11	23	56

FOOD	PORTION	CALS	PROT	FAT	CARB
Pizza Snack Cheese	6 pieces (7.5 oz)	200	9	8	24
Pizza Snack Pepperoni	6 pieces (7.5 oz)	230	8	11	23
Pizza Snack Pepperoni & Sausage	6 pieces (7.5 oz)	210	8	9	24
Di Giorno					
Rising Crust 12 inch Four Cheese	⅙ pie (4.9 oz)	320	16	11	39
Rising Crust 12 inch Italian Sausage	⅙ pie (5.3 oz)	360	18	14	40
Rising Crust 12 inch Pepperoni	⅙ pie (5.2 oz)	370	18	16	40
Rising Crust 12 inch Supreme	⅙ pie (5.8 oz)	380	18	17	40
Rising Crust 12 inch Three Meat	⅙ pie (5.4 oz)	380	19	16	40
Rising Crust 12 inch Vegetable	⅙ pie (5.6 oz)	310	15	10	41
Rising Crust 8 inch Chicken Supreme	⅓ pie (4.8 oz)	270	16	9	33
Rising Crust 8 inch Four Cheese	⅓ pie (4 oz)	260	14	9	33
Rising Crust 8 inch Italian Sausage	⅓ pie (4.4 oz)	300	15	12	33
Rising Crust 8 inch Pepperoni	⅓ pie (4.2 oz)	300	15	13	33
Rising Crust 8 inch Spinach	⅓ pie (4.3 oz)	250	15	8	33
Rising Crust 8 inch Supreme	⅓ pie (4.7 oz)	310	15	14	34
Rising Crust 8 inch Three Meat	⅓ pie (4.4 oz)	310	15	13	34
Rising Crust 8 inch Vegetable	⅓ pie (4.6 oz)	250	13	8	33
Health Is Wealth					
Pizza Munchees	6 (3 oz)	190	2	5	9
Healthy Choice					
French Bread Cheese	1 piece (6 oz)	340	22	5	51
French Bread Pepperoni	1 piece (6 oz)	340	24	5	49
French Bread Sausage	1 piece (6 oz)	320	21	5	48
French Bread Supreme	1 piece (6.35 oz)	330	21	5	51
French Bread Vegetable	1 piece (6 oz)	280	17	4	44
Jack's					
Great Combinations 12 inch Bacon Cheeseburger	¼ pie (4.7 oz)	360	20	18	31
Great Combinations 12 inch Double Cheese	¼ pie (4.9 oz)	380	21	19	32

FOOD	PORTION	CALS	PROT	FAT	CARB
Great Combinations 12 inch Pepperoni	¼ pie (5.2 oz)	410	19	19	42
Great Combinations 12 inch Pepperoni & Mushrooms	¼ pie (4.8 oz)	340	17	16	32
Great Combinations 12 inch Sausage	¼ pie (5.4 oz)	390	18	18	40
Great Combinations 12 inch Sausage & Mushroom	¼ pie (4.9 oz)	310	16	15	29
Great Combinations 12 inch Sausage & Pepperoni	¼ pie (4.8 oz)	350	17	19	29
Great Combinations 12 inch Supreme	¼ pie (5.2 oz)	350	17	18	30
Great Combinations 9 inch Double Cheese	½ pie (5.5 oz)	430	23	21	38
Great Combinations 9 inch Pepperoni & Sausage	½ pie (5.1 oz)	380	18	18	36
Naturally Rising 12 inch Bacon Cheeseburger	⅙ pie (5 oz)	350	18	15	35
Naturally Rising 12 inch Canadian Bacon	⅙ pie (4.9 oz)	280	16	9	34
Naturally Rising 12 inch Cheese	⅙ pie (4.5 oz)	290	15	10	35
Naturally Rising 12 inch Combination w/ Sausage & Pepperoni	⅙ pie (5.2 oz)	360	17	17	34
Naturally Rising 12 inch Pepperoni	⅙ pie (4.9 oz)	350	17	16	35
Naturally Rising 12 inch Pepperoni Supreme	⅙ pie (5.1 oz)	340	16	16	34
Naturally Rising 12 inch Sausage	⅙ pie (5.1 oz)	340	17	15	34
Naturally Rising 12 inch Spicy Italian Sausage	⅙ pie (5.1 oz)	330	17	14	34
Naturally Rising 12 inch The Works	⅙ pie (5.3 oz)	330	16	14	34
Naturally Rising 9 inch Cheese	⅓ pie (4.7 oz)	300	15	10	38
Naturally Rising 9 inch Combination w/ Sausage & Pepperoni	¼ pie (4.2 oz)	300	14	14	29
Naturally Rising 9 inch Pepperoni	⅓ pie (5.2 oz)	360	17	16	38
Naturally Rising 9 inch Sausage	⅓ pie (5.4 oz)	360	17	16	38

FOOD	PORTION	CALS	PROT	FAT	CARB
Naturally Rising 9 inch The Works	¼ pie (4.5 oz)	280	13	12	29
Original 12 inch Canadian Bacon	¼ pie (4.4 oz)	280	16	10	31
Original 12 inch Cheese	⅓ pie (5 oz)	360	19	13	41
Original 12 inch Hamburger	¼ pie (4.4 oz)	300	16	14	28
Original 12 inch Pepperoni	¼ pie (4.3 oz)	330	16	15	31
Original 12 inch Sausage	¼ pie (4.3 oz)	300	15	14	28
Original 12 inch Spicy Italian Sausage	¼ pie (4.3 oz)	290	15	13	29
Original 9 inch Pepperoni	½ pie (5 oz)	380	18	18	37
Original 9 inch Sausage	½ pie (5.1 oz)	360	17	16	36
Pizza Bursts Combination Sausage & Pepperoni	6 pieces (3 oz)	250	8	12	26
Pizza Bursts Pepperoni	6 pieces (3 oz)	260	9	14	25
Pizza Bursts Sausage	6 pieces (3 oz)	250	8	12	25
Pizza Bursts Supercheese	6 pieces (3 oz)	250	9	12	25
Pizza Bursts Supreme	6 pieces (3 oz)	250	8	13	26
Kid Cuisine					
Backpacking Pizza Snack	6 pieces	230	8	11	23
Big League Hamburger	1 meal (8.3 oz)	400	14	11	61
Fire Chief Cheese	1 pie (5.2 oz)	340	19	10	44
Pirate Pizza w/ Cheese	1 meal (8 oz)	430	12	11	71
Poolside Pepperoni	1 (5.2 oz)	380	18	14	44
Lean Cuisine					
Everyday Favorites French Bread Cheese	1 pkg (6 oz)	320	15	7	48
Everyday Favorites French Bread Deluxe	1 pkg (6.1 oz)	290	16	6	43
Everyday Favorites French Bread Pepperoni	1 pkg (5.25 oz)	300	15	8	43
Everyday Favorites French Bread Sun Dried Tomatoes	1 serv (6 oz)	340	19	8	48
Marie Callender's					
French Bread Cheese	1 (7.2 oz)	530	28	24	50
French Bread Pepperoni	1 (7.5 oz)	570	29	28	50
French Bread Supreme	1 (7.5 oz)	510	26	23	50
Pepperidge Farm					
Gourmet Crust Cheese	1 (4.4 oz)	390	12	20	39
Gourmet Crust Pepperoni	1 (4.5 oz)	420	15	23	39
Stouffer's					
French Bread Bacon Cheddar	1 piece (5.7 oz)	430	15	21	46
French Bread Cheese	1 piece (5.2 oz)	370	14	16	43
French Bread Cheeseburger	1 piece (6 oz)	420	17	20	44
French Bread Deluxe	1 piece (6.2 oz)	430	17	21	49

FOOD	PORTION	CALS	PROT	FAT	CARB
French Bread Double Cheese	1 piece (5.9 oz)	400	16	16	49
French Bread Pepperoni	1 piece (5.6 oz)	430	16	20	46
French Bread Pepperoni & Mushroom	1 piece (6.1 oz)	440	15	20	49
French Bread Sausage	1 piece (6 oz)	420	17	18	48
French Bread Sausage & Pepperoni	1 piece (6.25 oz)	470	18	23	47
French Bread Three Meat	1 piece (6.25 oz)	460	20	21	48
French Bread Vegetable Deluxe	1 piece (6.4 oz)	380	14	16	46
French Bread White Pizza	1 piece (5.1 oz)	460	18	23	45
Tombstone					
Double Top Pepperoni	⅙ pie (4.5 oz)	340	18	19	24
Double Top Sausage	⅙ pie (4.6 oz)	320	18	17	25
Double Top Sausage & Pepperoni	⅙ pie (4.6 oz)	340	19	19	25
Double Top Supreme	⅙ pie (4.7 oz)	330	18	18	25
Double Top Two Cheese	⅙ pie (5.2 oz)	380	22	19	29
For One ½ Less Fat Cheese	1 pie (6.5 oz)	460	23	10	43
For One ½ Less Fat Vegetable	1 pie (7.2 oz)	360	21	9	48
For One Extra Cheese	1 pie (6.9 oz)	520	26	28	47
For One Pepperoni	1 pie (6.9 oz)	550	25	32	41
For One Supreme	1 pie (7.5 oz)	550	24	32	42
Light Supreme	⅕ pie (4.8 oz)	270	17	9	30
Light Vegetable	⅕ pie (4.6 oz)	240	14	7	31
Original 12 inch Canadian Bacon	¼ pie (5.5 oz)	350	20	14	36
Original 12 inch Deluxe	⅕ pie (4.8 oz)	310	15	14	29
Original 12 inch Extra Cheese	¼ pie (5.1 oz)	350	18	15	35
Original 12 inch Hamburger	⅕ pie (4.4 oz)	310	15	15	29
Original 12 inch Pepperoni	¼ pie (5.3 oz)	400	19	21	35
Original 12 inch Sausage	⅕ pie (4.4 oz)	300	15	14	29
Original 12 inch Sausage & Mushroom	⅕ pie (4.6 oz)	300	15	14	29
Original 12 inch Sausage & Pepperoni	⅕ pie (4.4 oz)	320	15	16	29
Original 12 inch Supreme	⅕ pie (5.1 oz)	320	15	16	29
Original 9 inch Deluxe	⅓ pie (4.4 oz)	280	14	13	27
Original 9 inch Extra Cheese	½ pie (5.6 oz)	380	19	19	40
Original 9 inch Hamburger	⅓ pie (4 oz)	280	14	13	27
Original 9 inch Pepperoni	⅓ pie (4 oz)	300	14	15	27
Original 9 inch Pepperoni & Sausage	⅓ pie (4.1 oz)	300	14	15	27
Original 9 inch Sausage	⅓ pie (4 oz)	280	14	13	27

FOOD	PORTION	CALS	PROT	FAT	CARB
Original 9 inch Supreme	⅓ pie (4.4 oz)	310	15	16	27
Oven Rising Italian Sausage	⅙ pie (5.1 oz)	320	16	13	35
Oven Rising Pepperoni	⅙ pie (4.9 oz)	340	17	15	34
Oven Rising Supreme	⅙ pie (5.1 oz)	320	16	14	34
Oven Rising Three Cheese	⅙ pie (4.8 oz)	320	16	13	34
Oven Rising Three Meat	⅙ pie (5.1 oz)	340	17	15	34
Thin Crust Four Meat Combo	¼ pie (5 oz)	380	19	23	26
Thin Crust Italian Sausage	¼ pie (5 oz)	370	18	22	26
Thin Crust Pepperoni	¼ pie (4.8 oz)	400	18	25	25
Thin Crust Supreme	¼ pie (5 oz)	380	18	22	26
Thin Crust Supreme Taco	¼ pie (5.1 oz)	370	16	23	27
Thin Crust Three Cheese	¼ pie (4.7 oz)	360	19	21	25
Weight Watchers					
Smart Ones Deluxe Combo	1 (6.57 oz)	380	23	11	47
Smart Ones Pepperoni	1 (5.56 oz)	390	23	12	46
take-out					
cheese	12 in pie	1121	61	26	164
cheese	⅛ of 12 in pie	140	8	3	21
cheese deep dish individual	1 (5.5 oz)	460	15	24	47
cheese meat & vegetables	⅛ of 12 in pie	184	13	5	21
cheese meat & vegetables	12 in pie	1472	104	43	170
pepperoni	12 in pie	1445	81	56	157
pepperoni	⅛ of 12 in pie	181	10	7	20
PIZZA DOUGH					
crust	1 slice (1.7 oz)	130	4	2	25
Betty Crocker					
Italian Herb Crust Mix	¼ crust (1.6 oz)	180	4	2	32
Boboli					
Thin Crust	⅕ crust (2 oz)	160	6	4	24
Pillsbury					
Crust	⅕ crust (2 oz)	150	5	2	27
Robin Hood					
Crust	¼ crust	160	4	2	33
PIZZA SAUCE					
Hunt's					
Fully Prepared	¼ cup (2.2 oz)	21	1	1	4
Pizza Sauce	¼ cup (2.2 oz)	27	1	1	5
Prima Choice Supper Heavy	¼ cup (2.2 oz)	28	2	1	6
Muir Glen					
Organic	¼ cup (2.2 oz)	40	1	0	6
PLANTAINS					
fresh uncooked	1 (6.3 oz)	218	2	1	57
sliced cooked	½ cup	89	1	tr	24
take-out					
ripe fried	2.8 oz	214	1	7	38

FOOD	PORTION	CALS	PROT	FAT	CARB
PLUMS					
canned					
purple in heavy syrup	1 cup	320	1	tr	60
purple in light syrup	1 cup	158	1	tr	41
purple juice pack	1 cup	146	1	tr	38
purple water pack	1 cup	102	1	tr	27
Eden					
Umeboshi Paste	1 tsp	5	0	0	1
Umeboshi Plums	1	5	0	0	1
fresh					
plum	1	36	1	tr	9
sliced	1 cup	91	1	1	21
Chiquita					
Purple	2 med (4.6 oz)	80	1	1	19
POKEBERRY SHOOTS					
cooked	½ cup	16	2	tr	3
raw	½ cup	18	2	tr	3
POLENTA					
Frieda's					
Dried Tomato	4 oz	80	2	0	17
Italian Herb	4 oz	80	2	0	17
Mexicana	4 oz	80	2	0	17
Original	4 oz	80	2	0	16
Wild Mushroom	4 oz	80	2	0	17
Melissa's					
Original	4 oz	80	2	0	16
POLLACK					
atlantic fillet baked	5.3 oz	178	38	2	0
atlantic baked	3 oz	100	21	1	0
POMEGRANATE					
fresh	1	104	1	tr	26
Cortas					
Concentrated Juice	1 tbsp (0.6 oz)	40	0	0	9
POMPANO					
florida cooked	3 oz	179	20	10	0
florida raw	3 oz	140	16	8	0
POPCORN					
(*see also* CHIPS, POPCORN CAKES, PRETZELS, SNACKS)					
air-popped	1 cup (0.3 oz)	31	1	tr	6
air-popped	1 oz	108	3	1	22
caramel coated	1 oz	122	1	4	22
caramel coated	1 cup (1.2 oz)	152	1	5	28
carmel coated w/ peanuts	⅔ cup (1 oz)	114	2	2	23
cheese	1 oz	149	3	9	15
cheese	1 cup (0.4 oz)	58	1	4	6
oil popped	1 oz	142	3	8	16
oil popped	1 cup (0.4 oz)	55	1	3	6

FOOD	PORTION	CALS	PROT	FAT	CARB
Chester's					
Butter	3 cups	160	2	12	15
Caramel Craze	¾ cup	130	1	2	27
Cheddar Cheese	3 cups	190	3	13	17
Microwave Butter	5 cups	200	3	12	22
Cracker Jack					
Fat Free Butter Toffee	¾ cup	110	1	0	26
Original	½ cup (1 oz)	120	2	2	23
Herr's					
Regular	3 cups (1 oz)	140	2	11	11
Jolly Time					
Blast O Butter	1 cup	45	1	3	5
White Air Popped	5 cups	100	4	1	24
Yellow Air Popped	5 cups	100	4	1	24
Lance					
Cheese	1 pkg (0.6 oz)	90	2	5	9
Plain	1 pkg (0.5 oz)	70	1	3	10
White Cheddar	1 pkg (0.6 oz)	100	1	8	7
White Cheddar	1 pkg (0.9 oz)	150	2	11	10
Newman's Own					
Microwave Butter Flavor	3½ cups	170	2	11	16
Microwave Light Butter	3½ cups	110	2	3	20
Microwave Light Natural	3½ cups	110	2	3	20
Microwave Natural	3½ cups	170	2	11	16
Popcorn unpopped	3 tbsp	110	4	2	27
Orville Redenbacher's					
Gourmet Original	3 cups	92	3	1	22
Hot Air	3 cups	92	3	1	22
Microwave Butter	3 cups	168	2	13	15
Microwave Butter No Salt Added	3 cups	176	3	12	19
Microwave Butter Light	3 cups	122	3	6	20
Microwave Caramel	1 serv	179	1	10	23
Microwave Golden Cheddar	1 serv	169	2	13	15
Microwave Natural	3 cups	164	2	11	18
Microwave Natural No Salt Added	3 cups	174	3	12	19
Microwave Natural Light	3 cups	118	3	5	19
Microwave Smartpop	1 serv	96	3	3	20
Microwave Smartpop Butter Snack Size	1 bag	155	5	4	34
Microwave Snack Size Butter	1 bag	287	3	22	25
Microwave Snack Size Butter Light	1 bag	183	4	8	30
Microwave White Cheddar	1 serv	169	2	13	15
Redenbudders Microwave Herb & Garlic	1 serv	176	2	13	16

FOOD	PORTION	CALS	PROT	FAT	CARB
Redenbudders Microwave Zesty Butter	1 serv	177	2	13	16
Redenbudders Movie Theater Butter Light	1 serv	113	3	5	20
Redenbudders Movie Theater Microwave Butter	1 serv	176	2	13	16
Smart Pop Movie Theater Butter	1 serv	92	3	2	20
White	3 cups	92	3	1	22
Smartfood					
Butter	3 cups	150	2	9	15
Low Fat Toffee Crunch	¾ cup	110	1	1	25
Reduced Fat Golden Butter	3⅓ cups	130	3	4	21
Reduced Fat White Cheddar	3 cups	140	4	6	19
White Cheddar	2 cups	190	3	12	17
Snyder's Of Hanover					
Butter	⅝ oz	110	1	10	6
Tom's					
Caramel Corn	1 pkg (1.6 oz)	180	1	3	39
Utz					
Au Natural	3 cups (1 oz)	120	3	1	25
Butter	2 cups (1 oz)	170	2	12	13
Cheese	2 cups (1 oz)	150	2	10	14
Hulless Puff'N Corn	2 cups (1 oz)	180	1	15	11
Hulless Puff'N Corn Hot Cheese	1 pkg (1.75 oz)	290	3	22	21
Hulless Pull'N Corn Cheese	2 cups (1 oz)	170	2	12	13
White Cheddar	2 cups (1 oz)	150	3	9	15
Weight Watchers					
Butter	1 pkg (0.66 oz)	90	2	3	14
Butter Toffee	1 pkg (0.9 oz)	110	1	3	21
Caramel	1 pkg (0.9 oz)	100	1	1	22
Microwave	1 pkg (1 oz)	100	3	1	20
White Cheddar Cheese	1 pkg (0.66 oz)	90	2	4	12
POPCORN CAKES					
popcorn cake	1 (0.3 oz)	38	1	tr	8
Orville Redenbacher's					
BBQ Mini	8 (0.5 oz)	55	0	1	12
Butter	2 (0.6 oz)	134	2	1	13
Butter Mini	8 (0.5 oz)	56	2	1	11
Caramel	1 (0.4 oz)	34	1	tr	8
Caramel Mini	7 (0.5 oz)	50	1	tr	12
Nacho Cheese Mini	8 (0.5 oz)	56	2	1	11
Peanut Crunch Mini	7 (0.5 oz)	55	2	1	11
White Cheddar	2 (0.6 oz)	63	0	1	13
White Cheddar Mini	8 (0.5 oz)	56	2	1	12

FOOD	PORTION	CALS	PROT	FAT	CARB
POPOVER					
home recipe as prep w/ 2% milk	1 (1.4 oz)	87	4	3	11
home recipe as prep w/ whole milk	1 (1.4 oz)	90	4	3	11
mix as prep	1 (1.2 oz)	67	3	2	10
POPPY SEEDS					
poppy seeds	1 tsp	15	1	1	1
PORGY					
fresh	3 oz	77	18	tr	0
PORK					
(see also BACON, CANADIAN BACON, DELI MEATS/COLD CUTS, HAM, PORK DISHES, SAUSAGE)					
canned					
Hormel					
Pickled Tidbits	2 oz	100	8	8	0
fresh					
boston blade roast lean & fat cooked	3 oz	229	20	16	0
boston blade steak lean & fat cooked	3 oz	220	22	14	0
center loin roast lean bone in cooked	3 oz	169	23	8	0
center loin chop lean bone in cooked	3 oz	172	25	7	0
center rib chop lean & fat bone in cooked	3 oz	213	23	13	0
center rib roast lean & fat bone in cooked	3 oz	217	23	13	0
fresh ham rump lean roasted	3 oz	175	26	7	0
fresh ham rump lean & fat roasted	3 oz	214	25	12	0
fresh ham shank lean roasted	3 oz	183	24	9	0
fresh ham shank lean & fat roasted	3 oz	246	22	17	0
fresh ham whole lean roasted	3 oz	179	25	8	0
fresh ham whole lean roasted diced	1 cup	285	40	13	0
fresh ham whole lean & fat roasted	3 oz	232	23	15	0
fresh ham whole lean & fat roasted diced	1 cup	369	36	24	0
ground cooked	3 oz	252	22	18	0
loin chop lean bone in braised	3 oz	191	21	11	0

FOOD	PORTION	CALS	PROT	FAT	CARB
loin chop lean bone in broiled	3 oz	199	22	12	0
loin roast lean bone in roasted	3 oz	210	23	13	0
loin whole lean & fat braised	3 oz	203	23	12	0
loin whole lean & fat broiled	3 oz	206	23	12	0
loin whole lean & fat roasted	3 oz	211	23	12	0
lungs braised	3 oz	84	14	3	0
pancreas cooked	3 oz	186	24	9	0
ribs country style lean & fat braised	3 oz	252	20	18	0
shoulder arm picnic lean & fat roasted	3 oz	269	20	20	0
shoulder whole lean & fat roasted	3 oz	248	20	18	0
shoulder whole lean & fat roasted diced	1 cup	394	31	29	0
shoulder whole lean roasted	3 oz	196	22	12	0
shoulder whole lean roasted diced	1 cup	311	34	18	0
sirloin chop lean & fat bone in braised	3 oz	208	22	13	0
sirloin roast lean & fat bone in cooked	3 oz	222	23	14	0
spareribs braised	3 oz	338	25	26	0
spleen braised	3 oz	127	24	3	0
tail simmered	3 oz	336	15	30	0
tenderloin lean roasted	3 oz	139	24	4	0
top loin chop boneless lean & fat cooked	3 oz	198	24	11	0
top loin roast bonless lean & fat cooked	3 oz	192	24	10	0
Freirich					
Porkette	4 oz	220	16	18	1
Oscar Mayer					
Sweet Morsel Smoked Boneless Pork Shoulder Butt	3 oz	180	11	15	0
ready-to-eat					
Tyson					
Pork Pattie	1 (3.8 oz)	200	15	11	9
take-out					
chicharrones pork cracklings fried	1 cup	844	27	72	22
PORK DISHES					
Thomas E. Wilson					
Lemon Pepper Pork Roast	1 serv (3 oz)	110	19	3	2

FOOD	PORTION	CALS	PROT	FAT	CARB
take-out					
pork roast	2 oz	70	10	3	0
tourtiere	1 piece (4.9 oz)	451	15	34	21
POT PIE					
Amy's Organic					
Broccoli	1 (7.5 oz)	430	11	22	46
Country Vegetable	1 (7.5 oz)	370	12	16	47
Shepard's	1 (8 oz)	160	5	4	27
Vegetable	1 (7.5 oz)	360	7	18	44
Vegetable Non-Dairy	1 (7.5 oz)	320	9	9	50
Banquet					
Beef	1 (7 oz)	400	9	23	38
Cheesy Potato & Broccoli w/ Ham	1 (7 oz)	410	9	23	40
Chicken	1 (7 oz)	380	10	22	36
Chicken & Broccoli	1 (7 oz)	350	10	20	32
Family Size Hearty Chicken	1 cup	460	11	29	39
Macaroni & Cheese	1 pkg (6.5 oz)	210	7	5	34
Turkey	1 (7 oz)	370	10	20	38
Vegetable Cheese	1 (7 oz)	340	6	17	39
Healthy Choice					
Colonial Chicken	1 (9.5 oz)	310	22	7	40
Lean Cuisine					
Everyday Favorites Chicken Pie	1 pkg (9.5 oz)	300	19	8	38
Everyday Favorites Vegetable Eggroll	1 pkg (9 oz)	300	7	5	57
Marie Callender's					
Beef	1 (9.5 oz)	680	16	42	53
Chicken	1 (9.5 oz)	680	14	48	53
Chicken & Broccoli	1 (9.5 oz)	670	16	43	54
Chicken Au Gratin	1 (9.5 oz)	690	19	46	50
Turkey	1 (9.5 oz)	680	13	46	56
Morton					
Macaroni & Cheese	1 (6.5 oz)	210	7	5	34
Vegetable w/ Beef	1 (7 oz)	340	5	21	33
Vegetable w/ Chicken	1 (7 oz)	320	8	18	32
Vegetable w/ Turkey	1 (7 oz)	310	8	18	29
Mrs. Paterson's					
Aussie Pie Chicken	1 (5.5 oz)	460	12	25	45
Aussie Pie Chicken Low Fat	1 (5.5 oz)	380	13	17	44
Aussie Pie Philly Steak	1 (5.5 oz)	420	11	24	39
Stouffer's					
Beef Pie	1 pkg (10 oz)	450	19	26	36
Chicken Pie	1 pkg (10 oz)	540	23	33	38
Turkey	1 pkg (10 oz)	530	21	33	36

FOOD	PORTION	CALS	PROT	FAT	CARB
Swanson					
Beef	1 (7 oz)	376	12	19	39
Chicken	1 (7 oz)	416	9	22	45
Turkey	1 (7 oz)	440	12	24	44
take-out					
beef	⅛ of 9 in pie (7.4 oz)	515	21	30	39
chicken	⅛ of 9 in pie (8.1 oz)	545	23	31	42
POTATO					
(*see also* CHIPS, KNISH, PANCAKES)					
canned					
potatoes	½ cup	54	1	tr	12
Del Monte					
New Sliced	⅔ cup (5.4 oz)	60	1	0	13
New Whole	2 med (5.5 oz)	60	1	0	13
Hormel					
Au Gratin & Bacon	1 can (7.5 oz)	250	8	14	23
S&W					
Whole Small	2 (5.5 oz)	60	1	0	13
fresh					
baked skin only	1 skin (2 oz)	115	2	tr	27
baked w/ skin	1 (6.5 oz)	220	5	tr	51
baked w/o skin	1 (5 oz)	145	3	tr	34
baked w/o skin	½ cup	57	1	tr	13
boiled	½ cup	68	1	tr	16
microwaved	1 (7 oz)	212	5	tr	49
microwaved w/o skin	½ cup	78	2	tr	18
PurelyIdaho					
Oven Roasts	1 serv (3 oz)	70	2	0	17
frozen					
french fries	10 strips	111	2	4	17
french fries thick cut	10 strips	109	2	4	17
hashed brown	½ cup	170	2	9	22
potato puffs	½ cup	138	2	7	19
Birds Eye					
Baby Gourmet	7 (4 oz)	100	2	0	21
Whole	3 (2.6 oz)	50	1	0	13
Healthy Choice					
Cheddar Broccoli Potatoes	1 meal (10.5 oz)	330	13	7	53
Lean Cuisine					
Everyday Favorites Deluxe Cheddar Potato	1 pkg (10.4 oz)	250	13	6	37
Everyday Favorites Roasted Potatoes w/ Broccoli	1 pkg (10.25 oz)	260	12	6	39
Oh Boy!					
Stuffed w/ Cheddar Cheese	1 (5 oz)	130	3	4	22

FOOD	PORTION	CALS	PROT	FAT	CARB
Stouffer's					
Au Gratin	½ cup (5.75 oz)	130	4	6	15
Scalloped	½ cup (5.75 oz)	140	4	6	17
Tree Of Life					
Organic French Fries	20 pieces (3 oz)	110	2	3	19
Weight Watchers					
Smart Ones Baked Broccoli & Cheese	1 pkg (10 oz)	250	11	6	39
home recipe					
au gratin	½ cup	160	6	9	14
mashed w/ whole milk & margarine	⅓ cup	66	2	tr	13
scalloped	½ cup	105	4	5	13
mix					
au gratin as prep	4½ oz	127	3	6	18
instant mashed flakes as prep w/ whole milk & butter	½ cup	118	2	6	16
instant mashed flakes not prep	½ cup	78	2	tr	18
instant mashed granules as prep w/ whole milk & butter	½ cup	114	2	5	15
instant mashed granules not prep	½ cup	372	8	1	86
scalloped as prep	4½ oz	127	3	6	18
Barbara's					
Mashed not prep	⅓ cup (0.8 oz)	70	2	0	17
Betty Crocker					
Au Gratin Low Fat Recipe	½ cup	110	3	1	22
Au Gratin as prep	½ cup	150	3	6	22
Cheddar & Bacon	½ cup	150	3	6	21
Cheddar & Bacon Low Fat Recipe	½ cup	120	3	3	21
Cheddar & Sour Cream	½ cup	130	3	3	25
Chicken & Vegetable	⅔ cup	140	4	4	23
Chicken & Vegetable Low Fat Recipe	⅔ cup	120	4	3	23
Hash Browns	½ cup	190	3	8	30
Homestyle Broccoli Au Gratin	½ cup	140	3	6	21
Homestyle Broccoli Au Gratin Low Fat Recipe	½ cup	110	3	3	21
Homestyle Cheddar Cheese	½ cup	120	3	3	21
Homestyle Cheddar Cheese Stove Top Recipe	½ cup	140	3	5	21
Homestyle Cheesy Scalloped	½ cup	140	3	6	21

FOOD	PORTION	CALS	PROT	FAT	CARB
Homestyle Cheesy Scalloped Low Fat Recipe	½ cup	110	3	3	21
Julienne	½ cup	150	3	6	21
Mashed Butter & Herb	½ cup	160	3	8	20
Mashed Butter & Herb Reduced Fat Recipe	½ cup	130	3	5	20
Mashed Chicken & Herb	½ cup	150	3	7	21
Mashed Chicken & Herb Reduced Fat Recipe	½ cup	120	3	4	21
Mashed Four Cheese	½ cup	150	3	7	20
Mashed Four Cheese Reduced Fat Recipe	½ cup	120	3	4	20
Mashed Potato Buds	⅔ cup	160	3	8	19
Mashed Potato Buds Reduced Fat Recipe	⅔ cup	120	3	4	19
Mashed Roasted Garlic	½ cup	150	3	8	19
Mashed Roasted Garlic Reduced Fat Recipe	½ cup	130	3	5	19
Mashed Sour Cream & Chives	½ cup	150	3	7	21
Mashed Sour Cream & Chives Reduced Fat Recipe	½ cup	120	3	4	21
Potato Shakers Original	⅔ cup	140	3	4	23
Potato Shakers Original Low Fat Recipe	⅔ cup	120	3	2	23
Ranch	½ cup	160	3	6	25
Scalloped	½ cup	150	3	6	23
Scalloped Low Fat Recipe	⅔ cup	110	3	1	23
Sour Cream'n Chive	½ cup	160	3	7	22
Three Cheese	½ cup	150	3	6	23
Twice Baked Cheddar & Bacon Low Fat Recipe	⅔ cup	130	6	3	22
Twice Baked Cheddar & Bacon as prep	⅔ cup	210	6	11	22
Hungry Jack					
Au Gratin as prep	½ cup	150	3	5	24
Cheddar & Bacon as prep	½ cup	150	4	5	24
Chessy Scalloped as prep	½ cup	150	3	5	24
Creamy Scalloped as prep	½ cup	150	3	5	24
Mashed Butter Flavored as prep	½ cup	150	3	7	19
Mashed Flakes as prep	½ cup	160	3	7	20
Mashed Garlic Flavored as prep	½ cup	150	3	7	19
Mashed Parsley Butter as prep	½ cup	150	3	7	19

FOOD	PORTION	CALS	PROT	FAT	CARB
Mashed Sour Cream 'n Chives as prep	½ cup	150	3	7	19
Sour Cream & Chives as prep	½ cup	160	3	6	23
Idaho					
Mashed Potato Flakes as prep	½ cup	150	3	6	20
Mashed Potato Granules as prep	½ cup	160	3	7	22
Shake 'N Bake					
Perfect Potatoes Crispy Cheddar	⅛ pkg (7 g)	30	2	2	2
Perfect Potatoes Herb & Garlic	⅛ pkg (7 g)	20	0	0	5
Perfect Potatoes Home Fries	⅛ pkg (7 g)	20	0	0	5
Perfect Potatoes Parmesan Peppercorn	⅛ pkg (7 g)	25	1	1	3
Perfect Potatoes Savory Onion	⅛ pkg (7 g)	20	0	0	5
shelf-stable					
Lunch Bucket					
Scalloped w/ Ham Chunks	1 pkg (7.5 oz)	170	2	7	24
Micro Cup Meals					
Microcup Meals Scalloped Potatoes w/ Ham	1 cup (7.5 oz)	240	7	14	20
TastyBite					
Bombay Potatoes	½ pkg (5 oz)	190	9	8	22
Mumbai Pav Bhaji	½ pkg (5 oz)	229	2	6	23
Simla Potatoes	½ pkg (5 oz)	180	5	8	23
take-out					
au gratin w/ cheese	½ cup	178	7	10	17
baked topped w/ cheese sauce	1	475	15	29	47
baked topped w/ cheese sauce & bacon	1	451	18	26	44
baked topped w/ cheese sauce & broccoli	1	402	14	14	47
baked topped w/ cheese sauce & chili	1	481	23	22	56
baked topped w/ sour cream & chives	1	394	7	22	50
curry	1 serv (6 oz)	292	4	16	36
french fries	1 reg	235	3	12	29
french fries	1 lg	355	5	19	44
hash brown	½ cup (2.5 oz)	151	2	9	16
indian yogurt potatoes	1 serv	315	7	9	52
mashed	½ cup	111	2	4	18

FOOD	PORTION	CALS	PROT	FAT	CARB
mustard potato salad	3.5 oz	120	1	6	16
o'brien	1 cup	157	5	3	30
potato dumpling	3.5 oz	334	7	1	74
potato pancakes	1 (1.3 oz)	101	2	7	11
potato salad	½ cup	179	3	10	14
potato salad w/ vegetables	3.5 oz	120	2	3	20
scalloped	½ cup	127	4	5	18
POUT					
ocean baked	3 oz	86	18	1	0
ocean fillet baked	4.8 oz	139	29	2	0
PRETZELS					
chocolate covered	1 (0.4 oz)	50	1	2	8
chocolate covered	1 oz	130	2	5	20
dutch twist	4 (2.1 oz)	229	6	2	48
pretzels	1 oz	108	3	1	23
rods	4 (2 oz)	229	6	2	48
sticks	120 (2 oz)	229	6	2	48
twist	1 (½ oz)	65	2	1	13
twists	10 (2.1 oz)	229	6	2	48
whole wheat	2 sm (1 oz)	103	3	1	23
whole wheat	2 med (2 oz)	205	6	2	46
Bachman					
Thin'n Right	12 (1 oz)	120	3	1	23
Estee					
Chocolate Covered	7	130	2	6	19
Dutch	2 (1.1 oz)	130	3	1	26
Unsalted	23 (1 oz)	120	3	1	25
Gardetto's					
Mustard	1 pkg (0.5 oz)	50	1	1	10
Herr's					
Hard Sourdough	1 (1 oz)	100	3	0	23
Lance					
Pretzels	1 pkg (1.25 oz)	140	4	1	28
Little Debbie					
Mini Twists	1 pkg (1.2 oz)	140	4	1	28
Nabisco					
Air Crisps Fat Free	23 pieces (1 oz)	110	2	0	23
Nestle					
Flipz Milk Chocolate Covered	9 pieces (1 oz)	130	2	5	19
Flipz White Fudge Covered	9 pieces (1 oz)	130	2	6	19
Newman's Own					
Salted Rounds Organic	1 pkg (1.4 oz)	150	3	2	31
Rold Gold					
Crispy's Thins	4 (1 oz)	110	3	2	22
Fat Free Honey Mustard	17 (1 oz)	110	3	0	23
Fat Free Sticks	48 (1 oz)	110	3	0	23
Fat Free Thins	12 pieces (1 oz)	110	2	0	24

FOOD	PORTION	CALS	PROT	FAT	CARB
Fat Free Tiny Twists	18 pieces (1 oz)	110	3	0	23
Honey Mustard	16 (1 oz)	110	3	1	22
Rods	3 (1 oz)	110	3	1	22
Sharp Cheddar	22 (1 oz)	110	3	1	22
Sour Dough Nuggets	11 (1 oz)	110	2	0	24
Snyder's Of Hanover					
Dips White Fudge	1 oz	130	2	6	19
Hard Sourdough	1 oz	100	3	0	22
Hard Sourdough Unsalted	1 oz	100	3	0	22
Logs	1 oz	110	3	1	21
Mini	1 oz	120	3	0	25
Mini Unsalted	1 oz	110	3	0	25
Nibblers	1 oz	120	3	0	25
Nibblers Honey Mustard & Onions	1 oz	130	3	3	23
Nibblers Oat Bran	1 oz	130	3	3	23
Nibblers Unsalted	1 oz	120	3	0	25
Oat Bran	1 oz	100	3	3	22
Old Fashioned Dipping Stix	1 oz	100	3	0	22
Old Tyme Unsalted	1 oz	120	3	1	24
Olde Tyme	1 oz	120	3	1	24
Olde Tyme Stix	1 oz	120	3	1	23
Pieces Buttermilk Ranch	1 oz	130	3	5	19
Pieces Cheddar Cheese	1 oz	190	2	6	18
Pieces Honey Mustard & Onions	1 oz	140	2	7	18
Pieces Peppered Pizza	1 oz	150	2	8	16
Rods	1 oz	120	4	2	24
Snaps	24 (1 oz)	120	3	1	25
Thin	1 oz	130	3	0	23
Whole Wheat Honey	1 oz	120	3	1	24
Utz					
Country Store Stix	5 (1 oz)	110	3	1	22
Fat Free Hard	1 (0.8 oz)	90	2	0	18
Fat Free Hard No Salt Added	1 (0.8 oz)	90	2	0	19
Fat Free Sour Dough Nuggets	10 (1 oz)	100	2	0	22
Fat Free Stix	14 (1 oz)	100	3	0	23
Fat Free Thin	10 (1 oz)	100	2	0	22
Honey Mustard & Onion	⅓ cup (1 oz)	130	2	6	18
Rods	3 (1 oz)	120	3	1	24
Specials	5 (1 oz)	110	3	1	21
Specials Extra Dark	5 (1 oz)	110	3	1	21
Specials Unsalted	5 (1 oz)	110	3	1	21
Wheels	20 (1 oz)	100	2	0	22
Weight Watchers					
Oat Bran Nuggets	1 pkg (1.5 oz)	170	4	3	33

FOOD	PORTION	CALS	PROT	FAT	CARB
PRUNE JUICE					
canned	1 cup	181	2	tr	45
PRUNES					
canned in heavy syrup	5	90	1	tr	24
canned in heavy syrup	1 cup	245	2	tr	65
dried	10	201	2	tr	53
dried	1 cup	385	4	1	101
dried cooked w/ sugar	½ cup	147	1	tr	39
dried cooked w/o sugar	½ cup	113	1	tr	30
PUDDING					
(*see also* CUSTARD, PUDDING POPS)					
home recipe					
bread pudding	1 recipe 6 serv	1266	40	44	185
chocolate as prep w/ whole milk	½ cup (5.5 oz)	221	5	6	40
corn	⅔ cup	181	7	9	21
cornstarch	½ cup (4.4 oz)	137	5	5	20
rice	½ cup (5.3 oz)	217	6	4	40
mix					
banana as prep w/ 2% milk	½ cup (4.9 oz)	142	4	2	26
banana as prep w/ whole milk	½ cup (4.9 oz)	157	4	4	25
chocolate as prep w/ 2% milk	½ cup (5 oz)	150	5	3	28
chocolate as prep w/ whole milk	½ cup (5 oz)	158	5	5	26
coconut cream as prep w/ 2% milk	½ cup (4.9 oz)	148	4	4	25
coconut cream as prep w/ whole milk	½ cup (4.9 oz)	160	4	4	25
instant banana as prep w/ 2% milk	½ cup (5.2 oz)	152	4	3	29
instant banana as prep w/ whole milk	½ cup (5.2 oz)	167	4	4	27
instant chocolate as prep w/ 2% milk	½ cup (5.2 oz)	149	3	3	28
instant chocolate as prep w/ whole milk	½ cup (5.2 oz)	164	5	5	28
instant coconut cream as prep w/ 2% milk	½ cup (5.2 oz)	157	4	3	28
instant coconut cream as prep w/ whole milk	½ cup (5.2 oz)	172	4	5	28
instant lemon as prep w/ 2% milk	½ cup (5.2 oz)	155	4	4	30
instant lemon as prep w/ whole milk	½ cup (5.2 oz)	169	4	4	30
instant vanilla as prep w/ 2% milk	½ cup (5 oz)	147	2	2	28

FOOD	PORTION	CALS	PROT	FAT	CARB
instant vanilla as prep w/ whole milk	½ cup (5 oz)	181	4	4	28
lemon	½ cup (5.1 oz)	163	1	2	36
rice as prep w/ 2% milk	½ cup (5.1 oz)	161	5	2	30
rice as prep w/ whole milk	½ cup (5.1 oz)	175	5	4	30
tapioca as prep w/ 2% milk	½ cup (5 oz)	147	4	2	28
tapioca as prep w/ whole milk	½ cup (5 oz)	161	4	4	28
vanilla as prep w/ 2% milk	½ cup (4.9 oz)	141	4	2	26
vanilla as prep w/ whole milk	½ cup (4.9 oz)	155	2	4	26
Betty Crocker					
Rice as prep	1 serv	200	1	3	33
Jell-O					
Americana Rice as prep w/ skim milk	½ cup (5.2 oz)	140	5	0	29
Americana Tapioca as prep w/ skim milk	½ cup (5.1 oz)	130	4	0	28
Banana Cream as prep w/ 2% milk	½ cup (5.1 oz)	140	4	3	26
Butterscotch as prep w/ 2% milk	½ cup (5.2 oz)	160	4	3	30
Chocolate as prep w/ 2% milk	½ cup (5.2 oz)	150	5	3	28
Chocolate Fudge as prep w/ 2% milk	½ cup (5.2 oz)	150	5	3	28
Coconut Cream as prep w/ 2% milk	½ cup (5.1 oz)	150	4	5	24
Fat Free Chocolate as prep w/ skim milk	½ cup (5.2 oz)	130	5	0	29
Fat Free Vanilla as prep w/ skim milk	½ cup (5.1 oz)	130	4	0	28
Instant Banana Cream as prep w/ 2% milk	½ cup (5.2 oz)	150	4	3	29
Instant Butterscotch as prep w/ 2% milk	½ cup (5.2 oz)	150	4	3	29
Instant Chocolate as prep w/ 2% milk	½ cup (5.2 oz)	160	4	3	31
Instant Chocolate Fudge as prep w/ 2% milk	½ cup (4.2 oz)	160	5	3	31
Instant Coconut Cream as prep w/ 2% milk	½ cup (4.2 oz)	160	4	5	27
Instant French Vanilla as prep w/ 2% milk	½ cup (4.2 oz)	150	4	3	29
Instant Lemon as prep w/ 2% milk	½ cup (4.2 oz)	150	4	3	29
Instant Pistachio as prep w/ 2% milk	½ cup (4.2 oz)	160	4	3	29
Instant Vanilla as prep w/ 2% milk	½ cup (4.2 oz)	150	4	3	29

FOOD	PORTION	CALS	PROT	FAT	CARB
Instant Fat Free Chocolate as prep w/ skim milk	½ cup (5.3 oz)	140	5	0	31
Instant Fat Free Devil's Food as prep w/ skim milk	½ cup (5.3 oz)	140	5	0	31
Instant Fat Free Sugar Free Banana as prep w/ skim milk	½ cup (4.6 oz)	70	4	0	12
Instant Fat Free Sugar Free Butterscotch as prep w/ skim milk	½ cup (4.6 oz)	70	4	0	12
Instant Fat Free Sugar Free Chocolate Fudge as prep w/ skim milk	½ cup (4.7 oz)	80	5	0	14
Instant Fat Free Sugar Free Chocolate as prep w/ skim milk	½ cup (4.6 oz)	80	5	0	14
Instant Fat Free Sugar Free Vanilla as prep w/ skim milk	½ cup (4.6 oz)	70	4	0	12
Instant Fat Free Sugar Free White Chocolate as prep w/ skim milk	½ cup (4.6 oz)	70	4	0	12
Instant Fat Free Vanilla as prep w/ skim milk	½ cup (5.2 oz)	140	4	0	29
Instant Fat Free White Chocolate as prep w/ skim milk	½ cup (5.2 oz)	140	4	0	29
Milk Chocolate as prep w/ 2% milk	½ cup (5.2 oz)	150	4	3	28
Sugar Free Chocolate as prep w/ 2% milk	½ cup (4.6 oz)	90	5	3	13
Sugar Free Vanilla as prep w/ 2% milk	½ cup (4.5 oz)	80	4	3	11
Vanilla as prep w/ 2% milk	½ cup (5.1 oz)	150	0	3	30
Louisiana Purchase					
Bread	1 serv (1.3 oz)	150	3	3	28
Lundberg					
Elegant Rice Cinnamon Raisin	½ cup (3.9 oz)	70	0	0	16
Elegant Rice Coconut	½ cup (3.9 oz)	70	0	2	13
Elegant Rice Honey Almond	½ cup (3.9 oz)	70	2	1	15
Uncle Ben's					
Rice Pudding Cinnamon & Raisins as prep	½ cup (1.5 oz)	160	2	1	37
ready-to-eat					
banana	1 pkg (5 oz)	180	3	5	30

FOOD	PORTION	CALS	PROT	FAT	CARB
chocolate	1 pkg (5 oz)	189	4	6	32
rice	1 pkg (5 oz)	231	3	11	31
tapioca	1 pkg (5 oz)	169	3	5	28
vanilla	1 pkg (4 oz)	146	3	4	25
Handi-Snacks					
Banana	1 serv (3.5 oz)	120	1	4	22
Butterscotch	1 serv (3.5 oz)	120	1	4	22
Chocolate	1 serv (3.5 oz)	130	2	4	23
Chocolate Fudge	1 serv (3.5 oz)	130	2	4	23
Fat Free Chocolate	1 serv (3.5 oz)	90	2	0	21
Fat Free Vanilla	1 serv (3.5 oz)	90	1	0	21
Tapioca	1 serv (3.5 oz)	120	2	4	21
Vanilla	1 serv (3.5 oz)	120	1	4	21
Healthy Choice					
Low Fat Chocolate Raspberry	½ cup (3.5 oz)	102	3	2	19
Low Fat Chocolate Almond	½ cup (3.5 oz)	109	3	2	21
Low Fat Double Chocolate Fudge	½ cup (3.5 oz)	101	3	1	20
Low Fat French Vanilla	½ cup (3.5 oz)	98	2	1	20
Low Fat Tapioca	½ cup (3.5 oz)	101	2	1	21
Hunt's					
Snack Pack Banana	1 serv (3.5 oz)	119	2	4	18
Snack Pack Butterscotch	1 serv (3.5 oz)	130	2	4	21
Snack Pack Chocolate	1 serv (3.5 oz)	143	2	5	22
Snack Pack Chocolate Fudge	1 serv (3.5 oz)	147	2	5	23
Snack Pack Chocolate Marshmallow	1 serv (3.5 oz)	134	2	5	21
Snack Pack Fat Free Chocolate	1 serv (3.5 oz)	86	2	tr	19
Snack Pack Fat Free Tapioca	1 serv (3.5 oz)	82	2	tr	18
Snack Pack Fat Free Vanilla	1 serv (3.5 oz)	81	2	tr	18
Snack Pack Milk Chocolate Variety	1 serv (3.5 oz)	143	2	5	22
Snack Pack Swirl Chocolate Caramel	1 serv (3.5 oz)	143	2	5	23
Snack Pack Swirl Chocolate Peanut Butter	1 serv (3.5 oz)	146	3	6	21
Snack Pack Swirl Smores	1 serv (3.5 oz)	136	2	5	21
Snack Pack Tapioca	1 serv (3.5 oz)	125	1	4	21
Snack Pack Toppers Chocolate Fudge w/ Rainbow Sprinkles	1 serv (4 oz)	164	2	6	25
Snack Pack Toppers Chocolate w/ Dinosaurs	1 serv (4 oz)	161	2	6	25

FOOD	PORTION	CALS	PROT	FAT	CARB
Snack Pack Toppers Chocolate w/ Fun Chips	1 serv (4 oz)	176	2	6	28
Snack Pack Toppers Vanilla w/ Chocolate Sprinkles	1 serv (4 oz)	164	1	6	26
Snack Pack Vanilla	1 serv (3.5 oz)	135	2	5	21
Imagine					
Banana	1 pkg (4 oz)	150	1	3	30
Butterscotch	1 pkg (4 oz)	150	1	3	31
Chocolate	1 pkg (4 oz)	170	1	3	38
Lemon	1 pkg (4 oz)	150	1	3	33
Jell-O					
Chocolate	1 serv (4 oz)	160	3	5	28
Chocolate Marshmallow	1 serv (4 oz)	160	3	5	27
Chocolate Vanilla Swirls	1 serv (4 oz)	160	3	5	27
Free Chocolate	1 serv (4 oz)	100	3	0	23
Free Chocolate Vanilla Swirl	1 serv (4 oz)	100	3	0	23
Free Devil's Food	1 serv (4 oz)	100	3	0	23
Free Rocky Road	1 serv (4 oz)	100	3	0	23
Free Vanilla	1 serv (4 oz)	100	2	0	23
Tapioca	1 serv (4 oz)	140	2	4	26
Tapioca	1 serv (4 oz)	100	2	0	23
Vanilla	1 serv (4 oz)	160	2	5	25
NutraBalance					
Low Lactose All Flavors	1 serv (4 oz)	225	7	8	31
Swiss Miss					
Butterscotch	1 pkg (4 oz)	156	2	6	24
Chocolate	1 pkg (4 oz)	166	3	6	26
Chocolate Fudge	1 pkg (4 oz)	175	3	6	28
Fat Free Chocolate	1 pkg (4 oz)	98	2	tr	22
Fat Free Chocolate Fudge	1 pkg (4 oz)	101	2	tr	23
Fat Free Tapioca	1 pkg (4 oz)	98	2	tr	22
Fat Free Vanilla	1 pkg (4 oz)	93	2	tr	21
Fat Free Parfait Vanilla Chocolate	1 pkg (4 oz)	96	2	tr	21
Milk Chocolate	1 pkg (4 oz)	166	2	6	26
Parfait Vanilla Chocolate	1 pkg (4 oz)	164	3	6	25
Swirl Chocolate Caramel	1 pkg (4 oz)	169	2	6	26
Swirl Chocolate Vanilla	1 pkg (4 oz)	169	2	6	26
Swirl Chocolate Vanilla Chocolate	1 pkg (4 oz)	169	3	6	26
Tapioca	1 pkg (4 oz)	138	2	4	24
Vanilla	1 pkg (4 oz)	156	2	6	24
take-out					
blancmange	1 serv (4.7 oz)	154	4	5	25
bread pudding	1 serv (6.7 oz)	564	11	18	94
bread pudding	½ cup (4.4 oz)	212	7	7	31

FOOD	PORTION	CALS	PROT	FAT	CARB
bread w/ raisins	½ cup	180	5	5	31
chocolate	½ cup (5.5 oz)	206	5	4	41
queen of puddings	1 serv (4.4 oz)	266	6	10	41
rice pudding	1 serv (3 oz)	110	3	4	17
rice w/ raisins	½ cup	246	7	6	42
tapioca	½ cup (5.3 oz)	189	7	7	26
vanilla	½ cup (4.3 oz)	130	4	4	20
yorkshire	1 serv (3 oz)	177	6	8	22
PUDDING POPS					
chocolate	1 (1.6 oz)	72	2	2	12
vanilla	1 (1.6 oz)	75	2	2	13
PUMMELO					
fresh	1	228	5	tr	59
sections	1 cup	71	1	tr	18
PUMPKIN					
canned					
pumpkin	½ cup	41	1	tr	10
Libby					
Solid Pack	½ cup	40	2	1	9
fresh					
cooked mashed	½ cup	24	1	tr	6
flowers cooked	½ cup	10	1	tr	2
leaves cooked	½ cup	7	1	tr	1
leaves raw	½ cup	4	1	tr	tr
seeds					
dried	1 oz	154	7	13	5
roasted	1 oz	148	9	12	4
roasted	1 cup	1184	75	96	31
salted & roasted	1 oz	148	9	12	4
salted & roasted	1 cup	1184	75	96	31
whole roasted	1 oz	127	5	6	15
whole roasted	1 cup	285	12	12	34
whole salted roasted	1 oz	127	5	6	15
whole salted roasted	1 cup	285	12	12	34
PURSLANE					
cooked	1 cup	21	2	tr	4
raw	1 cup	7	1	tr	1
QUAIL					
breast w/o skin raw	1 (2 oz)	69	13	2	0
w/ skin raw	1 quail (3.8 oz)	210	21	13	0
w/o skin raw	1 quail (3.2 oz)	123	20	4	0
QUICHE					
take-out					
cheese	1 slice (3 oz)	283	11	20	16
lorraine	⅛ of 8 in pie	600	13	48	29
mushroom	1 slice (3 oz)	256	9	18	17
QUINOA					
quinoa not prep	1 cup (6 oz)	636	22	10	117

FOOD	PORTION	CALS	PROT	FAT	CARB
RABBIT					
domestic w/o bone roasted	3 oz	167	25	7	0
wild w/o bone stewed	3 oz	147	28	3	0
RACCOON					
roasted	3 oz	217	25	12	0
RADISHES					
chinese dried	½ cup	157	5	tr	37
chinese raw	1 (12 oz)	62	2	tr	14
daikon dried	½ cup	157	5	tr	37
daikon raw	1 (12 oz)	62	2	tr	14
white icicle raw sliced	½ cup	7	1	tr	1
Eden					
Daikon Dried Shredded	2 tbsp	45	1	0	9
Daikon Pickled	2 slices	5	0	0	1
take-out					
korean kimchee	½ cup	31	2	1	6
moo namul saengche korean salad	1 serv (3.7 oz)	34	1	tr	8
RAISINS					
chocolate coated	1 cup (6.7 oz)	741	8	28	130
golden seedless	1 cup	437	5	1	115
seedless	1 cup	434	5	1	115
sultanas	1 oz	88	1	0	23
Dole					
CinnaRaisins	1 pkg (1 oz)	95	1	0	22
Estee					
Chocolate Covered	¼ cup	180	3	6	27
Mariana					
Fruitn Yogurt Milk Chocolate Covered Raisins	32 pieces (1 oz)	130	1	5	20
Tree Of Life					
Organic	¼ cup (1.4 oz)	130	1	0	31
RASPBERRIES					
canned in heavy syrup	½ cup	117	1	tr	30
fresh	1 cup	61	1	1	14
fresh	1 pint	154	3	2	36
frozen sweetened	1 cup	256	2	tr	65
frozen sweetened	1 pkg (10 oz)	291	2	tr	74
Birds Eye					
Red	5 oz	90	1	0	22
Tree Of Life					
Organic	⅔ cup (5 oz)	50	1	0	12
RASPBERRY JUICE					
Crystal Light					
Raspberry Ice Drink	1 serv (8 oz)	5	0	0	0
Raspberry Ice Drink Mix as prep	1 serv (8 oz)	5	0	0	0

FOOD	PORTION	CALS	PROT	FAT	CARB
Dole					
Country Raspberry	8 fl oz	140	0	0	35
Fresh Samantha					
Raspberry Dream	1 cup (8 oz)	120	2	1	10
Kool-Aid					
Drink Mix as prep	1 serv (8 oz)	60	0	0	17
Raspberry Drink as prep w/ sugar	1 serv (8 oz)	100	0	0	25
Splash Blue Raspberry Drink	1 serv (8 oz)	120	0	0	30
RED BEANS					
canned					
Green Giant					
Red Beans	½ cup (4.5 oz)	100	6	1	19
Hunt's					
Small	½ cup (4.5 oz)	89	6	1	19
Van Camp					
Red Beans	½ cup (4.6 oz)	90	6	0	20
dried					
Hurst					
HamBeens w/ Ham	1 serv	120	8	1	20
mix					
Bean Cuisine					
Pasta & Beans Barcelona Red w/ Radiatore	1 serv	210	7	1	29
RELISH					
hamburger	½ cup	158	1	1	42
hot dog	½ cup	111	2	1	28
Claussen					
Sweet Pickle	1 tbsp (0.5 oz)	15	0	0	3
Green Giant					
Corn	1 tbsp (0.6 oz)	20	0	0	5
Vlasic					
Fancy Sweet	1 tbsp	15	0	0	4
RENNIN					
tablet	1 (0.9 g)	1	0	0	tr
RHUBARB					
fresh	½ cup	13	1	tr	3
RICE					
brown long grain cooked	1 cup (6.8 oz)	216	5	2	45
brown medium grain cooked	1 cup (6.8 oz)	218	5	2	46
glutinous cooked	1 cup (6.1 oz)	169	4	tr	37
white long grain cooked	1 cup (5.5 oz)	205	4	tr	45
white long grain instant cooked	1 cup (5.8 oz)	162	3	tr	35
white medium grain cooked	1 cup (6.5 oz)	242	4	tr	53
white short grain cooked	1 cup (6.5 oz)	242	4	tr	53

FOOD	PORTION	CALS	PROT	FAT	CARB
Birds Eye					
Rice & Broccoli In Cheese Sauce	1 pkg	290	8	9	15
White & Wild w/ Green Beans	1 cup (6.6 oz)	180	4	4	31
Carolina					
Red Beans & Rice as prep	¼ pkg	190	6	1	40
Chun King					
Fried Rice Mix	½ cup (1.4 oz)	126	4	tr	29
Goya					
Arroz Amarillo	¼ cup (1.6 oz)	170	4	0	37
Green Giant					
Rice & Broccoli	1 pkg (10 oz)	320	8	12	44
Rice Medley	1 pkg (10 oz)	240	6	3	46
Rice Pilaf	1 pkg (10 oz)	230	6	3	44
White & Wild	1 pkg (10 oz)	250	6	5	45
La Choy					
Fried Rice	1 cup (4.9 oz)	236	5	1	53
Lipton					
Oriental Stir Fry as prep	1 cup	270	5	8	47
Rice & Sauce Alfredo Broccoli as prep	1 cup	320	9	12	46
Rice & Sauce Beef as prep	1 cup	270	6	8	47
Rice & Sauce Cajun Style as prep	1 cup	270	7	7	46
Rice & Sauce Cajun Style w/ Beans as prep	1 cup	310	10	8	52
Rice & Sauce Cheddar Broccoli as prep	1 cup	280	7	9	46
Rice & Sauce Chicken & Parmesan Risotto as prep	1 cup	270	6	9	43
Rice & Sauce Chicken Broccoli as prep	1 cup	280	7	9	46
Rice & Sauce Chicken Flavor as prep	1 cup	280	7	9	45
Rice & Sauce Creamy Chicken as prep	1 cup	290	6	11	45
Rice & Sauce Herb & Butter as prep	1 cup	280	6	11	43
Rice & Sauce Medley as prep	1 cup	270	7	9	44
Rice & Sauce Mushroom as prep	1 cup	270	6	8	45
Rice & Sauce Mushroom & Herb as prep	1 cup	290	6	8	49
Rice & Sauce Oriental as prep	1 cup	280	7	8	48
Rice & Sauce Pilaf as prep	1 cup	260	6	11	44

FOOD	PORTION	CALS	PROT	FAT	CARB
Rice & Sauce Scampi Style as prep	1 cup	270	6	9	44
Rice & Sauce Spanish as prep	1 cup	270	6	8	47
Rice & Sauce Teriyaki as prep	1 cup	270	5	8	45
Roasted Chicken as prep	1 cup	260	4	8	46
Salsa Style as prep	1 cup	220	4	7	37
Southwestern Chicken Flavor as prep	1 cup	260	5	11	47
Lundberg					
One-Step Curry	1 cup (7.4 oz)	160	5	1	38
Quick Brown Rice Savory Vegetarian Chicken	1 cup (2.5 oz)	260	6	3	53
Risotto Tomato Basil	1 serv	140	4	1	30
Melting Pot					
Risotto Melanese w/ Saffron	1 cup	210	4	0	48
Risotto Primavera	1 cup	200	5	1	44
Risotto Sun-Dried Tomatoes & Peas	1 cup	200	5	1	45
Risotto Three Cheese	1 cup	200	5	2	44
Risotto Wild Mushroom	1 cup	200	5	1	44
Minute					
Boil-In-Bag White as prep	1 cup (5.7 oz)	190	4	0	42
Instant Brown as prep	⅔ cup	170	4	2	34
Instant White as prep	1 cup (5.7 oz)	160	3	0	36
Long Grain & Wild Seasoned w/ Herbs as prep	1 cup (7.8 oz)	230	6	1	50
Success					
Brown & Wild Mix as prep	½ cup	120	3	3	21
TastyBite					
Pilaf Curried Vegetable	½ pkg (4.5 oz)	180	5	6	26
Pilaf Green Peas	½ pkg (4.5 oz)	208	6	4	36
Pilaf Vegetable Kofta	½ pkg (4.5 oz)	229	7	5	39
Van Camp					
Spanish	½ cup (4.5 oz)	90	2	2	19
Zatarain's					
Dirty Rice Mix as prep w/o meat and oil	½ cup	130	3	0	29
Red Beans & Rice as prep w/o oil	½ cup	100	4	0	21
take-out					
nasi goreng indonesian rice & vegetables	1 cup (4.9 oz)	130	4	0	28
paella	1 serv (7 oz)	308	23	16	17
pilaf	½ cup	84	4	3	11
risotto	6.6 oz	426	6	18	65
spanish	¾ cup	363	11	27	19

FOOD	PORTION	CALS	PROT	FAT	CARB
RICE CAKES					
(*see also* POPCORN CAKES)					
brown rice	1 (0.3 oz)	35	1	tr	7
brown rice & buckwheat	1 (0.3 oz)	34	1	tr	7
brown rice & buckwheat unsalted	1 (0.3 oz)	34	1	tr	7
brown rice & corn	1 (0.3 oz)	35	1	tr	7
brown rice & rye	1 (0.3 oz)	35	1	tr	7
brown rice & sesame seed	1 (0.3 oz)	35	1	tr	7
brown rice multigrain	1 (0.3 oz)	35	1	tr	7
brown rice multigrain unsalted	1 (0.3 oz)	35	1	tr	7
brown rice unsalted	1 (0.3 oz)	35	1	tr	7
Estee					
Banana Nut	5	60	1	1	14
Cinnamon Spice	5	60	1	0	14
Granny Smith Apple	5	60	1	0	13
Mixed Berry	5	60	1	0	14
Peanut Butter Crunch	5	60	1	0	13
Lundberg					
Nutra Farmed Brown Rice	1 (0.7 oz)	70	1	0	15
Nutra Farmed Sesame Tamari	1 (0.7 oz)	70	2	1	16
Organic Koku Semsame	1 (0.7 oz)	80	2	0	17
Weight Watchers					
Apple Cinnamon	1 oz	110	2	1	25
Butter	1 oz	110	2	2	21
Caramel	1 oz	110	2	1	24
White Cheddar	1 oz	100	3	1	22
ROCKFISH					
pacific cooked	1 fillet (5.2 oz)	180	36	3	0
pacific cooked	3 oz	103	20	2	0
pacific raw	3 oz	80	16	1	0
ROE					
fish	1 oz	11	2	tr	tr
fresh baked	3 oz	173	24	7	2
fresh baked	1 oz	58	8	2	1
ROLL					
frozen					
New York					
Garlic	1 (2 oz)	210	3	10	26
Sara Lee					
Deluxe Cinnamon Rolls w/o Icing	1 (2.7 oz)	370	5	15	41
home recipe					
dinner as prep w/ 2% milk	1 (2½ in)	111	3	3	19
dinner as prep w/ whole milk	1 (2½ in)	112	3	3	19
raisin & nut	1 (2 oz)	196	4	7	30

FOOD	PORTION	CALS	PROT	FAT	CARB
ready-to-eat					
bialy	1 (2.2 oz)	138	14	0	32
brioche sweet roll	1 (3.5 oz)	410	10	23	41
brown & serve	1 (1 oz)	85	2	2	14
cheese	1 (2.3 oz)	238	5	12	29
cinnamon raisin	1 (2¾ in)	223	4	10	31
dinner	1 (1 oz)	85	2	2	14
egg	1 (2½ in)	107	3	2	18
french	1 (1.3 oz)	105	3	2	19
hamburger	1 (1½ oz)	123	4	2	22
hamburger multi-grain	1 (1½ oz)	113	4	2	19
hamburger reduced calorie	1 (1½ oz)	84	4	1	18
hard	1 (3½ in)	167	6	2	30
hot cross bun	1	202	5	4	38
hotdog	1 (1½ oz)	123	4	2	22
hotdog reduced calorie	1 (1½ oz)	84	4	1	18
hotdog whole wheat	1 (1.5 oz)	110	5	2	19
kaiser	1 (3½ in)	167	6	2	30
oat bran	1 (1.2 oz)	78	3	2	13
rye	1 (1 oz)	81	3	1	15
submarine	1 (4.7 oz)	155	5	2	30
wheat	1 (1 oz)	77	2	2	13
whole wheat	1 (1 oz)	75	3	1	15
Bread Du Jour					
Cracked Wheat	1 (1.2 oz)	100	3	1	17
Italian	1 (1.2 oz)	90	3	1	16
Sourdough	1 (1.2 oz)	90	3	1	17
Freihofer's					
Brown 'N Serve	1 (1 oz)	80	3	2	13
Pepperidge Farm					
Brown & Serve Club	1 (1.6 oz)	120	5	1	22
Dinner Rolls Finger Poppy	1 (0.9 oz)	80	3	2	12
Parker House	1 (0.9 oz)	80	2	2	13
Stroehmann					
Hamburger	1 (1.4 oz)	100	3	2	21
Hamburger Potato	1 (1.9 oz)	140	4	2	28
Hot Dog	1 (1.4 oz)	100	3	2	21
Hot Dog Potato	1 (1.9 oz)	140	4	2	28
Wonder					
Brown & Serve	1 (1 oz)	80	2	2	13
Brown & Serve Sourdough	1 (1 oz)	70	2	2	13
Brown & Serve Wheat	1 (1 oz)	80	2	2	13
Bun	3 (3 oz)	220	7	3	42
Club French	1 (1.6 oz)	120	4	2	23
Club Grain	1 (1.6 oz)	120	4	2	23
Club Sourdough	1 (1.6 oz)	120	4	2	23
Dinner	2 (1.6 oz)	130	4	1	25

FOOD	PORTION	CALS	PROT	FAT	CARB
Dinner Honey Rich	1 (1.3 oz)	100	3	2	17
Dinner Wheat	2 (1.6 oz)	140	3	3	24
Hamburger	1 (2.5 oz)	190	5	3	36
Hamburger	1 (2 oz)	150	4	2	28
Hamburger	1 (2.5 oz)	180	7	3	32
Hamburger	1 (1.5 oz)	110	3	2	21
Hamburger Wheat	1 (1.9 oz)	140	5	2	24
Hamburger Wheat	1 (1.5 oz)	120	4	2	21
Hoagie French	1 (3 oz)	220	7	3	41
Hoagie Grain	1 (3 oz)	220	7	3	41
Hoagie Sourdough	1 (3 oz)	220	8	3	41
Hot Dog	1 (2 oz)	160	4	3	29
Kaiser	1 (2.2 oz)	180	5	3	33
Kaiser Hoagie	1 (3 oz)	220	7	3	41
Multigrain	1 (1.8 oz)	140	4	2	25
Potato Bun	1 (1.5 oz)	110	4	1	22
Steak	1 (2.5 oz)	190	6	3	36
refrigerated					
cinnamon w/ frosting	1	109	2	4	17
crescent	1 (1 oz)	98	2	4	14
Pillsbury					
Apple Cinnamon	1 (1.5 oz)	150	2	6	23
Caramel	1 (1.7 oz)	170	2	7	24
Cinnamon w/ Icing	1 (1.5 oz)	150	2	6	23
Cinnamon w/ Icing Reduced Fat	1 (1.5 oz)	140	2	4	24
Cinnamon Raisin w/ Icing	1 (1.7 oz)	170	2	6	26
Cornbread Twists	1 (1.4 oz)	140	3	6	18
Crecents Reduced Fat	1 (1 oz)	100	2	5	12
Crescent	1 (1 oz)	110	2	6	11
Dinner	1 (1.4 oz)	110	4	2	18
Dinner Wheat	1 (1.4 oz)	110	4	2	18
Orange Sweet Roll w/ Icing	1 (1.7 oz)	150	2	7	25
ROSE APPLE					
fresh	3.5 oz	32	1	tr	7
ROSE HIP					
fresh	1 oz	26	1	0	5
ROSELLE					
fresh	1 cup	28	1	tr	6
ROUGHY					
orange baked	3 oz	75	16	1	0
RUTABAGA					
cooked mashed	½ cup	41	1	tr	9
SABLEFISH					
baked	3 oz	213	15	17	0
fillet baked	5.3 oz	378	26	30	0
smoked	1 oz	72	5	6	0
smoked	3 oz	218	15	17	0

FOOD	PORTION	CALS	PROT	FAT	CARB
SAFFLOWER					
seeds dried	1 oz	147	5	11	10
SALAD					
(see also LETTUCE, PASTA SALAD)					
mix					
Dole					
All American Toss	2 cups (3.5 oz)	50	4	1	7
American Blend	1½ cups (3 oz)	15	1	0	3
Classic	1½ cups (3 oz)	15	1	0	4
Classic Romaine Blend	1½ cups (3 oz)	15	1	0	3
Coleslaw	1½ cups (3 oz)	25	1	0	5
European Special Blend	2 cups (3 oz)	15	1	0	3
Garlic Caesar Complete w/ Dressing	1½ cups (3.5 oz)	180	3	15	8
Greek Marinade	1½ cups (3.5 oz)	100	2	8	5
Greener Selection	1½ cups (3 oz)	15	1	0	3
Light Caesar Complete w/ Dressing	1½ cups (3.5 oz)	60	3	1	10
Light Herb Ranch Complete w/ Dressing	1½ cups (3.5 oz)	50	2	1	10
Light Roasted Garlic Caesar Complete w/ Dressing	1½ cups (3.5 oz)	60	3	1	11
Light Zesty Italian Complete w/ Dressing	1½ cups (3.5 oz)	50	2	1	11
Mediterranean Marinade	2 cups (3.5 oz)	90	1	8	5
Oriental Complete w/ Dressing	1½ cups (3.5 oz)	120	2	6	13
Romano Complete w/ Dressing	1½ cups (3.5 oz)	150	3	12	9
Sunflower Ranch Complete w/ Dressing	1½ cups (3.5 oz)	160	2	16	5
Tomato & Mozzarella Medley	2 cups (3.5 oz)	60	4	2	7
Triple Cheese Toss	2 cups (3.5 oz)	80	5	5	4
Earthbound Farm					
Baby Caesar Mix	1 pkg (5 oz)	25	2	0	3
Baby Greens w/ Low Fat Honey Dijon Vinaigrette & Tomato Croutons	1 serv (3.5 oz)	90	3	3	15
Caesar w/ Garlic Croutons	1 serv (3.5 oz)	170	3	15	7
Italian Salad Organic	1⅔ cups (2.9 oz)	15	1	0	3
Mixed Baby Greens Organic	1 pkg (4 oz)	30	3	0	4
Organic Baby Greens w/ Vinaigrette & Garlic Croutons	1 serv (3.5 oz)	230	3	20	11
Organic Baby Spinach w/ Sesame Soy Vinaigrette & Peanuts	1 serv (3.5 oz)	150	5	11	8

FOOD	PORTION	CALS	PROT	FAT	CARB
Organic Italian Salad w/ Blue Cheese Dressing & Walnuts	1 serv (3.5 oz)	190	4	17	4
Romaine Blend Organic	1⅔ cups (2.9 oz)	15	1	0	3
Fresh Express					
Fancy Field Greens	1½ cups (3 oz)	15	1	0	3
Original Iceberg Garden w/ Zip	1½ cups (3 oz)	15	1	0	3
Veggie Lover's	1½ cups (3 oz)	20	1	0	4
Suddenly Salad					
Caesar	¾ cup	220	5	9	30
Caesar Low Fat Recipe	¾ cup	170	5	3	30
Italian Pepperoni	1 cup	190	6	4	35
Italian Pepperoni Low Fat Recipe	1 cup	180	6	2	35
Ranch & Bacon	¾ cup	330	7	20	30
Ranch & Bacon Low Fat Recipe	¾ cup	180	7	2	30
Weight Watchers					
Caesar Salad	1 serv (3.5 oz)	60	2	0	11
Caesar Salad w/ Cookies	1 pkg (4.3 oz)	160	4	3	29
European Salad	1 serv (3.5 oz)	60	2	0	13
European Salad w/ Cookies	1 pkg (4.3 oz)	160	3	3	31
Garden Salad	1 serv (3.5 oz)	60	2	0	12
Garden Salad w/ Cookies	1 pkg (4 oz)	120	3	2	24
take-out					
caesar	2 cups (5 oz)	235	5	20	11
chef w/o dressing	1½ cups	386	24	28	9
tossed w/o dressing	¾ cup	16	1	0	3
tossed w/o dressing	1½ cups	32	3	tr	7
tossed w/o dressing w/ cheese & egg	1½ cups	102	9	6	5
tossed w/o dressing w/ chicken	1½ cups	105	17	2	4
tossed w/o dressing w/ pasta & seafood	1½ cups (14.6 oz)	380	16	21	32
tossed w/o dressing w/ shrimp	1½ cups	107	15	2	7
waldorf	½ cup	79	1	6	6
SALAD DRESSING					
home recipe					
french	1 tbsp	88	0	10	1
vinegar & oil	1 tbsp	72	0	8	tr
mix					
Et Tu					
Caesar Salad Kit	1 serv	140	2	12	6
Good Seasons					
Cheese Garlic as prep	2 tbsp (1 oz)	140	0	16	1

FOOD	PORTION	CALS	PROT	FAT	CARB
Fat Free Honey Mustard as prep	2 tbsp (1.2 oz)	20	0	0	5
Fat Free Italian as prep	2 tbsp (1.1 oz)	10	0	0	2
Fat Free Ranch as prep	2 tbsp (1.2 oz)	20	0	0	5
Fat Free Zesty Herb as prep	2 tbsp (1.1 oz)	10	0	0	2
Garlic & Herbs as prep	2 tbsp (1 oz)	140	0	15	1
Gourmet Caesar as prep	2 tbsp (1.1 oz)	150	0	16	3
Gourmet Parmesan Italian as prep	2 tbsp (1.1 oz)	150	0	16	2
Honey French as prep	2 tbsp (1.2 oz)	160	0	15	5
Honey Mustard as prep	2 tbsp (1.1 oz)	150	0	15	3
Italian as prep	2 tbsp (1 oz)	140	0	15	1
Mexican Spice as prep	2 tbsp (1.1 oz)	140	0	15	2
Mild Italian as prep	2 tbsp (1.1 oz)	150	0	15	2
Oriental Sesame as prep	2 tbsp (1.1 oz)	150	0	16	3
Reduced Calorie Italian as prep	2 tbsp (1 oz)	50	0	5	2
Reduced Calorie Zesty Italian as prep	2 tbsp (1 oz)	50	0	5	2
Roasted Garlic as prep	2 tbsp (1.1 oz)	150	0	15	2
Zesty Italian as prep	2 tbsp (1 oz)	140	0	15	1
McCormick					
Pasta Salad Vinagarette	1 tsp (5 g)	15	0	0	2
ready-to-eat					
blue cheese	1 tbsp	77	1	8	1
french reduced calorie	1 tbsp	22	0	1	4
sesame seed	1 tbsp	68	1	7	1
Benecol					
Creamy Italian	2 tbsp	100	0	10	10
French	2 tbsp (0.8 oz)	130	0	11	6
Ranch	2 tbsp	130	0	13	3
Thousand Island	2 tbsp	130	0	12	5
Estee					
Creamy French	2 tbsp (1 oz)	10	0	0	2
Italian	2 tbsp	5	0	0	1
Hellmann's					
Citrus Splash Ruby Red Ginger	2 tbsp (1 oz)	90	0	7	8
Kraft					
⅓ Less Fat Catalina	2 tbsp (1.2 oz)	80	0	5	9
⅓ Less Fat Cucumber Ranch	2 tbsp (1.1 oz)	60	0	5	2
⅓ Less Fat Italian	2 tbsp (1.1 oz)	70	0	7	3
⅓ Less Fat Ranch	2 tbsp (1.1 oz)	110	0	11	1
⅓ Less Fat Thousand Island	2 tbsp (1.2 oz)	70	0	5	7
Buttermilk Ranch	2 tbsp (1.1 oz)	150	0	16	1
Caesar Ranch	2 tbsp (1.1 oz)	110	1	11	1

FOOD	PORTION	CALS	PROT	FAT	CARB
Catalina	2 tbsp (1.1 oz)	120	0	10	7
Catalina w/ Honey	2 tbsp (1.1 oz)	130	0	11	7
Classic Caesar	2 tbsp (1.1 oz)	110	1	11	1
Coleslaw	2 tbsp (1.1 oz)	130	0	11	7
Creamy French	2 tbsp (1.1 oz)	160	0	15	5
Creamy Garlic	2 tbsp (1.1 oz)	110	0	11	2
Creamy Italian	2 tbsp (1.1 oz)	110	0	11	2
Cucumber Ranch	2 tbsp (1.1 oz)	140	0	15	2
Free Blue Cheese	2 tbsp (1.2 oz)	45	0	0	11
Free Catalina	2 tbsp (1.2 oz)	35	0	0	8
Free Creamy Italian	2 tbsp (1.2 oz)	50	0	0	12
Free French	2 tbsp (1.2 oz)	45	0	0	11
Free Garlic Ranch	2 tbsp (1.2 oz)	45	0	0	11
Free Honey Dijon	2 tbsp (1.2 oz)	45	0	0	10
Free Italian	2 tbsp (1.2 oz)	20	0	0	4
Free Peppercorn Ranch	2 tbsp (1.2 oz)	45	0	0	11
Free Ranch	1 tbsp (1.2 oz)	50	0	0	11
Free Red Wine Vinegar	2 tbsp (1.1 oz)	15	0	0	3
Free Thousand Island	2 tbsp (1.2 oz)	40	0	0	9
Garlic Ranch	2 tbsp (1.1 oz)	180	0	19	1
Herb Vinaigrette	2 tbsp (1.1 oz)	140	0	15	tr
Honey Dijon	2 tbsp (1.1 oz)	110	0	10	6
Honey Mustard	2 tbsp (1.1 oz)	110	0	10	6
House Italian w/ Olive Oil Blend	2 tbsp (1.1 oz)	120	0	12	2
Pesto Italian	2 tbsp (1.1 oz)	90	0	9	2
Ranch	2 tbsp (1 oz)	170	0	18	1
Russian	2 tbsp (1.2 oz)	130	0	10	10
Sour Cream & Onion Ranch	2 tbsp (1 oz)	170	0	18	1
Thousand Island	2 tbsp (1.1 oz)	110	0	10	5
Thousand Island w/ Bacon	2 tbsp (1.1 oz)	130	0	12	5
Tomato & Herb Italian	2 tbsp (1.1 oz)	100	0	9	3
Zesty Italian	2 tbsp (1.1 oz)	110	0	11	2
LaMartinique					
Blue Cheese Vinaigrette	2 tbsp	160	2	17	0
Poppy Seed	2 tbsp	170	0	15	8
Nasoya					
Creamy Dill	2 tbsp	70	0	7	2
Creamy Italian	2 tbsp	60	0	6	2
Garden Herb	2 tbsp	70	0	7	2
Sesame Garlic	2 tbsp	60	0	6	2
Thousand Island	2 tbsp	70	0	6	3
Newman's Own					
Balsamic Vinaigrette	2 tbsp (1.1 oz)	90	0	9	3
Caesar	2 tbsp (1.1 oz)	150	1	16	1

FOOD	PORTION	CALS	PROT	FAT	CARB
Light Italian	2 tbsp (1.1 oz)	20	0	1	3
Olive Oil & Vinegar	2 tbsp (1 oz)	150	0	16	1
Ranch	2 tbsp (1 oz)	180	1	19	2
Old Dutch					
Sweet & Sour	2 tbsp	50	0	0	13
Seven Seas					
⅓ Less Fat Creamy Italian	2 tbsp (1.1 oz)	60	0	5	2
⅓ Less Fat Italian w/ Olive Oil Blend	2 tbsp (1.1 oz)	45	0	4	2
⅓ Less Fat Ranch	2 tbsp (1.1 oz)	100	0	9	5
⅓ Less Fat Red Wine Vinegar & Oil	2 tbsp (1.1 oz)	45	0	4	3
⅓ Less Fat Viva Italian	2 tbsp (1.1 oz)	45	0	4	2
2 Cheese Italian	2 tbsp (1.1 oz)	70	0	7	3
Creamy Italian	2 tbsp (1.1 oz)	120	0	12	1
Free Ranch	2 tbsp (1.2 oz)	45	0	0	11
Free Red Wine Vinegar	2 tbsp (1.1 oz)	15	0	0	3
Free Sour Cream & Onion Ranch	2 tbsp (1.2 oz)	50	0	0	11
Free Viva Italian	2 tbsp (1.1 oz)	10	0	0	2
Green Goddess	2 tbsp (1.1 oz)	130	0	13	1
Herbs & Spices	2 tbsp (1.1 oz)	90	0	9	1
Ranch	2 tbsp (1.1 oz)	160	0	17	2
Red Wine Vinegar & Oil	2 tbsp (1.1 oz)	90	0	9	2
Viva Italian	2 tbsp (1.1 oz)	90	0	9	2
Viva Russian	2 tbsp (1.1 oz)	150	0	16	3
Weight Watchers					
Fat Free Caesar	1 pkg (0.75 oz)	5	0	0	1
Fat Free Caesar	2 tbsp	10	0	0	1
Fat Free Creamy Italian	2 tbsp	30	0	0	7
Fat Free French Style	2 tbsp	40	0	0	9
Fat Free Honey Dijon	2 tbsp	45	0	0	11
Fat Free Italian	2 tbsp	10	0	0	2
Fat Free Ranch	1 pkg (0.75 oz)	25	0	0	6
Fat Free Ranch	2 tbsp	35	0	0	7
Wishbone					
Caesar	2 tbsp (1 oz)	90	1	10	2
Chunky Blue Cheese	2 tbsp (1 oz)	150	1	17	3
Classic House Italian	2 tbsp (1 oz)	140	0	14	2
Classic Olive Oil Italian	2 tbsp (1 oz)	60	0	5	4
Creamy Caesar	2 tbsp (1 oz)	180	1	18	1
Creamy Italian	2 tbsp (1 oz)	110	1	10	4
Creamy Roasted Garlic	2 tbsp (1 oz)	110	1	10	3
Deluxe French	2 tbsp (1 oz)	120	0	11	5
Fat Free Chunky Blue Cheese	2 tbsp (1 oz)	35	0	0	7
Fat Free Creamy Italian	2 tbsp (1 oz)	35	0	0	9

FOOD	PORTION	CALS	PROT	FAT	CARB
Fat Free Creamy Roasted Garlic	2 tbsp (1 oz)	40	0	0	9
Fat Free Deluxe French	2 tbsp (1 oz)	30	0	0	7
Fat Free Honey Dijon	2 tbsp (1 oz)	45	1	0	10
Fat Free Italian	2 tbsp (1 oz)	10	0	0	2
Fat Free Parmesan & Onion	2 tbsp (1 oz)	45	1	0	9
Fat Free Ranch	2 tbsp (1 oz)	40	0	0	9
Fat Free Red Wine Vinaigrette	2 tbsp (1 oz)	35	0	0	7
Fat Free Sweet N' Spicy French	2 tbsp (1 oz)	30	0	0	7
Fat Free Thousand Island	2 tbsp (1 oz)	35	0	0	9
Italian	2 tbsp (1 oz)	80	0	8	3
Lite French	2 tbsp (1 oz)	50	0	2	8
Lite Italian	2 tbsp (1 oz)	15	0	1	2
Lite Ranch	2 tbsp (1 oz)	100	0	8	5
Olive Oil Vinaigrette	2 tbsp (1 oz)	60	0	5	4
Oriental	2 tbsp (1 oz)	70	0	5	5
Parmesan & Onion	2 tbsp (1 oz)	110	1	10	5
Ranch	2 tbsp (1 oz)	160	0	17	1
Red Wine Vinaigrette	2 tbsp (1 oz)	80	0	5	9
Robusto Italian	2 tbsp (1 oz)	90	0	8	4
Russian	2 tbsp (1 oz)	110	0	6	15
Sweet N' Spicy French	2 tbsp (1 oz)	140	0	12	6
SALMON					
canned					
chum w/ bone	1 can (13.9 oz)	521	79	20	0
chum w/ bone	3 oz	120	18	5	0
pink w/ bone	3 oz	118	17	5	0
pink w/ bone	1 can (15.9 oz)	631	90	27	0
sockeye w/ bone	1 can (12.9 oz)	566	76	27	0
sockeye w/ bone	3 oz	130	17	6	0
Bumble Bee					
Keta	½ cup (3.5 oz)	160	20	8	0
Red	½ cup (3.5 oz)	180	20	10	0
fresh					
atlantic baked	3 oz	155	22	7	0
chinook baked	3 oz	196	22	11	0
chum baked	3 oz	131	22	4	0
coho cooked	½ fillet (5.4 oz)	286	42	12	0
coho cooked	3 oz	157	23	6	0
coho raw	3 oz	124	18	5	0
pink baked	3 oz	127	22	4	0
roe raw	1 oz	59	7	3	tr
sockeye cooked	3 oz	183	23	9	0
sockeye cooked	½ fillet (5.4 oz)	334	42	17	0
sockeye raw	3 oz	143	18	7	0

FOOD	PORTION	CALS	PROT	FAT	CARB
smoked					
chinook	3 oz	99	16	4	0
chinook	1 oz	33	5	1	0
Lascco					
Nova Sliced	2 oz	60	10	1	3
take-out					
roulette w/ spinach stuffing	1 serv (4 oz)	160	13	6	10
salmon cake	1 (3 oz)	241	18	15	6
SALSA					
black bean & corn	2 tbsp (1 oz)	15	1	0	3
citrus	2 tbsp (1 oz)	10	0	0	2
Chi-Chi's					
Con Queso	2 tbsp (1.1 oz)	90	3	7	4
Hot	2 tbsp (1 oz)	10	0	0	2
Medium	2 tbsp (1 oz)	10	0	0	2
Mild	2 tbsp (1 oz)	10	0	0	1
Picante Hot	2 tbsp (1 oz)	10	0	0	2
Picante Medium	2 tbsp (1 oz)	10	0	0	2
Picante Mild	2 tbsp (1 oz)	10	0	0	2
Verde Medium	2 tbsp (1.2 oz)	15	0	0	3
Verde Mild	2 tbsp (1.2 oz)	15	0	0	3
Guiltless Gourmet					
Roasted Red Pepper	2 tbsp (1 oz)	10	0	0	2
Southwestern Grill	2 tbsp (1 oz)	10	0	0	2
Hunt's					
Hot	2 tbsp (1.1 oz)	27	1	tr	6
Medium	2 tbsp (1.1 oz)	27	1	tr	6
Mild	2 tbsp (1.1 oz)	27	1	tr	6
Picante All Varieties	2 tbsp (1.1 oz)	11	1	tr	2
Squeeze Mild & Medium	2 tbsp (1.1 oz)	27	1	tr	6
Muir Glen					
Black Bean & Corn Medium	2 tbsp (1.1 oz)	15	1	0	3
Chipotle Medium	2 tbsp (1.1 oz)	10	0	0	2
Fire Roasted Tomato Medium	2 tbsp (1.1 oz)	10	0	0	2
Garlic Cilantro Medium	2 tbsp (1.1 oz)	10	0	0	2
Habanero Hot	2 tbsp (1.1 oz)	10	0	0	2
Organic Medium	2 tbsp (1.1 oz)	10	0	0	2
Organic Mild	2 tbsp (1.1 oz)	10	0	0	2
Roasted Garlic Medium	2 tbsp (1.1 oz)	10	0	0	2
Newman's Own					
Bandito Hot	2 tbsp (1.1 oz)	10	0	0	2
Bandito Medium	2 tbsp (1.1 oz)	10	0	0	2
Bandito Mild	2 tbsp (1.1 oz)	10	0	0	2
Peach	2 tbsp (1.1 oz)	25	0	0	6
Pineapple	2 tbsp (1.1 oz)	15	0	0	3
Roasted Garlic	2 tbsp (1.1 oz)	10	1	0	2

FOOD	PORTION	CALS	PROT	FAT	CARB
Pace					
Picante Mild or Medium	2 tbsp	10	0	0	2
Thick & Chunky Mild or Medium	2 tbsp	10	0	0	2
Rosarita					
Traditional Mild	2 tbsp (1 oz)	7	1	tr	1
Snyder's Of Hanover					
Mild	2 tbsp	10	0	0	2
Taco Bell					
Smooth 'N Zesty Picante Medium	2 tbsp (1.1 oz)	15	0	0	3
Smooth 'N Zesty Picante Mild	2 tbsp (1.1 oz)	15	0	0	3
Thick 'N Chunky Salsa Hot	2 tbsp (1.1 oz)	15	0	0	2
Thick 'N Chunky Salsa Medium	2 tbsp (1.1 oz)	15	0	0	2
Tostitos					
Con Queso	2.3 oz	80	2	5	10
Hot	2.3 oz	30	2	0	6
Low Fat Con Queso	2.5 oz	80	2	3	8
Medium	2.3 oz	30	2	0	6
Mild	2.3 oz	30	2	0	6
Restaurant Style	2.2 oz	30	<2	0	6
Ultimate Garden	2.4 oz	30	2	0	6
Tree Of Life					
Medium	2 tbsp (1 oz)	10	0	0	2
Mild	2 tbsp (1 oz)	10	0	0	2
Utz					
Chunky	2 tbsp (1 fl oz)	60	2	0	14
SALSIFY					
fresh sliced cooked	½ cup	46	2	tr	10
raw sliced	½ cup	55	2	tr	12
SALT SUBSTITUTES					
Eden					
Shiso Leaf Powder	1 tsp	0	0	0	0
Estee					
Salt-It	¼ tsp	0	0	0	0
Halsosalt					
All Flavors	¼ tsp (7 g)	1	0	0	0
Morton					
Salt Substitute	¼ tsp (1.2 g)	tr	0	0	tr
NoSalt					
Salt Alternative	1 pkg (0.75 g)	0	2	0	0
SALT/SEASONED SALT					
salt	1 tbsp (18 g)	0	0	0	0
salt	1 tsp (6 g)	0	0	0	0

FOOD	PORTION	CALS	PROT	FAT	CARB
Eden					
Atlantic Sea Salt	¼ tsp	0	0	0	0
Brittany Sea Salt	¼ tsp	0	0	0	0
Morton					
Lite	¼ tsp (1.4 g)	tr	0	0	tr
SANDWICHES					
Healthy Choice					
Bread Stuffs Chicken & Broccoli	1 (6.1 oz)	310	17	4	50
Bread Stuffs Ham & Cheese w/ Broccoli	1 (6.1 oz)	320	21	5	46
Bread Stuffs Italian Style Meatball	1 (6.1 oz)	330	16	5	52
Bread Stuffs Philly Beef Steak	1 (6.1 oz)	310	17	5	50
Smucker's					
Uncrustables Grape	1 (2 oz)	200	7	8	27
take-out					
chicken fillet plain	1	515	24	29	39
chicken fillet w/ cheese lettuce mayonnaise & tomato	1	632	29	39	42
croque monsieur	1 (12.4 oz)	765	41	46	43
fish fillet w/ tartar sauce	1	431	17	55	41
fish fillet w/ tartar sauce & cheese	1	524	21	29	48
fried egg w/ cheese	1	340	16	19	26
fried egg w/ cheese & ham	1	348	19	16	31
ham w/ cheese	1	353	21	15	33
roast beef submarine sandwich w/ tomato lettuce & mayonnaise	1	411	29	13	44
roast beef w/ cheese	1	402	32	18	27
roast beef plain	1	346	22	14	33
steak w/ tomato lettuce salt & mayonnaise	1	459	30	14	52
submarine w/ salami ham cheese lettuce tomato onion & oil	1	456	22	19	51
tuna salad submarine sandwich w/ lettuce & oil	1	584	30	28	55
SAPODILLA					
fresh	1	140	1	2	34
fresh cut up	1 cup	199	1	3	48
SAPOTES					
fresh	1	301	5	1	76

FOOD	PORTION	CALS	PROT	FAT	CARB
SARDINES					
canned					
atlantic in oil w/ bone	2	50	6	3	0
atlantic in oil w/ bone	1 can (3.2 oz)	192	23	11	0
pacific in tomato sauce w/ bone	1 can (13 oz)	658	61	44	0
pacific in tomato sauce w/ bone	1	68	6	5	0
Bumble Bee					
In Hot Sauce	½ can (2 oz)	109	9	8	tr
In Mustard	½ can (2 oz)	88	10	5	1
In Oil	½ can (2 oz)	125	15	7	0
In Water	½ can (2 oz)	83	15	3	0
SAUCE					
(*see also* BARBECUE SAUCE, GRAVY, PIZZA SAUCE, SALSA, SPAGHETTI SAUCE, TOMATO)					
jarred					
fish sauce chinese	1 tbsp	9	2	0	tr
fish sauce vietnamese nuoc mam	1 tbsp	6	1	0	1
hoisin	1 tbsp	35	1	1	7
teriyaki	1 oz	30	2	0	6
teriyaki	1 tbsp	15	1	0	3
Armour					
Chili Hot Dog	¼ cup (2.2 oz)	120	4	9	5
Meatless Sloppy Joe Sauce	¼ cup (2.2 oz)	30	0	0	7
Boar's Head					
Ham Glaze Brown Sugar & Spice	2 tbsp (1.4 oz)	120	0	0	30
Cheez Whiz					
Cheese	2 tbsp (1.2 oz)	90	4	7	3
Cheese Jalapeno Pepper	2 tbsp (1.2 oz)	90	4	7	3
Cheese Mild Salsa	2 tbsp (1.2 oz)	100	4	7	3
Chi-Chi's					
Enchilada	¼ cup (2.1 oz)	30	0	2	3
Taco	1 tbsp (0.5 oz)	10	0	0	1
Chun King					
Teriyaki	1 tbsp (0.6 oz)	17	1	tr	3
Teriyaki Hot	1 tbsp (0.6 oz)	17	2	tr	3
Del Monte					
Seafood Cocktail	¼ cup (2.7 oz)	100	1	0	24
Sloppy Joe Hickory Flavor	¼ cup (2.4 oz)	70	1	0	18
Sloppy Joe Original	¼ cup (2.4 oz)	70	1	0	16
Fritos					
Texas-Style Chili Hearty Topping	2.3 oz	50	2	2	8
Utimate Taco Hearty Topping	2.3 oz	50	2	2	8

FOOD	PORTION	CALS	PROT	FAT	CARB
Gebhardt					
Enchilada Sauce	¼ cup (2.2 oz)	35	1	2	4
Hot Dog Chili Sauce	¼ cup (2.2 oz)	60	3	3	6
Green Giant					
Sloppy Joe	¼ cup (2.6 oz)	50	2	0	11
Sloppy Joe as prep w/ meat	1 serv (4.4 oz)	200	14	11	11
Hormel					
Not-So-Sloppy-Joe Sauce	¼ cup (2.2 oz)	70	1	0	15
House Of Tsang					
Bangkok Padang	1 tbsp (0.6 oz)	45	1	3	4
Hoisin	1 tsp (6 g)	15	0	0	4
Mandarin Marinade	1 tbsp (0.6 oz)	25	0	0	6
Saigon Sizzle	1 tbsp (0.6 oz)	40	0	1	8
Spicy Brown Bean	1 tsp (6 g)	15	0	0	3
Stir Fry Classic	1 tbsp (0.6 oz)	25	0	1	4
Stir Fry Sweet & Sour	1 tbsp (0.6 oz)	30	0	0	7
Stir Fry Szechuan Spicy	1 tbsp (0.6 oz)	20	0	1	4
Sweet & Sour Concentrate	1 tsp (6 g)	10	0	0	3
Teriyaki Korean	1 tbsp (0.6 oz)	30	0	1	6
Hunt's					
Light w/ Mushrooms	½ cup (4.4 oz)	42	2	tr	8
Just Rite					
Hot Dog	¼ cup (2.2 oz)	50	2	3	5
Kraft					
Cocktail	¼ cup (2.3 oz)	60	1	1	13
Fat Free Tartar Sauce	2 tbsp (1.1 oz)	25	0	0	5
Lemon & Herb Tartar Sauce	2 tbsp (1 oz)	150	0	16	tr
Reduced Fat Sandwich Spread	1 tbsp (0.5 oz)	35	0	3	3
Sandwich Spread	1 tbsp (0.5 oz)	50	0	4	3
Sweet'n Sour	2 tbsp (1.2 oz)	60	0	0	14
Tartar	2 tbsp (1.1 oz)	90	0	9	4
La Choy					
Teriyaki	1 tbsp (0.6 oz)	17	1	tr	3
Lea & Perrins					
Worcestershire	1 tsp	5	0	0	1
Manwich					
BBQ Sloppy Joe	¼ cup (2.2 oz)	57	1	tr	14
Bold	¼ cup (2.2 oz)	62	1	1	13
Mexican	¼ cup (2.2 oz)	27	1	tr.	5
Original	¼ cup (2.2 oz)	32	1	tr	6
Taco Season	¼ cup (2.2 oz)	27	1	tr	6
Thick & Chunky	¼ cup (2.3 oz)	44	1	tr	9
McCormick					
Flavor Medleys Garlic & Herb	2 tbsp	50	0	5	5

FOOD	PORTION	CALS	PROT	FAT	CARB
Flavor Medleys Italian Herb	2 tbsp	50	0	4	4
Flavor Medleys Lemon Pepper	2 tbsp	50	0	4	4
Flavor Medleys Tomato & Basil	2 tbsp	50	0	3	4
Newman's Own					
Spicy Simmer Sauce Diavolo	½ cup (4.4 oz)	70	0	3	10
Open Range					
Hot Dog Chili	¼ cup (2.2 oz)	61	3	3	6
Pace					
Enchilada Sauce	¼ cup	36	0	0	6
Taco Sauce	¼ cup	32	0	2	4
Progresso					
Alfredo	½ cup (4.4 oz)	200	8	15	7
Sauce Arturo					
Original	¼ cup (2.2 fl oz)	50	1	1	8
Tabasco					
Caribbean Steak Sauce	1 tbsp (0.6 oz)	15	0	0	4
Garlic Basting Sauce	1 tbsp (0.6 oz)	20	0	0	4
Habanero Sauce	1 tsp (0.2 oz)	5	0	0	1
Hot Sauce w/ Garlic	1 tsp (0.2 oz)	0	0	0	0
New Orleans Steak Sauce	1 tbsp (0.6 oz)	15	0	0	4
Pepper Sauce	1 tsp (0.2 oz)	0	0	0	0
Taco Bell					
Taco Sauce Medium	2 tbsp (1.1 oz)	15	0	0	3
Taco Sauce Mild	2 tbsp (1.1 oz)	15	0	0	3
The Restaurant Hot Sauce	1 tsp (5 g)	0	0	0	0
Tostitos					
Beef Fiesta Nacho	2.4 oz	120	4	8	6
Chicken Quesadilla Topping	2.5 oz	90	4	6	6
mix					
cheese as prep w/ milk	1 cup	307	16	17	23
curry as prep w/ milk	1 cup	270	11	15	26
mushroom as prep w/ milk	1 cup	228	11	10	24
sourcream as prep w/ milk	1 cup	509	19	30	45
stroganoff as prep	1 cup	271	12	11	34
sweet & sour as prep	1 cup	294	1	tr	73
teriyaki as prep	1 cup	131	4	1	28
white as prep w/ milk	1 cup	241	10	13	21
Durkee					
A La King as prep	1 cup	60	1	4	8
Cheese as prep	¼ cup	25	1	2	4
Hollandaise as prep	2 tbsp	10	0	0	2
White as prep	¼ cup	20	0	1	5

FOOD	PORTION	CALS	PROT	FAT	CARB
French's					
Cheese as prep	¼ cup	25	1	1	4
Hollandaise as prep	2 tbsp	10	0	0	2
McCormick					
Bernaise Blend	1 tsp (3 g)	10	0	0	1
Grill Mates Mesquite Marinade as prep	1 tbsp	15	0	0	2
Grill Mates Southwest Marinade	2 tsp (5 g)	15	0	0	2
Hollandaise Blend	2 tsp (4 g)	15	0	0	1
Meat Marinade	1 tsp (4 g)	15	0	0	2
Pepper Medley Blend as prep	¼ cup	30	1	2	3
shelf-stable					
Cheez Whiz					
Cheese Sqeezable	2 tbsp (1.2 oz)	100	2	8	4
take-out					
bearnaise	1 oz	177	1	19	1
SAUERKRAUT					
canned	½ cup	22	1	tr	5
B&G					
Sauerkraut	2 tbsp (1 oz)	6	0	0	1
Boar's Head					
Sauerkraut	2 tbsp (1 oz)	5	0	0	1
Claussen					
Sauerkraut	¼ cup (1.1 oz)	5	0	0	1
Del Monte					
Bavarian Style	2 tbsp (1 oz)	15	0	0	4
Sauerkraut	2 tbsp (1 oz)	0	0	0	1
Eden					
Organic	½ cup	25	2	0	4
S&W					
Canned	2 tbsp (1 oz)	5	0	0	1
Red Cabbage	2 tbsp (1 oz)	15	0	0	3
SAUSAGE					
bierschinken	3.5 oz	174	18	11	tr
bierwurst	3.5 oz	258	16	21	0
blutwurst uncooked	3.5 oz	424	13	39	0
bockwurst	3.5 oz	276	12	25	0
bockwurst pork & veal raw	1 link (2.3 oz)	200	9	18	tr
bratwurst pork cooked	1 link (3 oz)	256	12	22	2
brotwurst pork	1 oz	92	4	8	1
brotwurst pork & beef	1 link (2.5 oz)	226	10	19	2
chipolata	3.5 oz	342	14	32	1
chorizo	3.5 oz	499	20	45	4
country-style pork cooked	1 patty (1 oz)	100	5	8	tr
country-style pork cooked	1 link (½ oz)	48	3	4	tr

FOOD	PORTION	CALS	PROT	FAT	CARB
fleischwurst	3.5 oz	305	12	29	0
gelbwurst uncooked	3.5 oz	363	12	33	0
italian pork cooked	1 (3 oz)	268	17	21	1
italian pork cooked	1 (2.4 oz)	216	13	17	1
jagdwurst	3.5 oz	211	16	16	0
kielbasa pork	1 oz	88	8	8	1
knockwurst pork & beef	1 (2.4 oz)	209	8	19	1
knockwurst pork & beef	1 oz	87	3	8	1
mettwurst uncooked	3.5 oz	483	13	45	0
plockwurst uncooked	3.5 oz	312	19	45	0
polish pork	1 (8 oz)	739	32	65	4
polish pork	1 oz	92	4	8	tr
pork & beef cooked	1 link (½ oz)	52	2	5	tr
pork & beef cooked	1 patty (1 oz)	107	4	10	1
pork cooked	1 link (½ oz)	48	3	4	tr
pork cooked	1 patty (1 oz)	100	5	8	tr
regensburger uncooked	3.5 oz	354	13	31	0
smoked pork	1 link (2.4 oz)	265	15	22	1
smoked pork	1 sm link (½ oz)	62	4	5	tr
smoked pork & beef	1 link (2.4 oz)	229	9	21	1
smoked pork & beef	1 sm link (½ oz)	54	2	5	tr
vienna canned	1 (½ oz)	45	2	4	tr
vienna canned	7 (4 oz)	315	12	28	2
weisswurst uncooked	3.5 oz	305	11	27	0
zungenwurst (tongue)	3.5 oz	285	17	24	0
Armour					
Vienna Sausage 25% Less Fat	3 (1.9 oz)	130	6	11	1
Vienna Sausage 50% Less Fat	3 (1.9 oz)	90	5	7	1
Vienna Sausage Chicken & Beef	3 (1.9 oz)	120	6	10	1
Vienna Sausage Hot'n Spicy	3 (2.1 oz)	150	5	13	2
Vienna Sausage In BBQ Sauce	3 (2.1 oz)	150	5	13	3
Vienna Sausage In Beef Stock	3 (1.9 oz)	150	5	14	0
Vienna Sausage Jalapeno In Beef Stock	3 (1.9 oz)	170	5	16	1
Banner					
Sausage Stomachs	2 oz	90	0	5	0
Sausage Tripe	2 oz	90	9	5	2
Boar's Head					
Bratwurst	1 (4 oz)	300	19	25	0
Hot Smoked	1 (3.2 oz)	280	12	25	1
Kielbasa	2 oz	120	9	10	0
Knockwurst	1 (4 oz)	310	15	27	1

FOOD	PORTION	CALS	PROT	FAT	CARB
Brown'N Serve					
Turkey	3 (2.1 oz)	120	10	8	2
Hormel					
Light & Lean 97 Dinner Smoked	2 oz	60	8	2	2
Pickled Hot	6 (2 oz)	140	8	11	1
Pickled Smoked	6 (2 oz)	140	8	11	1
Smoked Summer	2 oz	200	8	18	2
Vienna	2 oz	140	5	14	0
Vienna Chicken	2 oz	110	6	9	1
Little Sizzlers					
Brown & Serve	3 links (2.1 oz)	190	8	22	1
Brown & Serve	2 patties (1.8 oz)	190	7	18	1
Cooked	2 patties (1.8 oz)	230	8	22	0
Cooked	3 links (1.8 oz)	230	8	22	0
Heat & Serve Pork cooked	3 links (1.8 oz)	230	8	22	0
Louis Rich					
Polska Kielbasa	2 oz	90	8	5	2
Turkey Hot	2.5 oz	120	12	8	1
Turkey Original	2.5 oz	120	12	8	1
Turkey Smoked	2 oz	90	8	5	2
Old Smokehouse					
Summer Sausage	2 oz	200	8	18	2
Oscar Mayer					
Pork cooked	2 links (1.7 oz)	170	9	15	1
Smokies Beef	1 (1.5 oz)	120	5	11	1
Smokies Cheese	1 (1.5 oz)	130	6	12	1
Smokies Link	1 (1.5 oz)	130	5	12	1
Smokies Little	6 (2 oz)	170	7	15	1
Smokies Little Cheese	6 (2 oz)	180	7	16	1
Perdue					
Hot Italian Turkey Cooked	1 link (2.4 oz)	150	16	9	1
Sweet Italian Turkey Cooked	1 link (2.4 oz)	150	16	9	1
Turkey Store					
Breakfast	2 links (2 oz)	140	8	11	1
Wampler					
Breakfast Turkey	2 (2.4 oz)	110	13	6	1
Italian Turkey	1 (2.7 oz)	120	14	6	1
take-out					
pork	1 patty (1 oz)	100	5	8	tr
pork	1 link (0.5 oz)	48	3	4	tr
SAUSAGE DISHES					
take-out					
italian sausage w/ peppers & onions	1 cup	210	17	11	14
sausage roll	1 (2.3 oz)	311	5	24	22
SAUSAGE SUBSTITUTES					
nonmeat sausage	1 patty (38 g)	97	7	7	4
nonmeat sausage	1 link (25 g)	64	5	5	2

FOOD	PORTION	CALS	PROT	FAT	CARB
Boca Burgers					
Breakfast Patties	1 (1.3 oz)	70	9	3	4
GardenSausage					
Patty	1 (2.5 oz)	140	7	3	20
Lightlife					
Gimme Lean	2 oz	70	9	0	8
Lean Links Breakfast	1 (1.2 oz)	60	4	3	4
Lean Links Italian	1 (1.4 oz)	60	5	2	5
Light	2 patties (2.3 oz)	80	11	0	10
Loma Linda					
Linketts	1 (1.2 oz)	70	7	5	1
Little Links	2 (1.6 oz)	90	8	6	2
Morningstar Farms					
Breakfast Links	2 (1.6 oz)	60	8	2	2
Breakfast Patties	1 (1.3 oz)	80	10	3	3
Grillers	1 patty (2.2 oz)	140	14	7	5
Sausage Style Recipe Crumbles	⅔ cup (1.9 oz)	90	11	3	5
Natural Touch					
Vegan Sausage Crumbles	½ cup (1.9 oz)	60	10	0	4
Worthington					
Leanies	1 link (1.4 oz)	100	7	7	2
Prosage Links	2 (1.6 oz)	60	8	3	2
Saucettes	1 link (1.3 oz)	90	6	6	1
Super Links	1 (1.7 oz)	110	7	8	2
Veja Links	1 (1.1 oz)	50	5	3	1
Yves					
Veggie Breakfast Links	1 (1.6 oz)	60	11	0	3
Veggie Breakfast Patties	1 (2 oz)	70	11	2	4
SCALLOP					
take-out					
breaded & fried	2 lg	67	6	3	3
SCONE					
apricot scone	1	232	5	7	39
Finnegan's					
Cranberry	1 (2.7 oz)	90	2	2	20
Health Valley					
Apple Kiwi	1	180	4	0	43
Cinnamon Raisin	1	180	4	0	43
Cranberry Orange	1	180	4	0	43
Mountain Blueberry	1	180	4	0	43
Pineapple Banana	1	180	4	0	43
take-out					
blueberry	1 (3 oz)	270	7	9	41
cheese	1 (3.5 oz)	364	10	18	44
orange poppy	1 (3 oz)	260	6	6	47
plain	1 (3.5 oz)	362	8	14	54
raisin	1 (3 oz)	270	6	6	50

FOOD	PORTION	CALS	PROT	FAT	CARB
SCUP					
fresh baked	3 oz	115	21	3	0
SEA BASS					
(see BASS)					
SEA CUCUMBER					
dried	1 oz	74	14	1	1
fresh	1 oz	20	5	tr	tr
SEA TROUT					
(see TROUT)					
SEA URCHIN					
canned	1 oz	39	4	1	3
fresh	1 oz	36	4	1	3
roe paste	1 tbsp	19	2	tr	3
SEAWEED					
agar dried	1 oz	87	2	tr	23
hijiki dried	1 tbsp	9	1	0	2
laver fresh	1 oz	10	2	tr	1
nori fresh	1 oz	10	2	tr	1
nori sheet dried	1 (8 x 8 in)	5	1	0	1
seahair dried	1 tbsp	13	1	0	3
spirulina dried	1 oz	83	16	2	7
spirulina fresh	1 oz	7	2	tr	1
wakame fresh	1 oz	13	1	tr	3
SEITAN					
(see WHEAT)					
SEMOLINA					
dry	1 cup (5.9 oz)	601	21	2	122
SESAME					
seeds	1 tsp	16	1	2	tr
seeds dried	1 tbsp	52	2	5	2
seeds dried	1 cup	825	26	72	34
seeds roasted & toasted	1 oz	161	14	14	7
sesame butter	1 tbsp	95	3	8	4
sesame crunch candy	1 oz	146	3	9	14
sesame crunch candy	20 pieces (1.2 oz)	181	4	12	18
sesame sticks	1 oz	153	3	10	13
sesame sticks unsalted	1 oz	153	3	10	13
tahini from roasted & toasted kernels	1 tbsp	89	3	8	3
tahini from stone ground kernels	1 tbsp	86	3	7	4
tahini from unroasted kernels	1 tbsp	85	3	8	3
Eden					
Organic Seaweed Gomasio	1 serv (1.5 oz)	10	0	1	0
Organic Gomasio	½ tsp	10	0	1	0
Organic Gomasio Garlic	½ tsp	10	0	1	0

FOOD	PORTION	CALS	PROT	FAT	CARB
SESBANIA					
flowers cooked	1 cup	23	1	tr	5
SHAD					
american baked	3 oz	214	18	15	0
roe baked w/ butter & lemon	1 oz	36	6	1	tr
roe raw	1 oz	37	7	tr	tr
SHARK					
batter-dipped & fried	3 oz	194	16	12	5
SHEEPSHEAD FISH					
cooked	3 oz	107	22	1	0
cooked	1 fillet (6.5 oz)	234	48	3	0
SHELLFISH SUBSTITUTES					
crab imitation	3 oz	87	10	1	1
scallop imitation	3 oz	84	11	tr	9
shrimp imitation	3 oz	86	11	1	8
surimi	3 oz	84	13	1	6
surimi	1 oz	28	4	tr	2
Louis Kemp					
Crab Delights	½ cup (3 oz)	90	10	0	12
Lobster Delights	½ cup (3 oz)	80	8	0	12
Scallop Delights	13 pieces (3 oz)	80	9	0	12
SHELLIE BEANS					
canned	½ cup	37	2	tr	8
SHERBET					
(*see also* ICES AND ICE POPS)					
orange	½ cup (4 fl oz)	132	1	2	29
orange	½ gal	2158	17	31	469
orange	1 bar (2.75 fl oz)	91	1	1	20
orange home recipe	½ cup	120	2	2	24
Breyers					
Fat Free Orange	½ cup (3 oz)	110	2	0	27
Fat Free Rainbow	½ cup (3 oz)	110	1	0	28
Fat Free Raspberry	½ cup (3 oz)	120	2	0	28
Fat Free Tropical	½ cup (3 oz)	110	1	0	27
Orange	½ cup (3 oz)	120	1	1	26
Rainbow	½ cup (3 oz)	120	1	2	27
Raspberry	½ cup (3 oz)	120	1	2	28
Tropical	½ cup (3 oz)	120	1	1	27
SHRIMP					
canned	3 oz	102	20	2	1
canned	1 cup	154	30	3	1
chinese shrimp pasta	1 tbsp	15	3	tr	1
cooked	3 oz	84	18	1	0
cooked	4 large	22	5	tr	0
Bumble Bee					
Medium	⅓ can (2 oz)	45	10	tr	0

FOOD	PORTION	CALS	PROT	FAT	CARB
Gorton's					
Popcorn Garlic & Herb	22 pieces (3.6 oz)	270	11	14	24
Popcorn Original	20 pieces (3.2 oz)	240	9	13	22
take-out					
breaded & fried	3 oz	206	18	10	10
jambalaya	¾ cup	188	11	5	26
SMELT					
rainbow cooked	3 oz	106	19	3	0
rainbow raw	3 oz	83	15	2	0
SMOOTHIE					
(*see* FRUIT DRINKS)					
SNACKS					
cheese puffs	1 oz	157	2	10	15
corn puffs cheese	1 bag (8 oz)	1256	17	78	122
corn twists cheese	1 oz	157	2	10	15
corn twists cheese	1 bag (8 oz)	1256	17	78	122
oriental mix	1 oz	155	6	12	9
pork skins	1 oz	154	17	9	0
pork skins barbecue	1 oz	152	16	9	1
trail mix	1 oz	131	4	8	13
trail mix	1 cup (5.3 oz)	693	21	44	67
trail mix tropical	1 oz	115	2	5	19
trail mix w/ chocolate chips	1 cup (5.1 oz)	707	21	47	66
trail mix w/ chocolate chips	1 oz	137	4	9	13
Baken-ets					
BBQ	9 (0.5 oz)	70	7	5	tr
Hot N'Spicy	7 (0.5 oz)	70	8	5	tr
Hot N'Spicy Cracklins	8 (0.5 oz)	80	7	5	tr
Regular	9 (0.5 oz)	80	8	5	tr
Regular Cracklins	8 (0.5 oz)	40	7	6	tr
Barbara's Bakery					
Cheese Puffs Bakes	1½ cups (1 oz)	160	2	11	13
Cheese Puffs Jalapeno	¾ cup (1 oz)	150	2	10	16
Cheese Puffs Original	¾ cup (1 oz)	150	2	10	16
Bugles					
Baked Cheddar Cheese	1½ cups (1 oz)	130	2	4	23
Baked Original	1½ cups (1 oz)	130	2	4	23
Baked Original	1 pkg (1.4 oz)	170	2	5	30
Nacho	1⅓ cups (1 oz)	160	1	9	18
Nacho	1 pkg (0.9 oz)	130	1	7	15
Original	1 pkg (1.5 oz)	230	2	13	25
Original	1⅓ cups (1 oz)	160	1	9	18
Ranch	1⅓ cups (1 oz)	160	2	9	18
Smokin BBQ	1⅓ cups (1 oz)	150	1	8	19
Sour Cream & Onion	1⅓ cups (1 oz)	160	1	9	18
Cheetos					
Crunchy	21 pieces (1 oz)	160	2	10	15
Curls	15 pieces (1 oz)	150	2	10	15

FOOD	PORTION	CALS	PROT	FAT	CARB
Flamin' Hot	21 pieces (1 oz)	160	2	10	15
Nacho Cheese	23 pieces (1 oz)	160	2	10	15
Puffed Balls	38 pieces (1 oz)	150	2	10	15
Puffs	29 pieces (1 oz)	160	2	10	15
Zig Zags	17 pieces (1 oz)	170	2	11	17
Chex Mix					
Bold'n Zesty	1 pkg (1.7 oz)	230	4	9	33
Cheddar Cheese	1 pkg (1.7 oz)	220	5	9	33
Hot'n Spicy	⅔ cup (1 oz)	130	3	5	21
Hot'n Spicy	1 pkg (1.7 oz)	210	4	7	35
Traditional	1 pkg (1.7 oz)	210	4	7	35
Dakota Gourmet					
Amazing Corn Classic	1 pkg (1 oz)	360	10	7	78
Amazing Corn Cool Ranch	1 pkg (1 oz)	367	10	9	74
Amazing Corn Mesquite BBQ	1 pkg (1 oz)	369	11	8	76
Heart Smart Toasted Corn	⅓ cup (1 oz)	110	3	2	22
Toasted Corn Heart Smart	1 pkg (1.75 oz)	177	5	3	39
Trail Mix Heart Smart	1 pkg (1.75 oz)	172	4	0	39
Eden					
Rice Puffs Five Flavor Arare	1 oz	110	3	0	24
Frito Lay					
Funyuns	13 (1 oz)	140	2	7	18
Munchos	16 (1 oz)	160	1	10	16
Munchos BBQ	14 (1 oz)	160	1	10	15
Health Valley					
Cheddar Lites Green Onion	1¾ cups	120	3	3	21
Cheddar Lites Original	1¾ cups	120	3	3	21
Corn Puffs Caramel	2 cups	120	2	2	25
Low Fat Potato Puffs Cheddar Cheese	1½ cups	110	2	3	21
Low Fat Potato Puffs Garlic w/ Cheese	1½ cups	260	2	3	21
Low Fat Potato Puffs Zesty Ranch	1½ cups	110	2	3	21
Lance					
Cheese Balls	1 pkg (1 oz)	150	2	8	16
Crunchy Cheese Twists	1 pkg (1.25 oz)	190	2	4	15
Gold-N-Chees	1 pkg (1 oz)	130	3	5	18
Onion Rings	1 pkg (0.9 oz)	100	1	8	7
Pork Skins	1 pkg (0.4 oz)	65	6	4	1
Pork Skins BBQ	1 pkg (0.4 oz)	60	6	4	1
Old Dutch Foods					
Baked Cheese Curls	2 cups (1.1 oz)	180	2	12	15
Cheese Puffcorn Curls	2 cups (1.1 oz)	170	2	12	15
Planters					
Cheez Mania Original	42 pieces (1 oz)	150	2	10	15

FOOD	PORTION	CALS	PROT	FAT	CARB
Robert's American Gourmet					
Pirate's Booty Puffed Rice & Corn w/ Cheddar	1 oz	120	3	3	22
Rold Gold					
Snack Mix Colossal Cheddar	1 pkg (1 oz)	140	3	7	17
Snyder's Of Hanover					
Cheese Twists	1 oz	230	1	14	10
Fried Pork Skins	1 oz	80	8	4	1
Fried Pork Skins Barbecue	1 oz	80	8	4	1
Kruncheez	1.25 oz	200	2	10	19
Onion Toasters	1 oz	188	2	10	21
Utz					
Cheese Balls	50 (1 oz)	150	2	9	16
Cheese Curls	18 (1 oz)	150	2	9	16
Cheese Curls Crunchy	30 (1 oz)	160	2	10	16
Cheese Curls Reduced Fat	32 (1 oz)	140	3	6	18
Onion Rings	41 (1 oz)	140	1	7	18
Party Mix	¾ cup (1 oz)	140	2	6	19
Pork Cracklins	0.5 oz	90	6	7	0
Pork Cracklins Hot & Spicy	0.5 oz	80	8	5	0
Pork Rinds	0.5 oz	80	8	5	0
Pork Rinds BBQ	0.5 oz	80	8	5	0
Weight Watchers					
Cheese Curls	1 pkg (0.5 oz)	70	1	3	10
SNAIL					
cooked	3 oz	233	41	1	13
take-out					
escargot cooked	5	25	4	0	1
SNAKE					
fresh	3 oz	78	17	tr	3
SNAPPER					
cooked	3 oz	109	22	1	0
cooked	1 fillet (6 oz)	217	45	3	0
SODA					
club	12 oz	0	0	0	0
cream	12 oz	191	0	0	49
grape	12 oz	161	0	0	42
lemon lime	12 oz	149	0	0	38
orange	12 oz	177	0	0	46
pepper type	12 oz	151	0	tr	38
quinine	12 oz	125	0	0	32
tonic water	12 oz	125	0	0	32
7 Up					
Original	1 can	140	0	0	39
A & W					
Root Beer	1 can	180	0	0	46
Barritts					
Ginger Beer	1 bottle (12 oz)	200	0	0	49

FOOD	PORTION	CALS	PROT	FAT	CARB
Best Health					
Root Beer	1 bottle (12 oz)	165	0	0	42
Vanilla Cream	1 bottle (12 oz)	170	0	0	43
Canada Dry					
Ginger Ale	1 can	120	0	0	33
Tonic Water	8 fl oz	90	0	0	24
Dr Pepper					
Original	1 can	150	0	0	40
Health Valley					
Ginger Ale	1 bottle	160	0	0	40
Rootbeer Old Fashioned	1 bottle	160	0	0	40
Sarsaparilla Rootbeer	1 bottle	160	0	0	40
IBC					
Root Beer	1 can	160	0	0	43
Lucozade					
Soda	7 oz	136	0	0	36
Pepsi					
Blue Berry Cola Fusion	8 fl oz	100	0	0	28
Saranac					
Diet Root Beer	1 bottle (12 oz)	35	0	0	9
Ginger Beer	1 bottle (12 oz)	160	0	0	42
Root Beer	1 bottle (12 oz)	180	4	0	46
Shasta					
Black Cherry	1 can (12 oz)	170	0	0	41
Caffeine Free Cola	1 can (12 oz)	160	0	0	41
Cherry Cola	1 can (12 oz)	160	0	0	39
Club Soda	1 can (12 oz)	0	0	0	0
Cola	1 can (12 oz)	170	0	0	42
Creme	1 can (12 oz)	190	0	0	47
Diet Black Cherry	1 can (12 oz)	0	0	0	0
Diet Caffeine Free Cola	1 can (12 oz)	0	0	0	0
Diet Cherry Cola	1 can (12 oz)	0	0	0	0
Diet Cola	1 can (12 oz)	0	0	0	0
Diet Creme	1 can (12 oz)	0	0	0	0
Diet Doc Shasta	1 can (12 oz)	0	0	0	0
Diet Ginger Ale	1 can (12 oz)	0	0	0	0
Diet Grape	1 can (12 oz)	0	0	0	0
Diet Grapefruit	1 can (12 oz)	0	0	0	0
Diet Kiwi-Strawberry	1 can (12 oz)	0	0	0	0
Diet Lemon-Lime Twist	1 can (12 oz)	0	0	0	0
Diet Orange	1 can (12 oz)	0	0	0	0
Diet Pineapple-Orange	1 can (12 oz)	0	0	0	0
Diet Raspberry Creme	1 can (12 oz)	0	0	0	0
Diet Red Pop	1 can (12 oz)	0	0	0	0
Diet Root Beer	1 can (12 oz)	0	0	0	0
Diet Strawberry	1 can (12 oz)	0	0	0	0
Diet Strawberry-Peach	1 can (12 oz)	0	0	0	0

FOOD	PORTION	CALS	PROT	FAT	CARB
Doc Shasta					
Fruit Punch	1 can (12 oz)	160	0	0	39
Ginger Ale	1 can (12 oz)	200	0	0	50
Grape	1 can (12 oz)	130	0	0	32
Kiwi-Strawberry	1 can (12 oz)	190	0	0	48
Lemon-Lime Twist	1 can (12 oz)	170	0	0	43
Moon Mist	1 can (12 oz)	150	0	0	38
Orange	1 can (12 oz)	180	0	0	46
Peach	1 can (12 oz)	200	0	0	49
Pineapple	1 can (12 oz)	170	0	0	43
Pineapple-Orange	1 can (12 oz)	200	0	0	51
Quinine/Tonic	1 can (12 oz)	180	0	0	46
Raspberry Creme	1 can (12 oz)	130	0	0	32
Red Pop	1 can (12 oz)	170	0	0	44
Root Beer	1 can (12 oz)	170	0	0	43
Strawberry	1 can (12 oz)	170	0	0	42
Strawberry-Peach	1 can (12 oz)	190	0	0	46
	1 can (12 oz)	170	0	0	42
Stewart's					
Root Beer	1 bottle (12 oz)	160	0	0	41
Sunkist					
Orange	1 can	190	0	0	52
SOLE					
cooked	3 oz	99	21	1	0
cooked	1 fillet (4.5 oz)	148	31	2	0
lemon raw	3.5 oz	85	17	1	0
take-out					
battered & fried	3.2 oz	211	13	11	15
breaded & fried	3.2 oz	211	13	11	15
SORBET					
(*see* ICES AND ICE POPS)					
SORGHUM					
sorghum	1 cup (6.7 oz)	651	22	6	143
SOUFFLE					
lemon chilled	1 cup	176	9	tr	34
raspberry chilled	1 cup	173	10	tr	34
spinach	1 cup	218	11	18	3
SOUP					
canned					
asparagus cream of as prep w/ milk	1 cup	161	6	8	16
asparagus cream of as prep w/ water	1 cup	87	1	4	11
beef broth ready-to-serve	1 can (14 oz)	27	5	1	tr
beef broth ready-to-serve	1 cup	16	3	1	tr
beef noodle as prep w/water	1 cup	84	5	3	9
black bean turtle soup	1 cup	218	14	1	40
black bean as prep w/water	1 cup	116	6	2	20

FOOD	PORTION	CALS	PROT	FAT	CARB
celery cream of as prep w/ milk	1 cup	165	6	10	15
celery cream of as prep w/ water	1 cup	90	2	6	9
celery cream of not prep	1 can (10¾ oz)	219	4	14	21
cheese as prep w/ milk	1 cup	230	9	15	16
cheese as prep w/ water	1 cup	155	5	10	11
cheese not prep	1 can (11 oz)	377	13	25	26
chicken broth as prep w/ water	1 cup	39	5	1	1
chicken cream of as prep w/ milk	1 cup	191	7	11	15
chicken cream of as prep w/ water	1 cup	116	3	7	9
chicken gumbo as prep w/water	1 cup	56	3	1	8
chicken noodle as prep w/ water	1 cup	75	4	2	9
chicken rice as prep w/ water	1 cup	251	4	2	7
clam chowder manhattan as prep w/ water	1 cup	77	2	2	12
clam chowder new england as prep w/ water	1 cup	95	5	3	12
clam chowder new england as prep w/ milk	1 cup	163	9	7	17
consomme w/ gelatin not prep	1 can (10½ oz)	71	13	0	4
consomme w/ gelatin as prep w/ water	1 cup	29	5	0	2
escarole ready-to-serve	1 cup	27	2	2	2
french onion as prep w/ water	1 cup	57	4	2	8
gazpacho ready-to-serve	1 cup	57	9	2	1
minestrone as prep w/water	1 cup	83	4	3	11
mushroom cream of as prep w/ milk	1 cup	203	6	14	15
mushroom cream of as prep w/ water	1 cup	129	2	9	9
oyster stew as prep w/ milk	1 cup	134	6	8	10
oyster stew as prep w/ water	1 cup	59	2	4	4
pepperpot as prep w/ water	1 cup	103	6	5	9
potato cream of as prep w/ milk	1 cup	148	6	6	17

FOOD	PORTION	CALS	PROT	FAT	CARB
potato cream of as prep w/ water	1 cup	73	2	2	11
scotch broth as prep w/ water	1 cup	80	5	3	9
split pea w/ ham as prep w/ water	1 cup	189	10	4	28
tomato as prep w/ milk	1 cup	160	6	6	22
tomato as prep w/water	1 cup	86	2	2	17
vegetarian vegetable as prep w/ water	1 cup	72	2	2	12
vichyssoise	1 cup	148	6	6	17
Boston Market					
Chicken Broth Reduced Sodium	1 cup	15	1	1	1
Butterball					
Chicken Broth Reduced Sodium 99% Fat Free	1 cup	10	1	0	2
Campbell					
98% Fat Free Cream Of Chicken as prep	1 cup	80	3	3	10
Bean w/ Bacon as prep	1 cup	168	8	4	26
Beef Barley as prep	1 cup	81	6	2	11
Beef Noodle as prep	1 cup	73	5	2	8
Cheddar Cheese	1 cup	100	3	5	12
Cheddar Cheese as prep	1 cup	134	4	8	11
Chicken Vegetable as prep	1 cup	74	3	3	9
Chicken Gumbo as prep	1 cup	55	2	1	9
Chunky Savory Chicken w/ White & Wild Rice	1 cup	140	9	3	18
Chunky Classic Chicken Noodle	1 cup (8.4 oz)	130	8	4	15
Clam Chowder New England as prep	1 cup	89	4	3	13
Classic Chicken Noodle	1 cup	70	3	2	10
Classic Chicken Rice	1 cup (8.4 oz)	80	2	2	14
Consomme as prep	1 cup	24	5	tr	1
Cream Of Asparagus as prep	1 cup	72	2	4	9
Cream Of Mushroom as prep	1 cup	108	2	7	9
Cream Of Celery as prep	1 cup	107	2	7	9
Cream Of Chicken as prep	1 cup	120	3	8	10
Cream Of Potato as prep	1 cup	102	2	4	15
Fiesta Tomato as prep	1 cup	72	1	tr	16
Garden Vegetable as prep	1 cup	69	3	2	11
Green Pea as prep	1 cup	173	9	3	29
Healthy Request Chicken Noodle as prep	1 cup	60	2	2	8

FOOD	PORTION	CALS	PROT	FAT	CARB
Healthy Request Chicken Rice as prep	1 cup	60	2	2	8
Healthy Request Cream Of Mushroom as prep	1 cup	66	2	2	10
Healthy Request Cream Of Chicken & Broccoli as prep	1 cup	78	3	3	10
Healthy Request Cream Of Chicken as prep	1 cup	70	2	3	12
Healthy Request Hearty Pasta w/ Vegetables	1 cup	87	3	1	17
Healthy Request Tomato as prep	1 cup	91	2	2	18
Healthy Request Vegetable as prep	1 cup	84	3	1	17
Home Cookin' Chicken Vegetable	1 cup (8.4 oz)	130	6	4	20
Home Cookin' Chicken Rice	1 cup	110	6	1	20
Home Cookin' Chicken w/ Egg Noodles	1 cup (8.4 oz)	90	6	2	13
Home Cookin' Oriental Noodles w/ Vegetables	1 cup (8.4 oz)	100	4	1	18
Italian Tomato as prep	1 cup	105	2	tr	23
Low Sodium Chicken Broth	1 can (10.75 oz)	27	4	1	2
Low Sodium Chicken w/ Noodles	1 can (10.75 oz)	162	14	5	16
Low Sodium Chunky Vegetable Beef	1 can (10.75 oz)	159	13	4	17
Low Sodium Cream of Mushroom	1 can (10.75 oz)	200	3	13	18
Low Sodium Green Pea	1 can (10.75 oz)	235	12	4	38
Low Sodium Tomato w/ Pieces	1 can (10.75 oz)	170	4	5	28
Minestrone as prep	1 cup	81	3	2	12
Plus! Hearty Minestrone	2 cup (8.4 oz)	130	5	1	25
Plus! Roasted Vegetable w/ Barley & Wild Rice	1 cup (8.4 oz)	130	3	1	25
Ready To Serve Bean w/ Bacon 'N Ham	1 can (10.5 oz)	274	14	7	41
Ready To Serve Chicken Noodle	1 can (10.5 oz)	134	7	4	18
Ready To Serve Chicken w/ Rice	1 can (10.5 oz)	122	5	2	20
Ready-To-Serve Vegetable Beef	1 can (10.5 oz)	143	9	1	26
Savory Tomato & Dill as prep	1 cup	99	2	2	20

FOOD	PORTION	CALS	PROT	FAT	CARB
Select Chicken & Pasta w/ Roasted Garlic	1 cup (8.4 oz)	110	6	2	17
Select Chicken Rice	1 cup	110	7	1	18
Select Fiesta Vegetable	1 cup (8.4 oz)	120	4	1	24
Select Mushroom w/ White & Wild Rice	1 cup	90	6	1	16
Select Roasted Chicken w/ Rotini & Penne Pasta	1 cup	110	6	2	17
Select Split Pea w/ Ham	1 cup (8.4 oz)	170	10	2	30
Select Tuscany-Style Minestrone	1 cup (8.4 oz)	190	5	9	21
Simply Home Chicken Noodle	1 cup (8.4 oz)	80	5	1	12
Simply Home Chicken w/ Rice	1 cup (8.4 oz)	100	5	1	19
Tomato as prep	1 cup	80	2	0	18
Vegetable Beef as prep	1 cup	68	5	2	9
Vegetarian Vegetable as prep	1 cup	79	2	2	14
Gold's					
Russian Borscht	8 oz	70	1	0	17
Health Valley					
5 Bean Vegetable	1 cup	250	10	0	32
Beef Broth Fat Free	1 cup	20	5	0	0
Beef Broth Fat Free No Salt	1 cup	20	5	0	0
Black Bean & Vegetable	1 cup	110	11	0	24
Chicken Broth	1 cup	45	7	2	0
Chicken Broth Fat Free	1 cup	30	7	0	0
Chicken Broth No Salt	1 cup	45	7	2	0
Country Corn & Vegetable	1 cup	70	5	0	17
Garden Vegetable	1 cup	80	6	0	17
Italian Plus Carotene	1 cup	80	7	0	19
Lentil & Carrot	1 cup	100	10	0	25
Organic Black Bean	1 cup	110	8	0	28
Organic Lentil No Salt	1 cup	90	9	0	20
Organic Minestrone	1 cup	100	8	0	23
Organic Mushroom Barley No Salt	1 cup	60	5	0	15
Organic Potato Leek	1 cup	70	4	0	15
Organic Potato Leek No Salt	1 cup	70	4	0	15
Organic Split Pea	1 cup	110	10	0	23
Organic Split Pea No Salt	1 cup	110	10	0	23
Organic Tomato	1 cup	90	4	0	22
Organic Vegetable No Salt	1 cup	80	5	0	18
Pasta Bolognese	1 cup	100	4	0	20
Pasta Cacciatore	1 cup	100	4	0	20

FOOD	PORTION	CALS	PROT	FAT	CARB
Pasta Romano	1 cup	100	4	0	20
Real Italian Minestrone	1 cup	90	8	0	21
Rotini & Vegetable	1 cup	100	4	0	20
Split Pea & Carrots	1 cup	110	8	0	17
Super Broccoli Carotene	1 cup	70	6	0	16
Tomato Vegetable	1 cup	80	6	0	17
Vegetable Barley	1 cup	90	6	0	19
Vegetable Power Carotene	1 cup	70	5	0	17
Healthy Choice					
Bean & Ham	1 cup (8.7 oz)	166	9	1	31
Beef & Potato	1 cup (8.5 oz)	116	11	1	16
Broccoli Cheddar	1 cup (8.4 oz)	116	4	2	22
Chicken Corn Chowder	1 cup (8.8 oz)	176	8	3	30
Chicken Pasta	1 cup (8.6 oz)	119	7	3	18
Chicken Rice	1 cup (8.4 oz)	119	9	2	19
Chili Beef	1 cup (9.1 oz)	189	15	2	32
Clam Chowder	1 cup (8.8 oz)	123	6	1	23
Classic Italian Bean and Pasta	1 cup (8 oz)	100	6	2	17
Country Vegetable	1 cup (8.6 oz)	112	5	1	24
Cream Of Mushroom	1 cup (8.8 oz)	77	4	1	14
Cream Of Celery as prep	1 cup	73	1	2	14
Cream Of Chicken Vegetable	1 cup (8.9 oz)	127	7	2	21
Cream Of Roasted Chicken as prep	1 cup	80	2	3	13
Cream Of Roasted Garlic as prep	1 cup	57	1	1	13
Garden Tomato Herbs as prep	1 cup	80	2	1	18
Garden Vegetable	1 cup (8.6 oz)	108	5	1	22
Hearty Chicken	1 cup (8.7 oz)	136	9	3	20
Lentil	1 cup (8.7 oz)	135	10	1	28
Minestrone	1 cup (8.6 oz)	107	5	1	24
Old Fashion Chicken Noodle	1 cup (8.8 oz)	137	9	3	19
Split Pea & Ham	1 cup (8.8 oz)	164	11	2	26
Tomato Garden	1 cup (8.6 oz)	101	4	1	19
Turkey Wild Rice	1 cup (8.4 oz)	72	10	1	9
Vegetable Beef	1 cup (8.8 oz)	96	11	1	14
Herb-Ox					
Beef Liquid	2 tsp (0.4 oz)	20	2	0	2
Chicken Liquid	2 tsp (0.4 oz)	15	1	0	1
Imagine					
Creamy Broccoli	1 serv (8 oz)	70	3	2	10
Creamy Butternut Squash	1 serv (8 oz)	120	2	2	23
Creamy Mushroom	1 serv (8 oz)	80	4	3	10
Creamy Potato Leek	1 serv (8 oz)	90	2	3	14
Creamy Sweet Corn	1 serv (8 oz)	100	4	3	15

FOOD	PORTION	CALS	PROT	FAT	CARB
Creamy Tomato	1 serv (8 oz)	90	8	2	17
Vegetable Broth	1 serv (8 oz)	45	0	1	7
Natural Choice					
Organic Vegan Classic Tomato	1 cup	100	2	1	22
Organic Vegan Classic Mushroom	1 cup	50	2	2	9
Organic Vegan Country Corn	1 cup	100	3	1	24
Organic Vegan Kabocha Squash	1 cup	60	2	1	14
Organic Vegan Southern Greens	1 cup	80	2	3	13
Organic Vegan Split Pea	1 cup	120	7	1	21
Organic Vegan Vegetable Curry	1 cup	110	4	4	17
Pacific					
Free Range Organic Chicken Broth	1 cup	5	1	0	1
Progresso					
99% Fat Free Beef Barley	1 cup (8.5 oz)	140	11	2	20
99% Fat Free Beef Vegetable	1 cup (8.5 oz)	160	11	2	24
99% Fat Free Chicken Noodle	1 cup (8.3 oz)	90	7	2	13
99% Fat Free Chicken Rice w/ Vegetables	1 cup (8.4 oz)	110	7	2	16
99% Fat Free Creamy Mushroom Chicken	1 cup (8.3 oz)	90	7	2	12
99% Fat Free Lentil	1 cup (8.5 oz)	130	8	2	20
99% Fat Free Minestrone	1 cup (8.5 oz)	130	7	2	23
99% Fat Free Roasted Chicken w/ Italian Style Vegetable	1 cup (8 oz)	90	7	2	12
99% Fat Free Split Pea	1 cup (8.9 oz)	170	10	2	29
99% Fat Free Tomato Garden Vegetable	1 cup (8.6 oz)	100	3	2	19
99% Fat Free Vegetable	1 cup (8.4 oz)	70	2	1	13
99% Fat Free White Cheddar Potato	1 cup (8.6 oz)	140	4	3	26
Basil Rotini Tomato	1 cup (8.9 oz)	120	5	2	22
Bean & Ham	1 cup (8.4 oz)	160	10	2	25
Beef Barley	1 cup (8.5 oz)	130	10	4	13
Beef Minestrone	1 cup (8.5 oz)	140	10	3	18
Beef Noodle	1 cup (8.5 oz)	140	13	4	15
Beef Vegetable & Rotini	1 cup (8.4 oz)	130	13	3	14
Cheese & Herb Tortellini Tomato	1 cup (8.6 oz)	140	4	3	23
Chickarina	1 cup (8.3 oz)	130	8	5	12

FOOD	PORTION	CALS	PROT	FAT	CARB
Chicken Minestrone	1 cup (8.4 oz)	110	9	2	15
Chicken Vegetable	1 cup (8.4 oz)	90	7	2	13
Chicken & Wild Rice	1 cup (8.4 oz)	100	7	2	15
Chicken Barley	1 cup (8.5 oz)	110	8	2	16
Chicken Broth	1 cup (8.2 oz)	20	1	2	1
Chicken Noodle	1 cup (8.4 oz)	90	9	2	9
Chicken Rice w/ Vegetable	1 cup (8.4 oz)	90	6	2	13
Clam & Rotini Chowder	1 cup (8.8 oz)	190	7	9	21
Escarole In Chicken Broth	1 cup (8.1 oz)	25	1	1	3
Green Split Pea	1 cup (8.6 oz)	170	10	3	25
Hearty Black Bean	1 cup (8.5 oz)	170	8	2	30
Hearty Penne In Chicken Broth	1 cup (8.4 oz)	80	4	1	14
Hearty Tomato	1 cup (8.7 oz)	100	2	2	19
Herb Rotini Vegetable	1 cup (9.1 oz)	120	5	2	21
Homestyle Chicken w/ Vegetable	1 cup (8.4 oz)	90	7	2	11
Italian Herb Shells Minestrone	1 cup (9.1 oz)	120	5	2	22
Lentil	1 cup (8.5 oz)	140	9	2	22
Macaroni & Bean	1 cup (8.6 oz)	160	7	4	23
Manhattan Clam Chowder	1 cup (8.4 oz)	110	12	2	11
Meatballs & Pasta Pearls	1 cup (8.3 oz)	140	7	7	13
Minestrone	1 cup (8.4 oz)	120	5	2	21
Minestrone Parmesan	1 cup (8.3 oz)	100	3	3	16
New England Clam Chowder	1 cup (8.4 oz)	190	6	10	20
Oregano Penne Italian Style Vegetable	1 cup (8.7 oz)	90	3	2	15
Peppercorn Penne Vegetable	1 cup (9.1 oz)	100	3	1	20
Potato Broccoli & Cheese	1 cup (8.8 oz)	160	5	6	21
Potato Ham & Cheese	1 cup (8.6 oz)	170	6	7	21
Roasted Garlic Pasta Lentil	1 cup (9.3 oz)	120	7	2	20
Rotisserie Seasoned Chicken	1 cup (8.5 oz)	100	7	2	15
Spicy Chicken & Penne	1 cup (8.5 oz)	110	9	2	14
Split Pea w/ Ham	1 cup (8.4 oz)	150	9	4	20
Tomato	1 cup (8.5 oz)	100	2	2	19
Tomato Basil	1 cup (8.8 oz)	100	2	2	19
Tomato Vegetable	1 cup (8.5 oz)	90	3	2	15
Tortellini In Chicken Broth	1 cup (8.3 oz)	70	3	2	10
Turkey Noodle	1 cup (8.4 oz)	90	7	2	11
Turkey Rice w/ Vegetables	1 cup (8.5 oz)	110	7	1	18
Vegetable	1 cup (8.4 oz)	90	3	2	15
White Meat Roasted Chicken Rotini	1 cup (8.1 oz)	80	6	2	11

FOOD	PORTION	CALS	PROT	FAT	CARB
Swanson					
Beef Broth	1 cup	19	3	1	1
Beef Broth Onion Seasoned	1 cup (8.4 oz)	20	2	0	2
Chicken Broth 99% Fat Free	1 cup	15	1	1	1
Chicken Broth Seasoned Italian Herbs	1 cup (8.4 oz)	20	1	1	3
Vegetable Broth	1 cup	19	1	1	3
Ultra Slim-Fast					
Chicken Alfredo Pasta	1 cup (8.3 oz)	132	12	2	17
Walnut Acres					
Organic Country Corn Chowder	1 cup (8.8 oz)	150	4	3	28
Weight Watchers					
Chicken & Rice	1 can (10.5 oz)	110	6	2	17
Chicken Noodle	1 can (10.5 oz)	150	9	2	25
Minestrone	1 can (10.5 oz)	130	5	2	23
Vegetable	1 can (10.5 oz)	130	4	1	27
frozen					
Nature's Entree					
Chowder	1 pkg (12 oz)	230	16	6	26
Tortellini Minestrone	1 pkg (12 oz)	360	22	9	48
mix					
asparagus cream of as prep w/ water	1 cup	59	2	2	9
beef broth	1 pkg (0.2 oz)	14	1	1	1
beef broth as prep w/ water	1 cup	19	1	1	2
beef broth cube	1 cube (3.6 g)	6	1	tr	1
beef broth cube as prep w/ water	1 cup	8	1	tr	1
celery cream of as prep w/ water	1 cup	63	3	2	10
chicken broth	1 pkg (0.2 oz)	16	1	1	1
chicken broth as prep w/ water	1 cup	21	1	1	1
chicken broth cube	1 cube (4.8 g)	9	1	tr	1
chicken broth cube, as prep w/ water	1 cup	13	1	tr	2
chicken cream of as prep w/ water	1 cup	107	2	5	13
chicken noodle as prep w/ water	1 cup	53	3	1	7
french onion not prep	1 pkg (1.4 oz)	115	5	2	21
leek as prep w/ water	1 cup	71	2	2	11
onion as prep w/ water	1 cup	28	1	1	5
tomato as prep w/ water	1 cup	102	2	2	19
Armour					
Bouillon Cubes Beef	1 (4 g)	5	0	0	1
Bouillon Cubes Chicken	1 (4 g)	5	0	0	1

FOOD	PORTION	CALS	PROT	FAT	CARB
Azumaya					
Thin Cut Noodle	1 cup	120	5	0	24
Wide Cut Noodle	1 cup	120	5	0	24
Bean Cuisine					
13 Bean Bouillabisse	1 cup	220	6	0	17
Island Black Bean	1 cup	210	6	0	17
Lots of Lentil	1 cup	230	6	0	17
Mesa Malze	1 cup	160	6	0	18
White Bean Provencal	1 cup	250	10	1	32
Cup-a-Soup					
Broccoli & Cheese as prep	1 serv (6 oz)	70	2	3	9
Chicken Vegetable as prep	1 serv (6 oz)	50	1	1	10
Chicken Broth as prep	1 serv (6 oz)	20	1	0	3
Chicken Broth w/ Pasta Fat Free as prep	1 serv (6 oz)	45	2	0	8
Chicken Noodle as prep	1 serv (6 oz)	50	2	1	8
Cream Of Chicken as prep	1 serv (6 oz)	70	1	2	12
Creamy Chicken Vegetable as prep	1 serv (6 oz)	80	2	5	10
Creamy Mushroom as prep	1 serv (6 oz)	60	1	2	10
Green Pea as prep	1 serv (6 oz)	80	4	1	12
Hearty Chicken Noodle as prep	1 serv (6 oz)	60	3	1	10
Ring Noodle as prep	1 serv (6 oz)	50	2	1	9
Spring Vegetable as prep	1 serv (6 oz)	45	2	1	21
Tomato as prep	1 serv (6 oz)	100	2	1	20
Health Valley					
Chicken Noodles w/ Vegetables	1 serv	110	3	0	24
Corn Chowder w/ Tomatoes	1 serv	100	4	0	21
Creamy Potatoe w/ Broccoli	1 serv	70	4	0	17
Garden Split Pea w/ Carrots	1 serv	130	8	0	22
Lentil w/ Couscous	1 serv	130	7	0	28
Pasta Italiano	1 serv	140	5	0	31
Pasta Marinara	1 serv	100	5	0	20
Pasta Parmesan	1 serv	100	5	0	20
Spicy Black Bean w/ Couscous	1 serv	130	6	0	29
Zesty Black Bean w/ Rice	1 serv	100	5	0	22
Herb-Ox					
Beef Bouillon	1 cube (3.5 g)	5	0	0	tr
Beef Instant Bouillon Powder	1 tsp (4 g)	5	0	0	tr
Beef Instant Broth & Seasoning Pack	1 pkg (4.5 g)	5	0	0	tr
Beef Instant Broth & Seasoning Pack Low Sodium	1 pkg (4 g)	10	0	0	2

FOOD	PORTION	CALS	PROT	FAT	CARB
Chicken Bouillon	1 cube (4 g)	5	0	0	tr
Chicken Instant Bouillon Powder	1 tsp (4 g)	5	0	0	tr
Chicken Instant Broth & Seasoning Pack	1 pkg (4 g)	5	0	0	tr
Chicken Instant Broth & Seasoning Pack Low Sodium	1 pkg (4 g)	10	0	0	2
Vegetable Bouillon	1 cube (4 g)	5	0	0	tr
Hodgson Mill					
Choice Bean not prep	¼ cup (1.5 oz)	150	9	0	27
Hurst					
15 Bean Soup Beef	1 serv (6 oz)	120	8	1	20
15 Bean Soup Cajun	1 serv	120	8	1	20
15 Bean Soup Chicken	1 serv (6 oz)	120	8	1	20
15 Bean Soup Chili	1 serv (6 oz)	120	8	1	20
15 Bean Soup Ham	1 serv	120	8	1	20
HamBeens Great Northern Bean	1 serv	120	7	1	22
HamBeens Navy Bean	1 serv	120	8	1	21
Pasta Fagioli	1 serv	120	8	1	23
Spanish American Pinto Bean	1 serv	120	7	1	22
Spanish-American Black Bean	1 serv	120	7	1	22
Lipton					
Chicken Noodle w/ White Chicken Meat as prep	1 cup	80	3	2	11
Extra Noodle w/ Chicken Broth as prep	1 cup	90	3	2	15
Giggle Noodle w/ Chicken Broth as prep	1 cup	70	2	2	11
Recipe Secrets Beefy Mushroom	1½ tbsp (0.4 oz)	35	1	0	7
Recipe Secrets Beefy Onion	1 tbsp (0.3 oz)	25	1	1	5
Recipe Secrets Fiesta Herb w/ Red Pepper as prep	1 cup	30	1	0	6
Recipe Secrets Golden Onion	1⅔ tbsp (0.5 oz)	50	1	1	9
Recipe Secrets Onion as prep	1 cup	20	0	0	4
Recipe Secrets Onion Mushroom as prep	1 cup	30	1	1	5

FOOD	PORTION	CALS	PROT	FAT	CARB
Recipe Secrets Savory Herb w/ Garlic as prep	1 cup	30	1	0	6
Ring-O-Noodle w/ Chicken Broth as prep	1 cup	70	2	2	10
Soup Secrets Chicken 'N Onion as prep	1 cup	120	4	2	24
Soup Secrets Chicken w/ Pasta & Beans as prep	1 cup	110	5	2	19
Soup Secrets Country Chicken w/ Pasta & Herbs as prep	1 cup	100	4	2	18
Soup Secrets Homestyle Lentil w/ Bow Tie Pasta as prep	1 cup	130	7	1	22
Soup Secrets Minestrone as prep	1 cup	110	4	1	21
Spiral Pasta w/ Chicken Broth as prep	1 cup	60	2	1	11
Ramen Noodle					
Beef Low Fat as prep	1 pkg (2.2 oz)	216	6	1	45
Beef as prep	1 pkg (2.2 oz)	280	6	11	40
Chicken Low Fat as prep	1 pkg (2.2 oz)	216	7	1	44
Chicken as prep	1 pkg (2.2 oz)	279	6	11	40
Oriental Low Fat as prep	1 pkg (2.2 oz)	217	7	1	45
Shrimp Low Fat as prep	1 pkg (2.2 oz)	218	7	1	45
Shrimp as prep	1 pkg (2.2 oz)	294	6	13	39
Tomato as prep	1 pkg (2.2 oz)	295	6	13	39
Steero					
Beef Bouillon Cube	1 (3.5 g)	5	0	0	1
Beef Bouillon Cube Reduced Sodium	1 cube (3.5 oz)	5	0	0	1
Beef Bouillon Instant	1 tsp (3.5 oz)	5	0	0	1
Beef Bouillon Instant Reduced Sodium	1 tsp (3.5 oz)	5	0	0	1
Chicken Bouillon Cube	1 (3.5 g)	5	0	0	1
Chicken Bouillon Cube Reduced Sodium	1 (3.5 g)	5	0	0	1
Chicken Bouillon Instant	1 tsp (3.5 g)	5	0	0	1
Chicken Bouillon Instant Reduced Sodium	1 tsp (3.5 g)	5	0	0	1
Thai Kitchen					
Rice Noodle Bowl Roasted Garlic	1 bowl	170	3	2	35
Rice Noodle Bowl Spring Onion	1 bowl	170	3	2	35

FOOD	PORTION	CALS	PROT	FAT	CARB
Weight Watchers					
Instant Beef Broth	1 pkg (0.16 oz)	10	0	0	2
Instant Chicken Broth	1 pkg (0.16 oz)	10	0	0	2
Wyler's					
Beef Bouillon Cube	1 (3.5 g)	5	0	0	1
Beef Bouillon Cube Reduced Sodium	1 (3.5 g)	5	0	0	1
Beef Bouillon Instant	1 tsp (3.5 g)	5	0	0	1
Beef Bouillon Instant Reduced Sodium	1 tsp (3.5 g)	5	0	0	1
Chicken Bouillon Cube	1 (3.5 g)	5	0	0	1
Chicken Bouillon Cube Reduced Sodium	1 (3.5 g)	5	0	0	1
Chicken Bouillon Instant	1 tsp (3.5 g)	5	0	0	1
Chicken Bouillon Instant Reduced Sodium	1 tsp (3.5 g)	5	0	0	1
shelf-stable					
Hormel					
Micro Cup Bean & Ham	1 cup (7.5 oz)	190	9	4	29
Micro Cup Beef Vegetable	1 cup (7.5 oz)	90	6	1	15
Micro Cup Broccoli Cheese w/ Ham	1 cup (7.5 oz)	170	4	13	10
Micro Cup Chicken & Rice	1 cup (7.5 oz)	110	5	3	17
Micro Cup Chicken Noodle	1 cup (7.5 oz)	110	8	3	13
Micro Cup New England Clam Chowder	1 cup (7.5 oz)	130	5	5	17
Micro Cup Potato Cheese w/ Ham	1 cup (7.5 oz)	190	4	13	15
Lunch Bucket					
Chicken Noodle	1 pkg (7.25 oz)	80	2	2	13
Country Vegetable	1 pkg (7.25 oz)	60	1	1	14
TastyBite					
Tom Yum	½ pkg (5.3 oz)	92	2	7	6
take-out					
beef stew soup	1 cup (8.8 oz)	221	23	5	20
black bean turtle soup	1 cup	241	15	1	45
brunswick stew soup	1 cup (8.5 oz)	232	27	6	17
corn & cheese chowder	¾ cup	215	9	12	21
gazpacho	1 cup	46	1	tr	5
greek	¾ cup	63	4	2	7
hot & sour	1 serv (14 oz)	173	15	8	8
onion soup gratinee	1 serv	492	25	27	38
oxtail	5 oz	64	4	3	7
pasta e fagioli	1 cup (8.8 oz)	194	9	5	30
ratatouille	1 cup (7.5 oz)	266	2	25	12
vietnamese pho beef noodle	1 serv (7.8 oz)	480	15	12	78

FOOD	PORTION	CALS	PROT	FAT	CARB
SOUR CREAM					
sour cream	1 cup (8 oz)	493	7	48	10
Breakstone's					
Free	2 tbsp (1.1 oz)	35	2	0	6
Reduced Fat	2 tbsp (1.1 oz)	45	1	4	2
Knudsen					
Free	2 tbsp (1.1 oz)	35	2	0	6
Light	2 tbsp (1.1 oz)	50	2	3	2
Land O Lakes					
Fat Free	2 tbsp (1.1 oz)	25	2	0	4
Light	2 tbsp (1 oz)	40	1	3	3
SOUR CREAM SUBSTITUTES					
nondairy	1 cup	479	6	45	15
nondairy	1 oz	59	1	6	2
SOURSOP					
fresh	1	416	6	2	105
fresh cut up	1 cup	150	2	1	38
SOY					
(*see also* CHEESE SUBSTITUTES, ICE CREAM AND FROZEN DESSERTS, MILK SUBSTITUTES, MISO, SOY SAUCE, SOYBEANS, TEMPEH, TOFU, AND YOGURT FROZEN)					
lecithin	1 tbsp	104	0	14	0
soy milk	1 cup	79	7	5	4
soya cheese	1.4 oz	128	7	11	tr
I.M. Healthy					
SoyNut Butter Chocolate	2 tbsp (1.1 oz)	190	5	14	12
SoyNut Butter Honey Creamy	2 tbsp (1.1 oz)	170	7	11	12
SoyNut Butter Original Creamy	2 tbsp (1.1 oz)	170	8	11	10
SoyNut Butter Unsweetened Chunky	2 tbsp (1.1 oz)	160	7	13	5
SoyNut Butter Unsweetened Creamy	2 tbsp (1.1 oz)	160	7	13	5
Loma Linda					
Soyagen All Purpose	¼ cup (1 oz)	130	6	6	12
Soyagen Carob	¼ cup (1 oz)	130	6	6	13
Soyagen No Sucrose	¼ cup (1 oz)	130	6	6	12
Natural Touch					
Roasted Soy Butter	2 tbsp (1.1 oz)	170	6	11	10
Revival					
Chocolate Soy Nuts!	12–14 pieces (0.5 oz)	70	2	4	7
Soy Shake Plain as prep w/ water	1 pkg (1 oz)	110	20	2	2
Soy Shakes Chocolate Daydream Equal as prep w/ water	1 pkg (1.2 oz)	130	20	3	7

FOOD	PORTION	CALS	PROT	FAT	CARB
Soy Shakes Chocolate Daydream Unsweetened as prep w/ water	1 pkg (1.2 oz)	130	20	3	7
Soy Shakes Chocolate Daydreams as prep w/ water	1 pkg (2.2 oz)	240	20	3	36
Soy Shakes Vanilla Pleasures Equal as prep w/ water	1 pkg (1.2 oz)	120	20	2	6
Soy Shakes Vanilla Pleasures Unsweetened as prep w/ water	1 pkg (1.2 oz)	120	20	2	6
Soy Shakes Vanilla Pleasures as prep w/ water	1 pkg (2 oz)	220	20	2	31
Soy Wonder					
Creamy	2 tbsp	170	8	11	10
Crunchy	2 tbsp	170	8	11	10
SOY SAUCE					
shoyu	1 tbsp	9	1	tr	2
tamari	1 tbsp	11	2	tr	1
Chun King					
Lite	1 tbsp (0.5 oz)	15	2	tr	2
Soy Sauce	1 tbsp (0.6 oz)	11	2	tr	1
Eden					
Organic Shoyu Reduced Sodium	1 tbsp	10	2	0	2
Organic Tamari	1 tbsp	15	2	0	2
Ponzu Sauce	1 tbsp	5	0	0	1
Shoyu	1 tbsp	15	2	0	2
House Of Tsang					
Ginger Flavored	1 tbsp (0.6 oz)	20	1	0	4
Light	1 tbsp (0.6 oz)	5	1	0	0
Low Sodium	1 tbsp (0.6 oz)	5	0	0	0
Low Sodium Ginger	1 tbsp (0.6 oz)	10	0	0	2
Low Sodium Mushroom	1 tbsp (0.6 oz)	10	0	0	2
Just Rite					
Soy Sauce	1 tbsp (0.5 oz)	11	2	tr	1
Kikkoman					
Lite	1 tbsp (0.5 oz)	10	1	0	1
Soy Sauce	1 tbsp (0.5 oz)	10	2	0	0
La Choy					
Lite	1 tbsp (0.5 oz)	15	2	tr	2
Soy Sauce	1 tbsp (0.6 oz)	11	2	tr	1

FOOD	PORTION	CALS	PROT	FAT	CARB
Tree Of Life					
Shoyu	1 tbsp (0.5 oz)	15	2	0	1
Tamari Wheat Free	1 tbsp (0.5 oz)	15	2	0	1
SOYBEANS					
dried cooked	1 cup	298	29	15	17
dry roasted	½ cup	387	34	19	28
green cooked	½ cup	127	11	6	10
roasted	½ cup	405	30	22	29
roasted & toasted	1 oz	129	11	7	9
roasted & toasted	1 cup	490	40	26	33
roasted & toasted salted	1 oz	129	11	7	9
roasted & toasted salted	1 cup	490	40	26	33
sprouts raw	½ cup	43	5	2	3
sprouts steamed	½ cup	38	4	2	3
sprouts stir fried	1 cup	125	13	7	9
Dakota Gourmet					
Soy Nuts	1 oz	129	11	7	9
Eden					
Organic Black	½ cup (4.6 oz)	120	11	6	8
Seapoint Farms					
Edamame Organic	½ cup (2.6 oz)	100	8	3	9
Edamame In Pods frzn	½ cup (2.6 oz)	100	8	3	9
Edamame Rice Bowl Kung Pao Vegetable	1 pkg (12 oz)	420	15	6	72
Edamame Rice Bowl Szechwan Vegetables	1 pkg (12 oz)	420	13	4	80
Edamame Rice Bowl Teriyaki Vegetable	1 pkg (12 oz)	430	14	5	83
Edamame Rice Bowl Vegetable Fried Rice	1 pkg (11 oz)	220	11	6	31
Edamane Shelled	½ cup (2.6 oz)	100	8	3	9
SPAGHETTI					
(*see* PASTA, PASTA DINNERS, PASTA SALAD, SPAGHETTI SAUCE)					
SPAGHETTI SAUCE					
jarred					
marinara sauce	1 cup	171	4	8	25
spaghetti sauce	1 cup	272	12	12	40
Colavita					
Garden Style	½ cup (4.4 oz)	60	3	3	12
Del Monte					
Chunky Garlic & Herb	½ cup (4.4 oz)	60	2	2	11
Chunky Italian Herb	½ cup (4.4 oz)	60	2	1	12
Tomato & Basil	½ cup (4.4 oz)	70	2	1	16
Traditional	½ cup (4.4 oz)	60	2	1	15
With Garlic & Onion	½ cup (4.4 oz)	80	2	1	16
With Green Peppers & Mushrooms	½ cup (4.4 oz)	80	2	1	16
With Meat	½ cup (4.4 oz)	60	3	1	14

FOOD	PORTION	CALS	PROT	FAT	CARB
With Mushrooms	½ cup (4.4 oz)	60	2	1	14
Eden					
Organic Lightly Seasoned	½ cup (4.4 oz)	80	3	3	12
Francesco Rinaldi					
Alfredo	¼ cup (2.1 oz)	70	2	5	4
Chunky Garden Mushroom & Onion	½ cup (4.4 oz)	80	3	2	12
Chunky Garden Tomato Garlic & Onion	½ cup (4.4 oz)	80	3	2	12
Dolce Sweet & Tasty Tomato	½ cup (4.4 oz)	110	2	5	15
Dolce Three Cheese	½ cup (4.4 oz)	90	3	2	15
Dulce Super Mushroom	½ cup (4.4 oz)	110	3	5	15
Hearty Diavolo	½ cup (4.4 oz)	70	2	4	7
Hearty Mushroom Pepper & Onion	½ cup (4.4 oz)	80	3	3	10
Hearty Tomato & Basil	½ cup (4.4 oz)	80	2	3	11
Puttanesca	½ cup (4.3 oz)	70	2	4	8
Tomato Alfredo	¼ cup (2.1 oz)	60	2	4	4
Traditional Meat Flavored	½ cup (4.4 oz)	90	2	4	11
Traditional Mushroom	½ cup (4.4 oz)	90	2	4	11
Traditional No Salt Added	½ cup (4.4 oz)	70	2	3	10
Traditional Original	½ cup (4.4 oz)	90	2	4	11
Vodka Sauce	¼ cup (2.1 oz)	60	2	4	4
Healthy Choice					
Chunky Italian Vegetable	½ cup (4.4 oz)	40	2	tr	9
Chunky Mushroom	½ cup (4.4 oz)	42	2	tr	9
Garlic & Herbs	½ cup (4.4 oz)	49	2	tr	10
Garlic Lovers Garlic & Mushroom	½ cup (4.4 oz)	44	2	tr	10
Garlic Lovers Roasted Garlic	½ cup (4.4 oz)	52	2	tr	12
Garlic Lovers Roasted Garlic & Sun Dried Tomato	½ cup (4.4 oz)	52	2	tr	11
Super Chunky Mushroom & Sweet Peppers	½ cup (4.4 oz)	43	2	tr	9
Super Chunky Tomato Mushroom & Garlic	½ cup (4.4 oz)	45	2	tr	10
Super Chunky Vegetable Primavera	½ cup (4.4 oz)	43	2	tr	9
Traditional	½ cup (4.4 oz)	48	2	tr	11
With Mushrooms	½ cup (4.4 oz)	48	2	tr	11
Hunt's					
Angela Mia Marinara	¼ cup (2.2 oz)	24	1	1	4
Chunky	½ cup (4.4 oz)	38	1	1	8

FOOD	PORTION	CALS	PROT	FAT	CARB
Chunky Italian Sausage	½ cup (4.5 oz)	72	3	3	45
Chunky Italian Style Vegetable	½ cup (4.4 oz)	63	2	1	13
Chunky Marinara	½ cup (4.4 oz)	61	1	1	12
Chunky Tomato Garlic & Onion	½ cup (4.4 oz)	63	2	1	13
Classic Four Cheese	½ cup (4.4 oz)	50	3	1	9
Classic Garlic & Herb	½ cup (4.4 oz)	53	2	2	9
Classic Parmesan	½ cup (4.4 oz)	49	3	2	8
Classic Tomato & Basil	½ cup (4.4 oz)	48	2	1	9
Family Favorites Seasoned Diced Tomato Sauce	½ cup (4.3 oz)	50	2	1	11
Homestyle Meat Flavored	½ cup (4.4 oz)	51	2	2	9
Homestyle Mushrooms	½ cup (4.4 oz)	48	2	1	9
Homestyle Traditional	½ cup (4.4 oz)	49	2	1	9
Light Meat Flavored	½ cup (4.4 oz)	45	2	1	8
Light w/ Garlic & Herb	½ cup (4.5 oz)	40	2	1	7
Original Meat Flavored	½ cup (4.4 oz)	68	2	2	12
Original Traditional	½ cup (4.4 oz)	67	2	2	11
Original w/ Mushrooms	½ cup (4.4 oz)	62	2	2	11
Original w/ Italian Cheese & Garlic	½ cup (4.5 oz)	64	3	2	10
Tomato Bits	½ cup (4.5 oz)	49	2	tr	11
Traditional Light	½ cup (4.4 oz)	40	2	tr	7
Muir Glen					
Organic Balsamic Roasted Onion	½ cup (4.4 oz)	50	2	1	10
Organic Cabernet Marinara	½ cup (4.4 oz)	50	2	1	10
Organic Chunky Herb	½ cup (4.4 oz)	50	2	1	10
Organic Garden Vegetable	½ cup (4.4 oz)	50	2	1	10
Organic Garlic & Onion	½ cup (4.4 oz)	55	2	1	10
Organic Garlic Roasted Garlic	½ cup (4.4 oz)	50	2	1	10
Organic Green Olive	½ cup (4.4 oz)	60	2	2	10
Organic Italian Herb	½ cup (4.4 oz)	55	2	1	10
Organic Mushroom Marinara	½ cup (4.4 oz)	45	2	0	10
Organic Portabello Mushroom	½ cup (4.4 oz)	50	2	0	10
Organic Sun Dried Tomato	½ cup (4.4 oz)	55	2	1	10
Organic Tomato Basil	½ cup (4.4 oz)	50	2	1	12
Newman's Own					
Marinara Ventian	½ cup (4.4 oz)	60	2	2	9
Marinara Ventian w/ Mushrooms	½ cup (4.4 oz)	60	2	2	9
Pasta Sauce Bambolina	½ cup (4.5 oz)	100	1	5	15
Pasta Sauce Roasted Garlic & Red & Green Peppers	½ cup (4.7 oz)	70	2	3	11

FOOD	PORTION	CALS	PROT	FAT	CARB
Pasta Sauce Say Cheese	½ cup (4.4 oz)	90	3	3	14
Sockarooni	½ cup (4.4 oz)	60	2	2	9
Prego					
Pasta Bake Sauce Tomato Garlic & Basil	1 serv (3.4 oz)	80	1	4	11
Traditional	½ cup (4.2 oz)	140	2	5	23
Progresso					
Marinara	½ cup (4.3 oz)	80	2	5	8
Meat Flavored	½ cup (4.4 oz)	100	4	5	12
Sauce	½ cup (4.4 oz)	100	3	5	12
Ragu					
Chunky Garden Style Tomato Garlic & Onion	½ cup (4.5 oz)	110	2	3	18
Sara Lee					
Chunky Garden Mushroom & Peppers	½ cup (4.4 oz)	80	3	2	12
Tree Of Life					
Pasta Sauce	½ cup (4 oz)	50	2	2	9
Pasta Sauce Fat Free Classic	½ cup (3.9 oz)	40	2	0	8
Pasta Sauce Fat Free Mushroom & Basil	½ cup (3.9 oz)	30	1	0	7
Pasta Sauce Fat Free Onion & Garlic	½ cup (3.9 oz)	30	1	0	7
Pasta Sauce Fat Free Sweet Pepper	½ cup (3.9 oz)	30	1	0	7
Pasta Sauce No Salt Added	½ cup (3.9 oz)	50	2	2	9
mix					
Durkee					
Spaghetti Sauce as prep	½ cup	15	0	0	5
With Mushrooms as prep	½ cup	15	1	0	4
French's					
Italian as prep	½ cup	16	0	0	5
Mushroom as prep	½ cup	20	1	1	4
Thick as prep	½ cup	10	0	0	4
McCormick					
Pasta Rosa Blend	1 tbsp (10 g)	40	1	2	4
Primavera Pasta Blend	1 tbsp (7 g)	30	0	1	4
Spaghetti Sauce	1 tbsp (8 g)	25	0	0	5
refrigerated					
Di Giorno					
Alfredo	¼ cup (2.2 oz)	180	3	18	3
Basil Pesto	¼ cup (2.2 oz)	320	7	31	2
Four Cheese	¼ cup (2.2 oz)	160	5	15	3
Garlic Pesto	¼ cup (2.1 oz)	340	7	33	3
Light Alfredo Sauce	¼ cup (2.4 oz)	140	5	9	9
Marinara	½ cup (4.5 oz)	70	2	0	15
Plum Tomato Cream Sauce	½ cup (4.4 oz)	160	3	13	8

FOOD	PORTION	CALS	PROT	FAT	CARB
Plum Tomato & Mushroom	½ cup (4.4 oz)	60	2	0	13
Roasted Red Bell Pepper Cream Sauce	¼ cup (2.3 oz)	140	4	10	8
take-out					
bolognese	5 oz	195	11	15	4

SPANISH FOOD

(*see also* BEANS, CHIPS, CHILI, DINNER, PEPPERS, SALSA, SAUCE, SNACKS, TORTILLA)

FOOD	PORTION	CALS	PROT	FAT	CARB
canned					
Chi-Chi's					
Pico De Gallo	2 tbsp (1.2 oz)	10	0	0	2
Derby					
Tamales	3 (6.5 oz)	253	7	17	21
Gebhardt					
Enchiladas	2 (5.7 oz)	258	4	19	20
Tamales	2 (5.7 oz)	268	5	21	19
Tamales Jumbo	2 (6.9 oz)	332	6	25	24
Hormel					
Tamales Beef	3 (7.5 oz)	280	6	21	20
Tamales Chicken	3 (7.5 oz)	210	6	11	22
Tamales Hot Spicy Beef	3 (7.5 oz)	280	6	21	20
Tamales Jumbo Beef	2 (6.9 oz)	270	5	20	18
Rosarita					
Enchilada Sauce Mild	¼ cup (2.1 oz)	23	1	1	3
Van Camp					
Tamales	2 (5 oz)	210	5	13	20
frozen					
Amy's Organic					
Black Bean Vegetable Enchilada	1 (4.75 oz)	130	4	4	20
Burritos Bean & Cheese	1 (6 oz)	280	10	8	43
Burritos Bean & Rice Non-Dairy	1 (6 oz)	250	9	5	44
Burritos Black Bean Vegetable	1 (6 oz)	320	9	8	54
Burritos Breakfast	1 (6 oz)	230	9	5	38
Cheese Enchilada	1 (4.7 oz)	210	11	9	16
Mexican Tamale Pie	1 (8 oz)	220	10	3	41
Pocket Sandwich Tamale	1 (4.5 oz)	250	8	7	39
Whole Meals Cheese Enchilada	1 pkg (9 oz)	330	15	14	38
Whole Meals Enchilada	1 pkg (10 oz)	250	7	8	41
Banquet					
Chimichanga Meal	1 meal (9.5 oz)	500	13	24	56
Enchilada Beef	1 pkg (11 oz)	370	10	12	54
Enchilada Cheese	1 pkg (11 oz)	360	12	10	56
Enchilada Chicken	1 pkg (11 oz)	350	12	10	54
Enchilada Beef & Tamale Combo	1 pkg (11 oz)	450	10	20	50

FOOD	PORTION	CALS	PROT	FAT	CARB
Mexican Style Enchilada Combo	1 meal (11 oz)	360	10	11	55
Chi-Chi's					
Burro Beef	1 pkg (15.9 oz)	590	27	19	76
Burro Chicken	1 pkg (15.9 oz)	540	26	14	77
Chimichanga Beef	1 pkg (15.9 oz)	630	28	24	75
Chimichanga Chicken	1 pkg (15.9 oz)	580	25	19	78
Enchilada Chicken Suprema	1 pkg (15.9 oz)	600	26	20	80
Enchilida Baja	1 pkg (15.9 oz)	590	27	20	75
Health Is Wealth					
Burrito Munchees	10 (5 oz)	310	11	7	53
Mexican Munchees	2 (1 oz)	49	2	1	8
Healthy Choice					
Chicken Enchilada Supreme	1 meal (11.3 oz)	300	13	7	46
Chicken Enchiladas Suiz	1 meal (10 oz)	280	14	6	43
Chicken Breast Con Queso Burrito	1 meal (10.55 oz)	350	14	6	60
Lean Cuisine					
Everyday Favorites Chicken Enchilada Suiza	1 pkg (9 oz)	280	11	5	48
Patio					
Beef & Cheese Enchiladas Chili 'N Beans	1 meal (15.5 oz)	670	19	30	80
Beef Enchiladas Chili 'N Beans	1 meal (15.5 oz)	540	12	27	73
Burrito Bean & Cheese	1 (5 oz)	300	9	9	45
Burrito Beef & Bean Hot	1 (5 oz)	320	10	12	43
Burrito Beef & Bean Mild	1 (5 oz)	330	10	12	45
Burrito Chicken	1 (5 oz)	290	11	6	44
Burritos Beef & Bean Medium	1 (5 oz)	310	10	10	45
Burritos Beef & Bean Red Chili Pepper Red Hot	1 (5 oz)	320	10	12	42
Enchilada Beef	1 meal (12 oz)	320	12	12	52
Enchilada Cheese	1 meal (12 oz)	370	11	12	54
Enchilada Chicken	1 meal (12 oz)	400	13	12	60
Fiesta	1 meal (12 oz)	350	11	11	53
Mexican Style	1 meal (13.25 oz)	470	15	19	59
Stouffer's					
Chicken Enchilada	1 serv (4.8 oz)	230	7	11	25
Tyson					
Beef Fajita	3½ pieces (12.5 oz)	550	28	16	75
Chicken Fajita	3½ pieces (13.1 oz)	460	28	11	61
Weight Watchers					
Smart Ones Chicken Enchiladas Suiza	1 pkg (9 oz)	270	15	9	33

FOOD	PORTION	CALS	PROT	FAT	CARB
Smart Ones Santa Fe Style Rice & Beans	1 pkg (10 oz)	290	12	8	43
mix					
McCormick					
Fajitas Marinade Mix	2 tsp (4 g)	15	0	0	2
Taco Bell					
Home Originals Chicken Fajita Dinner as prep	2 (6.9 oz)	340	21	9	45
Home Originals Soft Taco Dinner as prep	2 (6.3 oz)	410	21	18	41
Home Originals Taco Dinner as prep	2 (4.4 oz)	280	16	15	19
Home Originals Ultimate Bean Burrito Dinner as prep	1 (4.4 oz)	200	6	5	34
Home Originals Ultimate Nachos as prep	12 pieces (4.6 oz)	240	6	11	31
ready-to-eat					
taco shell baked	1 med (0.5 oz)	61	1	3	8
taco shell baked w/o salt	1 med (½ oz)	61	1	3	8
Chi-Chi's					
Taco Shells White Corn	2 (1.2 oz)	170	3	8	22
Taco Shells Yellow Corn	2 shells (1.2 oz)	170	2	8	22
Gebhardt					
Taco Shells	3 (1.1 oz)	155	2	8	19
La Mexicana					
Flour Burritos	1 (1.6 oz)	160	4	5	26
Rosarita					
Taco Shells	3 (1.1 oz)	155	2	8	19
Tostada Shells	2 (1 oz)	125	2	5	17
Taco Bell					
Home Originals Taco Shells	3 (1.1 oz)	150	2	6	21
take-out					
burrito w/ apple	1 sm (2.6 oz)	231	3	10	35
burrito w/ apple	1 lg (5.4 oz)	484	5	20	73
burrito w/ beans	2 (7.6 oz)	448	14	14	71
burrito w/ beans & cheese	2 (6.5 oz)	377	15	12	55
burrito w/ beans & chili peppers	2 (7.2 oz)	413	16	15	58
burrito w/ beans & meat	2 (8.1 oz)	508	22	18	66
burrito w/ beans cheese & beef	2 (7.1 oz)	331	15	13	40
burrito w/ beans cheese & chili peppers	2 (11.8 oz)	663	33	23	85
burrito w/ beef	2 (7.7 oz)	523	27	21	59
burrito w/ beef & chili peppers	2 (7.1 oz)	426	22	17	49

FOOD	PORTION	CALS	PROT	FAT	CARB
burrito w/ beef cheese & chili peppers	2 (10.7 oz)	634	41	25	64
burrito w/ cherry	1 sm (2.6 oz)	231	3	10	35
burrito w/ cherry	1 lg (5.4 oz)	484	5	20	73
chimichanga w/ beef	1 (6.1 oz)	425	20	20	43
chimichanga w/ beef & cheese	1 (6.4 oz)	443	20	23	39
chimichanga w/ beef & red chili peppers	1 (6.7 oz)	424	18	19	46
chimichanga w/ beef cheese & red chili peppers	1 (6.3 oz)	364	15	18	38
enchilada w/ cheese	1 (5.7 oz)	320	10	19	29
enchilada w/ cheese & beef	1 (6.7 oz)	324	12	18	30
enchirito w/ cheese beef & beans	1 (6.8 oz)	344	18	16	34
frijoles w/ cheese	1 cup (5.9 oz)	226	11	8	29
nachos w/ cheese	6 to 8 (4 oz)	345	9	19	36
nachos w/ cheese & jalapeno peppers	6 to 8 (7.2 oz)	607	17	34	60
nachos w/ cheese beans ground beef & peppers	6 to 8 (8.9 oz)	568	20	31	56
nachos w/ cinnamon & sugar	6 to 8 (3.8 oz)	592	7	36	63
taco	1 sm (6 oz)	370	21	21	27
taco salad	1½ cups	279	13	15	24
taco salad w/ chili con carne	1½ cups	288	17	13	27
tostada w/ beans & cheese	1 (5.1 oz)	223	10	10	27
tostada w/ beans beef & cheese	1 (7.9 oz)	334	16	17	30
tostada w/ beef & cheese	1 (5.7 oz)	315	19	16	23
tostada w/ guacamole	2 (9.2 oz)	360	12	23	32

SPICES

(see individual names, HERBS/SPICES)

SPINACH

canned

spinach	½ cup	25	3	1	4
Del Monte					
Chopped	½ cup (4 oz)	30	2	0	4
No Salt Added	½ cup (4 oz)	30	2	0	4
Whole Leaf	½ cup (4 oz)	30	2	0	4
S&W					
Spinach	½ cup (4.5 oz)	30	3	0	4
fresh					
cooked	½ cup	21	3	tr	3
malabar cooked	1 cup (1.5 oz)	10	1	tr	1
mustard chopped cooked	½ cup	14	2	tr	3

FOOD	PORTION	CALS	PROT	FAT	CARB
mustard raw chopped	½ cup	17	2	tr	3
new zealand chopped cooked	½ cup	11	1	tr	2
raw chopped	½ cup	6	1	tr	1
Dole					
Baby Spinach	3½ cups (3 oz)	35	2	0	9
frozen					
cooked	½ cup	27	3	tr	5
Amy's Organic					
Pocket Sandwich Spinach Feta	1 (4.5 oz)	200	9	7	27
Birds Eye					
Creamed	½ cup (4.3 oz)	100	3	7	7
Cut Leaf	1 cup (2.8 oz)	20	2	0	2
Green Giant					
Butter Sauce	½ cup (3.4 oz)	40	2	2	5
Creamed	½ cup (3.8 oz)	80	4	3	10
Cut Leaf	¾ cup (2.6 oz)	25	3	0	3
Harvest Fresh	½ cup (3.5 oz)	25	3	0	3
Health Is Wealth					
Spinach Munchees	2 (1 oz)	60	2	3	9
Spinach Feta Munchees	2 (1 oz)	70	2	3	9
Stouffer's					
Creamed	1 serv (4.5 oz)	160	4	12	8
Souffle	1 serv (4 oz)	150	6	10	9
Tree Of Life					
Organic	1 cup (3 oz)	20	2	0	2
shelf-stable					
TastyBite					
Kashmir Spinach	½ pkg (5 oz)	170	10	10	8
take-out					
indian saag	1 serv	28	2	2	2
spanakopita spinach pie	1 cup (6 oz)	196	14	3	35
SPINACH JUICE					
juice	7 oz	14	2	0	2
SPORTS DRINKS					
(*see* ENERGY DRINKS)					
SPOT					
baked	3 oz	134	20	5	0
SPROUTS					
kidney bean	½ cup	27	4	tr	4
kidney bean cooked	1 lb	152	22	3	21
lentil sprouts	½ cup	40	3	tr	8
mung bean	½ cup	16	2	tr	3
mung bean canned	½ cup	8	1	tr	1
mung bean cooked	½ cup	13	1	tr	3
pea	½ cup	77	5	tr	17
radish	½ cup	8	1	tr	1

FOOD	PORTION	CALS	PROT	FAT	CARB
Chun King					
Bean Sprouts	1 cup (3 oz)	11	1	tr	1
Fresh Alternatives					
BroccoSprouts	½ cup (1 oz)	10	1	0	1
Deli Blend	½ cup (1 oz)	10	1	0	1
Salad Blend	½ cup (1 oz)	10	1	0	2
Sandwich Blend	½ cup (1 oz)	5	1	0	1
La Choy					
Bean Sprouts	1 cup (2.9 oz)	11	1	tr	1
take-out					
mung bean stir fried	½ cup	31	3	tr	7
SQUAB					
boneless baked	3.5 oz	175	37	3	0
breast w/o skin raw	1 (3.5 oz)	135	22	5	0
w/o skin raw	1 squab (5.9 oz)	239	29	13	0
SQUASH					
(*see also* ZUCCHINI)					
seeds dried	1 oz	154	7	13	5
seeds whole roasted	1 oz	127	5	6	15
canned					
crookneck sliced	½ cup	14	1	tr	3
fresh					
acorn cooked mashed	½ cup	41	1	tr	11
acorn cubed baked	½ cup	57	1	tr	15
butternut baked	½ cup	41	1	tr	11
crookneck raw sliced	½ cup	12	1	tr	3
crookneck sliced cooked	½ cup	18	1	tr	4
hubbard baked	½ cup	51	3	tr	11
hubbard cooked mashed	½ cup	35	2	tr	8
scallop raw sliced	½ cup	12	1	tr	3
scallop sliced cooked	½ cup	14	1	tr	3
spaghetti cooked	½ cup	23	1	tr	5
frozen					
butternut cooked mashed	½ cup	47	1	tr	12
crookneck sliced cooked	½ cup	24	1	tr	5
seeds					
dried	1 cup	747	34	63	25
roasted	1 cup	1184	75	96	31
roasted	1 oz	148	9	12	4
salted & roasted	1 oz	148	9	12	4
salted & roasted	1 cup	1184	75	96	31
whole roasted	1 cup	285	12	12	34
whole salted roasted	1 cup	285	12	12	34
whole salted roasted	1 oz	127	6	6	15
SQUID					
fried	3 oz	149	15	6	7
SQUIRREL					
roasted	3 oz	147	26	4	0

FOOD	PORTION	CALS	PROT	FAT	CARB
STARFRUIT					
fresh	1	42	1	tr	10
STRAWBERRIES					
canned					
in heavy syrup	½ cup	117	1	tr	30
fresh					
strawberries	1 cup	45	1	1	10
strawberries	1 pint	97	2	1	22
frozen					
sweetened sliced	1 cup	245	1	tr	66
sweetened sliced	1 pkg (10 oz)	273	2	tr	74
unsweetened	1 cup	52	1	tr	14
whole sweetened	1 cup	200	1	tr	54
whole sweetened	1 pkg (10 oz)	223	1	tr	60
Birds Eye					
In Syrup	½ cup (4.7 oz)	120	1	0	31
Lite Syrup	1 pkg (10 oz)	120	1	0	31
Tree Of Life					
Organic	¾ cup (5 oz)	50	1	0	13
STRAWBERRY JUICE					
Capri Sun					
Strawberry Cooler Drink	1 pkg (7 oz)	90	0	0	25
Kool-Aid					
Drink as prep w/ sugar	1 serv (8 oz)	100	0	0	25
Drink Mix as prep	1 serv (8 oz)	60	0	0	16
Veryfine					
Juice-Ups	8 fl oz	140	0	0	36
STUFFING/DRESSING					
bread as prep w/ water & fat	½ cup	251	5	15	25
bread as prep w/ water egg & fat	½ cup	107	3	7	9
bread dry as prep	½ cup	178	3	9	22
cornbread as prep	½ cup	179	3	9	22
Kellogg's					
Croutettes Mix	1 cup (1.2 oz)	120	5	0	25
Pepperidge Farm					
Corn Bread	¾ cup (1.5 oz)	170	4	2	33
Herb Seasoned	¾ cup (1.5 oz)	170	5	2	33
Herb Seasoned Cubed	¾ cup (1.3 oz)	140	4	2	28
One Step Chicken	½ cup (1.2 oz)	140	4	4	23
One Step Southwestern Corn Bread	½ cup (1.2 oz)	150	4	5	23
One Step Turkey	½ cup (1.2 oz)	150	4	5	22
Stove Top					
Chicken as prep w/ margarine	½ cup (3.6 oz)	170	4	9	20

FOOD	PORTION	CALS	PROT	FAT	CARB
Cornbread as prep w/ margarine	½ cup (3.6 oz)	170	3	8	21
Flexible Serve Chicken as prep w/ margarine	½ cup (3.3 oz)	170	3	8	19
Flexible Serve Cornbread as prep w/ margarine	½ cup (3.3 oz)	160	3	8	19
Flexible Serve Homestyle Herb as prep w/ margarine	½ cup (3.3 oz)	170	3	8	19
For Beef as prep w/ margarine	½ cup (3.7 oz)	180	4	9	22
For Pork as prep w/ margarine	½ cup (3.6 oz)	170	4	9	20
For Turkey as prep w/ margarine	½ cup (3.6 oz)	170	4	9	20
Long Grain & Wild Rice as prep w/ margarine	½ cup (3.7 oz)	180	4	9	22
Lower Sodium Chicken as prep w/ margarine	½ cup (3.6 oz)	180	4	9	21
Microwave Chicken as prep w/ margarine	½ cup (3.5 oz)	160	4	7	20
Microwave Homestyle Cornbread as prep w/ margarine	½ cup (3 oz)	160	3	7	20
Mushroom & Onion as prep w/ margarine	½ cup (3.6 oz)	180	4	9	20
San Francisco Style as prep w/ margarine	½ cup (3.6 oz)	170	4	9	20
Savory Herb as prep w/ margarine	½ cup (3.6 oz)	170	4	9	20
Traditional Sage as prep w/ margarine	½ cup (3.6 oz)	180	4	9	21
take-out					
bread	½ cup (3½ oz)	195	4	8	26
sausage	½ cup	292	8	11	40
STURGEON					
cooked	3 oz	115	18	4	0
roe raw	1 oz	59	7	3	tr
smoked	1 oz	48	9	1	0
smoked	3 oz	147	27	4	0
SUCKER					
white baked	3 oz	101	18	3	0
SUGAR					
brown packed	1 cup (7.7 oz)	828	0	0	214
brown unpacked	1 cup (5.1 oz)	546	0	0	141
maple	1 piece (1 oz)	100	0	tr	26
powdered	1 tbsp (0.3 oz)	31	0	0	8

FOOD	PORTION	CALS	PROT	FAT	CARB
sugarcane stem	3 oz	54	1	0	14
white	1 cup (7 oz)	773	0	0	200
white	1 tbsp	45	0	0	12
white	1 packet (6 g)	25	0	0	6
white	1 tsp (4 g)	15	0	0	4
Domino					
Dark Brown	1 tsp	15	0	0	4
White	1 tsp	16	0	0	4
Maui Brand					
Raw Sugar	1 tsp	15	0	0	4
SUGAR SUBSTITUTES					
(*see also* FRUCTOSE)					
Weight Watchers					
Sweetener	1 serv (1 g)	5	0	0	1
SUGAR-APPLE					
fresh	1	146	3	tr	37
fresh cut up	1 cup	236	5	1	59
SUNCHOKE					
fresh raw sliced	½ cup	57	2	tr	13
SUNFISH					
pumpkinseed baked	3 oz	97	21	1	0
SUNFLOWER					
seeds dried	1 oz	162	33	14	5
seeds dried	1 cup	821	33	71	27
seeds dry roasted	1 oz	165	5	14	7
seeds dry roasted	1 cup	745	25	64	31
seeds dry roasted salted	1 cup	745	25	64	31
seeds dry roasted salted	1 oz	165	5	14	7
seeds oil roasted	1 cup	830	29	78	20
seeds oil roasted salted	1 oz	175	6	16	4
seeds oil roasted salted	1 cup	830	29	78	20
seeds toasted	1 oz	176	5	16	6
seeds toasted	1 cup	826	23	76	28
seeds toasted salted	1 oz	176	5	16	6
seeds toasted salted	1 cup	826	23	76	28
sunflower butter	1 tbsp	93	3	8	4
sunflower butter w/o salt	1 tbsp	93	3	8	4
Dakota Gourmet					
Honey Roasted Kernels	1 pkg (1 oz)	158	6	12	8
Lightly Salted Kernels	1 pkg (1 oz)	168	6	14	5
Frito Lay					
Seeds	1 oz	180	7	15	5
Lance					
Seeds In Shell	⅔ cup (1.8 oz)	160	6	13	5
Seeds Roasted & Shelled	1 pkg (1⅛ oz)	190	7	16	6
SUSHI					
take-out					
california roll	1 piece (0.8 oz)	28	1	1	4

FOOD	PORTION	CALS	PROT	FAT	CARB
sashimi	1 serv (6 oz)	198	24	7	4
tuna roll	1 piece (0.7 oz)	23	2	tr	3
vegetable roll	1 piece (1.2 oz)	27	1	1	5
vinegared ginger	⅓ cup (1.6 oz)	48	1	tr	12
yellowtail roll	1 piece (0.6 oz)	25	1	1	3
SWAMP CABBAGE					
chopped cooked	½ cup	10	1	tr	2
raw chopped	1 cup	11	1	tr	2
SWEET POTATO					
(*see also* YAM)					
canned					
in syrup	½ cup	106	1	tr	25
pieces	1 cup	183	3	tr	42
fresh					
baked w/ skin	1 (3½ oz)	118	2	tr	28
leaves cooked	½ cup	11	1	tr	2
mashed	½ cup	172	3	tr	40
frozen					
cooked	½ cup	88	2	tr	21
take-out					
candied	3½ oz	144	1	3	29
SWEETBREADS					
beef braised	3 oz	230	23	15	0
lamb braised	3 oz	199	19	13	0
veal braised	3 oz	218	25	12	0
SWISS CHARD					
cooked	½ cup	18	2	tr	4
SWORDFISH					
cooked	3 oz	132	22	4	0
SYRUP					
corn	2 tbsp	122	0	0	32
corn dark	1 tbsp (0.7 oz)	56	0	0	15
corn dark	1 cup (11.5 oz)	925	0	tr	251
corn light	1 cup (11.5 oz)	925	0	tr	251
corn light	1 tbsp (0.7 oz)	56	0	0	15
malt	1 tbsp (0.8 oz)	76	2	0	17
malt	1 cup (13 oz)	1222	24	tr	274
maple	1 tbsp (0.8 oz)	52	0	0	13
rose hip	1 oz	9	0	0	2
sorghum	1 cup (11.6 oz)	957	0	0	247
sorghum	1 tbsp (0.7 oz)	61	0	0	16
Eden					
Organic Barley Malt	1 tbsp	60	1	0	14
Estee					
Blueberry	¼ cup	80	0	0	20
Hershey					
Strawberry	2 tbsp (1.4 oz)	100	0	0	26

FOOD	PORTION	CALS	PROT	FAT	CARB
Karo					
Corn Syrup Light	2 tbsp (1 oz)	120	0	0	31
Quik					
Strawberry	2 tbsp (1.5 oz)	110	0	0	27
Smucker's					
Apricot	¼ cup	210	0	0	52
Blackberry	¼ cup	210	0	0	52
Plate Scapers Kiwi Lime	2 tbsp (1.3 oz)	100	0	0	25
Plate Scapers Mango Orange	2 tbsp	100	0	0	24
Plate Scapers Raspberry	2 tbsp (1.3 oz)	100	0	0	25
TAHINI					
(*see* SESAME)					
TAMARIND					
fresh cut up	1 cup	287	3	1	75
TANGERINE					
canned					
in light syrup	½ cup	76	1	tr	20
juice pack	½ cup	46	1	tr	12
fresh					
sections	1 cup	86	1	tr	22
tangerine	1	37	1	tr	9
Chiquita					
Tangerine	1 med (3.5 oz)	50	1	1	15
TANGERINE JUICE					
canned sweetened	1 cup	125	1	1	30
fresh	1 cup	106	1	tr	25
frzn sweetened as prep	1 cup	110	1	tr	27
frzn sweetened not prep	6 oz	344	3	1	83
Fresh Samantha					
Fresh Juice	1 cup (8 oz)	110	2	0	8
TAPIOCA					
starch	1 oz	98	17	tr	24
Minute					
Minute Tapioca	1½ tsp (6 g)	20	0	0	5
TARO					
chips	10 (0.8 oz)	115	1	6	16
chips	1 oz	141	1	7	19
leaves cooked	½ cup	18	2	tr	3
shoots sliced cooked	½ cup	10	1	tr	2
tahitian sliced cooked	½ cup	30	3	tr	5
TARPON					
fresh	3 oz	87	17	2	0
TEA/HERBAL TEA					
(*see also* ICED TEA)					
herbal					
Celestial Seasonings					
Mandarin Orange Spice	1 tea bag	0	0	0	tr

FOOD	PORTION	CALS	PROT	FAT	CARB
Eden					
Organic Genmaicha Tea	1 cup	0	0	0	0
Organic Kukicha Tea	1 cup	0	0	0	0
Lipton					
Bedtime Story	1 tea bag	0	0	0	1
Cinnamon Apple	1 tea bag	0	0	0	1
Ginger Twist	1 tea bag	0	0	0	0
Lemon	1 tea bag	0	0	0	1
Orange	1 tea bag	0	0	0	1
Peppermint	1 tea bag	0	0	0	1
Quietly Chamomile	1 tea bag	0	0	0	1
Silk					
Chai	1 cup	140	6	4	19
regular					
brewed tea	6 oz	2	0	0	tr
Activitea					
Green Tea	1 cup	36	0	0	3
General Foods					
International Instant Tea Decaffeinated English Breakfast Creme	1 serv (8 oz)	70	0	2	13
International Instant Tea Decaffeinated Viennese Cinnamon Creme	1 serv (8 oz)	70	0	2	13
International Instant Tea English Breakfast Creme as prep	1 serv (8 oz)	70	0	2	13
International Instant Tea English Raspberry Creme as prep	1 serv (8 oz)	70	0	2	13
International Instant Tea Island Orange Creme as prep	1 serv (8 oz)	70	0	2	13
International Instant Tea Viennese Cinnamon Creme as prep	1 serv (8 oz)	70	0	2	13
Lipton					
Brisk Tea as prep	1 serv	0	0	0	0
Decaffeinated Brisk Tea as prep	1 serv	0	0	0	0
English Blend as prep	1 cup	0	0	0	0
Flavored Decaffeinated Orange & Spice	1 tea bag	0	0	0	0
Green Tea	1 tea bag	0	0	0	0
Loose Tea	1 tsp (2 g)	0	0	0	0
Paradise					
Tropical Tea	8 fl oz	1	0	0	tr

FOOD	PORTION	CALS	PROT	FAT	CARB
Tropical Tea Decafe	8 fl oz	1	0	0	tr
Tropical Tea Passion Fruit	8 fl oz	1	0	0	tr
Salada					
Green Tea	1 cup	0	0	0	0
Green Tea Decaffeinated	1 tea bag	0	0	0	0
Tetley					
British Blend Round Teabags	1 cup	0	0	0	0
Decaffeinated	1 tea bag	0	0	0	0
Tea Bag as prep	1	0	0	0	0
TEMPEH					
tempeh	½ cup	165	16	6	14
Lightlife					
Garden Vege	4 oz	200	21	8	12
Quinoa Sesame	4 oz	220	21	8	15
Smokey Strips	3 slices (2 oz)	80	8	3	6
Soy	4 oz	210	24	8	11
Three Grain	4 oz	200	20	7	13
Wild Rice	4 oz	190	19	7	13
Turtle Island					
Five Grain	3 oz	190	11	6	20
Low Fat Millet	3 oz	130	8	2	20
Soy	3 oz	160	13	4	20
Wild Rice Rhapsody	3 oz	160	13	4	20
White Wave					
Five Grain	⅓ block	140	12	4	15
Organic Original Soy	⅓ block	150	16	6	10
Organic Sea Veggie	⅓ block	120	12	3	11
Soy Rice	⅓ block	140	12	5	13
TILEFISH					
cooked	½ fillet (5.3 oz)	220	37	7	0
cooked	3 oz	125	21	4	0
TOFU					
firm	¼ block (3 oz)	118	13	7	3
firm	½ cup	183	20	11	5
fresh fried	1 piece (0.5 oz)	35	2	3	1
fuyu salted & fermented	1 block (⅓ oz)	13	1	1	1
koyadofu dried frozen	1 piece (½ oz)	82	8	5	2
okara	½ cup	47	2	1	8
regular	¼ block (4 oz)	88	9	6	2
regular	½ cup	94	6	6	2
Azumaya					
Baked Chili Picante	2 pieces	200	20	10	9
Baked Mesquite	2 pieces	100	20	10	6
Baked Spicy Thai Peanut	2 pieces	190	20	10	6
Baked Teriyaki	2 pieces	200	20	10	9
Extra Firm	1 serv (2.8 oz)	70	8	4	2
Firm	1 serv (2.8 oz)	70	7	4	2

FOOD	PORTION	CALS	PROT	FAT	CARB
Lite Extra Firm	1 serv (2.8 oz)	60	8	2	3
Lite Silken	1 serv (3.2 oz)	40	5	1	3
Silken	1 serv (3.2 oz)	40	4	2	1
Galaxy					
Slices Hickory Smoked	1 slice (1 oz)	50	2	2	5
Slices Italian Garlic Herb	1 slice (1 oz)	50	2	2	5
Slices Original	1 slice (1 oz)	50	2	2	5
Slices Savory	1 slice (1 oz)	50	2	2	5
Hinoichi					
Firm	1 inch slice (3 oz)	60	6	3	2
Long Life					
Tofu	3 oz	60	6	3	2
Nasoya					
5 Spice	1 serv (3 oz)	70	7	4	0
Baked Mesquite Smoke	2 pieces	220	21	9	17
Baked Teriyaki	2 pieces	230	20	9	21
Baked TexMex	2 pieces	230	21	9	21
Baked Thai Peanut	2 pieces	240	21	10	19
Extra Firm	1 serv (3 oz)	90	8	5	3
Firm	1 serv (3 oz)	70	7	4	2
Firm Enriched	1 serv (3 oz)	45	7	1	0
Garlic & Onion	1 serv (3 oz)	70	7	4	1
Silken	1 serv (3.2 oz)	45	4	3	2
Soft	1 serv (3 oz)	60	7	4	1
TofuMate Breakfast Scramble	¼ pkg	15	1	0	3
TofuMate Eggless Salad	¼ pkg	15	0	0	4
TofuMate Mandarin Stirfry	¼ pkg	30	1	0	6
TofuMate Mediterranean Herb	¼ pkg	15	1	0	3
TofuMate Szechwan StirFry	¼ pkg	25	1	0	4
TofuMate Texas Taco	¼ pkg	15	1	0	3
Tree Of Life					
30% Reduced Fat Firm	⅕ block (3.2 oz)	90	10	4	4
Easymeal Pasta Primavera as prep	1 serv	460	20	16	54
Easymeal Southwest Medley as prep	1 serv	380	15	14	44
Easymeal Teriyaki Stir Fry as prep	1 serv	270	13	14	24
Easymeal Thai Stir Fry as prep	1 serv	270	14	14	21
Organic Baked	⅓ block (2.7 oz)	150	16	8	5
Organic Baked Island Spice	⅓ pkg (2.7 oz)	130	15	7	3
Organic Baked Oriental	⅓ pkg (2.7 oz)	130	15	7	5

FOOD	PORTION	CALS	PROT	FAT	CARB
Organic Baked Savory	⅓ block (2.7 oz)	140	15	7	4
Organic Firm	⅕ block (3.2 oz)	100	9	5	2
Raw Firm	⅕ block (3.2 oz)	100	9	5	2
White Wave					
Baked Garlic Herb Italian	1 piece	120	13	6	3
Baked Hickory Smoke BBQ	1 piece	75	8	3	4
Baked Roma Italian Basil	1 piece	100	8	6	3
Baked Thai Style	1 piece	120	13	6	3
Baked Zesty Lemon Pepper	1 piece	120	8	8	3
Extra Firm	¼ block	80	10	5	1
Organic Extra Firm	⅕ block	90	10	6	1
Organic Soft	⅕ block	90	10	6	1
Reduced Fat	⅕ block	90	10	4	4
TOMATILLO					
fresh chopped	½ cup	21	1	1	4
TOMATO					
canned					
paste	½ cup	110	5	1	25
puree	1 cup	102	4	tr	25
puree w/o salt	1 cup	102	4	tr	25
red whole	½ cup	24	1	tr	5
sauce	½ cup	37	2	tr	9
sauce spanish style	½ cup	40	2	tr	9
sauce w/ mushrooms	½ cup	42	2	tr	10
sauce w/ onion	½ cup	52	1	tr	12
stewed	½ cup	34	1	tr	8
w/ green chiles	½ cup	18	1	tr	4
wedges in tomato juice	½ cup	34	1	tr	8
Amore					
Sun-Dried Tomato Paste	1 tsp (6 g)	15	0	1	tr
Big R					
Cajun Stewed	½ cup (4.2 oz)	25	1	0	4
Diced w/ Chilies	½ cup (4.2 oz)	25	1	0	4
Mexican Stewed	½ cups (4.2 oz)	25	1	0	5
Stewed	½ cup (4.2 oz)	25	1	0	5
Whole	½ cup (4.2 oz)	25	1	0	5
Claussen					
Halves	1 serv (1 oz)	5	0	0	1
Contadina					
Paste	2 tbsp (1.2 oz)	30	2	0	6
Recipe Ready Diced Roasted Garlic	½ cup (4.3 oz)	45	1	0	10
Del Monte					
Chunky Chili Style	½ cup (4.5 oz)	30	1	0	8
Chunky Pasta Style	½ cup (4.5 oz)	45	1	0	11
Crushed Italian Recipe	½ cup (4.4 oz)	45	2	0	9
Crushed Original Recipe	½ cup (4.4 oz)	45	2	0	9

FOOD	PORTION	CALS	PROT	FAT	CARB
Crushed w/ Garlic	½ cup (4.4 oz)	50	2	0	11
Diced	½ cup (4.4 oz)	25	1	0	6
Diced No Salt Added	½ cup (4.4 oz)	25	1	0	6
Diced w/ Basil Garlic & Oregano	½ cup (4.4 oz)	50	2	0	11
Diced w/ Garlic & Onion	½ cup (4.4 oz)	40	2	1	8
Diced w/ Green Pepper & Onion	½ cup (4.4 oz)	40	1	0	9
Paste	2 tbsp (1.2 oz)	30	1	0	7
Sauce	¼ cup (2.1 oz)	20	1	0	4
Sauce No Salt Added	¼ cup (2.1 oz)	20	0	0	4
Stewed Cajun Recipe	½ cup (4.4 oz)	35	1	0	9
Stewed Italian Recipe	½ cup (4.4 oz)	30	1	0	8
Stewed Mexican Recipe	½ cup (4.4 oz)	35	1	0	9
Stewed Original	½ cup (4.4 oz)	35	1	0	9
Stewed Original No Salt Added	½ cup (4.4 oz)	35	1	0	9
Wedges	½ cup (4.4 oz)	35	1	0	9
Zesty Diced w/ Mild Green Chilies	½ cup (4.4 oz)	30	1	0	6
Eden					
Organic Diced	½ cup	30	1	0	6
Organic Diced w/ Green Chilies	½ cup	30	2	0	5
Hunt's					
Angela Mia Puree	¼ cup (2.2 oz)	16	1	tr	3
Choice Cut	½ cup (4.2 oz)	23	1	tr	5
Choice Cut Diced Tomatoes & Italian Herb	½ cup (4.2 oz)	24	1	0	5
Choice Cut Diced Tomatoes & Roasted Garlic	½ cup (4.2 oz)	24	1	0	5
Choice Cut Diced Tomatoes w/ Red Pepper & Basil	¼ cup (4.2 oz)	27	1	tr	6
Crushed Pear Tomatoes	½ cup (4.2 oz)	29	1	tr	7
Diced In Juice	½ cup (4.2 oz)	20	1	tr	4
Diced In Puree	½ cup (4.3 oz)	23	1	tr	5
Paste	2 tbsp (1.2 oz)	30	1	tr	6
Paste Italian	2 tbsp (1.2 oz)	27	1	tr	6
Paste No Salt Added	2 tbsp (1.2 oz)	30	1	tr	6
Paste w/ Garlic	2 tbsp (1.2 oz)	28	2	tr	6
Puree	¼ cup (2.2 oz)	24	1	tr	5
Ready Sauce Chunky Chili	¼ cup (2.2 oz)	22	1	tr	4
Ready Sauce Chunky Italian	¼ cup (2.2 oz)	30	1	1	4

FOOD	PORTION	CALS	PROT	FAT	CARB
Ready Sauce Chunky Mexican	¼ cup (2.2 oz)	21	1	tr	4
Ready Sauce Chunky Salsa	¼ cup (2.2 oz)	18	1	tr	3
Ready Sauce Chunky Tomato	¼ cup (2.2 oz)	15	1	tr	3
Ready Sauce Garlic & Herb	¼ cup (2.2 oz)	26	1	tr	5
Sauce	¼ cup (2.2 oz)	16	1	tr	3
Sauce Herb	¼ cup (2.2 oz)	32	1	1	5
Sauce Italian	¼ cup (2.2 oz)	32	1	1	5
Sauce Meatloaf Fixins	¼ cup (2.2 oz)	23	1	tr	4
Sauce No Salt Added	¼ cup (2.2 oz)	16	1	tr	3
Sauce Special	¼ cup (2.2 oz)	21	1	1	4
Stewed	½ cup (4.2 oz)	33	1	tr	7
Stewed No Salt Added	½ cup (4.2 oz)	33	1	tr	7
Whole Peeled	2 (5.2 oz)	24	2	tr	5
Whole Peeled No Salt Added	2 (4.8 oz)	21	2	tr	4
Muir Glen					
Diced Fire Roasted	¼ cup	30	1	0	6
Diced w/ Green Chilies	½ cup (4.5 oz)	25	1	0	4
Organic Crushed Fire Roasted	¼ cup	20	1	0	5
Organic Diced	½ cup (4.5 oz)	25	1	0	4
Organic Diced No Salt Added	½ cup (4.5 oz)	25	1	0	4
Organic Diced w/ Basil & Garlic	½ cup (4.5 oz)	25	1	0	4
Organic Diced w/ Italian Herbs	½ cup (4.4 oz)	25	1	0	4
Organic Paste	2 tbsp (1.2 oz)	30	2	0	6
Organic Puree	¼ cup (2.2 oz)	20	1	0	5
Organic Stewed	½ cup (4.5 oz)	30	1	0	7
Organic Whole Peeled	½ cup (4.6 oz)	30	1	0	5
Whole Peeled w/ Basil	½ cup (4.6 oz)	30	1	0	5
Progresso					
Crushed	¼ cup (2.1 oz)	20	1	0	4
Italian Style Peeled	½ cup (4.2 oz)	20	1	0	4
Paste	2 tbsp (1.2 oz)	30	2	0	6
Puree	¼ cup (2.2 oz)	25	1	0	5
Sauce	¼ cup (2.1 oz)	20	1	0	4
Whole Peeled	½ cup (4.2 oz)	25	1	0	5
Red Pack					
Puree	¼ cup (2.2 oz)	25	1	0	5
dried					
sun dried	1 cup	140	8	2	30

FOOD	PORTION	CALS	PROT	FAT	CARB
sun-dried in oil	1 cup (4 oz)	235	6	15	26
sun-dried	5 pieces (0.5 oz)	40	2	0	7
fresh					
cooked	½ cup	32	1	1	7
green	1	30	1	tr	6
red	1 (4.5 oz)	26	1	tr	6
red chopped	1 cup	35	2	tr	8
Chiquita					
Tomato	1 med (5.2 oz)	35	1	1	7
take-out					
stewed	1 cup	80	2	3	13
TOMATO JUICE					
beef broth & tomato	5½ oz	61	1	tr	14
clam & tomato	1 can (5½ oz)	77	1	tr	18
tomato juice	6 oz	32	1	tr	8
tomato juice	½ cup	21	1	tr	5
Campbell					
Juice	8 oz	51	2	1	10
Del Monte					
Juice	8 fl oz	50	2	0	10
Snap-E-Tom Chile Cocktail	6 fl oz	40	2	0	8
Dole					
Juice	1 bottle (12 oz)	85	4	0	17
Hunt's					
Juice	1 can (6 oz)	22	1	tr	5
No Salt Added	8 fl oz	34	2	tr	8
Mott's					
Tomato Juice	8 fl oz	40	2	0	9
Muir Glen					
Organic	5.5 oz	40	1	0	8
TONGUE					
beef simmered	3 oz	241	19	18	tr
lamb braised	3 oz	234	18	17	0
pork braised	3 oz	230	20	16	0
TORTILLA					
corn	1 (6 in diam)	56	1	1	12
corn w/o salt	1 (6 in diam, 0.9 oz)	56	1	1	12
flour w/o salt	1 (8 in diam, 1.2 oz)	114	3	3	20
La Mexicana					
Corn	1 (0.8 oz)	50	1	1	10
Flour	1 (0.8 oz)	80	2	3	13
Tortillas de Trigo	1 (1 oz)	140	2	7	18
Mariachi					
Tortilla	1	112	3	3	20
Old El Paso					
Flour	1 (1.4 oz)	130	3	4	21

FOOD	PORTION	CALS	PROT	FAT	CARB
Tyson					
Flour	1 (1.7 oz)	150	3	4	24
Flour Heat Pressed	2 (2 oz)	170	4	4	30
White Corn	2 (1.8 oz)	100	2	1	21
Whole Wheat Heat Pressed	1 (1.4 oz)	120	4	3	20
Yellow Corn	3 (1.9 oz)	140	3	2	27
TRITICALE					
dry	1 cup (6.7 oz)	645	25	4	138
triticale not prep	1 oz	94	4	tr	18
TROUT					
baked	3 oz	162	23	7	0
rainbow cooked	3 oz	129	22	4	0
seatrout baked	3 oz	113	18	4	0
TRUFFLES					
fresh	0.5 oz	4	2	tr	9
TUNA					
canned					
light in oil	1 can (6 oz)	399	50	14	0
light in oil	3 oz	169	25	7	0
light in water	3 oz	99	22	1	0
light in water	1 can (5.8 oz)	192	42	1	0
white in oil	1 can (6.2 oz)	331	47	14	0
white in oil	3 oz	158	23	7	0
white in water	3 oz	116	23	2	0
white in water	1 can (6 oz)	234	46	4	0
Bumble Bee					
Albacore In Water	2 oz	60	12	1	0
Chunk Light In Water	2 oz	60	12	1	0
Chunk Light In Water Pouch	2 oz	60	13	1	0
Solid White In Water	2 oz	70	15	1	0
Progresso					
In Olive Oil drained	¼ cup (2 oz)	160	13	12	0
StarKist					
Chunk Light No Drain Package	¼ cup (2 oz)	60	13	1	0
Low Sodium Chunk White In Water	2 oz	60	14	1	0
Solid White Albacore In Spring Water	¼ cup (2 oz)	70	15	1	0
Tuna Fillet In Spring Water	¼ cup (2 oz)	60	13	1	0
fresh					
bluefin cooked	3 oz	157	25	5	0
bluefin raw	3 oz	122	20	4	0
skipjack baked	3 oz	112	24	1	0
yellowfin baked	3 oz	118	25	1	0

FOOD	PORTION	CALS	PROT	FAT	CARB
TUNA DISHES					
frozen					
Mrs. Paul's					
Microwave Tuna Sandwich	1	200	10	6	23
mix					
Tuna Helper					
AuGratin 50% Less Fat Recipe as prep	1 cup	240	13	6	37
AuGratin as prep	1 cup	300	13	11	37
Cheesy Broccoli 50% Less Fat Recipe as prep	1 cup	240	15	5	38
Cheesy Broccoli as prep	1 cup	290	15	9	38
Cheesy Pasta 50% Less Fat Recipe as prep	1 cup	230	14	5	32
Cheesy Pasta as prep	1 cup	280	14	11	32
Creamy Broccoli 50% Less Fat Recipe as prep	1 cup	240	14	5	35
Creamy Broccoli as prep	1 cup	310	14	12	35
Creamy Pasta 50% Less Fat Recipe as prep	1 cup	230	14	6	31
Creamy Pasta as prep	1 cup	300	14	13	31
Fettuccine Alfredo 50% Less Fat Recipe as prep	1 cup	240	14	6	32
Fettuccine Alfredo as prep	1 cup	310	14	14	32
Garden Cheddar 50% Less Fat Recipe as prep	1 cup	240	13	5	36
Garden Cheddar as prep	1 cup	290	13	11	36
Pasta Salad Low Fat Recipe as prep	⅔ cup	230	10	2	26
Pasta Salad as prep	⅔ cup	380	10	27	26
Tetrazzini 50% Less Fat Recipe as prep	1 cup	230	14	5	34
Tetrazzini as prep	1 cup	300	14	12	34
Tuna Melt Reduced Fat Recipe as prep	1 cup	240	12	6	34
Tuna Melt as prep	1 cup	300	12	12	34
Tuna Pot Pie as prep	1 cup	440	18	24	40
Tuna Romanoff 50% Less Fat Recipe as prep	1 cup	240	15	3	38
Tuna Romanoff as prep	1 cup	280	15	8	38

FOOD	PORTION	CALS	PROT	FAT	CARB
ready-to-eat					
Bumble Bee					
Tuna Salad Fat Free	1 pkg (3.5 oz)	190	9	2	25
Tuna Salad Kit	1 pkg (3.8 oz)	250	17	13	15
StarKist					
Lunch To-Go	1 pkg	310	22	13	26
Ready-Mixed Tuna Salad Kit	1 pkg (3.5 oz)	190	9	6	25
Tuna Salad Lunch Kit	1 pkg (4.3 oz)	230	20	9	17
Wampler					
Salad	⅓ cup	180	6	12	9
take-out					
tuna salad	1 cup	383	33	19	19
tuna salad	3 oz	159	14	8	8
TURBOT					
european baked	3 oz	104	17	3	0
TURKEY					
(*see also* DINNER, HOT DOG, TURKEY DISHES, TURKEY SUBSTITUTES)					
canned					
w/ broth	1 can (5 oz)	231	34	10	0
w/ broth	½ can (2.5 oz)	116	17	5	0
Mary Kitchen					
Roast Turkey Hash	1 can (14.9 oz)	420	39	11	42
fresh					
back w/ skin roasted	½ back (9 oz)	637	70	38	0
breast w/ skin roasted	4 oz	212	32	8	0
dark meat w/ skin roasted	3.6 oz	230	29	12	0
dark meat w/o skin roasted	3 oz	170	26	7	0
dark meat w/o skin roasted	1 cup (5 oz)	262	40	10	0
ground cooked	3 oz	188	20	11	0
leg w/ skin roasted	1 (1.2 lbs)	1133	152	54	0
leg w/ skin roasted	2.5 oz	147	20	7	0
light meat w/ skin roasted	4.7 oz	268	39	11	0
light meat w/ skin roasted	from ½ turkey (2.3 lbs)	2069	87	87	0
light meat w/o skin roasted	4 oz	183	35	4	0
neck simmered	1 (5.3 oz)	274	41	11	0
skin roasted	1 oz	141	13	13	0
skin roasted	from ½ turkey	1096	49	98	0
w/ skin roasted	½ turkey (4 lbs)	3857	522	181	0
w/ skin roasted	8.4 oz	498	67	23	0
w/ skin neck & giblets roasted	½ turkey (8.8 lbs)	4123	190	190	1
w/o skin roasted	1 cup (5 oz)	238	41	7	0
w/o skin roasted	7.3 oz	354	61	10	0
wing w/ skin roasted	1 (6.5 oz)	426	51	23	0
Louis Rich					
Ground	4 oz	190	20	12	0
Patties White	1 (4 oz)	170	19	10	0

FOOD	PORTION	CALS	PROT	FAT	CARB
Perdue					
Breast Tenderloins Butter Garlic	3 oz	100	20	1	2
Burger Cooked	1 (4 oz)	160	20	9	0
Dark Cooked	3 oz	180	20	11	0
Drumsticks Cooked	1 (2.2 oz)	110	14	6	0
Ground Cooked	3 oz	160	20	9	0
Tenderloins Black Pepper Cooked	3 oz	90	20	1	1
Thighs Cooked	1 (3.2 oz)	240	17	19	0
White Cooked	3 oz	150	22	7	0
Shady Brook					
Ground Breast	4 oz	120	28	1	0
Turkey Store					
Breakfast Sausage Patties Mild	2 patties (2.3 oz)	160	10	13	1
Lean Ground Italian Style	4 oz	190	20	10	4
Wampler					
Boneless Breast Roast	4 oz	160	25	6	0
Breast Half	4 oz	160	25	6	0
Breast Steaks	4 oz	120	28	1	0
Drumsticks	4 oz	180	22	10	0
Ground	4 oz	210	18	15	0
Ground Breast	4 oz	130	28	1	0
Ground Lean	4 oz	160	20	8	0
Thighs	4 oz	170	22	10	0
Wings	4 oz	220	23	14	0
Woodfire Grill Burger	1 (3 oz)	180	21	9	2
frozen					
roast boneless seasoned light & dark meat roasted	1 pkg (1.7 lbs)	1213	167	45	24
Wampler					
Burger BBQ	1 (4 oz)	240	19	17	3
Burgers Cracked Peppercorn & Garlic	1 (3 oz)	170	21	9	0
Seasoned Burgers Cracker Peppercorn & Garlic	1 (3 oz)	170	21	9	0
ready-to-eat					
bologna	1 oz	57	4	4	tr
breast	1 slice (0.75 oz)	23	5	tr	0
diced light & dark seasoned	½ lb	313	42	14	2
diced light & dark seasoned	1 oz	39	5	2	tr
ham thigh meat	2 oz	73	11	3	tr
ham thigh meat	1 pkg (8 oz)	291	43	12	1
pastrami	2 oz	80	10	4	1
pastrami	1 pkg (8 oz)	320	42	14	4
patties battered & fried	1 (3.3 oz)	266	13	17	15
patties battered & fried	1 (2.3 oz)	181	9	12	10

FOOD	PORTION	CALS	PROT	FAT	CARB
patties breaded & fried	1 (3.3 oz)	266	13	17	15
patties breaded & fried	1 (2.3 oz)	181	9	12	10
poultry salad sandwich spread	1 tbsp	109	2	2	1
poultry salad sandwich spread	1 oz	238	4	4	2
prebasted breast w/ skin roasted	1 breast (3.8 lbs)	2175	383	60	0
prebasted breast w/ skin roasted	½ breast (1.9 lbs)	1087	191	30	0
prebasted thigh w/ skin roasted	1 thigh (11 oz)	494	59	27	0
roll light & dark meat	1 oz	42	5	2	1
roll light meat	1 oz	42	5	2	2
salami cooked	2 oz	111	9	8	tr
salami cooked	1 pkg (8 oz)	446	37	31	1
turkey loaf breast meat	1 pkg (6 oz)	187	38	3	0
turkey loaf breast meat	2 slices (1.5 oz)	47	10	1	0
turkey sticks battered & fried	1 stick (2.3 oz)	178	9	11	11
turkey sticks breaded & fried	1 stick (2.3 oz)	178	9	11	11
Alpine Lace					
Breast Fat Free	2 oz	45	10	0	0
Boar's Head					
Breast Cracked Pepper Smoked	2 oz	60	13	1	1
Breast Golden Skin On	2 oz	60	11	2	0
Breast Golden Skinless	2 oz	60	12	1	tr
Breast Hickory Smoked	2 oz	70	12	2	tr
Breast Low Sodium Skinless	2 oz	60	12	1	tr
Breast Lower Sodium Skin On	2 oz	60	11	2	tr
Breast Maple Glazed Honey Coat	2 oz	70	14	1	2
Breast Ovengold Skin On	2 oz	60	12	2	1
Breast Ovengold Skinless	2 oz	60	13	1	0
Breast Roasted Mesquite Smoked Skinless	2 oz	60	13	1	0
Breast Roasted Salsalito	2 oz	60	13	1	1
Pastrami Seasoned	2 oz	60	13	1	1
Carl Buddig					
Honey Roasted Turkey Breast	1 pkg (2.5 oz)	120	12	7	3
Lean Slices Honey Roasted Breast	1 pkg (2.5 oz)	70	13	1	4

FOOD	PORTION	CALS	PROT	FAT	CARB
Lean Slices Oven Roasted Breast	1 pkg (2.5 oz)	70	15	1	1
Lean Slices Smoked Breast	1 pkg (2.5 oz)	70	15	1	1
Oven Roasted Breast	1 pkg (2.5 oz)	110	12	7	1
Smoked Breast	1 pkg (2.5 oz)	110	12	7	1
Turkey Ham	1 pkg (2.5 oz)	100	13	5	1
Hormel					
Light & Lean 97 Breast Sliced	1 slice (1 oz)	30	5	1	0
Light & Lean 97 Mesquite Smoked Breast	1 slice (1 oz)	30	5	1	0
turkey pepperoni	17 slices (1 oz)	80	9	4	0
Louis Rich					
Bologna	1 slice (28 g)	50	3	4	1
Breaded Nuggets	4 (3.2 oz)	260	13	16	15
Breaded Patties	1 (3 oz)	220	12	13	13
Breaded Sticks	3 (3 oz)	230	12	15	12
Breast Skinless Hickory Smoked	2 oz	50	11	0	1
Breast Skinless Honey Roasted	2 oz	60	11	0	3
Breast Skinless Oven Roasted	2 oz	50	11	0	1
Breast Skinless Rotisserie	2 oz	50	11	0	1
Breast Slices Hickory Smoked	1 slice (2 oz)	50	11	0	1
Breast Slices Honey Roasted	1 slice (2 oz)	60	11	0	3
Breast Slices Oven Roasted	1 slice (2 oz)	50	11	0	1
Breast Slices Rotisserie	1 slice (2 oz)	50	11	0	1
Carving Board Hickory Smoked	2 slices (1.6 oz)	40	9	1	0
Carving Board Oven Roasted Thin	6 slices (2.1 oz)	60	12	1	1
Carving Board Oven Roasted Traditional	2 slices (1.6 oz)	40	9	1	0
Carving Board Rotisserie	2 slices (1.6 oz)	40	9	1	0
Cotto Salami	1 slice (28 g)	40	4	3	0
Deli-Thin Oven Roasted	4 slices (1.8 oz)	50	9	1	2
Deli-Thin Smoked	4 slices (1.8 oz)	50	9	2	1
Fat Free Hickory Smoked Breast	1 slice (1 oz)	25	4	0	1
Fat Free Oven Roasted Breast	1 slice (1 oz)	25	4	0	1
Fat Free Oven Roasted Deli-Thin Breast	4 slices (1.8 oz)	45	8	0	2

FOOD	PORTION	CALS	PROT	FAT	CARB
Fat Free Turkey Ham Honey	2 slices (1.7 oz)	35	7	0	2
Fat Free Turkey Ham Smoked	2 slices (1.7 oz)	35	7	0	1
Hickory Smoked	1 slice (1 oz)	30	5	1	1
Oven Roasted	1 slice (1 oz)	30	5	1	1
Pastrami	1 slice (1 oz)	30	5	1	1
Smoked	1 slice (1 oz)	30	5	1	0
Turkey Ham	1 slice (1 oz)	30	5	1	1
Turkey Ham Chopped	1 slice (1 oz)	45	5	3	1
Turkey Ham Honey Cured	1 slice (1 oz)	30	5	1	1
Oscar Mayer					
Free Oven Roasted Breast	4 slices (1.8 oz)	40	8	0	2
Free Smoked Breast	4 slices (1.8 oz)	40	8	0	2
Oven Roasted White	1 slice (1 oz)	30	4	1	1
Smoked White	1 slice (1 oz)	30	4	1	1
Perdue					
Breast Sliced Cajun Style	2 oz	50	9	1	1
Breast Sliced Honey Smoked	2 oz	50	10	0	2
Breast Sliced Pan Roasted	2 oz	70	14	2	0
Ham Hickory Smoked	2 oz	60	9	3	1
Healthsense Breast Sliced Oven Roasted	2 oz	60	10	0	3
Pastrami Hickory Smoked	2 oz	70	9	3	2
Shady Brook					
Meatballs Italian Style	3 (3 oz)	130	12	7	5
Wampler					
Bologna	2 oz	130	8	11	1
Dark Cured	2 oz	80	8	5	2
Deli Roast Breast	2 oz	50	12	1	0
Deli Roast Classic Spiced Breast	2 oz	70	16	1	1
Deli Roast Pan Roasted Breast	2 oz	70	13	2	1
Deli Roast Pan Roasted Skinless Breast	2 oz	50	12	0	1
Deli Roast Peppered Breast	21 oz	40	8	0	1
Deli Roast Rotisserie Breast	2 oz	50	9	2	1
Pastrami	2 oz	90	9	5	1
Salami	2 oz	90	9	6	1
Turkey Ham	2 oz	60	10	3	0
TURKEY DISHES					
gravy & turkey	1 cup (8.4 oz)	160	14	6	11
gravy & turkey	1 pkg (5 oz)	95	8	4	7

FOOD	PORTION	CALS	PROT	FAT	CARB
Banquet					
Sandwich Toppers Gravy & Sliced Turkey	1 pkg (5 oz)	160	8	11	6
Dinty Moore					
Microwave Cup Stew	1 pkg (7.5 oz)	130	9	3	16
Stew	1 cup (8.5 oz)	140	10	3	19
Mosey's					
Turkey Breast w/ Gravy	1 serv (5 oz)	140	30	1	4
Wampler					
Turkey Ham Salad	⅓ cup	150	7	10	9
TURKEY SUBSTITUTES					
Lightlife					
Smart Deli Turkey	3 slices (1.5 oz)	40	9	0	1
Tofurkey					
Deli Slices Hickory	1.5 oz	120	13	2	14
Deli Slices Original	1.5 oz	120	13	2	14
Deli Slices Peppered	1.5 oz	120	13	2	14
Drummettes	1 (3 oz)	105	11	2	11
Giblet Gravy	1 serv (3.5 oz)	42	4	2	5
Stuffed Tofu Roast	1 serv (4 oz)	193	26	5	10
Worthington					
Smoked Turkey Meatless	3 slices (2 oz)	140	10	10	3
Turkee Slices	3 slices (3.3 oz)	130	13	14	3
Yves					
Veggie Turkey Deli Slices	1 serv (2.2 oz)	85	18	0	4
TURNIPS					
canned					
greens	½ cup	17	2	tr	3
fresh					
cooked mashed	½ cup (4.2 oz)	47	2	tr	10
cubed cooked	½ cup (3 oz)	33	1	tr	7
greens chopped cooked	½ cup	15	1	tr	3
frozen					
greens cooked	½ cup	24	3	tr	4
Birds Eye					
Greens w/ Diced Turnip	1 cup (3 oz)	25	2	0	2
VEAL					
(*see also* DINNER, VEAL DISHES)					
cutlet lean only braised	3 oz	172	31	4	0
cutlet lean only fried	3 oz	156	28	4	0
ground broiled	3 oz	146	21	6	0
loin chop w/ bone lean & fat braised	1 chop (2.8 oz)	227	24	14	0
loin chop w/ bone lean only braised	1 chop (2.4 oz)	155	23	6	0
shoulder w/ bone lean only braised	3 oz	169	29	5	0

FOOD	PORTION	CALS	PROT	FAT	CARB
sirloin w/ bone lean & fat roasted	3 oz	171	21	9	0
sirloin w/ bone lean only roasted	3 oz	143	22	5	0
VEAL DISHES					
take-out					
parmigiana	4.2 oz	279	22	18	6
VEGETABLE JUICE					
vegetable juice cocktail	6 fl oz	34	1	tr	8
vegetable juice cocktail	½ cup	22	1	tr	6
Dole					
Vegetable Blend	1 bottle (12 oz)	90	4	0	19
Hunt's					
Cocktail	1 can (6 oz)	20	2	0	7
Muir Glen					
Organic	5.5 oz	50	1	0	10
V8					
Lightly Tangy	8 oz	58	2	1	11
Low Sodium	8 oz	53	2	tr	11
Original	8 oz	51	2	1	10
Picante Vegetable	8 oz	51	2	tr	10
Spicy Hot	8 oz	49	2	tr	10
Splash Tropical Blend	8 fl oz	120	0	0	30
VEGETABLES MIXED					
canned					
mixed vegetables	½ cup	39	2	tr	8
peas & carrots	½ cup	48	3	tr	11
peas & carrots low sodium	½ cup	48	3	tr	11
peas & onions	½ cup	30	2	tr	5
succotash	½ cup	102	4	1	23
Chi-Chi's					
Diced Tomatoes & Green Chilies	¼ cup (2.5 oz)	20	0	0	4
Chun King					
Chow Mein Vegetables	⅔ cup (3 oz)	14	1	tr	3
Del Monte					
Mixed	½ cup (4.4 oz)	40	2	0	8
Mixed No Salt Added	½ cup (4.4 oz)	40	2	0	8
Peas And Carrots	½ cup (4.5 oz)	60	2	0	11
Green Giant					
Garden Medley	½ cup (4.2 oz)	40	1	0	9
Mixed	½ cup (4.3 oz)	60	2	0	12
Sweet Peas & Carrots	½ cup (4.3 oz)	50	2	0	11
Sweet Peas & Tiny Pearl Onions	½ cup (4.4 oz)	60	4	0	11
House Of Tsang					
Vegetables & Sauce Cantonese Classic	½ cup (4.2 oz)	70	1	1	14

FOOD	PORTION	CALS	PROT	FAT	CARB
Vegetables & Sauce Hong Kong Sweet & Sour	½ cup (4.5 oz)	160	0	0	40
Vegetables & Sauce Szechuan Hot & Spicy	½ cup (4.2 oz)	70	1	1	14
Vegetables & Sauce Tokyo Teriyaki	½ cup (4.4 oz)	100	1	0	23
La Choy					
Chop Suey Vegetables	½ cup (2.2 oz)	10	1	tr	2
LeSueur					
Early Peas w/ Mushrooms & Pearl Onions	½ cup (4.3 oz)	60	3	0	11
S&W					
Mixed	½ cup (4.4 oz)	35	1	0	7
Peas & Carrots	½ cup (4.5 oz)	60	2	0	11
Peas & Onions	½ cup (4.3 oz)	40	3	0	11
frozen					
mixed vegetables cooked	½ cup	54	3	tr	12
peas & carrots cooked	½ cup	38	3	tr	8
peas & onions cooked	½ cup	40	2	tr	8
succotash cooked	½ cup	79	4	1	17
Amy's Organic					
Pocket Sandwich Mediterranean Vegetables	1 (4.5 oz)	220	9	7	33
Pocket Sandwich Roasted Vegetables	1 (4.5 oz)	220	6	8	35
Pocket Sandwich Vegetable Pie	1 (5 oz)	230	7	6	37
Birds Eye					
Baby Sweet Peas & Pearl Onions	⅔ cup (3.2 oz)	60	4	1	12
Bavarian Vegetables	1 cup (5.5 oz)	150	5	8	15
Broccoli Cauliflower Carrots w/ Cheese	½ cup (3.9 oz)	70	3	4	7
Broccoli Cauliflower & Red Peppers	½ cup	20	2	0	5
Broccoli & Cauliflower	½ cup	20	2	0	4
Broccoli Carrots & Water Chestnuts	½ cup (3.3 oz)	30	2	0	7
Broccoli Corn & Red Peppers	½ cup	50	3	0	12
Broccoli Red Peppers Onions & Mushrooms	½ cup	25	2	0	5
Broccoli & Cauliflower & Carrots	½ cup	25	2	0	5
Brussels Sprouts Cauliflower & Carrots	½ cup	30	2	0	7

FOOD	PORTION	CALS	PROT	FAT	CARB
California Style Vegetables	½ cup (3 oz)	100	3	5	9
Cauliflower Nuggets Corn Carrots & Snow Pea Pods	½ cup (3.2 oz)	30	2	0	6
Chicken Viola! Italian Pesto Chicken	2 cups (6.6 oz)	240	15	9	24
Chicken Viola! Three Cheese Chicken	1¾ cups (5.6 oz)	220	14	8	24
French Style	⅔ cup (4.4 oz)	110	2	6	10
Gumbo Blend	¾ cup (3 oz)	40	2	0	10
Italian Style Vegetables & Bow Tie Pasta	1 cup (5.8 oz)	150	3	9	13
New England Style Vegetables & Pasta Shells	1 pkg (7.9 oz)	260	6	14	29
Peas & Pearl Onions	⅔ cup (4.2 oz)	90	5	1	18
Peas & Potatoes In Cream Sauce	½ cup (4.4 oz)	90	4	3	13
Radiatore Pasta & Vegetables	1 cup (4.6 oz)	200	6	8	27
Roasted Potatoes & Broccoli	⅔ cup (3.9 oz)	100	3	4	15
Roletti Pasta & Vegetables	1 cup (4.4 oz)	190	5	8	11
Stir Fry Asparagus	2 cups (5.8 oz)	90	5	1	16
Stir Fry Broccoli	1 cup (3.4 oz)	30	2	0	5
Stir Fry Pepper	1 cup (3 oz)	25	1	0	5
Stir Fry Sugar Snap	¾ cup	35	1	0	5
Stir Fry Whole Green Bean	1¾ cup (5.3 oz)	100	4	1	19
Stir Fry Style Vegetables	½ cup (3.6 oz)	60	2	4	5
Vegetables For Stew	⅔ cup (2.9 oz)	40	1	0	9
Green Giant					
Alfredo Vegetables	¾ cup	70	4	3	9
American Mixtures Broccoli Carrots Cauliflower	¾ cup (2.6 oz)	25	1	0	5
American Mixtures Broccoli Carrots Waterchestnuts	¾ cup (3 oz)	30	1	0	6
American Mixtures Carrots Green Bean Cauliflower	¾ cup (2.7 oz)	25	1	0	5
American Mixtures Cauliflower Broccoli Sugar Snap & Sweet Peas	¾ cup (2.8 oz)	35	2	0	7
American Mixtures Corn Broccoli Red Pepper	¾ cup (3.1 oz)	60	2	0	13

FOOD	PORTION	CALS	PROT	FAT	CARB
American Mixtures Green Beans Potatoes Onions Red Peppers	¾ cup (2.8 oz)	45	1	1	8
American Mixtures Sweet Peas Potatoes Carrots	⅔ cup (3 oz)	70	2	2	12
Butter Sauce Broccoli Cauliflower Carrots Corn Sweet Peas	¾ cup (3.6 oz)	60	2	2	8
Butter Sauce Broccoli Pasta Sweet Peas Corn Red Peppers	¾ cup (3.5 oz)	70	3	2	11
Butter Sauce Mixed	¾ cup (3.6 oz)	70	2	2	11
Cheese Sauce Broccoli Cauliflower Carrots	1 cup (4.1 oz)	60	3	3	7
Harvest Fresh Broccoli Cauliflower Carrots	1 cup (3.4 oz)	30	2	0	5
Harvest Fresh Mixed Vegetables	⅔ cup (3.1 oz)	50	2	0	10
Harvest Fresh Sweet Peas & Pearl Onions	½ cup (2.7 oz)	55	3	0	10
Mixed	¾ cup (2.9 oz)	50	2	0	11
Select Sweet Peas & Pearl Onions	⅔ cup (3.1 oz)	60	4	0	12
Health Is Wealth					
Veggie Munchees	2 (1 oz)	50	2	1	9
La Choy					
Fancy Chinese Mixed Vegetables	½ cup (2.9 oz)	9	1	tr	1
Tree Of Life					
Mixed	½ cup (3 oz)	65	2	0	13
shelf-stable					
TastyBite					
Curry Bangkok Red	½ pkg (5.3 oz)	88	2	6	7
Curry Patong Yellow	½ pkg (5.3 oz)	118	2	7	12
Curry Siam Green	½ pkg (5.3 oz)	63	2	3	6
Jaipur Vegetables	½ pkg (5 oz)	220	9	15	13
Malabar Mixed	½ pkg (5 oz)	67	1	1	15
take-out					
buddha's delight	1 serv (16 oz)	174	17	5	17
curry	1 serv (7.7 oz)	398	4	33	22
gyoza potstickers vegetable	8 (4.9 oz)	210	8	4	34
pakoras	1 (2 oz)	108	5	5	12
ratatouille	1 serv (3.5 oz)	96	2	7	7
samosa	2 (4 oz)	519	3	46	25
succotash	½ cup	111	5	1	23

FOOD	PORTION	CALS	PROT	FAT	CARB
VENISON					
roasted	3 oz	134	26	3	0
VINEGAR					
balsamic	1 tbsp (0.5 oz)	5	0	0	2
Eden					
Organic Brown Rice	1 tbsp	2	0	0	0
Ume Plum	1 tsp	2	0	0	0
Progresso					
Balsamic	2 tbsp (0.5 oz)	10	0	0	2
Victoria					
Balsamic	1 tbsp (0.5 oz)	5	0	0	2
White House					
Apple Cider	1 tbsp (0.5 oz)	0	0	0	0
White	1 tbsp (0.5 oz)	0	0	0	0
WAFFLES					
frozen					
buttermilk	1 4 in sq (1.2 oz)	88	2	3	14
plain	1 4 in sq (1.2 oz)	88	2	3	14
Eggo					
Apple Cinnamon	2 (2.7 oz)	220	5	8	33
Banana Bread	2 (2.7 oz)	200	5	7	32
Blueberry	2 (2.7 oz)	220	5	9	32
Buttermilk	2 (2.7 oz)	220	5	8	31
Golden Oat	2 (2.7 oz)	150	6	3	29
Homestyle	2 (2.7 oz)	220	5	8	32
Minis Cinnamon Toast	12 (3.2 oz)	290	5	10	45
Minis Homestyle	12 (3.3 oz)	260	7	9	38
Nut & Honey	2 (2.7 oz)	240	6	10	31
Nutri-Grain	2 (2.7 oz)	190	5	6	30
Nutri-Grain Multi-Bran	2 (2.7 oz)	180	5	6	32
Nutri-Grain Raisin & Bran	2 (2.9 oz)	210	5	6	36
Special K	2 (2 oz)	120	6	0	26
Strawberry	2 (2.7 oz)	220	6	8	32
Kellogg's					
Homestyle Low Fat	2 (2.7 oz)	180	6	3	34
Nutri-Grain Low Fat	2 (2.7 oz)	160	5	3	31
Nutri-Grain Low Fat Blueberry	2 (2.7 oz)	160	5	2	33
Kid Cuisine					
Wave Rider Waffle Sticks	1 meal (6.6 oz)	380	3	8	75
home recipe					
plain	1 (7 in diam)	218	6	11	25
mix					
plain as prep	1 7 in diam (2.6 oz)	218	5	10	26
ready-to-eat					
Thomas'					
Buttermilk	1 (1.6 oz)	130	3	5	18

FOOD	PORTION	CALS	PROT	FAT	CARB
WALNUTS					
black dried chopped	1 cup	759	30	71	15
english dried	1 oz	182	4	18	5
english dried chopped	1 cup	770	17	74	22
halves	14 (1 oz)	190	4	19	4
WASABI					
(see HORESERADISH)					
WATER					
Absopure					
Natural Spring	8 fl oz	0	0	0	0
Aquafina					
Essentials B-Power Wild Berry	8 fl oz	40	0	0	11
Essentials Calcium + Tangerine Pineapple	8 fl oz	40	0	0	11
Essentials Daily C Citrus	8 fl oz	40	0	0	11
Essentials Multi-V Watermelon	8 fl oz	40	0	0	11
Water	8 fl oz	0	0	0	0
Aquess					
Purified Water w/ Soluble Fiber	1 bottle (18 oz)	30	0	0	8
Castellina					
Sparking Spring	8 fl oz	0	0	0	0
Crystal Geyser					
Spring Water	8 fl oz	0	0	0	0
Dasani					
Purfied Water	8 oz	0	0	0	0
Diamond Spring					
Water	1 qt	0	0	0	0
Evian					
Spring Water	1 bottle (11.5 oz)	0	0	0	0
Ferrarelle					
Sparkling	8 fl oz	0	0	0	0
Gerolsteiner					
Sparkling Mineral	8 fl oz	0	0	0	0
Glaceau					
Smartwater	8 oz	0	0	0	0
Vitamin Water Tropical Citrus	1 cup (8 oz)	40	0	0	9
Glacier Springs					
Drinking Water	8 fl oz	0	0	0	0
LaCroix					
Spring	1 bottle (12 oz)	0	0	0	0
Meridian					
Clear All Flavors	8 oz	100	0	0	25
Mountain Valley					
Mineral Water	1 qt	0	0	0	0

FOOD	PORTION	CALS	PROT	FAT	CARB
Mt Shasta					
Natural Spring	1 bottle (20 oz)	0	0	0	0
Propel					
Fitness Water Berry	8 fl oz	10	0	0	3
Fitness Water Black Cherry	8 fl oz	10	0	0	3
Reebok					
Fitness Water Berry	1 bottle (24 oz)	30	0	0	0
Fitness Water Natural	1 bottle (24 oz)	0	0	0	0
San Pellegrino					
Acqua Panna	8 fl oz	0	0	0	0
Saratoga					
Spring	8 oz	0	0	0	0
Snapple					
Natural Spring	8 fl oz	0	0	0	0
Veryfine					
Fruit 2 O Lemon	8 oz	0	0	0	0
Fruit 2 O Lemon Lime	8 fl oz	0	0	0	0
Fruit 2 O Orange	8 fl oz	0	0	0	0
Fruit 2 O Raspberry	8 fl oz	0	0	0	0
Volvic					
Spring Water	8 oz	0	0	0	0
WATER CHESTNUTS					
chinese sliced canned	½ cup	35	1	tr	9
fresh sliced	½ cup	66	1	tr	15
WATERMELON					
cut up	1 cup	50	1	1	11
seeds dried	1 oz	158	8	13	4
seeds dried	1 cup	602	8	51	17
wedge	⅛	152	3	2	35
WATERMELON JUICE					
Kool-Aid					
Splash Drink	1 serv (8 oz)	110	0	0	30
WAX BEANS					
canned					
Del Monte					
Cut Golden	½ cup (4.2 oz)	20	1	0	4
S&W					
Cut	½ cup (4.2 oz)	20	1	0	4
WHEAT					
(*see also* BULGUR, BRAN, CEREAL, COUSCOUS, FLOUR, WHEAT GERM)					
sprouted	1 cup (3.8 oz)	214	8	1	46
Lightlife					
Savory Seitan Barbecue	4 oz	160	24	2	12
Savory Seitan Teriyaki	4 oz	160	26	2	10
WHEAT GERM					
plain toasted	¼ cup (1 oz)	108	8	3	14
plain toasted	1 cup	431	33	12	56

FOOD	PORTION	CALS	PROT	FAT	CARB
w/ brown sugar & honey toasted	1 oz	107	6	2	17
w/ brown sugar & honey toasted	1 cup	426	25	9	69
Kretschmer					
Original Toasted	2 tbsp (0.5 oz)	50	4	1	6
WHEY					
acid fluid	1 cup (8 fl oz)	59	25	tr	13
sweet dry	1 tbsp (8 g)	26	1	tr	6
sweet fluid	1 cup (8 fl oz)	66	2	1	13
whey cheese	1 oz	126	4	8	9
WHIPPED TOPPINGS					
cream pressurized	1 cup (2.1 oz)	154	2	13	7
nondairy powdered as prep w/ whole milk	1 cup	151	3	10	13
nondairy pressurized	1 cup	184	1	16	11
Cool Whip					
Extra Creamy	2 tbsp (0.3 oz)	25	0	2	2
Free	2 tbsp (0.3 oz)	15	0	0	3
Lite	2 tbsp (0.3 oz)	20	0	1	2
Original	2 tbsp (0.3 oz)	25	0	2	2
Dream Whip					
Mix as prep	2 tbsp (0.3 oz)	20	0	1	2
Estee					
Whipped Topping	1 serv	10	0	1	1
Kraft					
Dairy Whip Light Cream	2 tbsp (0.2 oz)	10	0	1	tr
Fat Free	1 tbsp (0.3 oz)	15	0	0	2
WHITE BEANS					
canned					
white beans	1 cup	306	19	1	58
Progresso					
Cannellini	½ cup (4.6 oz)	100	5	1	18
dried					
regular cooked	1 cup	249	17	1	45
small cooked	1 cup	253	16	1	46
WHITEFISH					
baked	3 oz	146	21	6	0
smoked	1 oz	39	7	tr	0
smoked	3 oz	92	20	1	0
WHITING					
cooked	3 oz	98	20	1	0
WILD RICE					
cooked	1 cup (5.7 oz)	166	7	1	35
WINE					
madeira	3.5 oz	169	0	0	10
Eden					
Mirin Rice Cooking Wine	1 tbsp	25	0	0	7

FOOD	PORTION	CALS	PROT	FAT	CARB
WINGED BEANS					
dried cooked	1 cup	252	18	10	26
WOLFFISH					
atlantic baked	3 oz	105	19	3	0
WRAPS					
(*see* BREAD)					
YAM					
(*see also* SWEET POTATO)					
canned					
S&W					
Candied	½ cup (4.9 oz)	170	2	0	46
fresh					
mountain yam hawaii cooked	½ cup	59	1	tr	14
yam cubed cooked	½ cup	79	1	tr	19
YAMBEAN					
cooked	¾ cup	38	1	tr	9
YARDLONG BEANS					
dried cooked	1 cup	202	14	1	36
YAUTIA (TANNIER)					
raw sliced	1 cup (4.7 oz)	132	2	1	32
root raw	1 (10.7 oz)	299	4	1	72
YEAST					
baker's compressed	1 cake (0.6 oz)	18	1	tr	3
baker's dry	1 pkg (¼ oz)	21	3	tr	3
baker's dry	1 tbsp	35	5	1	5
brewer's dry	1 tbsp	25	3	tr	3
Hodgson Mill					
Fast Rise	1 tsp (9 g)	25	3	0	4
YELLOW BEANS					
canned	½ cup	13	1	tr	3
canned low sodium	½ cup	13	1	tr	3
dried cooked	1 cup	254	16	2	45
fresh cooked	½ cup	22	1	tr	5
fresh raw	½ cup	17	1	tr	4
frozen cooked	½ cup	18	1	tr	4
YELLOWTAIL					
baked	3 oz	159	25	6	0
YOGURT					
(*see also* YOGURT FROZEN)					
coffee lowfat	8 oz	194	11	3	31
fruit lowfat	8 oz	225	9	3	42
fruit lowfat	4 oz	113	5	1	21
plain	8 oz	139	8	7	11
plain lowfat	8 oz	144	12	4	16
plain no fat	8 oz	127	13	tr	17
vanilla lowfat	8 oz	194	11	3	31

FOOD	PORTION	CALS	PROT	FAT	CARB
Breyers					
Blended Blueberry	4.4 oz	130	4	1	25
Blended Peach	4.4 oz	130	4	1	26
Blended Strawberry	4.4 oz	130	4	1	26
Light Nonfat Apple Pie A La Mode	8 oz	120	7	0	22
Light Nonfat Berry Banana Split	8 oz	120	8	0	21
Light Nonfat Black Cherry Jubilee	8 oz	120	8	0	23
Light Nonfat Blueberries N' Cream	8 oz	120	8	0	23
Light Nonfat Cherry Bon-Bon	8 oz	120	8	0	22
Light Nonfat Cherry Vanilla Cream	8 oz	120	8	0	22
Light Nonfat Classic Strawberry	8 oz	120	8	0	22
Light Nonfat Key Lime Pie	8 oz	120	8	0	22
Light Nonfat Lemon Chiffon	8 oz	120	7	0	22
Light Nonfat Peaches N' Cream	8 oz	120	8	0	22
Light Nonfat Raspberries N' Cream	8 oz	120	8	0	22
Light Nonfat Strawberry Cheesecake	8 oz	120	8	0	22
Lowfat Black Cherry	8 oz	240	9	3	44
Lowfat Blueberry	8 oz	230	9	3	43
Lowfat Mixed Berry	8 oz	320	9	3	43
Lowfat Peach	8 oz	240	9	3	43
Lowfat Pineapple	8 oz	240	9	3	45
Lowfat Red Raspberry	8 oz	230	9	3	43
Lowfat Strawberry	8 oz	230	9	3	43
Lowfat Strawberry Banana	8 oz	240	9	3	44
Lowfat Vanilla	8 oz	220	10	3	38
Smooth & Creamy Apple Cobbler	8 oz	230	8	2	46
Smooth & Creamy Black Cherry Parfait	8 oz	240	9	2	46
Smooth & Creamy Black Cherry Parfait	4.4 oz	130	5	1	26
Smooth & Creamy Blueberries 'N Cream	8 oz	240	9	2	46
Smooth & Creamy Blueberries 'N Cream	4.4 oz	130	5	1	26
Smooth & Creamy Classic Strawberry	8 oz	230	9	2	45

FOOD	PORTION	CALS	PROT	FAT	CARB
Smooth & Creamy Classic Strawberry	4.4 oz	130	5	1	25
Smooth & Creamy Orange Vanilla Cream	8 oz	230	9	2	45
Smooth & Creamy Peaches 'N Cream	4.4 oz	130	5	1	25
Smooth & Creamy Peaches 'N Cream	8 oz	230	9	2	46
Smooth & Creamy Raspberries 'N Cream	8 oz	230	9	2	45
Smooth & Creamy Strawberry Banana Split	8 oz	240	8	2	48
Smooth & Creamy Strawberry Cheesecake	8 oz	240	9	2	46
Colombo					
99% Fat Free Peach	4 oz	110	3	1	22
99% Fat Free Strawberry	4 oz	110	3	1	22
Dannon					
Chunky Fruit Nonfat Apple Cinnamon	6 oz	160	7	0	33
Chunky Fruit Nonfat Blueberry	6 oz	160	7	0	32
Chunky Fruit Nonfat Cherry Vanilla	6 oz	160	7	0	31
Chunky Fruit Nonfat Peach	6 oz	160	7	0	33
Chunky Fruit Nonfat Strawberry	6 oz	160	7	0	32
Chunky Fruit Nonfat Strawberry Banana	6 oz	160	7	0	32
Danimals Lowfat Tropical Punch	4.4 oz	130	6	1	25
Danimals Lowfat Blueberry	4.4 oz	130	6	1	24
Danimals Lowfat Grape Lemonade	4.4 oz	120	6	1	22
Danimals Lowfat Lemon Ice	4.4 oz	120	6	1	22
Danimals Lowfat Orange Banana	4.4 oz	130	6	1	24
Danimals Lowfat Strawberry	4.4 oz	130	6	1	24
Danimals Lowfat Vanilla	4.4 oz	120	6	1	23
Danimals Lowfat Wild Raspberry	4.4 oz	120	6	1	22
Double Delights Banana Creme Strawberry	6 oz	160	7	1	32

FOOD	PORTION	CALS	PROT	FAT	CARB
Double Delights Bavarian Creme Raspberry	6 oz	170	7	1	34
Double Delights Cheesecake Cherry	6 oz	170	7	1	34
Double Delights Cheesecake Strawberry	6 oz	170	7	1	33
Double Delights Chocolate Cheesecake	6 oz	220	8	1	45
Double Delights Chocolate Dipped Strawberry	6 oz	210	8	1	45
Double Delights Chocolate Eclair	6 oz	220	8	1	45
Double Delights Vanilla Strawberry	6 oz	170	7	1	33
Double Delights Vanilla Peach & Apricot	6 oz	170	7	1	33
Fruit On The Bottom Lowfat Apple Cinnamon	8 oz	240	9	3	46
Fruit On The Bottom Lowfat Blueberry	8 oz	240	9	3	46
Fruit On The Bottom Lowfat Boysenberry	8 oz	240	9	3	45
Fruit On The Bottom Lowfat Cherry	8 oz	240	9	3	46
Fruit On The Bottom Lowfat Minipack Mixed Berry	4.4 oz	130	5	2	25
Fruit On The Bottom Lowfat Minipack Strawberry	4.4 oz	130	5	2	25
Fruit On The Bottom Lowfat Mixed Berries	8 oz	240	9	3	45
Fruit On The Bottom Lowfat Orange	8 oz	240	9	3	45
Fruit On The Bottom Lowfat Peach	8 oz	240	9	3	45
Fruit On The Bottom Lowfat Raspberry	8 oz	240	9	3	45
Fruit On The Bottom Lowfat Strawberry	8 oz	240	9	3	46
Fruit On The Bottom Lowfat Strawberry Banana	8 oz	240	9	3	43
LaCreme Vanilla	1 pkg (4.4 oz)	140	5	5	20
Light 'N Crunchy Mint Chocolate Chip	8 oz	140	8	0	27
Light 'N Crunchy Nonfat Caramel Apple Crunch	8 oz	140	8	0	26

FOOD	PORTION	CALS	PROT	FAT	CARB
Light 'N Crunchy Nonfat Lemon Blueberry Cobbler	8 oz	140	8	0	25
Light 'N Crunchy Nonfat Mocha Cappuccino	8 oz	140	8	0	26
Light 'N Crunchy Nonfat Raspberry w/ Granola	8 oz	140	9	0	26
Light 'N Crunchy Nonfat Vanilla Chocolate Crunch	8 oz	130	8	0	23
Light Duets Cherry Cheesecake	6 oz	90	5	0	18
Light Duets Peaches N' Cream	6 oz	90	5	0	18
Light Duets Raspberry Royale	6 oz	90	5	0	17
Light Duets Strawberry Cheesecake	6 oz	90	5	0	18
Light Nonfat Banana Cream Pie	8 oz	100	8	0	15
Light Nonfat Blueberry	8 oz	100	8	0	18
Light Nonfat Cappuccino	8 oz	100	8	0	16
Light Nonfat Cherry Vanilla	8 oz	100	8	0	18
Light Nonfat Coconut Cream Pie	8 oz	100	8	0	16
Light Nonfat Creme Caramel	8 oz	100	8	0	15
Light Nonfat Lemon Chiffon	8 oz	100	8	0	15
Light Nonfat Mint Chocolate Cream Pie	8 oz	100	8	0	17
Light Nonfat Peach	8 oz	100	8	0	16
Light Nonfat Raspberry	8 oz	100	8	0	17
Light Nonfat Strawberry	8 oz	100	8	0	16
Light Nonfat Strawberry Banana	8 oz	100	8	0	17
Light Nonfat Strawberry Kiwi	8 oz	100	8	0	16
Light Nonfat Tangerine Chiffon	8 oz	100	8	0	15
Light Nonfat Vanilla	8 oz	100	8	0	15
Lowfat Coffee	8 oz	210	10	3	36
Lowfat Cranberry Raspberry	8 oz	210	10	3	36
Lowfat Lemon	8 oz	210	10	3	36
Lowfat Vanilla	8 oz	210	10	3	36
Minipack Blended Nonfat Blueberry	4.4 oz	120	5	0	25
Minipack Blended Nonfat Cherry	4.4 oz	110	5	0	24

FOOD	PORTION	CALS	PROT	FAT	CARB
Minipack Blended Nonfat Peach	4.4 oz	120	5	0	23
Minipack Blended Nonfat Raspberry	4.4 oz	120	5	0	24
Minipack Blended Nonfat Strawberry	4.4 oz	120	5	0	23
Minipack Blended Nonfat Strawberry Banana	4.4 oz	120	5	0	23
Sprinkl'ins Cherry Vanilla	1 (4.1 oz)	130	5	2	24
Sprinkl'ins Strawberry	1 (4.1 oz)	130	5	2	24
Sprinkl'ins Strawberry Banana	1 (4.1 oz)	130	5	2	24
Sprinkl'ins Vanilla w/ Cherry Crystals	1 (4.1 oz)	110	5	1	21
Sprinkl'ins Vanilla w/ Orange Crystals	1 (4.1 oz)	110	5	1	21
Horizon Organic					
Fat Free Apricot Mango	¾ cup (6 oz)	120	7	0	23
Fat Free Honey	1 cup (8 oz)	160	9	0	32
Jell-O					
Lowfat Cherry	4.4 oz	130	4	1	25
Lowfat Grape	4.4 oz	130	4	1	25
Lowfat Raspberry	4.4 oz	130	4	1	25
Lowfat Tropical Berry Twist	4.4 oz	130	4	1	25
Lowfat Tropical Punch	4.4 oz	130	4	1	25
Lowfat Watermelon	4.4 oz	130	4	1	25
Lowfat Wild Berry	4.4 oz	130	4	1	25
Lowfat Wild Strawberry	4.4 oz	130	4	1	25
Light N'Lively					
Free Blueberry	4.4 oz	70	4	0	13
Free Peach	4.4 oz	70	4	0	12
Free Strawberry	4.4 oz	70	4	0	12
Free Strawberry Banana Cream	4.4 oz	70	4	0	13
Free Strawberry Fruit Cup	4.4 oz	70	4	0	13
Lowfat Blueberry	4.4 oz	130	4	1	25
Lowfat Peach	4.4 oz	130	4	1	26
Lowfat Pineapple	4.4 oz	130	4	1	26
Lowfat Red Raspberry	4.4 oz	120	5	1	23
Lowfat Strawberry	4.4 oz	130	4	1	26
Lowfat Strawberry Banana Cream	4.4 oz	130	4	1	25
Lowfat Strawberry Fruit Cup	4.4 oz	130	4	1	25

FOOD	PORTION	CALS	PROT	FAT	CARB
Oberweis					
Peach	1 pkg (8 oz)	210	10	3	39
Pascual					
Nonfat Cherries & Berries	1 pkg (4.4 oz)	100	4	0	19
Nonfat Peach	1 pkg (4.4 oz)	100	4	0	19
Silk					
Organic Soy Strawberry	1 pkg (6 oz)	160	4	2	31
Soy Apricot Mango	1 pkg	160	4	2	30
Soy Banana Strawberry	1 pkg	160	4	2	30
Soy Black Cherry	1 pkg	160	4	2	29
Soy Blueberry	1 pkg	160	4	2	29
Soy Key Lime	1 pkg	170	4	2	30
Soy Lemon	1 pkg	160	4	2	31
Soy Lemon Kiwi	1 pkg	150	4	2	29
Soy Peach	1 pkg	170	4	2	32
Soy Plain	8 oz	120	5	3	22
Soy Raspberry	1 pkg	160	4	2	30
Soy Vanilla	1 pkg (8 oz)	120	4	2	23
Stonyfield Farm					
Creamy Maple	1 pkg	160	6	6	19
Mocha-ccino	1 pkg	170	6	6	23
Nonfat Apricot Mango	1 pkg (8 oz)	160	8	0	31
Nonfat Black Cherry	1 pkg (8 oz)	160	8	0	31
Nonfat Cappuccino	1 pkg (8 oz)	160	9	0	31
Nonfat Cherry Vanilla	1 pkg (8 oz)	190	7	0	43
Nonfat Chocolate Underground	1 pkg (8 oz)	200	8	0	46
Nonfat French Vanilla	1 pkg (8 oz)	180	9	0	30
Nonfat Lotsa Lemon	1 pkg (8 oz)	160	9	0	30
Nonfat Peach	1 pkg (8 oz)	150	8	0	30
Nonfat Plain	1 pkg (8 oz)	100	10	8	15
Nonfat Raspberry	1 pkg (8 oz)	160	8	0	31
Nonfat Strawberry	1 pkg (8 oz)	180	8	0	32
Organic French Vanilla	1 pkg	170	6	6	23
Organic Wild Blueberry	1 pkg	160	5	6	22
Organic Lowfat Blueberry	1 pkg (6 oz)	130	5	2	23
Organic Lowfat Luscious Lemon	1 pkg (6 oz)	130	5	2	23
Organic Lowfat Maple Vanilla	1 pkg (6 oz)	120	6	2	19
Organic Lowfat Mocha Latte	1 pkg (6 oz)	120	6	2	20
Organic Lowfat Plain	1 cup (8 oz)	110	9	2	14
Organic Lowfat Raspberry	1 pkg (6 oz)	130	6	2	23
Organic Lowfat Strawberry	1 pkg (6 oz)	130	5	2	23
Organic Lowfat Vanilla	1 pkg (6 oz)	120	6	2	20
Strawberries & Cream	1 pkg	160	5	5	23
Vanilla Truffle	1 pkg	220	7	5	37
YoSelf Organic Chocolate	1 (4 oz)	110	4	1	21

FOOD	PORTION	CALS	PROT	FAT	CARB
YoSelf Organic Creme Carmel	1 (4 oz)	110	4	1	21
YoSqueeze Strawberry	1 tube (2 oz)	60	2	1	11
Total					
Greek Yogurt	1 pkg (5 oz)	180	10	12	10
Greek Yogurt 0% Fat	1 pkg (5 oz)	80	15	0	6
Greek Yogurt 1% Fat	1 pkg (5 oz)	120	8	8	8
Yoplait					
99% Fat Free Blueberry	6 oz	180	6	2	34
99% Fat Free Boysenberry	6 oz	180	6	2	34
99% Fat Free Cherry	6 oz	180	6	2	34
99% Fat Free Harvest Peach	6 oz	120	4	1	23
99% Fat Free Harvest Peach	6 oz	180	6	2	34
99% Fat Free Key Lime Pie	6 oz	180	6	2	34
99% Fat Free Lemon	6 oz	180	6	2	34
99% Fat Free Mixed Berry	6 oz	120	4	1	23
99% Fat Free Mixed Berry	6 oz	180	6	2	34
99% Fat Free Orange	6 oz	180	6	2	34
99% Fat Free Pina Colada	6 oz	180	6	2	34
99% Fat Free Pineapple	6 oz	180	6	2	34
99% Fat Free Raspberry	6 oz	180	6	2	34
99% Fat Free Strawberry	6 oz	180	6	2	43
99% Fat Free Strawberry	6 oz	120	4	1	23
99% Fat Free Strawberry Banana	6 oz	180	6	2	34
99% Fat Free Strawberry Banana	6 oz	120	4	1	23
99% Fat Free Strawberry Cheesecake	6 oz	180	6	2	34
Custard Style Banana	6 oz	190	7	4	32
Custard Style Blueberry	6 oz	190	7	4	32
Custard Style Cherry Vanilla	6 oz	190	7	4	32
Custard Style Key Lime Pie	6 oz	190	7	4	32
Custard Style Lemon	6 oz	190	7	4	32
Custard Style Peaches'n Cream	6 oz	190	7	4	32
Custard Style Raspberry	6 oz	190	7	4	32
Custard Style Raspberry Cheesecake	6 oz	190	7	4	32
Custard Style Strawberry	6 oz	190	7	4	32
Custard Style Strawberry Banana	6 oz	190	7	4	32
Custard Style Strawberry Vanilla	4 oz	120	5	2	21
Custard Style Vanilla	6 oz	190	8	4	32

FOOD	PORTION	CALS	PROT	FAT	CARB
Go-Gurt Strawberry Banana Burst	1 pkg (2.25 oz)	80	2	2	12
Go-Gurt Watermelon Meltdown	1 pkg (2.25 oz)	80	2	2	12
Light Amaretto Cheesecake	6 oz	90	6	0	16
Light Apricot Mango	6 oz	90	5	0	16
Light Banana Cream	6 oz	90	6	0	16
Light Blueberry	6 oz	90	5	0	16
Light Boston Cream Pie	6 oz	90	6	0	16
Light Caramel Apple	6 oz	90	6	0	16
Light Cherry	6 oz	90	5	0	16
Light Key Lime Pie	6 oz	90	6	0	16
Light Lemon Cream Pie	6 oz	90	6	0	16
Light Peach	6 oz	90	5	0	16
Light Peach Melba	6 oz	90	5	0	16
Light Raspberry	6 oz	90	5	0	16
Light Strawberry	6 oz	90	5	0	16
Light Strawberry Banana	6 oz	90	5	0	16
Light White Chocolate Strawberry	6 oz	90	5	0	16
Original Cafe Au Lait	6 oz	170	6	2	31
Original Coconut Cream Pie	6 oz	200	6	4	35
Original French Vanilla	6 oz	180	6	2	34
Trix Rainbow Punch	6 oz	190	6	2	36
Trix Raspberry Rainbow	6 oz	190	6	2	36
Trix Strawberry Banana Bash	6 oz	190	6	2	36
Trix Strawberry Punch	4 oz	130	4	2	24
Trix Triple Cherry	6 oz	190	6	2	36
Trix Watermelon Burst	4 oz	130	4	2	24
Trix Wild Berry Blue	4 oz	130	4	2	24
Whips! Orange Creme	1 pkg (4 oz)	140	5	3	23
Whips! Raspberry Mousse	1 pkg (4 oz)	140	5	3	23
YOGURT FROZEN					
chocolate soft serve	½ cup (4 fl oz)	115	3	4	18
vanilla soft serve	½ cup (4 fl oz)	114	3	4	17
Ben & Jerry's					
Cherry Garcia	½ cup	170	4	3	32
Chocolate Cherry Garcia	½ cup	190	5	4	35
Chocolate Chip Cookie Dough	½ cup	200	4	5	35
Chocolate Fudge Brownie	½ cup	190	5	3	36
Chocolate Heath Bar Crunch	½ cup	210	5	6	35

FOOD	PORTION	CALS	PROT	FAT	CARB
Chunky Monkey	½ cup	200	4	6	34
Pop Cherry Garcia	1	260	5	14	31
Breyers					
Chocolate	½ cup (2.6 oz)	130	3	3	23
Fat Free Chocolate	½ cup (2.6 oz)	100	3	0	23
Fat Free Cookies N Cream	½ cup (2.6 oz)	110	3	0	25
Fat Free Peach	½ cup (2.6 oz)	90	3	0	20
Fat Free Strawberry	½ cup (2.6 oz)	100	2	0	22
Fat Free Take Two Vanilla Chocolate	½ cup (2.6 oz)	100	2	0	23
Fat Free Vanilla	½ cup (2.6 oz)	100	3	0	23
Fat Free Vanilla Fudge Twirl	½ cup (2.6 oz)	110	3	0	25
Vanilla	½ cup (2.6 oz)	120	3	3	22
Vanilla Chocolate Strawberry	½ cup (2.6 oz)	120	3	3	22
Dannon					
Light Cappuccino	½ cup (2.8 oz)	80	4	0	20
Light Cherry Vanilla Swirl	½ cup (2.8 oz)	90	4	0	21
Light Chocolate	½ cup (2.7 oz)	80	4	0	21
Light Mint Chocolate Fudge	½ cup (2.8 oz)	90	4	0	23
Light Peach Raspberry Melba	½ cup (2.8 oz)	90	4	0	20
Light Strawberry Cheesecake	½ cup (2.8 oz)	90	3	0	21
Light Vanilla	½ cup (2.8 oz)	80	4	0	20
Light Duets Strawberry Sundae	6 oz	90	5	0	18
Light'N Crunchy Banana Cream Pie	½ cup (2.8 oz)	110	3	1	23
Light'N Crunchy Carmel Toffee Crunch	½ cup (2.8 oz)	110	3	1	26
Light'N Crunchy Mocha Chocolate Chunk	½ cup (2.8 oz)	110	4	1	23
Light'N Crunchy Peanut Chocolate Crunch	½ cup (2.8 oz)	110	4	1	24
Light'N Crunchy Rocky Road	½ cup (2.8 oz)	110	3	1	27
Light'N Crunchy Triple Chocolate	½ cup (2.8 oz)	110	4	1	25
Light'N Crunchy Vanilla Streusel	½ cup (2.8 oz)	110	3	1	25
Edy's					
Black Cherry Vanilla Swirl	½ cup	90	3	0	20
Caramel Fudge Cosmo	½ cup	140	2	4	23
Caramel Praline Crunch	½ cup	100	3	0	23
Chocolate Decadence	½ cup	120	2	4	20
Chocolate Fudge	½ cup	100	3	0	22

FOOD	PORTION	CALS	PROT	FAT	CARB
Coffee Fudge Sundae	½ cup	100	3	0	22
Cookies'N Cream	½ cup	120	2	4	19
Heath Toffee Crunch	½ cup	120	2	4	18
Raspberry	½ cup	90	2	3	16
Ultimate Tin Roof Sundae	½ cup	130	3	4	20
Vanilla	½ cup	90	3	0	19
Vanilla Chocolate Swirl	½ cup	90	3	0	19
Haagen-Dazs					
Lowfat Dulce De Leche	½ cup	190	6	3	35
Nonfat Chocolate	½ cup	140	7	0	28
Nonfat Coffee	½ cup	140	7	0	29
Nonfat Strawberry	½ cup	140	5	0	31
Nonfat Vanilla	½ cup	140	6	0	29
Nonfat Vanilla Raspberry Swirl	½ cup	130	4	0	29
Nonfat Vanilla Fudge	½ cup	160	6	0	34
Turkey Hill					
Chocolate Chip Cookie Dough	½ cup	140	3	5	23
Fat Free Chocolate Cherry Cordial	½ cup	100	4	0	24
Fat Free Chocolate Marshmallow	½ cup	130	3	0	30
Fat Free Mint Cookie 'N Cream	½ cup	110	4	0	24
Fat Free Neapolitan	½ cup	100	3	0	22
Fat Free Vanilla Fudge	½ cup	110	3	0	24
Peach Raspberry	½ cup	110	3	2	20
Tin Roof Sundae	½ cup	140	4	5	21
Vanilla & Chocolate	½ cup	110	3	3	19
Vanilla Bean	½ cup	110	4	3	17
ZUCCHINI					
canned					
italian style	½ cup	33	1	tr	8
Progresso					
Italian Style	½ cup (4.2 oz)	50	2	2	7
fresh					
raw sliced	½ cup	9	1	tr	2
sliced cooked	½ cup	14	1	tr	4
frozen					
cooked	½ cup	19	1	tr	4
take-out					
indian paalkora	1 serv	46	2	2	7

PART II

Restaurant Chains

FOOD	PORTION	CALS	PROT	FAT	CARB
APPLEBEE'S					
desserts					
Apple Betty Cobbler Ala Mode	1 serv	598	7	22	94
Fudge Brownie Sundae	1 serv	739	9	40	87
Low Fat Bikini Banana Strawberry Shortcake	1 serv	248	6	2	48
Low Fat Brownie Sundae	1 serv	415	11	2	82
Low Fat Marble Cheesecake	1 serv	261	10	2	50
main menu selections					
Applebee's Burger w/ Fries	1 serv	1274	55	79	90
Basic Hamburger w/ Fries	1 serv	980	31	58	86
Beef Fajita Quesadilla	1 serv	1205	51	86	58
Bourbon Street Steak w/ Fried New Potatoes	1 serv	1115	60	94	50
Low Fat Asian Chicken Salad	1 med serv (2.5 oz)	370	19	6	64
Low Fat Asian Chicken Salad	1 reg serv (5 oz)	623	35	9	107
Low Fat Blackened Chicken Salad	1 med serv (2.5 oz)	287	40	3	27
Low Fat Blackened ChickenSalad	1 reg serv (5 oz)	411	56	5	39
Low Fat Garlic Chicken Pasta	1 serv	587	41	8	89
Low Fat Lemon Chicken Pasta	1 serv	528	33	11	78
Low Fat Quesadilla Chicken Fajita	1 serv	518	42	11	63
Low Fat Quesadilla Veggie	1 serv	344	27	8	46
Mozzarella Stix	8 pieces	963	41	57	74
Quesadillas	1 serv	684	31	46	40
Riblet Basket w/ Fries	1 serv	1317	78	92	45
Salad Dinner w/o Dressing	1 serv	303	22	18	13
Salad Santa Fe Chicken	1 med	724	33	42	56
Sandwich Bacon Cheese Chicken Grill w/o Fries	1	746	46	46	36
Sandwich Gyro	1	880	24	69	44
Stir Fry Chicken	1 serv	566	38	7	89
ARBY'S					
beverages					
Chocolate Shake	1 (14 oz)	480	10	16	84
Hot Chocolate	1 serv (8.6 oz)	110	2	1	23
Jamocha Shake	1 (14 oz)	470	10	15	82
Orange Juice	1 serv (10 oz)	140	1	0	34
Strawberry Shake	1 (14 oz)	500	11	13	87
Vanilla Shake	1 (14 oz)	470	10	15	83

FOOD	PORTION	CALS	PROT	FAT	CARB
breakfast selections					
Add Egg To Breakfast	1 serv (2 oz)	110	5	9	2
Biscuit w/ Bacon	1 (3.4 oz)	360	9	24	27
Biscuit w/ Butter	1 (2.9 oz)	280	5	17	27
Biscuit w/ Ham	1 (4.3 oz)	330	12	20	28
Biscuit w/ Sausage	1 (4.2)	460	12	33	28
Croissant w/ Bacon	1 (2.7 oz)	340	10	23	28
Croissant w/ Ham	1 (3.7 oz)	310	13	19	29
Croissant w/ Sausage	1 (3.6 oz)	440	13	32	29
Maple Syrup	1 serv (0.5 oz)	130	0	0	32
Sourdough w/ Bacon	1 (5.1 oz)	420	16	10	66
Sourdough w/ Ham	1 (6.1 oz)	390	19	6	67
Sourdough w/ Sausage	1 (5.9 oz)	520	19	19	67
Toastix w/o Syrup	6 pieces (4.4 oz)	370	7	17	48
desserts					
Apple Turnover Iced	1 (4.5 oz)	420	4	16	65
Cherry Turnover Iced	1 (4.5 oz)	410	4	16	63
main menu selections					
Arby's Sauce	1 serv (0.5 oz)	15	0	0	4
BBQ Dipping Sauce	1 serv (1 oz)	40	0	0	10
Baked Potato Broccoli'N Cheddar	1 (14 oz)	540	12	24	71
Baked Potato Deluxe	1 (13 oz)	650	20	34	67
Baked Potato w/ Butter & Sour Cream	1 (11.2 oz)	500	8	24	65
Bronco Berry Sauce	1 serv (1.5 oz)	90	0	0	23
Caesar Salad w/o Dressing	1 serv (8 oz)	90	7	4	8
Cheddar Curly Fries	1 serv (6 oz)	460	6	24	54
Chicken Finger 4-Pak	1 serv (6.77 oz)	640	31	38	42
Chicken Finger Salad w/o Dressing	1 serv (13 oz)	570	30	34	39
Chicken Finger Snack	1 serv (6.4 oz)	580	19	32	55
Curly Fries	1 med (4.5 oz)	400	5	20	50
Curly Fries	1 lg (7 oz)	620	8	30	78
Curly Fries	1 sm (3.8 oz)	310	4	15	39
German Mustard	1 pkg (0.25 oz)	5	0	0	0
Grilled Chicken Caesar Salad w/o Dressing	1 serv (12 oz)	230	33	8	8
Homestyle Fries	1 lg (7.5 oz)	560	6	24	79
Homestyle Fries	1 med (5 oz)	370	4	16	53
Homestyle Fries	1 sm (4 oz)	300	3	13	42
Homestyle Fries Child-Size	1 serv (3 oz)	220	3	10	32
Honey Mustard	1 serv (1 oz)	130	0	12	5
Horsey Sauce	1 pkg (0.5 oz)	60	0	5	3
Jalapeno Bites	1 serv (4 oz)	330	7	21	29
Ketchup	1 pkg (0.3 oz)	10	0	0	2
Light Grilled Chicken Salad	1 (16.3 oz)	210	30	5	14
Marinara Sauce	1 serv (1.5 oz)	35	1	1	4

FOOD	PORTION	CALS	PROT	FAT	CARB
Mayonnaise	1 pkg (0.4 oz)	90	0	10	0
Mayonnaise Light Cholesterol Free	1 pkg (0.4 oz)	20	0	2	1
Mozzarella Sticks	1 serv (4.8 oz)	470	18	29	34
Onion Petals	1 serv (4 oz)	410	4	24	43
Potato Cakes	2 (3.5 oz)	250	2	16	26
Roast Beef Sandwich Arby's Melt w/ Cheddar	1 (5.2 oz)	320	16	14	36
Roast Beef Sandwich Arby-Q	1 (6.4 oz)	360	16	14	40
Roast Beef Sandwich Beef'N Cheddar	1 (6.9 oz)	460	23	23	43
Roast Beef Sandwich Big Montana	1 (11 oz)	560	47	27	42
Roast Beef Sandwich Giant	1 (7.9 oz)	440	32	20	42
Roast Beef Sandwich Junior	1 (4.4 oz)	290	16	12	34
Roast Beef Sandwich Regular	1 (5.4 oz)	330	21	14	35
Roast Beef Sandwich Super	1 (8.5 oz)	450	22	21	48
Sandwich Chicken Bacon'N Swiss	1 (7.4 oz)	610	31	33	49
Sandwich Chicken Breast Fillet	1 (7.2 oz)	550	24	30	47
Sandwich Chicken Cordon Bleu	1 (8.4 oz)	630	34	35	47
Sandwich Grilled Chicken Deluxe	1 (8.7 oz)	450	29	22	37
Sandwich Hot Ham 'N Swiss	1 (5.9 oz)	340	23	13	35
Sandwich Light Roast Chicken Deluxe	1 (7.2 oz)	260	23	5	33
Sandwich Light Roast Turkey Deluxe	1 (7.2 oz)	260	23	5	33
Sandwich Market Fresh Roast Beef & Swiss	1 (12.5 oz)	780	37	40	74
Sandwich Market Fresh Roast Chicken Caesar	1 (12.7 oz)	820	43	38	75
Sandwich Market Fresh Roast Ham & Swiss	1 (12.5 oz)	730	36	34	74
Sandwich Market Fresh Roast Turkey & Swiss	1 (12.5 oz)	760	43	33	75
Sandwich Roast Chicken Club	1 (8.4 oz)	520	29	28	38
Sub Sandwich French Dip	1 (10 oz)	410	26	16	43
Sub Sandwich Hot Ham'N Swiss	1 (9.7 oz)	530	29	27	45
Sub Sandwich Italian	1 (11 oz)	780	29	53	49

FOOD	PORTION	CALS	PROT	FAT	CARB
Sub Sandwich Pilly Beef'N Swiss	1 (10.8 oz)	670	36	40	46
Sub Sandwich Roast Beef	1 (11.6 oz)	730	35	46	48
Sub Sandwich Turkey	1 (10.6 oz)	630	29	37	51
Tangy Southwest Sauce	1 serv (1.5 oz)	250	0	26	3
salad dressings					
Bleu Cheese	1 serv (2 oz)	300	2	31	3
Buttermilk Ranch	1 serv (2 oz)	360	1	39	2
Buttermilk Ranch Reduced Calorie	1 serv (2 oz)	60	1	0	13
Caesar	1 serv (2 oz)	310	1	34	1
Honey French	1 serv (2 oz)	290	0	24	18
Italian Reduced Calorie	1 serv (2 oz)	25	0	1	3
Thousand Island	1 serv (2 oz)	290	1	28	9
salads and salad bars					
Croutons Seasoned	1 serv (0.25 oz)	30	1	1	5
Croutons Cheese & Garlic	1 serv (0.63 oz)	100	3	6	10
Garden Salad	1 (12.3 oz)	70	4	1	14
Light Roast Chicken Salad	1 (14.8 oz)	160	20	3	15
Side Salad	1 (6.1 oz)	30	2	0	6
Turkey Club Salad w/o Dressing	1 serv (12 oz)	350	33	21	9
AU BON PAIN					
baked selections					
Apple Coffee Cake	1 piece (4.6 oz)	480	6	24	60
Bagel Chocolate Chip	1 (5 oz)	380	12	7	69
Bagel Dutch Apple w/ Walnut Streussel	1 (5 oz)	360	11	5	77
Baguette Loaf	1 slice (1.8 oz)	140	5	5	29
Biscotti	1 (1.5 oz)	200	4	10	24
Biscotti Chocolate	1 (1.7 oz)	240	5	13	28
Braided Roll	1 (1.8 oz)	170	5	5	26
Cinnamon Roll	1 (7 oz)	710	12	26	110
Cookie Chocolate Chip	1 (2.1 oz)	280	3	13	40
Cookie Oatmeal Raisin	1 (2.1 oz)	250	3	10	40
Cookie Shortbread	1 (2.4 oz)	390	3	25	39
Croissant Almond	1 (4.3 oz)	560	12	37	50
Croissant Apple	1 (3.4 oz)	280	4	10	46
Croissant Chocolate	1 (3.4 oz)	440	7	23	53
Croissant Cinnamon Raisin	1 (3.7 oz)	380	7	13	61
Croissant Plain	1 (2.1 oz)	270	6	15	30
Croissant Raspberry Cheese	1 (3.5 oz)	380	6	19	47
Croissant Sweet Cheese	1 (3.6 oz)	390	7	22	42
Danish Cheese Swirl	1 (3.8 oz)	450	7	28	46
Danish Lemon Swirl	1 (4 oz)	450	7	24	53
Four Grain Loaf	1 slice (1.8 oz)	130	5	1	25

FOOD	PORTION	CALS	PROT	FAT	CARB
French Sandwich Roll	1 (1.8 oz)	120	4	5	25
Hazelnut Fudge Brownie	1 (4 oz)	380	5	18	56
Mochaccino Bar	1 (4 oz)	404	5	24	44
Muffin Blueberry	1 (4.5 oz)	410	8	15	64
Muffin Carrot	1 (5 oz)	480	8	23	61
Muffin Chocolate Chip	1 (4.5 oz)	490	8	20	70
Muffin Corn	1 (4.6 oz)	470	8	18	70
Muffin Pumpkin w/ Streusel Topping	1 (5.5 oz)	470	8	18	74
Muffin Low Fat Chocolate Cake	1 (4 oz)	290	4	3	68
Muffin Low Fat Triple Berry	1 (4.2 oz)	270	5	3	60
Multigrain Loaf	1 slice (1.8 oz)	130	5	1	26
Parisienne Loaf	1 slice (1.8 oz)	120	4	5	25
Pear Ginger Tea Cake	1 piece (4 oz)	380	3	20	47
Pecan Roll	1 (6.8 oz)	900	11	48	111
Roll 3 Seed Pecan Raisin	1 (2.7 oz)	250	9	6	43
Roll Hearth Sandwich	1 (2.8 oz)	220	9	2	43
Roll Petit Pan	1 (2.5 oz)	200	7	1	41
Rye Loaf	1 slice (1.8 oz)	110	5	2	21
Scone Cinnamon	1 (4.1 oz)	520	10	28	60
Scone Current	1 (3.7 oz)	430	10	23	47
Scone Orange	1 (4.1 oz)	440	10	23	53
Sourdough Bagel Asiago Cheese	1 (4.2 oz)	380	17	6	66
Sourdough Bagel Cinnamon Raisin	1 (4.5 oz)	390	14	1	83
Sourdough Bagel Cranberry Walnut	1 (5 oz)	460	15	4	93
Sourdough Bagel Everything	1 (4.2 oz)	360	14	3	72
Sourdough Bagel Honey 8 Grain	1 (4.2 oz)	360	14	2	72
Sourdough Bagel Mocha Chip Swirl	1 (5 oz)	370	12	4	72
Sourdough Bagel Plain	1 (4 oz)	350	13	1	71
Sourdough Bagel Sesame	1 (4.2 oz)	380	15	4	71
Sourdough Bagel Wild Blueberry	1 (4.5 oz)	380	14	2	80
beverages					
Frozen Java Blast	1 serv (16 oz)	220	7	2	42
Frozen Mocha Blast	1 serv (16 oz)	320	9	3	64
Hot Hazelnut Blast	1 serv (16 oz)	310	11	6	57
Hot Mocha Blast	1 lg (17 oz)	310	14	8	45
Hot Strawberry Chocolate Blast	1 serv (16 oz)	330	11	6	57
Hot Vanilla Chocolate Blast	1 serv (16 oz)	310	11	6	57
Iced Hazelnut Blast	1 serv (16 oz)	310	11	6	54
Iced Mocha Blast	1 med (12 oz)	260	11	6	41

FOOD	PORTION	CALS	PROT	FAT	CARB
Iced Raspberry Mocha Blast	1 serv (16 oz)	310	11	6	54
Iced Strawberry Chocolate Blast	1 serv (16 oz)	310	11	6	54
Iced Vanilla Chocolate Blast	1 serv (16 oz)	310	11	6	54
Iced Tea Peach	1 med (16 oz)	130	0	0	33
Iced Tea Peach	1 sm (12 oz)	90	0	0	22
Iced Tea Raspberry	1 lg (16 oz)	150	0	0	38
salad dressings					
Bleu Cheese	1 serv (3 oz)	370	4	41	8
Buttermilk Ranch	1 serv (3 oz)	310	3	32	4
Caesar	1 serv (3 oz)	380	5	39	3
Fat Free Tomato Basil	1 serv (3 oz)	70	1	0	17
Greek	1 serv (3 oz)	440	0	50	2
Lemon Basil Vinaigrette	1 serv (3 oz)	330	0	32	15
Lite Honey Mustard	1 serv (3 oz)	280	2	17	30
Lite Italian	1 serv (3 oz)	230	0	20	15
Sesame French	1 serv (3 oz)	370	1	30	26
salads and salad bars					
Caesar	1 serv (8.9 oz)	270	19	10	27
Chicken Caesar	1 serv (11.4 oz)	360	36	11	28
Garden	1 lg (10.6 oz)	160	7	2	34
Garden	1 sm (7.5 oz)	100	5	1	20
Mozzarella & Roasted Pepper Salad	1 serv (13.7 oz)	340	22	18	25
Pesto Chicken Salad	1 serv (10.7 oz)	230	20	11	11
Tuna	1 serv (15 oz)	490	26	27	40
sandwiches and fillings					
Bagel Spreads Lite Strawberry	1 serv (2 oz)	150	5	11	6
Bagel Spreads Lite Vanilla Hazelnut	1 serv (2 oz)	150	5	11	6
Cheddar	½ serv (1.5 oz)	170	11	14	1
Chicken Tarragon	1 serv (4 oz)	240	20	17	1
Club Sandwich Hot Roasted Turkey	1 (14.9 oz)	950	50	50	80
Country Ham	1 serv (3.7 oz)	150	21	7	1
Cracked Pepper Chicken	1 serv (3.9 oz)	140	27	2	2
Cream Cheese Lite	1 serv (2 oz)	130	5	12	2
Cream Cheese Lite Honey Walnut	1 serv (2 oz)	260	4	12	8
Cream Cheese Lite Raspberry	1 serv (2 oz)	200	6	8	10
Cream Cheese Lite Sun-Dried Tomato	1 serv (2 oz)	130	5	11	6
Cream Cheese Plain	1 serv (2 oz)	190	3	18	2
Cream Cheese Veggie Lite	1 serv (2 oz)	100	6	10	6
Grilled Chicken	1 serv (3.9 oz)	140	27	2	2

FOOD	PORTION	CALS	PROT	FAT	CARB
Hot Croissant Ham & Cheese	1 (4.2 oz)	380	16	20	36
Hot Croissant Spinach & Cheese	1 (3.6 oz)	270	9	16	27
Provolone	½ serv (1.5 oz)	150	11	11	1
Roast Beef	1 serv (3.7 oz)	140	22	5	1
Sandwich Arizona Chicken	1 (12.7 oz)	720	49	33	57
Sandwich Buffalo Chicken	1 (13.7 oz)	640	41	19	76
Sandwich California Chicken	1 (13.2 oz)	820	51	44	55
Sandwich Fresh Mozzarella Tomato & Pesto	1 (10.5 oz)	650	30	30	69
Sandwich Honey Dijon Chicken	1 (15.3 oz)	730	57	18	85
Sandwich Parmesan Chicken	1 (11.1 oz)	740	42	24	91
Sandwich Steak & Cheese Melt	1 (11.7 oz)	750	40	32	79
Sandwich Thai Chicken	1 (8.3 oz)	420	20	6	72
Swiss	½ serv (1.5 oz)	160	12	12	1
Tuna Salad	1 serv (4.5 oz)	360	21	29	3
Turkey Breast	1 serv (3.7 oz)	120	24	1	1
Wraps Chicken Caesar	1 (9.9 oz)	630	36	31	46
Wraps Southwestern Tuna	1 (14.4 oz)	950	41	64	53
Wraps Summer Turkey	1 (11.7 oz)	340	29	9	36
soups					
Beef Barley	1 serv (12 oz)	112	9	3	16
Beef Barley	1 serv (16 oz)	150	12	4	22
Beef Barley	1 serv (8 oz)	75	6	2	11
Bohemian Cabbage	1 serv (8 oz)	70	3	3	11
Bohemian Cabbage	1 serv (12 oz)	110	4	5	17
Bohemian Cabbage	1 serv (16 oz)	140	5	6	22
Bread Bowl	1 (9 oz)	640	27	4	131
Caribbean Black Bean	1 serv (16 oz)	250	13	2	43
Caribbean Black Bean	1 serv (12 oz)	180	10	2	32
Caribbean Black Bean	1 serv (8 oz)	120	7	1	22
Chicken Chili	1 serv (12 oz)	350	21	18	31
Chicken Chili	1 serv (8 oz)	240	14	12	21
Chicken Chili	1 serv (16 oz)	470	28	24	41
Chicken Noodle	1 serv (16 oz)	170	16	3	19
Chicken Noodle	1 serv (8 oz)	80	8	2	10
Chicken Noodle	1 serv (12 oz)	120	12	2	14
Clam Chowder	1 serv (12 oz)	400	16	29	24
Clam Chowder	1 serv (16 oz)	540	22	39	32
Clam Chowder	1 serv (8 oz)	270	11	19	16
Cream Of Broccoli	1 serv (16 oz)	440	10	37	28
Cream Of Broccoli	1 serv (8 oz)	220	5	18	14

FOOD	PORTION	CALS	PROT	FAT	CARB
French Onion	1 serv (12 oz)	120	4	5	17
French Onion	1 serv (16 oz)	170	5	7	23
French Onion	1 serv (8 oz)	80	2	4	12
In A Bread Bowl Beef Barley	1 serv (21 oz)	760	36	7	147
In A Bread Bowl Carribean Black Bean	1 serv (21 oz)	830	36	5	163
In A Bread Bowl Chicken Chili	1 serv (21 oz)	990	48	22	162
In A Bread Bowl Chicken Noodle	1 serv (21 oz)	760	39	6	146
In A Bread Bowl Clam Chowder	1 serv (21 oz)	1050	43	32	155
In A Bread Bowl Cream of Broccoli	1 serv (21 oz)	970	34	31	152
In A Bread Bowl French Onion	1 serv (21 oz)	760	30	8	148
In A Bread Bowl New England Potato & Cheese w/ Ham	1 serv (21 oz)	860	34	15	152
In A Bread Bowl Tomato Florentine	1 serv (21 oz)	760	33	5	150
In A Bread Bowl Vegetarian Chili	1 serv (21 oz)	870	36	7	171
Louisiana Beans & Rice	1 serv (16 oz)	360	18	9	50
Louisiana Beans & Rice	1 serv (8 oz)	180	9	5	25
Louisiana Beans & Rice	1 serv (12 oz)	280	13	7	37
New England Potato & Cheese w/ Ham	1 serv (8 oz)	150	5	8	14
New England Potato & Cheese w/ Ham	1 serv (12 oz)	220	7	12	21
New England Potato & Cheese w/ Ham	1 serv (16 oz)	290	10	15	28
Potato Leek	1 serv (12 oz)	320	6	20	28
Potato Leek	1 serv (8 oz)	200	4	13	18
Potato Leek	1 serv (16 oz)	400	7	25	36
Sante Fe Chicken Tortilla	1 serv (16 oz)	300	12	13	42
Sante Fe Chicken Tortilla	1 serv (8 oz)	150	6	7	21
Sante Fe Chicken Tortilla	1 serv (12 oz)	230	9	10	32
Tomato Florentine	1 serv (8 oz)	61	4	1	13
Tomato Florentine	1 serv (12 oz)	90	6	2	20
Tomato Florentine	1 serv (16 oz)	122	8	2	27
Vegetarian Chili	1 serv (12 oz)	210	9	4	40
Vegetarian Chili	1 serv (8 oz)	139	6	3	27
Vegetarian Chili	1 serv (16 oz)	278	13	5	53
Vegetarian Corn & Green Chili Bisque	1 serv (8 oz)	190	4	10	21

FOOD	PORTION	CALS	PROT	FAT	CARB
Vegetarian Corn & Green Chili Bisque	1 serv (16 oz)	380	8	20	41
Vegetarian Corn & Green Chili Bisque	1 serv (12 oz)	300	7	16	30
AUNTIE ANNE'S					
Caramel Dip	1 serv (1.5 oz)	135	1	3	27
Cheese Sauce	1 serv (1 oz)	70	3	5	2
Chocolate Dip	1 serv (1.25 oz)	130	1	4	24
Cream Cheese Light	1 serv (.75 oz)	45	2	4	1
Dutch Ice Kiwi Banana	1 (18 oz)	250	0	0	57
Dutch Ice Kiwi Banana	1 (12 oz)	160	0	0	38
Dutch Ice Lemonade	1 (12 oz)	270	0	0	66
Dutch Ice Lemonade	1 (18 oz)	405	0	0	99
Dutch Ice Mocha	1 (18 oz)	500	0	14	95
Dutch Ice Mocha	1 (12 oz)	340	0	9	63
Dutch Ice Orange Creme	1 (12 oz)	240	0	0	55
Dutch Ice Orange Creme	1 (18 oz)	360	0	0	83
Dutch Ice Raspberry	1 (18 oz)	220	0	0	51
Dutch Ice Raspberry	1 (12 oz)	150	0	0	34
Dutch Ice Strawberry	1 (12 oz)	190	0	0	43
Dutch Ice Strawberry	1 (18 oz)	280	0	0	65
Marinara Sauce	1 serv (1 oz)	10	0	0	3
Pretzel Almond w/ Butter	1	400	9	8	72
Pretzel Almond w/o Butter	1	350	9	2	72
Pretzel Cinnamon Raisin w/o Butter	1	350	9	2	74
Pretzel Cinnamon Sugar w/ Butter	1	450	8	9	83
Pretzel Garlic w/ Butter	1	350	9	5	68
Pretzel Garlic w/o Butter	1	320	9	1	66
Pretzel Glazin' Raisin w/ Butter	1	510	11	4	107
Pretzel Glazin' Raisin w/o Butter	1	470	11	1	104
Pretzel Jalapeno w/ Butter	1	310	8	5	59
Pretzel Jalapeno w/o Butter	1	270	8	1	58
Pretzel Original w/ Butter	1	370	10	4	72
Pretzel Original w/o Butter	1	340	10	1	72
Pretzel Sesame w/ Butter	1	410	12	12	64
Pretzel Sesame w/o Butter	1	350	11	6	63
Pretzel Sour Cream & Onion w/ Butter	1	340	9	5	66
Pretzel Sour Cream & Onion w/o Butter	1	310	9	1	66
Pretzel Whole Wheat w/ Butter	1	370	11	5	72
Pretzel Whole Wheat w/o Butter	1	350	11	2	72

FOOD	PORTION	CALS	PROT	FAT	CARB
BASKIN-ROBBINS					
frozen yogurt					
Maui Brownie Madness	½ cup	140	4	3	26
Perils Of Pauline	½ cup	140	4	3	25
ice cream					
Banana Strawberry	½ cup	130	2	7	17
Baseball Nut	½ cup	160	2	9	18
Black Walnut	½ cup	160	3	11	13
Cherries Jubilee	½ cup	140	2	7	16
Chocolate	½ cup	150	2	9	18
Chocolate Almond	½ cup	180	3	11	17
Chocolate Chip	½ cup	150	2	10	15
Chocolate Chip Cookie Dough	½ cup	170	2	9	20
Chocolate Fudge	½ cup	160	2	9	21
Chocolate Mousse Royale	½ cup	170	2	10	20
Chocolate Raspberry Truffle	½ cup	180	3	9	23
Chunky Heath Bar	½ cup	170	2	10	19
Cookies N Cream	½ cup	170	2	11	16
Dirt'N Worms	½ cup	160	2	8	22
Egg Nog	½ cup	150	2	8	16
Everybody's Favorite Candy Bar	½ cup	170	2	9	20
French Vanilla	½ cup	160	2	10	14
Fudge Brownie	½ cup	170	3	11	19
German Chocolate Cake	½ cup	180	3	10	20
Gold Medal Ribbon	½ cup	150	2	8	20
Jamoca	½ cup	140	2	9	14
Jomoca Almond Fudge	½ cup	140	3	9	17
Lemon Custard	½ cup	150	2	8	16
Lowfat Carmel Apple Ala Mode	½ cup	100	3	2	20
Lowfat Espresso'N Cream	½ cup	100	3	3	18
Mint Chocolate Chip	½ cup	150	3	10	15
No Sugar Added Call Me Nuts	½ cup	110	3	2	21
No Sugar Added Cherry Cordial	½ cup	100	3	2	18
No Sugar Added Mad About Chocolate	½ cup	100	3	2	19
No Sugar Added Pineapple Coconut	½ cup	90	3	2	16
No Sugar Added Thin Mint	½ cup	100	3	3	16
Nonfat Berry Innocent Cheese	½ cup	110	3	0	24
Nonfat Check-It-Out Cherry	½ cup	100	3	0	22

FOOD	PORTION	CALS	PROT	FAT	CARB
Nonfat Jamoca Swirl	½ cup	110	3	0	23
Ocean Commotion	½ cup	150	1	7	20
Old Fashion Butter Pecan	½ cup	160	2	11	13
Oregon Blueberry	½ cup	140	2	8	16
Peanut Butter 'N Chocolate	½ cup	180	3	12	16
Pink Bubblegum	½ cup	150	2	8	19
Pistachio Almond	½ cup	170	3	12	13
Pralines N Cream	½ cup	160	2	9	19
Pumpkin Pie	½ cup	130	2	7	16
Quarterback Crunch	½ cup	160	2	10	18
Reeses Peanut Butter	½ cup	180	3	11	17
Rocky Road	½ cup	170	3	10	19
Rum Raisin	½ cup	140	2	7	18
Strawberry Cheesecake	½ cup	150	2	9	17
Triple Chocolate Passion	½ cup	180	3	11	21
Vanilla	½ cup	140	3	8	14
Very Berry Strawberry	½ cup	130	1	7	16
Winter White Chocolate	½ cup	150	2	9	18
World Class Chocolate	½ cup	160	2	9	18
ices and ice pops					
Daiquiri Ice	½ cup	110	0	0	28
Sherbet Blue Raspberry	½ cup	120	1	2	25
Sherbet Orange	½ cup	120	1	2	26
Sherbet Rainbow	½ cup	120	1	2	26
Sorbet Pink Raspberry Lemon	½ cup	120	0	0	29
The Mask Ice	½ cup	120	0	0	29
Watermelon Ice	½ cup	110	0	0	28
BEN & JERRY'S					
Sugar Cone	1	48	1	tr	10
frozen yogurt					
Cherry Garcia	½ cup (3.3 oz)	150	4	3	29
Chocolate Cherry Garcia	½ cup (3.3 oz)	170	4	4	37
Chocolate Fudge Brownie	½ cup (3.3 oz)	180	5	3	32
No Fat Black Raspberry	½ cup (3.4 oz)	140	4	0	30
No Fat Coffee Fudge	½ cup (3.4 oz)	140	4	0	30
No Fat Vanilla	½ cup (3.4 oz)	140	5	0	28
No Fat Vanilla Fudge Swirl	½ cup (3.4 oz)	130	3	0	29
ice cream					
Bovinity Divinity	½ cup (3.1 oz)	240	3	14	24
Butter Pecan	½ cup (3.1 oz)	270	4	21	17
Cherry Garcia	½ cup (3.1 oz)	210	3	12	20
Chocolate Chip Cookie Dough	½ cup (3.1 oz)	180	3	11	17
Chocolate Fudge Brownie	½ cup (3.1 oz)	230	4	11	28
Chubby Hubby	½ cup (3.1 oz)	280	5	17	26
Chunky Monkey	½ cup (3.1 oz)	220	3	13	25

FOOD	PORTION	CALS	PROT	FAT	CARB
Coconut Almond Fudge Chip	½ cup (3.1 oz)	250	4	18	19
Coffee Coffee Buzz Buzz	½ cup (3.1 oz)	240	3	16	23
Coffee Ole	½ cup (3.1 oz)	200	3	13	18
Coffee w/ Heath Bar Crunch	½ cup (3.1 oz)	250	3	16	25
Deep Dark Chocolate	½ cup (3.1 oz)	210	4	12	22
Dilbert's World Totally Nuts	½ cup (3.1 oz)	260	4	18	21
Low Fat Blackberry Cobbler	½ cup (3.2 oz)	160	3	2	32
Low Fat Chocolate Comfort	½ cup (3.2 oz)	150	4	2	27
Low Fat Coconut Creme Pie	½ cup (3.2 oz)	160	4	3	29
Low Fat Mocha Latte	½ cup (3.2 oz)	150	4	2	27
Low Fat Rockin Road	½ cup (3.2 oz)	180	5	3	34
Low Fat Smore's	½ cup (3.2 oz)	180	4	2	34
Low Fat Vanilla & Chocolate Mint Patty	½ cup (3.2 oz)	170	4	3	32
Maple Walnut	½ cup (3.1 oz)	240	3	13	19
Mint Chocolate Chunk	½ cup (3.1 oz)	240	3	16	24
Mint Chocolate Cookie	½ cup (3.1 oz)	230	4	14	24
New York Super Fudge Chunk	½ cup (3.1 oz)	250	4	16	25
Peanut Butter Cup	½ cup (3.1 oz)	270	5	18	21
Phish Food	½ cup (3.1 oz)	230	3	12	30
Pistachio Pistachio	½ cup (3.1 oz)	190	3	13	17
Praline Pecan	½ cup (3.1 oz)	230	3	14	24
Southern Pecan Pie	½ cup (3.1 oz)	240	3	16	21
Strawberry	½ cup (3.1 oz)	180	3	10	20
Sweet Cream Cookie	½ cup (3.1 oz)	230	4	14	23
Triple Caramel Chunk	½ cup (3.1 oz)	240	4	13	28
Vanilla Caramel Fudge	½ cup (3.1 oz)	230	3	13	25
Vanilla Chocolate Chunk	½ cup (3.1 oz)	240	3	16	23
Vanilla World's Best	½ cup (3.1 oz)	200	3	13	17
Wavy Gravy	½ cup (3.1 oz)	260	5	17	24
White Russian	½ cup (3.1 oz)	200	3	13	18
sorbets					
Doonesberry	½ cup (3.2 oz)	100	0	0	27
Lemon Swirl	½ cup (3.2 oz)	100	0	0	25
Purple Passion Fruit	½ cup (3.2 oz)	100	0	0	27
Strawberry Kiwi	½ cup (3.2 oz)	110	0	0	27
BIG BOY					
desserts					
Frozen Yogurt Fat Free	1 serv	118	3	0	27
Frozen Yogurt Shake	1	156	7	1	33
main menu selections					
Baked Cod w/ Salad Baked Potato Roll & Margarine	1 meal	744	57	21	82
Baked Potato	1	163	6	2	37

FOOD	PORTION	CALS	PROT	FAT	CARB
Breast of Chicken Pita w/ Mozzarella & Ranch Dressing	1	361	41	11	23
Breast of Chicken w/ Mozzarella Salad Baked Potato Roll & Margarine	1 meal	697	50	20	80
Cabbage Soup	1 bowl	40	1	5	7
Cabbage Soup	1 cup	34	1	4	6
Cajun Cod w/ Salad Baked Potato Roll & Margarine	1 meal	736	56	21	80
Chicken & Pasta Primavera w/ Salad Roll & Margarine	1 meal	676	53	14	83
Chicken 'n Vegetable Stir Fry w/ Salad Baked Potato Roll & Margarine	1 meal	795	51	18	109
Dinner Roll	1	210	0	5	36
Plain Egg Beaters Omelette w/ Whole Wheat Bread & Margarine	1 meal	305	19	10	36
Promise Margarine	1 pat	25	0	3	0
Rice Pilaf	1 serv	153	3	4	25
Scrambled Egg Beaters w/ Whole Wheat Bread & Margarine	1 meal	305	19	10	36
Southwest Chicken w/ Salad Baked Potato Roll & Margarine	1 meal	702	50	18	85
Spaghetti Marinara w/ Salad Roll & Margarine	1 meal	754	17	11	105
Turkey Pita w/ Ranch Dressing	1	245	25	6	23
Vegetable Stir Fry w/ Salad Baked Potato Roll & Margarine	1 meal	616	17	14	109
Vegetarian Egg Beaters Omelette w/ Whole Wheat Bread & Margarine	1 meal	330	21	10	40

FOOD	PORTION	CALS	PROT	FAT	CARB
salad dressings					
Italian Fat Free	1 oz	11	0	0	3
Lo Cal Oriental	1 oz	20	1	2	4
Lo Cal Ranch	1 oz	41	1	3	3
salads and salad bars					
Chicken Breast Salad w/ Roll & Margarine	1 serv	523	44	16	50
Oriental Chicken Breast Salad w/ Dinner Roll & Margarine	1 serv	660	48	20	73
Tossed Salad	1	35	2	2	7
BLIMPIE					
6 inch sub					
5 Meatball	1 (7.8 oz)	500	23	22	52
Blimpie Best	1 (8.5 oz)	410	26	13	47
Cheese Trio	1 (8.2 oz)	510	26	23	51
Club	1 (9.8 oz)	450	30	13	53
Grilled Chicken	1 (9.1 oz)	400	28	9	52
Ham & Swiss	1 (8.2 oz)	400	25	13	47
Ham Salami Provolone	1 (9.8 oz)	590	32	28	52
Roast Beef	1 (8.5 oz)	340	27	5	47
Steak & Cheese	1 (7.1 oz)	550	27	26	51
Tuna	1 (10.2 oz)	570	21	32	50
Turkey	1 (8.2 oz)	320	19	5	51
salads and salad bars					
Grilled Chicken Salad	1 serv (16.2 oz)	350	47	12	13
BOJANGLES					
baked selections					
Biscuit	1	243	4	12	29
Multi-Grain Roll	1	150	6	3	26
Sweet Biscuit Apple Cinnamon	1	330	4	13	48
Sweet Biscuit Bo*Berry	1	220	3	10	29
Sweet Biscuit Cinnamon	1	320	4	18	37
main menu selections					
Biscuit Sandwich Bacon	1	290	8	17	26
Biscuit Sandwich Bacon Egg & Cheese	1	550	17	42	27
Biscuit Sandwich Cajun Filet	1	454	20	21	46
Biscuit Sandwich Country Ham	1	270	9	15	26
Biscuit Sandwich Egg	1	400	8	30	26
Biscuit Sandwich Sausage	1	350	9	23	26
Biscuit Sandwich Smoked Sausage	1	380	10	26	27
Biscuit Sandwich Steak	1	649	14	49	13

FOOD	PORTION	CALS	PROT	FAT	CARB
Bo Rounds	1 serv	235	3	11	31
Buffalo Bites	1 serv	180	27	5	5
Cajun Pintos	1 serv	110	6	0	18
Cajun Roast Skinfree Breast	1 serv	143	24	5	tr
Cajun Roast Skinfree Leg	1 serv	161	23	8	tr
Cajun Roast Skinfree Thigh	1 serv	215	20	15	tr
Cajun Roast Wing	1 serv	231	22	15	3
Cajun Spiced Breast	1 serv	278	18	17	12
Cajun Spiced Leg	1 serv	310	15	23	11
Cajun Spiced Thigh	1 serv	264	19	16	11
Cajun Spiced Wing	1 serv	355	21	25	11
Chicken Supremes	1 serv	337	21	16	26
Corn On The Cob	1 serv	140	5	2	34
Dirty Rice	1 serv	166	5	6	24
Green Beans	1 serv	25	5	0	25
Macaroni & Cheese	1 serv	198	7	14	12
Marinated Cole Slaw	1 serv	136	1	3	26
Potatoes w/o Gravy	1 serv	80	2	1	16
Sandwich Cajun Filet w/ Mayonnaise	1	437	22	22	41
Sandwich Cajun Filet w/o Mayonnaise	1	337	22	11	41
Sandwich Cajun Steak w/ Horseradish Sauce & Pickles	1	434	18	26	39
Sandwich Grilled Filet w/ Mayonnaise	1	335	23	16	25
Seasoned Fries	1 serv	344	5	19	39
Southern Style Breast	1 serv	261	16	16	12
Southern Style Leg	1 serv	254	19	15	11
Southern Style Thigh	1 serv	308	16	21	14
Southern Style Wing	1 serv	337	17	21	19
BOSTON MARKET					
baked selections					
Brownie	1 (3.3 oz)	450	6	27	47
Cinnamon Apple Pie	⅛ pie (4.8 oz)	390	2	23	46
Cookie Chocolate Chip	1 (2.8 oz)	340	4	17	48
main menu selections					
½ Chicken w/ Skin	1 serv (9.7 oz)	590	70	33	4
¼ Dark Meat Chicken No Skin	1 serv (3.3 oz)	190	22	10	1
¼ Dark Meat Chicken w/ Skin	1 serv (4.4 oz)	320	30	21	2
¼ White Meat Chicken No Skin Or Wing	1 serv (4.9 oz)	170	23	4	2
¼ White Meat Chicken w/ Skin And Wing	1 serv (5.3 oz)	280	40	12	2

FOOD	PORTION	CALS	PROT	FAT	CARB
BBQ Baked Beans	¾ cup (7.1 oz)	270	8	5	48
BBQ Chicken Sandwich	1 (9.9 oz)	540	30	9	84
Baked Sweet Potato Low Fat	1 (12.5 oz)	460	6	7	94
Black Beans And Rice	1 cup (8 oz)	300	8	10	45
Boston Hearth Ham Lean	1 serv (5 oz)	210	25	9	9
Broccoli Cauliflower Au Gratin	¾ cup (6.1 oz)	200	9	11	14
Broccoli Rice Casserole	¾ cup (6 oz)	240	5	12	26
Broccoli w/ Red Peppers	¾ cup (3.4 oz)	60	3	4	5
Butternut Squash Low Fat	¾ cup (6.8 oz)	160	2	6	25
Chicken Gravy	1 serv (1 oz)	15	0	1	2
Chicken Salad Sandwich	1 (11.5 oz)	680	39	30	63
Chicken Sandwich w/ Cheese & Sauce	1 (12.4 oz)	750	41	33	72
Chicken Sandwich w/o Cheese & Sauce Low Fat	1 (10 oz)	430	34	5	62
Chunky Chicken Salad	¾ cup (5.5 oz)	370	28	27	3
Chunky Cinnamon Apple Sauce No Fat	¾ cup (6.4 oz)	250	1	0	62
Cole Slaw	¾ cup (6.5 oz)	300	2	19	30
Corn Bread	1 (2.4 oz)	200	3	6	33
Coyote Bean Salad	¾ cup (5.3 oz)	190	4	9	24
Cranberry Relish Low Fat	¾ cup (7.9 oz)	370	2	5	84
Creamed Spinach	¾ cup (6.4 oz)	260	9	20	11
Fruit Salad Low Fat	¾ cup (5.5 oz)	70	1	1	15
Green Bean Casserole	¾ cup (6 oz)	130	2	9	10
Green Beans	¾ cup (3 oz)	80	1	6	5
Ham Sandwich w/ Cheese & Sauce	1 (11.8 oz)	760	38	34	72
Ham Sandwich w/o Cheese & Sauce	1 (9.3 oz)	440	25	8	66
Homestyle Mashed Potatoes & Gravy	¾ cup (6.6 oz)	210	4	10	26
Honey Glazed Carrots	¾ cup (5.4 oz)	280	1	15	35
Hot Cinnamon Apples	¾ cup (6.4 oz)	250	0	5	56
Macaroni & Cheese	¾ cup (6.7 oz)	280	13	11	32
Mashed Potatoes	⅔ cup (5.6 oz)	190	3	9	24
Meat Loaf & Brown Gravy	1 serv (7 oz)	390	30	22	19
Meat Loaf & Chunky Tomato Sauce	1 serv (8 oz)	370	30	18	22
Meat Loaf Sandwich w/ Cheese	1 (13.8 oz)	860	46	33	95
Meat Loaf Sandwich w/o Cheese	1 (12.3 oz)	690	40	21	86
New Potatoes Low Fat	¾ cup (4.6 oz)	130	3	3	25

FOOD	PORTION	CALS	PROT	FAT	CARB
Old Fashioned Potato Salad	¾ cup (6.2 oz)	340	2	24	30
Open Face Turkey Sandwich	1 (13.4 oz)	500	37	12	61
Original Chicken Pot Pie	1 pie (14.9 oz)	780	32	46	61
Oven Roasted Potato Planks Low Fat	5 pieces (5.8 oz)	180	3	5	32
Pastry Sandwich BBQ Chicken	1 (7.2 oz)	640	17	39	56
Pastry Sandwich Broccoli Chicken Cheddar	1 (7.2 oz)	690	21	47	45
Pastry Sandwich Ham & Cheddar	1 (6.6 oz)	640	19	41	47
Pastry Sandwich Italian Chicken	1 (7.2 oz)	630	21	41	43
Red Beans And Rice Low Fat	1 cup (8 oz)	260	8	5	45
Rice Pilaf	⅔ cup (5.1 oz)	180	5	5	32
Rotisserie Turkey Breast Skinless Low Fat	1 serv (5 oz)	170	36	1	1
Savory Stuffing	¾ cup (6.1 oz)	310	6	12	44
Southwest Savory Chicken	1 serv (9.6 oz)	400	40	15	26
Squash Casserole	¾ cup (6.6 oz)	330	7	24	20
Steamed Vegetables Low Fat	⅔ cup (3.7 oz)	35	2	1	7
Sweet Potato Casserole	¾ cup (6.4 oz)	280	3	18	39
Tabasco BBQ Drumstick	1 (2.4 oz)	130	14	6	4
Tabasco BBQ Wing	1 (1.8 oz)	110	9	7	4
Teriyaki Chicken ¼ White w/ Skin	1 serv (6.8 oz)	340	40	12	17
Teriyaki Chicken ¼ w/ Skin	1 serv (5.9 oz)	380	30	21	17
Tossed Salad w/ Caesar Dressing	1 serv (8 oz)	380	5	31	18
Triple Topped Chicken	1 serv (9.2 oz)	470	50	22	20
Turkey Club Sandwich	1 (11.1 oz)	650	39	26	64
Turkey Sandwich w/ Cheese & Sauce	1 (11.8 oz)	710	45	28	68
Turkey Sandwich w/o Cheese & Sauce	1 (9.3 oz)	400	45	4	61
Whole Kernel Corn	¾ cup (5.8 oz)	180	5	4	30
Zucchini Marinara Low Fat	¾ cup (6.6 oz)	60	1	3	7
salads and salad bars					
Caesar Salad Entree	1 serv (10 oz)	510	17	42	17
Caesar Salad w/o Dressing	1 serv (8 oz)	230	16	12	14
Caesar Side Salad	1 (4 oz)	200	7	17	7
Chicken Caesar Salad	1 serv (13 oz)	650	43	45	17
Tossed Salad w/ Fat Free Ranch	1 serv (8 oz)	160	5	3	29

FOOD	PORTION	CALS	PROT	FAT	CARB
Tossed Salad w/ Old Venice Dressing	1 serv (8 oz)	340	4	27	20
soups					
Chicken Chili	1 cup (8.7 oz)	220	18	7	21
Chicken Noodle	1 cup (8.4 oz)	130	11	5	12
Chicken Tortilla	1 cup (8.4 oz)	220	10	11	19
Potato	1 cup (8 oz)	270	8	16	24
Tomato Bisque	1 cup (8 oz)	280	4	23	16
BOSTON PIZZA					
children's menu selections					
Dino Fingers & Fries w/ Ketchup	1 serv	680	22	35	87
Grill Cheese Sandwich w/ Fries & Ketchup	1 serv	770	25	32	103
Mini Lasagna	1 serv	400	19	14	48
Pint Sized Ham Pizza	1 serv	430	22	8	66
Potato Smiles	1 serv	580	8	30	84
Stuffed Pizza w/ Fries & Ketchup	1 serv	850	30	31	124
Super Spaghetti	1 serv	340	10	6	61
main menu selections					
BBQ Ribs w/ Fries	1 serv	2220	71	148	140
BBQ Ribs w/ Garlic Mashed Potatoes	1 serv	1760	65	122	94
BBQ Ribs w/ Spaghetti	1 serv	1870	74	121	113
Baked Onion Soup	1 serv	210	11	7	28
Bayou Chicken Strips w/ Dipping Sauce	1 serv	370	43	16	6
Boston's Extreme Double Order	1 serv	1660	159	107	15
Boston's Extreme Starter Order	1 serv	940	90	61	10
Bruschetta	1 serv	640	17	39	55
Buffalo Chicken Fingers w/ Caesar Salad	1 serv	650	37	38	42
Buffalo Chicken Fingers w/ Fries	1 serv	1430	45	82	122
Buffalo Chicken Fingers w/ Light Ranch	1 serv	600	35	34	40
Cactus Cuts & Dip	1 serv	1380	21	83	136
Carne Amore	1 full order	1250	50	50	144
Cheese Toast	1 basket	800	36	41	64
Cheese Toast	1 serv	400	18	21	32
Chicken & Rib Combo	1 serv	1470	68	90	94
Chicken & Rib Combo w/ Fries	1 serv	1920	74	116	140
Chicken & Rib Combo w/ Spaghetti	1 serv	1590	78	90	113

FOOD	PORTION	CALS	PROT	FAT	CARB
Chicken Fingers w/ Caesar Salad	1 serv	640	37	38	38
Chicken Fingers w/ Fries	1 serv	1420	45	82	118
Chicken Fingers w/ Light Ranch	1 serv	590	34	34	36
Chips & Salsa	1 serv	830	11	41	109
Deluxe Cheese Bread	1 basket	890	37	42	84
Deluxe Cheese Toast	1 serv	420	19	21	35
Fettuccini Four Cheese	1 full order	1370	54	64	140
Fettuccini Jambalaya	1 full order	1360	68	50	151
Fettuccini Spicy Chicken & Spinach	1 full order	1330	53	53	146
Fries	1 serv	700	10	33	87
Garlic Toast w/ Garlic Margarine	1 slice	170	4	6	22
Garlic Twist Bread	1 basket	1080	33	30	168
Garlic Twist Bread	1 serv	540	17	15	84
Homestyle Macaroni	1 full order	1490	62	83	119
Italian Pizza Bread w/ Dip	1 serv	1000	32	53	98
Ketchup	1 serv (2 oz)	20	1	1	16
Lasagna Mediterranean	1 full order	870	41	35	97
Lasagna Seafood	1 full order	970	41	45	95
Linguini Chicken & Mushroom	1 full order	1320	59	53	144
Mashed Potatoes	1 serv	240	4	8	41
Mexican Beef w/ Sour Cream	1 serv	970	49	57	66
NY Steak Sandwich w/ Fries	1 serv	1580	54	96	118
Nachos	1 full order	1540	52	95	127
Nachos Beef	1 full order	1760	73	106	129
Nachos Chicken	1 full order	1630	68	96	129
Penne Baked 3 Cheese	1 full order	990	43	37	118
Penne Italiano	1 full order	1160	50	46	137
Penne Pisa Pesto	1 full order	1270	49	63	110
Penne Roast Veggie	1 full order	900	25	31	146
Pizza Bread w/o Meat Sauce	1 serv	520	15	14	84
Plain Pasta w/ Alfredo Sauce	1 full order	1200	36	52	141
Plain Pasta w/ Creamy Tomato Sauce	1 full order	1070	33	38	142
Plain Pasta w/ Marinara Sauce	1 full order	870	26	20	144
Plain Pasta w/ Meatsauce	1 full order	910	33	22	142
Plain Pasta w/ Seafood Sauce	1 full order	1050	34	36	141

FOOD	PORTION	CALS	PROT	FAT	CARB
Plain Pasta w/ Spicy Tomato Sauce	1 full order	880	27	20	145
Plain Pasta w/ Tex Mex Sauce	1 full order	940	37	23	141
Potato Skins	1 full order	860	28	53	70
Quesadilla Chicken w/ Sour Cream	1 serv	770	36	40	67
Quesadilla Garden Veggie w/ Sour Cream	1 serv	750	29	40	70
Quesadilla Sundried Tomato w/ Sour Cream	1 serv	890	67	50	39
Shrimp Dinner w/ Fries	1 serv	1510	51	82	135
Shrimp Dinner w/ Garlic Mashed Potatoes	1 serv	1050	45	57	89
Shrimp Dinner w/ Spaghetti	1 serv	1180	55	56	108
Side Tossed Salad w/ House Dressing	1 serv	170	2	14	10
Sirloin Steak Dinner w/ Fries	1 serv	1910	95	113	117
Sirloin Steak Dinner w/ Garlic Mashed Potatoes	1 serv	1450	89	88	71
Sirloin Steak Dinner w/ Spaghetti	1 serv	1580	100	87	90
Smokey Mountain Spaghetti	1 full order	1860	83	71	211
Spaghetti w/ Meatsauce	1 serv	370	14	8	60
Spinach & Artichoke Dip w/ Tortilla Chips	1 serv	890	21	57	81
Steak & Shrimp Dinner w/ Fries	1 serv	1760	65	108	129
Steak & Shrimp Dinner w/ Garlic Mashed Potatoes	1 serv	1310	59	83	83
Steak & Shrimp Dinner w/ Spaghetti	1 serv	1430	69	82	102
The Ribber w/ Fries	1 serv	1470	46	85	121
The Ribber w/ Garlic Mashed Potatoes	1 serv	1010	40	60	74
The Ribber w/ Spaghetti	1 serv	1140	50	60	94
Tortellini w/ Alfredo Sauce	1 full order	1220	46	40	165
Tortellini w/ Creamy Tomato Sauce	1 full order	1370	46	57	166
Tortellini w/ Marinara Sauce	1 full order	1180	40	39	167
Tortellini w/ Meatsauce	1 full order	1500	50	71	164
Tortellini w/ Seafood Sauce	1 full order	1360	48	55	164

FOOD	PORTION	CALS	PROT	FAT	CARB
Tortellini w/ Spicy Tomato Sauce	1 full order	1180	40	39	168
Tortellini w/ Tex Mex Sauce	1 full order	1240	51	42	164
Veal Parmigan w/ Fries	1 serv	1550	46	88	138
Veal Parmigan w/ Garlic Mashed Potatoes	1 serv	1090	40	63	92
Veal Parmigan w/ Spaghetti	1 serv	1220	50	62	112
Wings BBQ Double Order	1 serv	1700	159	107	26
Wings BBQ Starter Size	1 serv	960	90	61	13
Wings Cajun Double Order	1 serv	1610	158	107	5
Wings Cajun Starter Size	1 serv	910	89	60	3
Wings Honey Garlic Double Order	1 serv	1720	158	107	32
Wings Honey Garlic Starter Size	1 serv	970	89	60	17
Wings Screamin' Hot Double Order	1 serv	1630	158	107	10
Wings Screamin' Hot Starter Size	1 serv	920	89	60	5
Wings Teriyaki Double Order	1 serv	1690	159	107	21
Wings Teriyaki Starter Size	1 serv	950	90	60	11
Wings Thai Double Order	1 serv	1870	164	123	27
Wings Thai Starter Size	1 serv	1040	92	69	14
pizza					
Bacon Double Cheeseburger Individual	1 pie	1210	77	56	94
Bacon Double Cheeseburger Large	1 slice	350	23	15	30
Bacon Double Cheeseburger Medium	1 slice	300	19	13	25
Boston Royal Individual	1 pie	770	45	23	96
Boston Royal Large	1 slice	230	13	6	31
Boston Royal Medium	1 slice	200	11	6	26
Cajun Chicken Individual	1 pie	780	41	25	99
Cajun Chicken Large	1 slice	250	13	8	31
Cajun Chicken Medium	1 slice	200	10	7	26
Californian Individual	1 pie	580	23	8	109
Californian Large	1 slice	190	8	3	35
Californian Medium	1 slice	160	6	2	30
Four Cheese Individual	1 pie	800	45	29	89
Four Cheese Large	1 slice	260	14	10	29
Four Cheese Medium	1 slice	240	14	10	24
Great White Individual	1 pie	880	53	34	89
Great White Large	1 slice	260	16	9	29
Great White Medium	1 slice	220	13	8	24
Hawaiian Individual	1 pie	690	39	16	97

FOOD	PORTION	CALS	PROT	FAT	CARB
Hawaiian Large	1 slice	220	13	5	31
Hawaiian Medium	1 slice	180	10	4	26
Meat Lovers Individual	1 pie	1120	64	55	89
Meat Lovers Large	1 slice	330	19	15	28
Meat Lovers Medium	1 slice	280	15	14	24
Pepperoni Individual	1 pie	760	39	27	89
Pepperoni Large	1 slice	240	13	9	28
Pepperoni Medium	1 slice	200	10	7	24
Pepperoni & Mushroom Individual	1 pie	760	90	27	40
Pepperoni & Mushroom Large	1 slice	250	13	9	29
Pepperoni & Mushroom Medium	1 slice	200	10	7	24
Perogy Individual	1 pie	1010	50	45	102
Perogy Large	1 slice	330	16	15	33
Perogy Medium	1 slice	280	13	13	28
Popeye Individual	1 pie	730	41	21	94
Popeye Large	1 slice	240	14	7	30
Popeye Medium	1 slice	200	11	6	26
Rustic Italian Individual	1 pie	940	50	37	102
Rustic Italian Large	1 slice	310	16	12	33
Rustic Italian Medium	1 slice	250	13	10	28
Sante Fe Chicken Individual	1 pie	800	47	27	94
Sante Fe Chicken Large	1 slice	260	15	9	30
Sante Fe Chicken Medium	1 slice	220	12	7	25
Super Veggie Individual	1 pie	850	42	29	108
Super Veggie Large	1 slice	280	14	10	35
Super Veggie Medium	1 slice	230	11	7	30
Thai Chicken Individual	1 pie	870	45	29	106
Thai Chicken Large	1 slice	280	15	10	34
Thai Chicken Medium	1 slice	240	12	8	29
The Basic Individual	1 pie	620	34	15	89
The Basic Large	1 slice	200	11	5	28
The Basic Medium	1 slice	160	9	4	24
The Deluxe Individual	1 pie	780	43	26	92
The Deluxe Large	1 slice	240	14	7	30
The Deluxe Medium	1 slice	190	11	6	25
Tropical Chicken Individual	1 pie	1060	57	50	94
Tropical Chicken Large	1 slice	340	18	16	30
Tropical Chicken Medium	1 slice	280	15	13	25
Tuscan Individual	1 pie	900	49	32	108
Tuscan Large	1 slice	290	16	11	35
Tuscan Medium	1 slice	240	13	8	30
Vegetarian Individual	1 pie	670	36	15	100
Vegetarian Large	1 slice	220	12	5	31
Vegetarian Medium	1 slice	170	9	4	26
Zorba The Greek Individual	1 pie	810	43	27	99

FOOD	PORTION	CALS	PROT	FAT	CARB
Zorba The Greek Large	1 slice	270	14	9	32
Zorba The Greek Medium	1 slice	220	11	7	27
salads and salad bars					
Boston's Cobb Salad	1 serv	1100	25	80	66
Caesar Salad	1 reg	260	5	21	15
Caesar Salad Meal Sized	1 serv	690	13	48	52
Greek Salad	1 serv	500	10	44	19
Greek Salad Meal Sized	1 serv	1110	22	90	53
Spinach Salad Meal Sized	1 serv	500	20	31	32
Taco Salad Beef w/ Sour Cream & Salsa	1 serv	640	33	41	40
Taco Salad Chicken w/ Sour Cream & Salsa	1 serv	520	28	28	39
Thai Chicken Salad	1 serv	730	44	21	90
Tossed Garden Greens w/ House Dressing	1 serv	170	2	14	10
Veggie Plate w/ Low Fat Ranch Dressing	1 serv	180	6	7	26
sandwiches					
BBQ Beef w/ Fries	1 serv	1580	66	62	179
Beef Dip w/ Fries & Au Jus	1 serv	1560	64	72	151
Boston Cheesesteak w/ Fries & Au Jus	1 serv	1790	80	87	172
Boston Brute w/ Fries	1 serv	1420	48	60	163
Buffalo Chicken w/ Fries	1 serv	1720	85	80	187
Chicken Foccacia w/ Fries	1 serv	1350	45	65	140
Spicy Italian Sausage w/ Caesar Salad	1 serv	1070	47	51	104
Stromboli Chicken w/ Caesar Salad	1 serv	1020	53	44	101
Stromboli Perogy w/ Caesar Salad	1 serv	1120	41	58	109
Stromboli Sante Fe w/ Caesar Salad	1 serv	1000	44	45	104
Super Ham & Cheese w/ Fries	1 serv	1370	39	71	137
Tango Chicken Wrap w/ Caesar Salad	1 serv	740	37	42	55
BROWN'S CHICKEN					
Breadsticks w/ Garlic Butter	1	199	6	4	36
Breast	3.5 oz	284	26	15	12
Coleslaw	3.5 oz	131	2	10	9
Corn Fritters	3.5 oz	415	5	25	42
Corn On Cob	1 ear (3 inch)	126	3	3	22
Fettucini Alfredo	1 serv (12 oz)	1507	56	64	173
French Fries	3.5 oz	503	5	22	44
Gizzard	3.5 oz	387	24	20	26

FOOD	PORTION	CALS	PROT	FAT	CARB
Leg	3.5 oz	287	26	16	9
Liver	3.5 oz	341	23	19	19
Mostaccioli w/ Meat	1 serv (12 oz)	835	27	14	44
Mostaccioli w/o Meat	1 serv (12 oz)	792	24	10	146
Mushrooms	3.5 oz	289	6	16	30
Potato Salad	3.5 oz	94	2	4	13
Ravioli w/ Meat	1 serv (12 oz)	865	30	20	138
Ravioli w/o Meat	1 serv (12 oz)	822	27	16	140
Shrimp	3.5 oz	277	13	10	34
Thigh	3.5 oz	355	21	24	13
Wing	3.5 oz	385	23	25	17
BRUEGGER'S BAGELS					
Blueberry	1	300	10	2	60
Cinnamon Raisin	1	290	10	2	60
Egg	1	280	10	1	67
Everything	1	290	11	2	55
Garlic	1	280	10	2	57
Honey Grain	1	300	11	3	58
Onion	1	280	10	2	57
Orange Cranberry	1	290	10	1	61
Pesto	1	280	10	2	55
Plain	1	280	10	2	56
Poppy Seed	1	280	11	2	57
Pumpernickel	1	280	11	2	56
Salt	1	270	10	2	55
Sesame	1	290	11	3	57
Spinach	1	280	11	1	56
Sun Dried Tomato	1	280	10	2	58
Wheat Bran	1	280	10	2	55
BURGER KING					
beverages					
Coca Cola Classic	1 med (22 fl oz)	280	0	0	70
Coffee	1 serv (12 oz)	5	0	0	1
Diet Coke	1 med (22 fl oz)	1	0	0	tr
Shake Chocolate	1 med (13.9 oz)	440	12	10	75
Shake Vanilla	1 med (13.9 oz)	430	13	9	73
Sprite	1 med (22 fl oz)	260	0	0	66
Tropicana Orange Juice	1 serv (10 oz)	140	2	0	33
breakfast selections					
AM Express Grape Jam	1 serv (0.4 oz)	30	0	0	7
AM Express Strawberry Jam	1 serv (0.4 oz)	30	0	0	8
Bacon	3 strips (0.3 oz)	40	3	3	0
Biscuit	1 (3.3 oz)	300	6	15	35
Biscuit w/ Bacon Egg & Cheese	1 (6.6 oz)	620	20	43	37
Biscuit w/ Egg	1 (4.6 oz)	380	11	21	37
Biscuit w/ Sausage	1 (4.6 oz)	490	13	33	36

FOOD	PORTION	CALS	PROT	FAT	CARB
Cini-Minis w/o Icing	4 (3.8 oz)	440	6	23	51
Croissan'wich Sausage Egg & Cheese	1 (5.3 oz)	530	18	41	23
Croissan'wich w/ Sausage & Cheese	1 (3.7 oz)	450	13	35	21
French Toast Sticks	5 sticks (4 oz)	440	7	23	51
Ham	1 serv (1.2 oz)	35	6	1	0
Hash Browns	1 sm (2.6 oz)	240	2	15	25
Land O'Lakes Whipped Classic Blend	1 serv (0.4 oz)	65	0	7	0
Vanilla Icing Cini-Minis	1 serv (1 oz)	110	0	3	20
main menu selections					
American Cheese	2 slices (0.9 oz)	90	6	8	0
BK Big Fish Sandwich	1 (8.8 oz)	720	23	43	59
BK Broiler Chicken Breast Patty	1 (3.5 oz)	140	21	4	4
BK Broiler Chicken Sandwich	1 (8.7 oz)	530	29	16	45
BK Broiler Chicken Sandwich w/o Mayo	1 (8.7 oz)	370	29	9	45
Bacon Cheeseburger	1 (4.9 oz)	400	24	22	27
Bacon Double Cheeseburger	1 (7.2 oz)	630	41	38	28
Big King Sandwich	1 (7.6 oz)	640	38	42	28
Bull's Eye Barbecue Sauce	1 serv (0.5 oz)	20	0	0	5
Cheeseburger	1 (4.7 oz)	360	21	19	27
Chick'N Crisp Sandwich	1 (4.9 oz)	460	16	27	37
Chick'N Crisp Sandwich w/o Mayo	1 (4.9 oz)	360	16	16	37
Chicken Sandwich	1 (8 oz)	710	26	43	54
Chicken Sandwich w/o Mayo	1 (8 oz)	500	26	20	54
Chicken Tenders	4 (2.2 oz)	180	11	11	9
Chicken Tenders	8 (4.3 oz)	350	22	22	17
Chicken Tenders	5 (2.7 oz)	230	14	14	11
Dipping Sauce Barbecue	1 serv (1 oz)	35	0	0	9
Dipping Sauce Honey	1 serv (1 oz)	90	0	0	23
Dipping Sauce Honey Mustard	1 serv (1 oz)	90	0	6	10
Dipping Sauce Ranch	1 serv (1 oz)	170	0	17	2
Dipping Sauce Sweet & Sour	1 serv (1 oz)	45	0	0	11
Double Cheeseburger	1 (6.9 oz)	580	38	36	27
Double Whopper	1 (12.2 oz)	920	49	59	47
Double Whopper w/ Cheese	1 (13.1 oz)	1010	55	67	47
Double Whopper w/o Mayo	1 (12.2 oz)	760	49	42	47
Double Whopper w/o Mayo	1 (13.1 oz)	850	55	50	47
Dutch Apple Pie	1 serv (4 oz)	300	3	15	39
French Fries Salted	1 med (4.1 oz)	400	3	21	50

FOOD	PORTION	CALS	PROT	FAT	CARB
French Fries Salted	1 sm (2.6 oz)	250	2	13	32
French Fries Salted	1 king size (6 oz)	590	5	30	74
Hamburger	1 (4.2 oz)	320	19	15	27
Hamburger Bun	1 (4.6 oz)	130	5	2	24
Hamburger Patty	1 (1.9 oz)	170	14	13	0
Hash Browns	1 lg (4.5 oz)	410	3	26	42
Ketchup	1 serv (0.5 oz)	15	0	0	4
King Sauce	1 serv (0.5 oz)	70	0	7	2
Lettuce	1 leaf (0.7 oz)	0	0	0	0
Mustard	1 serv (3 g)	0	0	0	0
Onion	1 serv (0.5 oz)	5	0	0	1
Onion Rings	1 med serv (3.3 oz)	380	5	19	46
Onion Rings	1 king serv (5.3 oz)	600	8	30	74
Pickles	4 slices (0.5 oz)	0	0	0	0
Tartar Sauce	1 serv (1.5 oz)	260	0	29	0
Tomato	2 slices (1 oz)	5	0	0	1
Whopper	1 (9.5 oz)	660	29	40	47
Whopper Bun	1 (2.7 oz)	220	8	4	39
Whopper Jr.	1 (5.5 oz)	400	19	24	28
Whopper Jr. w/ Cheese	1 (6 oz)	450	22	28	28
Whopper Jr. w/ Cheese w/o Mayo	1 (6 oz)	370	22	19	28
Whopper Jr. w/o Mayo	1 (5.5 oz)	320	19	15	28
Whopper Patty	1 (2.8 oz)	250	20	19	0
Whopper w/ Cheese	1 (10.4 oz)	760	35	48	47
Whopper w/ Cheese w/o Mayo	1 (10.4 oz)	600	35	31	47
Whopper w/o Mayo	1 (9.5 oz)	510	29	23	47
CARVEL					
frozen yogurt					
Vanilla Low Fat No Sugar Added	4 fl oz	110	4	2	22
ice cream					
Brown Bonnet Cone	1 (4.7 oz)	380	6	21	43
Brown Bonnet Cone No Fat Vanilla	1 (4.7 oz)	300	5	11	47
Cake	1 pkg (7 oz)	450	8	23	54
Cake	1 pkg (4 oz)	270	5	14	33
Cake Cheesecake	1 serv (4 oz)	280	5	14	34
Cake Chocolate Vanilla Chocolate Crunchies	1/15 cake (3.4 oz)	230	4	12	27
Cake Cookies & Cream	1 serv (4 oz)	270	5	14	32
Cake Fudge Drizzle	1/8 cake (4 oz)	310	6	17	35
Cake Fudgie The Whale	1/14 cake (3.6 oz)	290	5	16	33
Cake Holiday	1/15 cake (3.4 oz)	240	4	12	30
Cake S'mores	1 serv (4 oz)	270	5	14	33
Cake Sinfully Chocolate	1 serv (4 oz)	280	5	14	34
Cake Strawberries & Cream	1/8 cake (3.8 oz)	240	4	12	31

FOOD	PORTION	CALS	PROT	FAT	CARB
Chocolate	4 fl oz	190	4	10	22
Chocolate No Fat	4 fl oz	120	2	0	28
Flying Saucer Chocolate	1 (4 oz)	230	5	9	33
Flying Saucer Chocolate w/ Sprinkles	1 (4 oz)	330	5	14	49
Flying Saucer Low Fat Chocolate	1 (4 oz)	190	3	3	38
Flying Saucer Low Fat Vanilla	1 (4 oz)	180	4	3	36
Flying Saucer Vanilla	1 (4 oz)	240	5	10	33
Flying Saucer Vanilla w/ Sprinkles	1 (4 oz)	340	5	14	49
Lil'Love Cake All Vanilla	1 piece (4.4 oz)	330	6	16	41
Lil'Love Cake Chocolate & Vanilla	1 piece (4 oz)	260	5	13	31
Nature's Crunch	1 (4.2 g)	450	5	25	55
Olde Fashion Sundae Butterscotch	1 (8 oz)	500	7	17	80
Olde Fashion Sundae Chocolate	1 (8 oz)	470	8	19	71
Olde Fashion Sundae Strawberry	1 (8 oz)	420	7	15	64
Sheet Cake Chocolate Vanilla Chocolate Crunchies	1/26 cake (3.3 oz)	230	4	12	27
Sinful Love Bar	1 (4.2 oz)	460	8	29	48
Thick Shake Chocolate	1 (16 oz)	719	18	31	96
Thick Shake Low Fat Chocolate	1 (16 oz)	490	16	1	108
Thick Shake Low Fat Strawberry	1 (16 oz)	460	15	1	96
Thick Shake Low Fat Vanilla	1 (16 oz)	460	15	1	98
Thick Shake No Fat Chocolate	1 (16 oz)	524	17	8	100
Thick Shake No Fat Strawberry	1 (16 oz)	453	16	7	82
Thick Shake No Fat Vanilla	1 (16 oz)	462	16	7	84
Thick Shake Strawberry	1 (16 oz)	648	17	30	77
Thick Shake Vanilla	1 (16 oz)	657	17	30	79
Vanilla	4 fl oz	200	5	10	21
Vanilla No Fat	4 fl oz	120	4	0	25
sherbet					
Black Raspberry	1/2 cup (3.4 oz)	150	1	1	33
Blueberry	1/2 cup (3.4 oz)	150	1	1	33
Lemon	1/2 cup (3.5 oz)	150	1	1	31
Lime	1/2 cup (3.5 oz)	150	1	1	31

FOOD	PORTION	CALS	PROT	FAT	CARB
Mango	½ cup (3.5 oz)	140	1	1	30
Orange	½ cup (3.5 oz)	150	1	1	31
Peach	½ cup (3.4 oz)	150	1	1	32
Pineapple	½ cup (3.5 oz)	150	1	1	33
Strawberry	½ cup (3.5 oz)	150	1	1	32
CHICK-FIL-A					
beverages					
Coca-Cola Classic	1 serv (9 oz)	110	0	0	28
Diet Coke	1 serv (9 oz)	0	0	0	0
Diet Lemonade	1 serv (9 oz)	5	0	0	2
Ice Tea Sweetened	1 serv (9 oz)	150	0	0	38
Iced Tea Unsweetened	1 serv (9 oz)	0	0	0	0
Lemonade	1 sm (9 oz)	90	0	0	23
desserts					
Cheesecake + One Side	1 slice (3.1 oz)	300	6	21	23
Fudge Nut Brownie	1 (2.6 oz)	350	10	16	41
Icedream Cone	1 sm (4.5 oz)	140	11	4	16
Lemon Pie	1 slice (3.5 oz)	280	1	22	19
main menu selections					
Barbecue Sauce	1 serv (1 oz)	45	0	0	11
Carrot & Raisin Salad	1 sm (2.7 oz)	150	5	2	28
Chargrilled Chicken Club Sandwich	1 (8.2 oz)	390	33	12	38
Chargrilled Chicken Garden Salad	1 serv (9.8 oz)	190	26	5	12
Chargrilled Chicken Sandwich	1 (5.3 oz)	280	27	3	36
Chick-n-Strips	4 (4.2 oz)	230	29	8	10
Chick-n-Strips Salad	1 serv (11.7 oz)	370	32	17	21
Chicken Sandwich	1 (5.9 oz)	290	24	9	29
Chicken Caesar Salad	1 serv (8.1 oz)	230	31	10	5
Chicken Salad Sandwich	1 (5.9 oz)	320	25	5	42
Cole Slaw	1 sm (2.8 oz)	130	6	6	11
Dijon Honey Sauce	1 serv (0.4 oz)	60	0	1	2
Hearty Breast of Chicken Soup	1 cup (7.6 oz)	110	16	1	10
Honey Mustard Sauce	1 serv (1 oz)	45	0	0	11
Nuggets	8 (3.9 oz)	290	28	14	12
Polynesian Sauce	1 serv (1 oz)	110	0	6	13
Side Salad	1 serv (4.6 oz)	70	5	0	13
Waffle Potato Fries	1 sm (3 oz)	290	1	10	49
salad dressings					
Basil Vinaigrette	1 serv (1.5 oz)	250	0	26	5
Blue Cheese	1 serv (1.5 oz)	230	0	24	2
Buttermilk Ranch	1 serv (1.5 oz)	220	1	24	2
Fat Free Dijon Honey Mustard	1 serv (1.5 oz)	70	1	1	17
House	1 serv (1.6 oz)	190	0	17	9

FOOD	PORTION	CALS	PROT	FAT	CARB
Light Italian	1 serv (1.5 oz)	20	0	1	2
Spicy	1 serv (1.2 oz)	210	0	22	2
Thousand Island	1 serv (1.5 oz)	210	0	20	6
DAIRY QUEEN					
food selections					
Chicken Breast Fillet Sandwich	1 (6.7 oz)	430	24	20	37
Chicken Strip Basket	1 serv (14.5 oz)	1000	35	50	102
Chili 'n' Cheese Dog	1 (5 oz)	330	14	21	22
DQ Homestyle Bacon Double Cheeseburger	1 (8.9 oz)	610	41	36	31
DQ Homestyle Cheeseburger	1 (5.3 oz)	340	20	17	29
DQ Homestyle Double Cheeseburger	1 (7.7 oz)	540	35	31	30
DQ Homestyle Hamburger	1 (4.8 oz)	290	17	12	29
DQ Ultimate Burger	1 (9.4 oz)	670	40	43	29
French Fries	1 sm (4 oz)	350	4	18	42
French Fries	1 med (3.9 oz)	440	5	23	53
Grilled Chicken Sandwich	1 (6.5 oz)	310	24	10	30
Hot Dog	1 (3.5 oz)	240	9	14	19
Onion Rings	1 serv (4 oz)	320	5	16	39
The Great Steakmelt Basket	1 serv (13.2 oz)	770	32	38	72
ice cream					
Banana Split	1 (12.9 oz)	510	8	12	96
Blizzard Chocolate Sandwich Cookie	1 med (11.4 oz)	640	12	23	97
Blizzard Chocolate Sandwich Cookie	1 sm (12 oz)	520	10	18	79
Blizzard Chocolate Chip Cookie Dough	1 med (15.4 oz)	950	17	36	143
Blizzard Chocolate Chip Cookie Dough	1 sm (12 oz)	660	12	24	99
Breeze Heath	1 med (14.2 oz)	710	15	18	123
Breeze Heath	1 sm (10.2 oz)	470	11	10	85
Breeze Strawberry	1 sm (12 oz)	320	10	1	68
Breeze Strawberry	1 med (13.4 oz)	460	13	1	99
Buster Bar	1 (5.2 oz)	450	10	28	41
Chocolate Malt	1 sm (14.7 oz)	650	15	16	111
Chocolate Malt	1 med (19.9 oz)	880	19	22	153
Cone Chocolate	1 med (6.9 oz)	340	8	11	53
Cone Chocolate	1 sm (5 oz)	240	6	8	37
Cone Vanilla	1 med (6.9 oz)	330	8	9	53
Cone Vanilla	1 lg (8.9 oz)	410	10	12	65
Cone Vanilla	1 sm (5 oz)	230	6	7	38
Cone Yogurt	1 med (6.9 oz)	260	9	1	56
Cone Dipped	1 med (7.7 oz)	490	9	24	59

FOOD	PORTION	CALS	PROT	FAT	CARB
Cone Dipped	1 sm (5.5 oz)	340	6	17	42
Cup Of Yogurt	1 med (6.7 oz)	230	8	1	48
DQ 8 Inch Round Cake Undecorated	⅛ of cake (6.2 oz)	340	7	13	56
DQ Fudge Bar No Sugar Added	1 (2.3 oz)	50	4	0	13
DQ Lemon Freez'r	½ cup (3.2 oz)	80	0	0	20
DQ Nonfat Frozen Yogurt	½ cup (3 oz)	100	3	0	21
DQ Sandwich	1 (2.1 oz)	200	4	6	31
DQ Soft Serve Chocolate	½ cup (3.3 oz)	150	4	5	22
DQ Soft Serve Vanilla	½ cup (3.3 oz)	140	3	5	22
DQ Treatzza Pizza Heath	⅛ of pie (2.3 oz)	180	3	7	28
DQ Treatzza Pizza M&M	⅛ of pie (2.4 oz)	190	3	7	29
DQ Vanilla Orange Bar No Sugar Added	1 (2.3 oz)	60	2	0	17
Dilly Bar Chocolate	1 (3 oz)	210	3	13	21
Frozen Hot Chocolate	1 (20.9 oz)	860	14	35	127
Misty Slush	1 sm (15.9 oz)	220	0	0	56
Misty Slush	1 med (20.9 oz)	290	0	0	74
Peanut Buster Parfait	1 (10.7 oz)	730	16	31	99
Pecan Mudslide Treat	1 (4.6 oz)	650	11	30	85
S'more Galore Parfait	1 (10.7 oz)	730	11	30	111
Shake Chocolate	1 sm (13.9 oz)	560	13	15	94
Shake Chocolate	1 med (18.9 oz)	770	17	20	130
Starkiss	1 (3 oz)	80	0	0	21
Strawberry Shortcake	1 (8.5 oz)	430	7	14	70
Sundae Chocolate	1 med (8.2 oz)	400	8	10	71
Sundae Chocolate	1 sm (5.7 oz)	280	5	7	49
Yogurt Sundae Strawberry	1 med (8.2 oz)	280	8	1	61
DELTACO					
beverages					
Coffee	1 serv (8 oz)	0	0	0	1
Coke Classic	1 med (12 oz)	150	0	0	37
Diet Coke	1 med (12 oz)	0	0	0	0
Iced Tea	1 med (12 oz)	0	0	0	1
Mr Pibb	1 med (12 oz)	150	0	0	37
Orange Juice	1 serv (11 oz)	140	2	0	34
Shake Chocolate	1 sm (11.4 oz)	520	12	12	89
Shake Strawberry	1 sm (11.4 oz)	410	11	6	76
Shake Vanilla	1 sm (11.4 oz)	420	12	7	75
Sprite	1 med (12 oz)	140	0	0	37
breakfast selections					
Burrito Breakfast	1 (3.8 oz)	250	10	11	24
Burrito Egg & Cheese	1 (7.5 oz)	450	23	24	39
Burrito Macho Bacon & Egg	1 (15.9 oz)	1030	40	60	82
Burrito Steak & Egg	1 (9 oz)	580	33	34	41
Quesadilla Bacon & Egg	1 (6.1 oz)	450	21	23	40
Side of Bacon	2 strips (0.3 oz)	50	3	4	0

FOOD	PORTION	CALS	PROT	FAT	CARB
main menu selections					
Beans 'n Cheese Cup	1 serv (7.7 oz)	260	16	3	44
Burrito Combo	1 (8.2 oz)	490	26	21	53
Burrito Del Beef	1 (8 oz)	550	31	30	42
Burrito Del Classic Chicken	1 (8.5 oz)	580	24	38	42
Burrito Deluxe Combo	1 (10.7 oz)	530	27	25	56
Burrito Deluxe Del Beef	1 (10.5 oz)	590	32	33	45
Burrito Green	1 (5 oz)	280	11	8	38
Burrito Macho Beef	1 (18.9 oz)	1170	60	62	89
Burrito Macho Combo	1 (19.4 oz)	1050	49	44	113
Burrito Red	1 (5 oz)	270	11	8	38
Burrito Red Regular	1 (7.5 oz)	390	18	12	59
Burrito Regular Green	1 (7.5 oz)	400	18	12	59
Burrito Spicy Chicken	1 (8.7 oz)	480	23	16	65
Burrito The Works	1 (10.2 oz)	480	18	18	69
Cheeseburger	1 (4.6 oz)	330	16	13	37
Del Cheeseburger	1 (5.6 oz)	430	16	25	35
Double Del Cheeseburger	1 (7.1 oz)	560	26	35	35
Fries	1 sm (3 oz)	210	2	14	20
Fries	1 reg (5 oz)	350	3	23	34
Fries Best Value	1 serv (7 oz)	490	5	32	47
Fries Chili Cheese	1 serv (10.5 oz)	670	17	46	51
Fries Deluxe Chili Cheese	1 serv (11.9 oz)	710	17	49	53
Get A Lot Meals #1 Combo Burrito Fries Drink	1 meal	980	29	44	124
Get A Lot Meals #2 Del Classic Chicken Burrito Fries Drink	1 meal	1080	28	61	113
Get A Lot Meals #3 Regular Red Burrito Fries Drink	1 meal	890	21	35	130
Get A Lot Meals #4 Two Chicken Soft Tacos Fries Drink	1 meal	910	25	46	102
Get A Lot Meals #5 Taco Combo Burrito Drink	1 meal	790	32	31	101
Get A Lot Meals #6 Two Tacos Quesadilla Drink	1 meal	960	37	47	98
Get A Lot Meals #7 Macho Combo Burrito Fries Drink	1 meal	1530	52	67	183

FOOD	PORTION	CALS	PROT	FAT	CARB
Get A Lot Meals #8 Two Big Fat Tacos Fries Drink	1 meal	802	35	45	148
Get A Lot Meals #9 Double Del Cheeseburger Fries Drink	1 meal	1050	29	58	106
Nachos	1 serv (4 oz)	380	5	24	40
Nachos Macho	1 serv (17 oz)	1200	33	66	130
Quesadilla Chicken	1 (6.8 oz)	580	33	31	41
Quesadilla Regular	1 (5.3 oz)	500	23	27	39
Quesadilla Spicy Jack Chicken	1 (6.8 oz)	570	32	30	40
Quesadilla Spicy Jack Regular	1 (5.3 oz)	490	23	26	38
Rice Cup	1 serv (4 oz)	150	3	2	28
Soft Taco	1 (2.8 oz)	160	8	8	16
Soft Taco Chicken	1 (3.3 oz)	210	11	12	16
Taco	1 (2.2 oz)	160	7	10	11
Taco Big Fat	1 (5.4 oz)	320	16	11	39
Taco Big Fat Chicken	1 (5.4 oz)	340	18	13	38
Taco Big Fat Steak	1 (5.4 oz)	390	18	19	38
Taco Salad Deluxe	1 (18.8 oz)	760	31	37	76
Tostada Salad	1 (4.5 oz)	210	9	9	24
DENNY'S					
beverages					
Chocolate Milk	1 serv (10 oz)	235	9	9	30
Coffee French Vanilla	1 serv (8 oz)	76	0	1	16
Coffee Hazelnut	1 serv (8 oz)	66	0	1	14
Coffee Irish Cream	1 serv (8 oz)	73	0	1	16
Grapefruit Juice	1 serv (10 oz)	115	0	0	29
Hot Chocolate	1 serv (8 oz)	90	4	2	18
Lemonade	1 serv (16 oz)	150	0	0	35
Orange Juice	1 serv (10 oz)	126	2	0	31
Raspberry Ice Tea	1 serv (16 oz)	78	0	0	21
Tomato Juice	1 serv (10 oz)	56	2	0	11
breakfast selections					
All American Slam	1 serv (15 oz)	1028	48	87	24
Applesauce	1 serv (3 oz)	60	0	0	15
Bacon	4 strips (1 oz)	162	12	18	1
Bagel Dry	1 (3 oz)	235	9	1	46
Banana	1 (4 oz)	110	1	0	29
Banana Strawberry Medley	1 serv (4 oz)	108	1	1	27
Biscuit Plain	1 (3 oz)	375	5	22	40
Biscuit w/ Sausage Gravy	1 serv (7 oz)	570	11	38	45
Blueberry Topping	1 serv (3 oz)	106	0	0	26
Canadian Bacon	1 serv (3 oz)	110	17	5	1

FOOD	PORTION	CALS	PROT	FAT	CARB
Cantaloup	1 serv (3 oz)	32	1	0	8
Cheddar Cheese Omelette	1 serv (13 oz)	770	34	62	24
Cherry Topping	1 serv (3 oz)	86	0	0	21
Chicken Fried Steak & Eggs	1 serv (14 oz)	723	28	56	31
Country Scramble	1 serv (16 oz)	795	20	50	67
Cream Cheese	1 oz	100	2	10	1
Egg	1 (2 oz)	134	6	12	1
Egg Beaters	1 serv (2.3 oz)	71	5	5	1
Eggs Benedict	1 serv (19 oz)	860	35	56	55
English Muffin Dry	1 (4 oz)	125	5	1	24
Farmer's Omelette	1 serv (18 oz)	912	34	69	38
French Slam	1 serv (14 oz)	1029	44	71	58
French Toast	2 pieces (8 oz)	510	19	25	51
Fresh Fruit Mix	1 serv (3 oz)	36	1	0	9
Grapefruit	½ (5 oz)	60	1	0	16
Grapes	1 serv (3 oz)	55	1	1	15
Grits	1 serv (4 oz)	80	2	0	18
Ham	1 serv (3 oz)	94	15	3	2
Ham'n'Cheddar Omelette	1 serv (14 oz)	743	36	55	24
Hashed Browns	1 serv (4 oz)	218	2	14	20
Hashed Browns Covered	1 serv (6 oz)	318	9	23	21
Hashed Browns Covered & Smothered	1 serv (8 oz)	359	9	26	26
Honeydew	1 serv (3 oz)	31	1	0	8
Junior Meals Basic Breakfast	1 serv (9 oz)	558	18	39	38
Junior Meals Junior French Slam	1 serv (7 oz)	461	21	35	18
Junior Meals Junior Grand Slam	1 serv (5 oz)	397	17	25	33
Junior Meals Junior Waffle Supreme	1 serv (4 oz)	190	3	11	20
Meat Lover's Sampler	1 serv (14 oz)	806	42	62	24
Moon Over My Hammy	1 serv (12 oz)	807	44	48	46
Muffin Blueberry	1 (3 oz)	309	4	14	42
Oatmeal	1 serv (4 oz)	100	5	2	18
Original Grand Slam	1 serv (10 oz)	795	34	50	65
Pancakes	3 (5 oz)	491	12	7	95
Pork Chop & Eggs	1 serv (12 oz)	555	33	36	21
Porterhouse Steak & Eggs	1 serv (18 oz)	1223	70	95	21
Ready To Eat Cereal	1 serv (1 oz)	100	2	0	23
Sausage	4 links (3 oz)	354	16	32	0
Sausage Cheddar Omelette	1 serv (16 oz)	1036	46	86	24
Scram Slam	1 serv (18 oz)	974	42	80	30
Senior Belgian Waffle Slam	1 serv (6 oz)	399	16	33	12
Senior Omelette	1 serv (12 oz)	623	23	47	27
Senior Starter	1 serv (7 oz)	336	11	24	36

FOOD	PORTION	CALS	PROT	FAT	CARB
Senior Triple Play	1 serv (8 oz)	537	20	25	64
Sirloin Steak & Eggs	1 serv (13 oz)	808	37	64	21
Slim Slam	1 serv (14 oz)	638	34	12	98
Southern Slam	1 serv (13 oz)	1065	37	84	47
Strawberries w/ Sugar	1 serv (3 oz)	115	1	1	26
Strawberry Topping	1 serv (3 oz)	115	1	1	26
Sunshine Slam	1 serv (8 oz)	537	20	25	64
Super Play It Again Slam	1 serv (15 oz)	1192	51	75	98
Syrup	3 tbsp (1.5 oz)	143	0	0	36
Syrup Reduced Calorie	1 serv (1.5 oz)	25	0	0	6
T-Bone Steak & Eggs	1 serv (16 oz)	1045	56	82	21
Toast Dry	1 slice (1 oz)	92	3	1	17
Ultimate Omelette	1 serv (17 oz)	780	31	62	29
Veggie Cheese Omelette	1 serv (16 oz)	714	28	53	29
Waffle	1 (6 oz)	304	7	21	23
Whipped Margarine	1 serv (0.5 oz)	87	0	10	0
desserts					
Apple Pie	1 serv (7 oz)	430	3	20	59
Apple Pie w/ Equal	1 serv (7 oz)	370	3	20	43
Banana Split	1 serv (19 oz)	894	15	43	121
Blueberry Topping	1 serv (3 oz)	106	0	0	26
Cheesecake Pie	1 serv (4 oz)	470	8	27	48
Cherry Topping	1 serv (3 oz)	86	0	0	21
Cherry Pie	1 serv (7 oz)	540	5	21	83
Chocolate Topping	1 serv (2 oz)	317	2	25	27
Chocolate Cake	1 serv (4 oz)	370	4	17	53
Chocolate Pecan Pie	1 serv (6 oz)	790	6	37	107
Chocolate Shake	1 serv (10 oz)	579	12	27	77
Coconut Cream Pie	1 serv (7 oz)	480	5	26	58
Double Scoop Sundae	1 serv (6 oz)	375	6	27	29
Dutch Apple Pie	1 serv (7 oz)	440	3	19	65
French Silk Pie	1 serv (6 oz)	650	6	43	60
Fudge Topping	1 serv (2 oz)	201	1	10	30
German Chocolate Pie	1 serv (7 oz)	580	7	33	66
Hot Fudge Cake Sundae	1 serv (8 oz)	687	9	38	83
Ice Cream Float	1 serv (12 oz)	280	3	10	47
Key Lime Pie	1 serv (6 oz)	600	10	27	79
Lemon Meringue Pie	1 serv (7 oz)	460	5	17	71
Pecan Pie	1 serv (6 oz)	600	5	28	81
Single Scoop Sundae	1 serv (3 oz)	188	3	14	14
Strawberry Topping	1 serv (3 oz)	115	1	1	26
Vanilla Shake	1 serv (11 oz)	581	11	27	77
main menu selections					
BBQ Sauce	1 serv (1.5 oz)	47	0	1	11
Bacon Cheddar Burger	1 (14 oz)	935	53	63	43
Bacon Lettuce & Tomato Sandwich	1 (6 oz)	634	18	46	37

FOOD	PORTION	CALS	PROT	FAT	CARB
Baked Potato Plain	1 (6 oz)	186	4	0	43
Battered Cod Dinner w/ Tartar Sauce	1 serv (9 oz)	732	30	47	48
Broccoli In Butter Sauce	2 serv (4 oz)	50	3	2	7
Brown Gravy	1 serv (1 oz)	13	0	0	2
Buffalo Chicken Strips	1 serv (10 oz)	734	48	42	43
Buffalo Wings	12 pieces (15 oz)	856	92	54	1
Carrots In Honey Glaze	2 serv (4 oz)	80	1	3	12
Charleston Chicken Sandwich	1 (11 oz)	632	35	32	53
Chicken Fried Chicken	1 serv (6 oz)	327	25	18	16
Chicken Fried Steak w/ Gravy	1 serv (4 oz)	265	15	17	14
Chicken Gravy	1 serv (1 oz)	14	0	1	2
Chicken Melt Sandwich	1 (7 oz)	520	26	29	43
Chicken Strip w/ Dressing	1 serv (10 oz)	635	47	25	55
Chicken Strips	5 pieces (10 oz)	720	47	33	56
Classic Burger	1 (11 oz)	673	37	40	42
Classic Burger w/ Cheese	1 (13 oz)	836	47	53	43
Corn In Butter Sauce	2 serv (4 oz)	120	3	4	19
Cornbread Stuffing Plain	1 serv (2 oz)	182	4	9	20
Cottage Cheese	1 serv (3 oz)	72	9	3	2
Country Gravy	1 serv (1 oz)	17	0	1	2
Delidinger Sandwich	1 (14 oz)	852	56	45	62
Deluxe Grilled Cheese Sandwich	1 (7 oz)	482	18	26	44
Dinner Roll	1 (1.5 oz)	132	4	2	26
French Fries Unsalted	1 serv (4 oz)	323	5	14	44
Fried Fish Sandwich	1 (11 oz)	905	29	56	74
Gardenburger Patty	1 patty (3.4 oz)	160	11	3	22
Gardenburger Patty w/ Bun & Fat Free Honey Mustard Dressing	1 serv (11.1 oz)	653	21	32	72
Green Beans w/ Bacon	2 serv (4 oz)	60	1	4	6
Green Peas In Butter Sauce	2 serv (4 oz)	100	5	2	14
Grilled Alaskan Salmon	1 serv (7 oz)	296	43	14	1
Grilled Chicken Breast	1 serv (4 oz)	130	24	4	0
Grilled Chicken Dinner	1 serv (4 oz)	130	24	4	0
Grilled Chicken Sandwich	1 (11 oz)	509	34	19	52
Grilled Chopped Steak w/ Gravy	1 serv (10 oz)	400	30	26	12
Ham & Swiss On Rye	1 (9 oz)	533	23	31	40
Hashed Browns	1 serv (4 oz)	218	2	14	20
Herb Toast	1 serv (2 oz)	200	4	11	21
Horseradish Sauce	1 serv (1.5 oz)	170	1	20	3
Junior Meals Junior Burger	1 serv (3 oz)	261	14	15	16
Junior Meals Junior Chicken Strips	1 serv (5 oz)	318	25	12	28

FOOD	PORTION	CALS	PROT	FAT	CARB
Junior Meals Junior Fried Fish	1 serv (5 oz)	465	15	34	25
Junior Meals Junior Grilled Cheese	1 serv (4 oz)	375	12	22	35
Junior Meals Junior Shrimp Basket	1 serv (4 oz)	291	10	16	27
Lunch Basket Charleston Chicken Ranch Melt	1 serv (14 oz)	975	47	59	68
Lunch Basket Chicken Strips	1 serv (8 oz)	568	34	26	45
Lunch Basket Classic Burger	1 serv (12 oz)	674	38	39	42
Lunch Basket Delidinger	1 serv (14 oz)	852	56	45	62
Lunch Basket Five Star Philly	1 serv (10 oz)	657	41	29	55
Lunch Basket Patty Melt	1 serv (8 oz)	696	39	42	39
Mashed Potatoes Plain	1 serv (6 oz)	105	3	1	21
Mayonnaise	2 tbsp (1 oz)	200	0	22	1
Mozzarella Sticks w/ Sauce	8 pieces (10 oz)	756	37	43	56
Onion Ring Basket	1 serv (5 oz)	439	6	27	44
Onion Rings	1 serv (3 oz)	264	3	16	27
Patty Melt Sandwich	1 (8 oz)	695	38	44	39
Pork Chop Dinner w/ Gravy	1 serv (8 oz)	386	39	24	0
Porterhouse Steak	1 (14 oz)	708	56	54	0
Pot Roast Dinner w/ Gravy	1 serv (7 oz)	260	39	11	5
Rice Pilaf	1 serv (3 oz)	112	2	2	21
Roast Turkey & Stuffing	1 serv (12 oz)	701	47	27	63
Sampler	1 serv (15 oz)	1120	44	59	104
Seasoned Fries	1 serv (4 oz)	261	5	12	35
Senior Battered Cod	1 serv (5 oz)	465	15	34	25
Senior Chicken Fried Steak	1 serv (8 oz)	341	16	18	29
Senior Grilled Chicken Breast	1 serv (6 oz)	219	26	6	16
Senior Liver w/ Bacon & Onions	1 serv (8 oz)	322	22	19	20
Senior Pork Chop	1 serv (4 oz)	193	19	12	0
Senior Pot Roast	1 serv (5 oz)	149	20	6	6
Senior Roast Turkey & Stuffing	1 serv (8 oz)	596	29	25	61
Senior Sandwich Ham & Swiss	1 serv (9 oz)	497	22	30	34
Shrimp Dinner	1 serv (8 oz)	558	19	32	49
Sirloin Steak Dinner	1 serv (5.5 oz)	271	22	21	0
Sliced Tomatoes	3 slices (2 oz)	13	1	0	3
Sour Cream	1 serv (1.5 oz)	91	1	9	2
Steak & Shrimp Dinner w/ Gravy	1 serv (9 oz)	645	36	42	31

FOOD	PORTION	CALS	PROT	FAT	CARB
Super Bird Sandwich	1 (9 oz)	620	35	32	48
T-Bone Steak Dinner	1 serv (10 oz)	530	42	40	0
Turkey Breast On Multigrain	1 (9 oz)	476	23	26	39
salad dressings					
Bleu Cheese	1 oz	124	4	12	4
Caesar	1 oz	142	1	15	1
Creamy Italian	1 oz	106	0	10	4
Fat Free Honey Mustard	1 oz	38	0	0	9
French	1 oz	106	0	10	3
Oriental Peanut Dressing	1 serv (1 oz)	106	1	8	6
Ranch	1 oz	101	1	11	1
Reduced Calorie French	1 oz	76	0	5	8
Reduced Calorie Italian	1 oz	32	0	1	3
Thousand Island	1 oz	104	0	10	2
salads and salad bars					
Buffalo Chicken Salad	1 serv (17 oz)	615	39	37	36
Fried Chicken Salad	1 serv (13 oz)	506	38	31	30
Garden Chicken Delight Salad	1 serv (16 oz)	277	30	5	30
Grilled Chicken Caesar Salad w/ Dressing	1 serv (13 oz)	655	37	47	23
Oriental Chicken Salad w/ Dressing	1 serv (20 oz)	568	33	26	49
Side Caesar w/ Dressing	1 serv (6 oz)	338	8	25	20
Side Garden Salad w/ Dressing	1 serv (7 oz)	113	3	4	16
soups					
Cheese	1 serv (8 oz)	293	6	23	13
Chicken Noodle	1 serv (8 oz)	60	2	2	8
Clam Chowder	1 serv (8 oz)	214	5	11	22
Cream Of Broccoli	1 serv (8 oz)	193	4	12	15
Cream of Potato	1 serv (8 oz)	222	4	12	23
Split Pea	1 serv (8 oz)	146	8	6	18
Vegetable Beef	1 serv (8 oz)	79	6	1	11
DOMINO'S PIZZA					
12 inch medium pizzas					
Add A Topping Anchovies	1 topping serv	23	3	1	0
Add A Topping Bacon	1 topping serv	81	4	7	tr
Add A Topping Cheddar Cheese	1 topping serv	57	4	5	tr
Add A Topping Cooked Beef	1 topping serv	56	3	5	tr
Add A Topping Extra Cheese	1 topping serv	48	3	4	1
Add A Topping Ham	1 topping serv	18	2	1	tr
Add A Topping Italian Sausage	1 topping serv	55	2	4	2
Add A Topping Pepperoni	1 topping serv	62	3	6	tr

FOOD	PORTION	CALS	PROT	FAT	CARB
Deep Dish Cheese	2 slices (6.3 oz)	477	18	22	50
Hand Tossed Cheese	2 slices (5.2 oz)	347	14	11	49
Thin Crust Cheese	¼ pie (3.7 oz)	271	12	12	31
14 inch large pizzas					
Add A Topping Anchovies	1 topping serv	23	3	1	0
Add A Topping Bacon	1 topping serv	75	4	6	tr
Add A Topping Cheddar Cheese	1 topping serv	48	3	4	tr
Add A Topping Cooked Beef	1 topping serv	44	2	4	tr
Add A Topping Extra Cheese	1 topping serv	45	3	4	1
Add A Topping Ham	1 topping serv	17	2	1	tr
Add A Topping Italian Sausage	1 topping serv	44	2	3	1
Add A Topping Pepperoni	1 topping serv	55	2	5	tr
Add A Topping Pineapple Tidbits	1 topping serv	8	2	0	tr
Deep Dish Cheese	2 slices (6.1 oz)	455	18	20	54
Hand-Tossed Cheese	2 slices (4.8 oz)	317	13	10	45
Thin Crust Cheese	⅛ pie (3.5 oz)	253	11	11	29
6 inch deep dish pizzas					
Add A Topping Anchovies	1 topping serv	45	6	2	0
Add A Topping Bacon	1 topping serv	82	4	7	tr
Add A Topping Cheddar Cheese	1 topping serv	86	5	7	tr
Add A Topping Cooked Beef	1 topping serv	44	2	4	tr
Add A Topping Extra Cheese	1 topping serv	57	4	5	1
Add A Topping Ham	1 topping serv	17	2	1	tr
Add A Topping Italian Sausage	1 topping serv	44	1	3	1
Add A Topping Pepperoni	1 topping serv	50	2	5	tr
Cheese	1 pie (7.6 oz)	595	23	27	68
main menu selections					
Breadstick	1 (0.8 oz)	78	2	3	11
Buffalo Wings Barbeque	1 piece (0.9 oz)	50	6	2	2
Buffalo Wings Hot	1 piece (0.9 oz)	45	5	2	1
Cheesy Bread	1 piece (1 oz)	103	3	5	11
Garden Salad	1 lg (7.7 oz)	39	2	tr	8
Garden Salad	1 sm (4.3 oz)	22	1	tr	4
salad dressings					
Marzetti Blue Cheese	1 serv (1.5 oz)	220	2	24	2
Marzetti Creamy Caesar	1 serv (1.5 oz)	200	1	22	2
Marzetti Fat Free Ranch	1 serv (1.5 oz)	40	0	0	10
Marzetti Honey French	1 serv (1.5 oz)	210	0	18	14
Marzetti House Italian	1 serv (1.5 oz)	220	0	24	1
Marzetti Ranch	1 serv (1.5 oz)	260	0	29	1

FOOD	PORTION	CALS	PROT	FAT	CARB
Marzetti Thousand Island	1 serv (1.5 oz)	200	0	20	5
DUNKIN' DONUTS					
bagels and cream cheese					
Bagel Blueberry	1	340	10	1	75
Bagel Cinnamon Raisin	1	340	10	1	74
Bagel Egg	1	350	11	2	72
Bagel Everything	1	360	11	2	74
Bagel Garlic	1	360	11	1	76
Bagel Onion	1	330	10	1	70
Bagel Plain	1	340	10	1	73
Bagel Poppyseed	1	360	11	3	74
Bagel Pumpernickel	1	350	11	2	75
Bagel Salt	1	340	10	1	73
Bagel Sesame	1	380	12	5	74
Bagel Wheat	1	330	12	2	73
Cream Cheese Chive	1 pkg	190	3	19	3
Cream Cheese Garden Vegetable	1 pkg	180	3	17	3
Cream Cheese Lite	1 pkg	130	5	11	3
Cream Cheese Plain	1 pkg	200	4	19	3
Cream Cheese Salmon	1 pkg	180	5	17	2
baked selections					
Bow Tie Donut	1	300	4	17	34
Cake Donut Blueberry	1	290	3	16	35
Cake Donut Butternut	1	300	3	16	36
Cake Donut Chocolate Coconut	1	300	4	19	31
Cake Donut Chocolate Frosted	1	300	3	16	38
Cake Donut Chocolate Glazed	1	290	3	16	33
Cake Donut Cinnamon	1	270	3	15	31
Cake Donut Coconut	1	290	3	17	33
Cake Donut Double Chocolate	1	310	3	17	37
Cake Donut Glazed	1	270	3	15	33
Cake Donut Old Fashioned	1	250	3	15	26
Cake Donut Powdered	1	270	3	15	32
Cake Donut Toasted Coconut	1	300	3	17	35
Cake Donut Whole Wheat Glazed	1	310	4	19	32
Chocolate Frosted Donut	1	200	3	9	29
Chocolate Kreme Filled Donut	1	270	3	13	35
Cinnamon Bun	1	510	8	15	85
Coffee Roll	1	270	4	14	33

FOOD	PORTION	CALS	PROT	FAT	CARB
Coffee Roll Chocolate Frosted	1	290	4	15	36
Coffee Roll Maple Frosted	1	290	4	14	36
Coffee Roll Vanilla Frosted	1	290	4	14	36
Cookie Chocolate Chocolate Chunk	1	210	3	11	26
Cookie Chocolate Chunk	1	220	3	11	28
Cookie Chocolate Chunk w/ Nut	1	230	3	12	27
Cookie Chocolate White Chocolate Chunk	1	230	3	12	28
Cookie Oatmeal Raisin Pecan	1	220	3	10	29
Cookie Peanut Butter Chocolate Chunk w/ Nuts	1	240	4	14	24
Cookie Peanut Butter w/ Nuts	1	240	5	14	24
Croissant Almond	1	350	6	22	34
Croissant Chocolate	1	400	5	25	37
Croissant Plain	1	290	5	18	26
Cruller Plain	1	240	3	15	25
Cruller Powdered	1	270	3	15	30
Cruller Sugar	1	250	3	15	27
Donut Apple Crumb	1	230	3	10	34
Donut Apple N' Spice	1	200	3	8	29
Donut Bavarian Kreme	1	210	3	9	30
Donut Black Raspberry	1	210	3	8	32
Donut Blueberry Crumb	1	240	3	10	36
Donut Boston Kreme	1	240	3	9	36
Donut Chocolate Iced Bismark	1	340	3	15	50
Dunkin' Donut	1	240	3	15	25
Eclair Donut	1	270	3	11	39
Fritter Glazed	1	260	4	14	31
Glazed Donut	1	180	3	8	25
Jelly Filled Donut	1	210	3	8	32
Jelly Stick	1	290	3	12	44
Lemon Donut	1	200	3	9	28
Maple Frosted Donut	1	210	3	9	30
Marble Frosted Donut	1	200	3	9	29
Muffin Apple Cinnamon Pecan	1	510	8	21	74
Muffin Apple N'Spice	1	350	5	12	57
Muffin Banana Nut	1	360	7	15	52
Muffin Blueberry	1	490	8	17	78
Muffin Bran	1	390	11	12	60
Muffin Cherry	1	340	6	12	53
Muffin Chocolate Hazelnut	1	610	10	26	87

FOOD	PORTION	CALS	PROT	FAT	CARB
Muffin Chocolate Chip	1	590	8	24	88
Muffin Corn	1	500	10	16	78
Muffin Cranberry Orange	1	470	8	15	76
Muffin Cranberry Orange Nut	1	350	6	15	52
Muffin Lemon Poppyseed	1	360	5	13	56
Muffin Oat Bran	1	370	11	13	55
Muffin Lowfat Apple & Spice	1	240	4	2	54
Muffin Lowfat Banana	1	250	4	2	57
Muffin Lowfat Blueberry	1	250	4	2	55
Muffin Lowfat Bran	1	240	4	1	57
Muffin Lowfat Cherry	1	250	4	2	56
Muffin Lowfat Chocolate	1	250	4	3	53
Muffin Lowfat Corn	1	240	3	3	52
Muffin Lowfat Cranberry Orange	1	240	4	2	55
Muffin Reduced Fat Blueberry	1	450	8	12	77
Muffin Reduced Fat Corn	1	460	10	11	79
Munchkins Chocolate Cake Glazed	3	200	2	10	26
Munchkins Cake Butternut	3	200	2	11	25
Munchkins Cake Cinnamon	4	250	3	14	29
Munchkins Cake Coconut	3	200	2	12	23
Munchkins Cake Glazed	3	200	2	10	27
Munchkins Cake Plain	4	220	2	14	22
Munchkins Cake Powdered	4	250	2	14	29
Munchkins Cake Sugared	4	240	2	14	28
Munchkins Cake Toasted Coconut	3	200	2	11	24
Munchkins Yeast Glazed	5	200	3	9	27
Munchkins Yeast Jelly Filled	5	210	3	9	30
Munchkins Yeast Lemon Filled	4	170	2	8	23
Munchkins Yeast Sugar Raised	7	220	4	12	26
Strawberry Frosted Donut	1	210	3	9	30
Strawberry Donut	1	210	3	8	32
Sugar Raised Donut	1	170	3	8	22
Sugared Cake Donut	1	250	3	15	27
Vanilla Frosted Donut	1	210	3	9	30
Vanilla Kreme Filled Donut	1	270	3	13	36
beverages					
Coffee Coolatta w/ 2% Milk	1 (16 oz)	240	4	2	52
Coffee Coolatta w/ Cream	1 (16 oz)	410	3	22	51
Coffee Coolatta w/ Milk	1 (16 oz)	260	4	4	52
Coffee Coolatta w/ Skim Milk	1 (16 oz)	230	4	0	52
Coolatta Pink Lemonade	1 (16 oz)	350	7	0	88

FOOD	PORTION	CALS	PROT	FAT	CARB
Fruit					
Coolatta Raspberry Lemonade	1 (16 oz)	280	0	0	68
Coolatta Vanilla	1 (16 oz)	450	1	7	94
Coolatta Strawberry Fruit	1 (16 oz)	280	0	0	70
Dunkaccino	1 (10 oz)	250	2	11	34
Hot Cocoa	1 (10 oz)	230	2	8	38
sandwiches					
Breakfast Sandwich Ham Egg Cheese	1	320	22	12	31
Omwich Bagel Bacon Cheddar	1	600	26	21	79
Omwich Bagel Spanish Cheese	1	570	24	18	79
Omwich Bagel Three Cheese	1	610	25	22	78
Omwich Croissant Spanish Cheese	1	530	19	36	33
Omwich Croissant Bacon Cheddar	1	560	21	38	33
Omwich Croissant Three Cheese	1	560	20	39	33
Omwich English Muffin Bacon Cheddar	1	400	21	21	33
Omwich English Muffin Spanish Cheese	1	370	18	18	34
Omwich English Muffin Three Cheese	1	400	19	22	33

EINSTEIN BROS BAGELS

FOOD	PORTION	CALS	PROT	FAT	CARB
bagels					
Bagel Chips Cinnamon Raisin Swirl	1 serv (1 oz)	90	3	1	19
Bagel Chips Plain	1 serv (1 oz)	90	3	0	18
Bagel Chips Sourdough Dill	1 serv (1 oz)	90	3	1	18
Bagel Chips Sun Dried Tomato	1 serv (1 oz)	90	3	1	17
Bagel Chips Sunflower	1 serv (1 oz)	100	3	2	8
Bagel Chips Wild Blueberry	1 serv (1 oz)	90	3	1	19
Chocolate Chip	1 (4 oz)	380	11	3	78
Chopped Garlic	1 (4.2 oz)	377	14	4	81
Chopped Onion	1 (4 oz)	340	11	3	72
Cinnamon Raisin Swirl	1 (4 oz)	360	11	1	78
Cinnamon Sugar	1	330	10	0	72
Dark Pumpernickel	1 (3.8 oz)	330	11	1	72
Everything	1 (4 oz)	342	13	2	74
Honey 8 Grain	1 (4 oz)	320	11	1	71

FOOD	PORTION	CALS	PROT	FAT	CARB
Nutty Banana	1 (4 oz)	370	11	3	77
Plain	1 (3.7 oz)	330	11	1	72
Poppy Dip'd	1 (3.9 oz)	346	12	2	73
Salt	1 (3.9 oz)	330	11	1	72
Sesame Dip'd	1 (4.1 oz)	381	11	5	74
Spinach Herb	1 (3.8 oz)	320	11	1	71
Sun Dried Tomato	1 (3.8 oz)	320	11	1	70
Veggie Confetti	1 (3.8 oz)	330	10	1	71
Wild Blueberry	1 (4 oz)	360	11	1	79
sandwiches and fillings					
Butter & Margarine Blend	1 serv (0.4 oz)	60	0	7	0
Capers	1 tbsp	0	0	0	0
Cheddar Cheese	1 serv (0.75 oz)	110	7	9	1
Classic New York Lox & Bagel	1 (11.4 oz)	560	24	24	31
Cream Cheese Cheddarpeno	1 serv (1 oz)	90	2	8	2
Cream Cheese Chive	1 serv (1 oz)	90	1	9	2
Cream Cheese Maple Walnut Raisin	1 serv (1 oz)	100	1	8	7
Cream Cheese Plain	1 serv (1 oz)	100	1	9	2
Cream Cheese Smoked Salmon	1 serv (1 oz)	90	2	8	2
Cream Cheese Strawberry	1 serv (1 oz)	90	1	8	4
Cream Cheese Sun Dried Tomato	1 serv (1 oz)	90	1	8	3
Cucumbers	1 serv (1 oz)	0	0	0	1
Fruit Spreads	1 tbsp	40	0	0	10
Ham	1 serv (2.5 oz)	75	10	2	1
Ham & Cheese Sandwich	1 (9.9 oz)	520	31	15	63
Honey	1 tbsp	64	0	0	18
Hummus	2 tbsp	60	2	3	4
Hummus Sandwich	1 (6 oz)	440	13	7	62
Lettuce	1 leaf	0	0	0	0
Lite Cream Cheese Plain	1 serv (1 oz)	60	2	5	2
Lite Cream Cheese Spinach Dill	1 serv (1 oz)	60	2	5	2
Lite Cream Cheese Veggie	1 serv (1 oz)	60	2	5	3
Lite Cream Cheese Wildberry	1 serv (1 oz)	70	2	4	7
Lowfat Chicken Salad Sandwich	1 (11.6 oz)	440	26	9	63
Lowfat Tuna Salad Sandwich	1 (11.6 oz)	440	29	8	62
Marshall's Lox	1 serv (2 oz)	90	12	4	2
Mayonnaise Lite Reduced Calorie	1 serv (0.5 oz)	50	0	5	1
Peanut Butter	1 serv (1.1 oz)	190	7	16	8

FOOD	PORTION	CALS	PROT	FAT	CARB
Peanut Butter & Jelly Sandwich	1 (6 oz)	595	18	17	99
Scrambled Egg Sandwich	1 (7.7 oz)	480	25	17	56
Scrambled Egg Sandwich w/ Meat & Cheese	1 (8.9 oz)	520	32	31	57
Smoked Turkey	1 serv (2.5 oz)	75	13	1	0
Smoked Turkey Sandwich	1 (9.9 oz)	480	28	14	59
Spouts Alfalfa	1 serv (0.5 oz)	0	0	0	3
Sweet Onions	1 serv (1 oz)	0	0	0	2
Swiss Cheese	1 serv (0.75 oz)	100	8	8	0
Tasty Turkey Sandwich	1 (10 oz)	530	25	22	61
Tomato	1 serv (1.5 oz)	0	0	0	2
Turkey Pastrami 99% Fat Free	1 serv (2.5 oz)	75	12	6	2
Turkey Pastrami Sandwich	1 (9.7 oz)	460	29	12	60
Veg Out Sandwich	1 (8.9 oz)	350	12	17	62
Whitefish Salad Sandwich	1 (9.2 oz)	630	22	23	59

EL POLLO LOCO
main menu selections

FOOD	PORTION	CALS	PROT	FAT	CARB
Broccoli Slaw	1 serv (5 oz)	203	3	17	14
Burrito BRC	1 (9.3 oz)	482	16	15	72
Burrito Classic Chicken	1 (9.3 oz)	556	30	22	61
Burrito Grilled Steak	1 (11.3 oz)	705	39	32	68
Burrito Loco Grande	1 (13.1 oz)	632	33	26	67
Burrito Smokey Black Bean	1 (9.3 oz)	566	16	22	78
Burrito Spicy Hot Chicken	1 (9.8 oz)	559	30	22	61
Burrito Whole Wheat Chicken	1 (10.8 oz)	592	31	26	60
Chicken Breast	1 piece (3 oz)	160	26	6	0
Chicken Leg	1 piece (1.75 oz)	90	11	5	0
Chicken Soft Taco	1 (4 oz)	224	16	12	15
Chicken Thigh	1 piece (2 oz)	180	16	12	0
Chicken Wing	1 (1.5 oz)	110	12	6	0
Chicken Tamale	1 (3.5 oz)	190	6	8	23
Cole Slaw	1 serv (5 oz)	206	2	16	12
Corn-On-Cob	1 ear (5.5 oz)	146	5	2	33
Cornbread Stuffing	1 serv (6 oz)	281	6	12	40
Crispy Green Beans	1 serv (5 oz)	41	1	2	6
Cucumber Salad	1 serv (4.2 oz)	34	2	0	7
Fiesta Corn	1 serv (5 oz)	152	4	6	25
Flame Broiled Chicken Salad	1 serv (14.9 oz)	167	27	5	11
French Fries	1 serv (4.4 oz)	323	5	14	44
Garden Salad	1 serv (6.4 oz)	29	3	0	6
Gravy	1 serv (1 oz)	14	0	0	2
Honey Glazed Carrots	1 serv (5 oz)	104	1	6	14
Lime Parfait	1 serv (5 oz)	125	1	3	25
Macaroni & Cheese	1 serv (6 oz)	238	10	12	22

FOOD	PORTION	CALS	PROT	FAT	CARB
Mashed Potatoes	1 serv (5 oz)	97	3	1	21
Pinto Beans	1 serv (6 oz)	185	11	4	29
Polo Bowl	1 serv (19 oz)	504	37	13	69
Potato Salad	1 serv (6 oz)	256	3	14	30
Rainbow Pasta Salad	1 serv (5 oz)	157	6	1	30
Salad Shell	1 (5.6 oz)	440	7	27	42
Smokey Black Beans	1 serv (5 oz)	255	6	13	29
Southwest Cole Slaw	1 serv (5 oz)	178	2	13	15
Spanish Rice	1 serv (4 oz)	130	2	3	24
Spiced Apples	1 serv (5 oz)	146	0	0	39
Steak Bowl	1 serv (15.2 oz)	616	37	26	62
Taco Al Carbon Chicken	1 serv (4.4 oz)	265	10	12	30
Taco Al Carbon Steak	1 (4.4 oz)	394	20	22	30
Taquito	1 serv (5 oz)	370	15	17	43
Tortilla Corn	1 (1.1 oz)	70	1	1	14
Tortilla Flour	1 (1 oz)	90	3	3	13
Tortilla Wrap Chicken Caesar	1 (10.47 oz)	518	28	19	59
Tortilla Wrap Southwest	1 (11.97 oz)	632	30	27	69
Tostada Salad Chicken	1 serv (14.7 oz)	332	35	14	26
Tostado Salad Steak	1 serv (13.2 oz)	525	40	31	26
salad dressings					
Blue Cheese	1 serv (2 oz)	300	2	32	2
Light Italian	1 serv (2 oz)	25	0	1	3
Ranch	1 serv (2 oz)	350	1	39	2
Thousand Island	1 serv (2 oz)	270	1	27	9
FAZOLI'S					
desserts					
Cheesecake	1 slice	290	6	22	17
Cheesecake Turtle	1 slice	420	8	34	24
Cookie Milk Chocolate Chunk	1	360	6	15	54
Lemon Ice	1 serv	190	0	0	45
Specialty Cheesecake	1 serv	300	7	22	22
Strawberry Topping	1 serv	35	0	0	8
main menu selections					
Baked Chicken Parmesan	1 serv	740	42	20	99
Baked Spaghetti Parmesan	1 serv	700	38	25	76
Baked Ziti	1 reg	750	36	26	87
Baked Ziti	1 sm	490	23	17	56
Breadstick	1	140	4	6	18
Breadstick Dry	1	90	4	1	17
Broccoli Fettuccine Alfredo	1 sm	560	19	15	85
Broccoli Fettuccine Alfredo	1 reg	830	27	23	125
Cheese Ravioli w/ Marinara Sauce	1 serv	480	21	15	65
Cheese Ravioli w/ Meat Sauce	1 serv	510	20	17	65
Classic Sampler	1 serv	710	26	21	97

FOOD	PORTION	CALS	PROT	FAT	CARB
Fettuccine Alfredo	1 reg	800	25	22	119
Fettuccine Alfredo	1 sm	530	17	15	80
Fettuccine w/ Shrimp & Scallop	1 serv	590	32	16	81
Homestyle Lasagna	1 serv	440	22	19	41
Homestyle Lasagna w/ Broccoli	1 serv	420	21	18	45
Minestrone Soup	1 serv	120	1	1	23
Peppery Chicken Alfredo	1 serv	610	31	16	80
Pizza Cheese	1 serv	460	24	15	58
Pizza Combination Double Slice	1 serv	570	29	25	63
Pizza Pepperoni	1 serv	530	27	22	61
Pizza Baked Spaghetti	1 serv	750	40	31	78
Spaghetti w/ Marinara Sauce	1 sm	420	15	6	74
Spaghetti w/ Marinara Sauce	1 reg	620	21	8	111
Spaghetti w/ Meat Sauce	1 reg	670	21	11	111
Spaghetti w/ Meat Sauce	1 sm	450	14	8	74
Spaghetti w/ Meatballs	1 reg	1020	39	42	119
Spaghetti w/ Meatballs	1 sm	730	28	31	80
salad dressings					
Honey French	1 serv	150	0	12	9
House Italian	1 serv	110	0	9	5
Ranch	1 serv	150	0	17	1
Reduced Calorie Italian	1 serv	50	0	5	3
Thousand Island	1 serv	130	0	13	4
salads and salad bars					
Caesar Side Salad	1	220	7	17	13
Chicken & Pasta Caesar Salad	1	500	28	27	35
Chicken Caesar Salad	1	420	22	29	17
Chicken Finger Salad	1	190	20	9	8
Chicken Finger Salad w/ Bacon & Honey Mustard	1	400	20	28	17
Garden Salad	1	25	2	0	4
Garden Salad w/ Balsamic Vinaigrette	1	120	2	9	10
Italian Chef Salad	1	260	15	21	13
Pasta Salad	1 serv	590	18	25	70
sandwiches					
Panini Chicken Caesar Club	1	660	39	35	51
Panini Chicken Pesto	1	510	33	20	51
Panini Four Cheese & Tomato	1	720	28	43	55
Panini Ham & Swiss	1	600	31	30	53
Panini Italian Club	1	670	30	37	54
Panini Italian Deli	1	660	34	35	61
Panini Smoked Turkey	1	710	32	38	57
Submarinos Club	half	1100	51	44	121

FOOD	PORTION	CALS	PROT	FAT	CARB
Submarinos Ham & Swiss	1	1000	44	37	120
Submarinos Meatball	half	1260	55	59	128
Submarinos Original	half	1160	45	55	124
Submarinos Pepperoni Pizza	half	1060	55	40	133
Submarinos Turkey	half	990	43	34	121
GODFATHER'S PIZZA					
Golden Crust Cheese	1/10 lg (3.5 oz)	242	12	9	28
Golden Crust Cheese	1/8 med (3.1 oz)	212	10	8	26
Golden Crust Combo	1/8 med (4.4 oz)	271	13	12	28
Golden Crust Combo	1/10 lg (4.9 oz)	305	16	14	31
Original Crust Cheese	1/10 jumbo (5.8 oz)	382	22	9	53
Original Crust Cheese	1/4 mini (1.9 oz)	131	7	3	19
Original Crust Cheese	1/8 med (3.5 oz)	231	13	5	24
Original Crust Cheese	1/10 lg (4 oz)	258	15	6	36
Original Crust Combo	1/4 mini (2.9 oz)	176	10	7	21
Original Crust Combo	1/10 lg (5.6 oz)	338	19	12	38
Original Crust Combo	1/8 med (5.1 oz)	306	17	11	36
Original Crust Combo	1/10 jumbo (8.3 oz)	503	29	18	56
GODIVA					
Chocolatier Dark Chocolate w/ Raspberry	1 bar (1.5 oz)	220	2	11	28
Chocolatier Milk Chocolate	1 bar (1.5 oz)	230	3	13	26
Mochaccino Mousse	2 pieces (1.25 oz)	210	2	15	17
Truffle Assorted	2 pieces (1.5 oz)	220	2	13	24
HAAGEN-DAZS					
frozen yogurt					
Pinapple Coconut	1/2 cup	230	4	13	25
Soft Serve Nonfat Chocolate	1/2 cup	110	4	0	23
Soft Serve Nonfat Chocolate Mousse	1/2 cup	80	5	0	24
Soft Serve Nonfat Coffee	1/2 cup	110	5	0	22
Soft Serve Nonfat Strawberry	1/2 cup	110	4	0	24
Soft Serve Nonfat Vanilla	1/2 cup	110	5	0	22
Soft Serve Nonfat Vanilla Mousse	1/2 cup	70	4	0	23
Soft Serve Nonfat White Chocolate	1/2 cup	110	5	0	22
Vanilla Fudge	1/2 cup	160	6	0	34
Vanilla Raspberry Swirl	1/2 cup	130	4	0	29
ice cream					
Bailey's Irish Cream	1/2 cup	270	5	17	23
Bar Chocolate	1 (2.7 oz)	200	4	12	16
Bar Chocolate & Dark Chocolate	1 (3.6 oz)	350	5	24	28
Bar Coffee	1 (2.7 oz)	190	3	13	15

FOOD	PORTION	CALS	PROT	FAT	CARB
Bar Coffee & Almond Crunch	1 (3.7 oz)	370	5	27	27
Bar Vanilla	1 (2.7 oz)	190	3	13	15
Bar Vanilla & Almonds	1 (3.7 oz)	380	6	28	26
Bar Vanilla & Milk Chocolate	1 (3.5 oz)	340	5	24	25
Belgian Chocolate Chocolate	½ cup	330	5	21	29
Brownies A La Mode	½ cup	280	5	16	28
Butter Pecan	½ cup	300	5	22	20
Cappuccino Commotion	½ cup	310	5	21	25
Chocolate	½ cup	269	5	17	21
Chocolate Chocolate Chip	½ cup	300	5	19	26
Chocolate Chocolate Mint	½ cup	300	5	20	25
Chocolate Swiss Almond	½ cup	300	5	20	24
Coffee	½ cup	250	5	17	20
Coffee Mocha Chip	½ cup	270	4	19	24
Cookie Dough Dynamo	½ cup	310	4	20	29
Cookies & Cream	½ cup	270	5	17	23
Cookies & Fudge	½ cup	180	7	3	33
Deep Chocolate Peanut Butter	½ cup	350	8	24	26
Dulce De Leche Caramel	½ cup	270	5	16	27
Lowfat Coffee Fudge	½ cup	170	5	3	32
Macadamia Brittle	½ cup	280	4	19	24
Macadamia Nut	½ cup	320	5	24	20
Mint Chip	½ cup	280	4	18	25
Pistachio	½ cup	280	5	19	21
Pralines & Cream	½ cup	280	4	17	28
Rum Raisin	½ cup	260	4	17	21
Strawberry	½ cup	250	4	16	22
Vanilla	½ cup	250	4	17	20
Vanilla Chocolate Chip	½ cup	290	5	19	25
Vanilla Swiss Almond	½ cup	290	5	20	23
sorbet					
Bar Raspberry & Vanilla	1 (2.5 oz)	90	2	0	21
Mango	½ cup	120	0	0	31
Orange	½ cup	120	0	0	30
Raspberry	½ cup	120	0	0	30
Soft Serve Raspberry	½ cup	110	0	0	28
Strawberry	½ cup	120	0	0	30
Zesty Lemon	½ cup	120	0	0	31
HARDEE'S					
beverages					
Orange Juice	1 serv (11 oz)	140	2	tr	34
Shake Chocolate	1 (12.2 oz)	370	13	5	67
Shake Peach	1 (12.1 oz)	390	10	4	77
Shake Strawberry	1 (12.7 oz)	420	11	4	83
Shake Vanilla	1 (12.2 oz)	350	12	5	65

FOOD	PORTION	CALS	PROT	FAT	CARB
breakfast selections					
Apple Cinnamon 'N' Raisin Biscuit	1 (2.18 oz)	200	2	8	30
Bacon & Egg Biscuit	1 (5.5 oz)	570	22	33	45
Bacon Egg & Cheese Biscuit	1 (5.9 oz)	610	24	37	45
Big Country Breakfast Bacon	1 serv (9.4 oz)	820	33	49	62
Big Country Breakfast Sausage	1 serv (11.4 oz)	1000	41	66	62
Biscuit 'N' Gravy	1 (7.8 oz)	510	10	28	55
Country Ham Biscuit	1 (3.8 oz)	430	15	22	45
Frisco Breakfast Sandwich Ham	1 (7.4 oz)	500	24	25	46
Ham Biscuit	1 (4 oz)	400	9	20	47
Ham Egg & Cheese Biscuit	1 (6.5 oz)	540	20	30	48
Hash Rounds	1 serv (2.8 oz)	230	3	14	24
Jelly Biscuit	1 (3.5 oz)	440	6	21	57
Rise 'N' Shine Biscuit	1 (2.9 oz)	390	6	21	44
Sausage Biscuit	1 (4.1 oz)	510	14	31	44
Sausage & Egg Biscuit	1 (6.3 oz)	630	23	40	45
Three Pancakes	1 serv (4.8 oz)	280	8	2	56
Ultimate Omelet Biscuit	1 (5.8 oz)	570	22	33	45
desserts					
Big Cookie	1 (2.0 oz)	280	4	12	41
Cone Chocolate	1 (4.1 oz)	180	5	2	34
Cone Vanilla	1 (4.1 oz)	170	4	2	34
Cool Twist Cone Vanilla/Chocolate	1 (4.1 oz)	180	4	2	34
Peach Cobbler	1 serv (6 oz)	310	2	7	60
Sundae Hot Fudge	1 (5.5 oz)	290	7	6	51
Sundae Strawberry	1 (5.8 oz)	210	5	2	43
main menu selections					
Baked Beans	1 serv (5 oz)	170	8	1	32
Big Roast Beef Sandwich	1 (6.5 oz)	460	26	24	35
Cheeseburger	1 (4.3 oz)	310	16	14	30
Chicken Fillet Sandwich	1 (7.5 oz)	480	26	18	54
Cole Slaw	1 serv (4 oz)	240	2	20	13
Cravin' Bacon Cheeseburger	1 (8.1 oz)	690	30	46	38
Fisherman's Fillet	1 (8.3 oz)	560	26	27	54
French Fries	1 lg (6 oz)	430	6	18	59
French Fries	1 sm (3.4 oz)	240	4	10	33
French Fries	1 med (5 oz)	350	5	15	49
Fried Chicken Breast	1 piece (5.2 oz)	370	29	15	29
Fried Chicken Leg	1 piece (2.4 oz)	170	13	7	15
Fried Chicken Thigh	1 piece (4.2 oz)	330	19	15	30
Fried Chicken Wing	1 piece (2.3 oz)	200	10	8	23

FOOD	PORTION	CALS	PROT	FAT	CARB
Frisco Burger	1 (8.1 oz)	720	33	46	43
Grilled Chicken Sandwich	1 (7.1 oz)	350	25	11	38
Hamburger	1 (3.9 oz)	270	14	11	29
Hot Ham 'N' Cheese	1 (5.1 oz)	310	16	12	34
Mashed Potatoes	1 serv (4 oz)	70	2	tr	14
Mesquite Bacon Cheeseburger	1 (4.5 oz)	370	19	18	32
Mushroom 'N' Swiss Burger	1 (6.8 oz)	490	28	25	39
Quarter Pound Double Cheeseburger	1 (6 oz)	470	27	27	31
Regular Roast Beef	1 (4.3 oz)	320	17	16	26
The Boss	1 (7 oz)	570	37	33	42
The Works Burger	1 (8.1 oz)	530	25	30	41
salad dressings					
French Fat Free	1 serv (2 oz)	70	0	0	18
Ranch	1 serv (2 oz)	290	1	29	6
Thousand Island	1 serv (2 oz)	250	1	23	9
salads and salad bars					
Garden Salad	1 (10.2 oz)	220	12	13	11
Grilled Chicken Salad	1 (11.5 oz)	150	20	3	11
Side Salad	1 (4.6 oz)	25	1	tr	4
HOT SAM'S PRETZELS					
Bavarian	1 lg (5.1 oz)	390	14	0	83
Bavarian	1 reg (2.5 oz)	200	7	0	42
Bavarian Stix	10 (5 oz)	390	14	0	83
Sweet Dough	1 (4.5 oz)	360	11	3	73
Sweet Dough Blueberry	1 (4.5 oz)	400	11	4	81
HUNGRY HOWIE'S					
main menu selections					
Howie Wings	6 (3 oz)	180	12	14	0
Three Cheeser Bread	1 serv	370	15	14	47
pizza					
Large Cheese	1 slice	175	10	4	24
Large Cheese + Bacon	1 slice	208	17	5	25
Large Cheese + Beef	1 slice	197	11	6	24
Large Cheese + Black Olives	1 slice	181	10	5	24
Large Cheese + Green Olives	1 slice	181	10	5	24
Large Cheese + Green Peppers	1 slice	175	10	4	24
Large Cheese + Ham	1 slice	179	11	6	24
Large Cheese + Mushrooms	1 slice	175	10	4	24
Large Cheese + Onions	1 slice	175	10	5	24
Large Cheese + Pepperoni	1 slice	191	11	4	24
Large Cheese + Pineapple	1 slice	388	11	5	25
Large Cheese + Sausage	1 slice	195	12	6	24
Medium Cheese	1 slice	153	9	5	21
Medium Cheese + Bacon	1 slice	179	14	5	21

FOOD	PORTION	CALS	PROT	FAT	CARB
Medium Cheese + Beef	1 slice	177	10	6	21
Medium Cheese + Black Olives	1 slice	159	9	5	21
Medium Cheese + Green Olives	1 slice	159	9	4	21
Medium Cheese + Green Peppers	1 slice	155	9	5	21
Medium Cheese + Ham	1 slice	159	10	6	21
Medium Cheese + Mushrooms	1 slice	155	9	5	21
Medium Cheese + Onions	1 slice	155	9	5	21
Medium Cheese + Pepperoni	1 slice	171	10	6	21
Medium Cheese + Pineapple	1 slice	158	9	5	22
Medium Cheese + Sausage	1 slice	175	10	6	21
Small Cheese	1 slice	121	7	3	37
Small Cheese + Bacon	1 slice	138	10	3	17
Small Cheese + Beef	1 slice	137	8	4	17
Small Cheese + Black Olives	1 slice	125	7	3	17
Small Cheese + Green Olives	1 slice	125	7	3	17
Small Cheese + Green Peppers	1 slice	122	7	3	17
Small Cheese + Ham	1 slice	126	8	3	17
Small Cheese + Mushrooms	1 slice	123	7	3	17
Small Cheese + Onions	1 slice	122	7	3	17
Small Cheese + Pepperoni	1 slice	136	8	4	17
Small Cheese + Pineapple	1 slice	124	7	3	18
Small Cheese + Sausage	1 slice	136	8	3	17
salads and salad bars					
Antipasto Salad w/o Dressing	1 lg	101	8	7	3
Chef Salad w/o Dressing	1 lg	99	8	6	4
Garden Salad w/o Dressing	1 lg	17	1	tr	3
Greek Salad w/o Dressing	1 lg	109	6	7	7
sandwiches					
Sub Deluxe Italian	½ sub	506	24	18	61
Sub Ham & Cheese	½ sub	475	26	15	61
Sub Pizza	½ sub	689	30	34	67
Sub Pizza Special	½ sub	606	29	24	68
Sub Steak Cheese Mushroom	½ sub	491	27	15	64
Sub Turkey	½ sub	466	25	13	63
Sub Turkey Club	½ sub	556	42	18	62
Sub Vegetarian	½ sub	530	22	21	64

FOOD	PORTION	CALS	PROT	FAT	CARB
JACK IN THE BOX					
beverages					
Barq's Root Beer	1 reg (20 fl oz)	180	0	0	50
Classic Ice Cream Shake Chocolate	1 reg (11 fl oz)	630	11	27	85
Classic Ice Cream Shake Oreo Cookie	1 reg (12 oz)	740	13	36	91
Classic Ice Cream Shake Strawberry	1 reg (10 fl oz)	640	10	28	85
Classic Ice Cream Shake Vanilla	1 reg (11 oz)	610	12	31	73
Classice Ice Cream Shake Cappuccino	1 reg (11 oz)	630	11	29	80
Coca-Cola Classic	1 reg (20 fl oz)	170	0	0	46
Coffee	1 reg (12 fl oz)	5	0	0	1
Diet Coke	1 reg (20 fl oz)	0	0	0	0
Dr Pepper	1 reg (20 fl oz)	190	0	0	49
Iced Tea	1 reg (20 fl oz)	0	0	0	0
Minute Maid Lemonade	1 reg (20 fl oz)	190	0	0	48
Orange Juice	1 serv (10 oz)	150	2	0	34
Sprite	1 reg (20 fl oz)	160	0	0	41
breakfast selections					
Breakfast Jack	1 (4.2 oz)	300	18	12	30
Country Crock Spread	1 pat (5 g)	25	0	3	0
Grape Jelly	1 serv (0.5 oz)	40	0	0	9
Hash Browns	1 serv (2 oz)	160	1	11	14
Pancake Syrup	1 serv (1.5 oz)	120	0	0	30
Pancakes w/ Bacon	1 serv (5.6 oz)	400	13	12	59
Sausage Croissant	1 (6.4 oz)	670	21	48	39
Sourdough Breakfast Sandwich	1 (5.2 oz)	380	21	21	31
Supreme Croissant	1 (6 oz)	570	21	20	39
Ultimate Breakfast Sandwich	1 (8.5 oz)	620	36	36	39
desserts					
Carrot Cake	1 serv (3.5 oz)	370	3	16	54
Cheesecake	1 serv (3.5 oz)	310	8	18	29
Double Fudge Cake	1 serv (3 oz)	300	3	10	50
Hot Apple Turnover	1 (3.8 oz)	340	4	18	41
main menu selections					
¼ lb Burger	1 (6 oz)	510	26	27	39
American Cheese	1 slice (0.4 oz)	45	2	4	0
Bacon & Cheddar Potato Wedges	1 serv (9.3 oz)	800	20	58	49
Bacon Ultimate Cheeseburger	1 (10.4 oz)	1150	57	89	31
Barbeque Dipping Sauce	1 serv (1 fl oz)	45	1	0	11
Cheeseburger	1 (4 oz)	330	15	15	32

FOOD	PORTION	CALS	PROT	FAT	CARB
Chicken & Fries	1 serv (9.3 oz)	730	26	34	79
Chicken Caesar Sandwich	1 (8.3 oz)	520	27	26	44
Chicken Fajita Pita	1 (6.6 oz)	280	24	9	25
Chicken Sandwich	1 (5.9 oz)	450	16	26	38
Chicken Strips Breaded	5 pieces (5.3 oz)	360	27	17	24
Chicken Supreme Sandwich	1 (8.2 oz)	680	23	45	46
Chili Cheese Curly Fries	1 serv (8.1 oz)	650	12	41	60
Double Cheeseburger	1 (5.3 oz)	450	24	24	35
Egg Rolls	3 pieces (6 oz)	440	15	24	40
Egg Rolls	5 pieces (10 oz)	730	25	41	67
Fish & Chips	1 serv (9 oz)	720	19	35	81
French Fries	1 reg (4.1 oz)	360	4	17	48
Grilled Chicken Fillet Sandwich	1 (8.1 oz)	520	27	26	42
Hamburger	1 (3.6 oz)	280	13	12	32
Jumbo Fries	1 serv (5 oz)	430	4	20	58
Jumbo Jack	1 (7.8 oz)	560	28	36	31
Jumbo Jack w/ Cheese	1 (8.6 oz)	650	32	43	32
Ketchup	1 pkg (0.3 oz)	10	0	0	3
Monster Taco	1 (4 oz)	290	11	18	21
Onion Rings	1 serv (4.2 oz)	460	7	25	50
Philly Cheesesteak Sandwich	1 (7.6 oz)	520	33	25	41
Salsa	1 serv (1 oz)	10	0	0	2
Seasoned Curly Fries	1 serv (4.5 oz)	420	6	24	46
Sour Cream	1 serv (1 oz)	60	1	6	1
Sourdough Jack	1 (7.8 oz)	670	32	43	39
Spicy Crispy Chicken Sandwich	1 (7.9 oz)	560	24	27	55
Stuffed Jalapenos	10 pieces (7.6 oz)	680	20	40	59
Stuffed Jalapenos	7 pieces (5.3 oz)	470	14	28	41
Super Scoop French Fries	1 serv (7 oz)	610	6	28	82
Swiss-Style Cheese	1 slice (0.4 oz)	40	3	3	0
Taco	1 (2.7 oz)	190	7	11	15
Tartar Dipping Sauce	1 pkg (1.5 oz)	220	1	23	2
Teriyaki Bowl Chicken	1 serv (17.6 oz)	670	29	4	128
Ultimate Cheeseburger	1 (9.8 oz)	1030	50	79	30
salad dressings					
Blue Cheese	1 serv (2 fl oz)	210	1	18	11
Buttermilk House	1 serv (2 fl oz)	290	1	30	6
Low Calorie Italian	1 serv (2 fl oz)	25	0	2	2
Thousand Island	1 serv (2 fl oz)	250	1	24	10
salads and salad bars					
Croutons	1 serv (0.4 oz)	50	1	2	8
Garden Chicken Salad	1 serv (8.9 oz)	200	23	9	8
Side Salad	1 (3 oz)	50	2	3	3

FOOD	PORTION	CALS	PROT	FAT	CARB
KFC					
BBQ Baked Beans	1 serv (5.5 oz)	190	6	3	33
Biscuit	1 (2 oz)	180	4	10	20
Chicken Pot Pie	1 (13 oz)	770	29	42	69
Chicken Twister	1 (8.7 oz)	550	26	32	40
Cole Slaw	1 serv (5 oz)	180	2	9	21
Corn On The Cob	1 ear (5.7 oz)	150	5	2	35
Cornbread	1 (2 oz)	228	3	13	25
Crispy Strips Colonel's	3 (3.25 oz)	261	20	16	10
Crispy Strips Spicy Buffalo	3 (4.2 oz)	350	22	19	22
Extra Tasty Crispy Breast	1 (5.9 oz)	470	31	28	25
Extra Tasty Crispy Drumstick	1 (2.4 oz)	190	13	11	8
Extra Tasty Crispy Thigh	1 (4.2 oz)	370	19	25	18
Extra Tasty Crispy Whole Wing	1 (1.9 oz)	200	10	13	10
Green Beans	1 serv (4.7 oz)	45	1	2	7
Hot & Spicy Breast	1 (6.5 oz)	530	32	35	23
Hot & Spicy Drumstick	1 (2.3 oz)	190	13	11	10
Hot & Spicy Thigh	1 (3.8 oz)	370	18	27	13
Hot & Spicy Whole Wing	1 (1.9 oz)	210	10	15	9
Hot Wings	6 (4.8 oz)	471	27	33	18
Macaroni & Cheese	1 serv (5.4 oz)	180	7	8	21
Mashed Potatoes w/ Gravy	1 serv (4.8 oz)	120	1	6	17
Mean Greens	1 serv (5.4 oz)	70	4	3	11
Original Recipe Breast	1 (5.4 oz)	400	29	24	16
Original Recipe Chicken Sandwich	1 (7.3 oz)	497	29	22	46
Original Recipe Drumstick	1 (2.2 oz)	140	13	9	4
Original Recipe Thigh	1 (3.2 oz)	250	16	18	6
Original Recipe Whole Wing	1 (1.6 oz)	140	9	10	5
Potato Salad	1 serv (5.6 oz)	230	4	14	23
Potato Wedges	1 serv (4.8 oz)	280	5	13	28
Tender Roast Breast w/ Skin	1 (4.9 oz)	251	37	11	1
Tender Roast Breast w/o Skin	1 (4.2 oz)	169	31	4	1
Tender Roast Drumstick w/ Skin	1 (1.9 oz)	97	15	4	tr
Tender Roast Drumstick w/o Skin	1 (1.2 oz)	67	11	2	tr
Tender Roast Thigh w/ Skin	1 (3.2 oz)	207	19	12	<2
Tender Roast Thigh w/o Skin	1 (2.1 oz)	106	13	6	tr
Tender Roast Wing w/ Skin	1 (1.8 oz)	121	12	8	1
Value BBQ Chicken Sandwich	1 (5.3 oz)	256	17	8	28
KRISPY KREME					
Chocolate Iced	1 (2 oz)	260	3	14	30
Chocolate Iced Cake	1 (2 oz)	230	3	12	28

FOOD	PORTION	CALS	PROT	FAT	CARB
Chocolate Iced Creme Filled	1 (2.3 oz)	270	4	14	32
Chocolate Iced Cruller	1 (1.7 oz)	240	2	14	26
Chocolate Iced Custard Filled	1 (2.7 oz)	250	4	9	38
Chocolated Iced w/ Sprinkles	1 (2 oz)	220	2	10	31
Cinnamon Apple Filled	1 (2.3 oz)	210	4	9	29
Cinnamon Bun	1 (2.1 oz)	220	5	11	26
Glazed Blueberry	1 (2.4 oz)	300	2	15	37
Glazed Creme Filled	1 (2.3 oz)	270	4	14	32
Glazed Cruller	1 (1.5 oz)	220	2	14	22
Glazed Devil's Food	1 (1.9 oz)	240	2	13	29
Lemon Filled	1 (2.2 oz)	210	4	10	28
Maple Iced	1 (1.8 oz)	200	3	9	28
Original Glazed	1 (1.3 oz)	180	2	10	17
Powdered Blueberry Filled	1 (2.1 oz)	200	4	9	26
Powdered Cake	1 (1.8 oz)	220	3	11	26
Raspberry Filled	1 (2 oz)	210	4	10	27
Traditional Cake	1 (1.7 oz)	200	3	11	22
LONG JOHN SILVER'S **main menu selections**					
Breaded Chicken Strips	1 piece (1.15 oz)	100	6	5	6
Breaded Clams	1 serv (3 oz)	300	11	17	31
Breaded Fish	1 piece (1.6 oz)	110	5	5	11
Cheese Sticks	1 serv (1.6 oz)	160	6	9	12
Chicken Salsa	1 reg (11 oz)	690	18	32	81
Corn Cobbette w/ Butter	1 piece (3.3 oz)	140	3	8	19
Corn Cobbette w/o Butter	1 (3.1 oz)	80	3	1	19
Fish Cajun	1 lg (23 oz)	1450	18	70	85
Flavorbaked Chicken	1 piece (2.6 oz)	110	19	3	tr
Flavorbaked Fish	1 piece (2.3 oz)	90	14	3	1
Fries	1 reg (3 oz)	250	3	15	28
Fries	1 lg (5 oz)	420	5	24	46
Honey Mustard Sauce	1 serv (0.4 oz)	20	0	0	5
Hushpuppy	1 (0.8 oz)	60	1	3	9
Ketchup	1 serv (.32 oz)	10	0	0	2
Popcorn Chicken Munchers	1 serv (4 oz)	380	23	23	20
Popcorn Fish Munchers	1 serv (4 oz)	300	14	14	29
Popcorn Shrimp Munchers	1 serv (4 oz)	320	15	15	33
Rice	1 serv (3 oz)	140	3	3	26
Sandwich Batter Dipped Fish No Sauce	1 (5.4 oz)	320	17	13	40
Sandwich Flavorbaked Chicken	1 (5.8 oz)	290	24	10	27
Sandwich Flavorbaked Fish	1 (6 oz)	320	23	14	28
Sandwich Ultimate Fish	1 (6.4 oz)	430	18	21	44
Shrimp Sauce	1 serv (0.4 oz)	15	0	0	3
Side Salad	1 (4.3 oz)	25	1	0	4
Slaw	1 serv (3.4 oz)	140	1	6	20
Sweet 'N' Sour Sauce	1 serv (0.4 oz)	20	0	0	5

FOOD	PORTION	CALS	PROT	FAT	CARB
Tartar Sauce	1 serv (0.4 oz)	35	0	2	5
Wraps Chicken Cajun	1 reg (11 oz)	720	18	35	83
Wraps Chicken Cajun	1 lg (22 oz)	1440	37	71	165
Wraps Chicken Ranch	1 reg (11 oz)	730	18	36	82
Wraps Chicken Ranch	1 lg (22 oz)	1450	36	72	165
Wraps Chicken Salsa	1 lg (22 oz)	1370	36	64	162
Wraps Chicken Tartar	1 lg (22 oz)	1450	36	72	165
Wraps Chicken Tartar	1 reg (11 oz)	730	18	36	83
Wraps Fish Cajun	1 reg (11.5 oz)	730	18	35	85
Wraps Fish Ranch	1 lg (23 oz)	1460	35	72	170
Wraps Fish Ranch	1 reg (11.5 oz)	730	18	36	85
Wraps Fish Salsa	1 reg (11.5 oz)	690	18	32	84
Wraps Fish Salsa	1 lg (23 oz)	1380	35	64	167
Wraps Fish Tartar	1 lg (23 oz)	1470	35	72	170
Wraps Fish Tartar	1 reg (11.5 oz)	730	18	36	85
Wraps Popcorn Shrimp Cajun	1 reg (11 oz)	720	16	35	86
Wraps Popcorn Shrimp Cajun	1 lg (22 oz)	1450	32	71	172
Wraps Popcorn Shrimp Ranch	1 lg (22 oz)	1460	32	72	171
Wraps Popcorn Shrimp Ranch	1 reg (11 oz)	720	16	35	86
Wraps Popcorn Shrimp Salsa	1 reg (11 oz)	690	16	32	84
Wraps Popcorn Shrimp Salsa	1 lg (22 oz)	1380	32	64	169
Wraps Popcorn Shrimp Tartar	1 reg (11 oz)	730	16	36	86
Wraps Popcorn Shrimp Tartar	1 lg (22 oz)	1460	32	72	172
salad dressings					
Fat-Free French	1 serv (1.5 oz)	50	0	0	14
Fat-Free Ranch	1 serv (1.5 oz)	50	2	0	13
Italian	1 serv (1 oz)	130	0	14	2
Malt Vinegar	1 serv (0.3 oz)	0	0	0	0
Ranch Dressing	1 serv (1 oz)	170	0	18	1
Thousand Island	1 serv (1 oz)	110	0	10	5
MANHATTAN BAGEL					
Blueberry	1	260	9	tr	54
Cheddar Cheese	1	270	11	4	48
Chocolate Chip	1	290	9	3	56
Cinnamon Raisin	1	280	10	tr	57
Egg	1	270	10	2	53
Everything	1	290	11	3	54
Jalapeno Cheddar	1	260	16	2	53
Marble	1	260	10	tr	52
Oat Bran	1	260	10	1	53

FOOD	PORTION	CALS	PROT	FAT	CARB
Oat Bran Raisin Walnut	1	270	10	3	54
Onion	1	270	10	tr	55
Plain	1	260	10	tr	52
Poppy	1	300	11	4	54
Pumpernickel	1	250	10	1	52
Rye	1	260	10	1	52
Salt	1	260	10	tr	53
Sesame	1	310	11	5	55
Spinach	1	270	10	tr	54
Sun-Dried Tomato	1	260	10	1	53
Whole Wheat	1	260	10	tr	52
MCDONALD'S					
baked selections					
Apple Pie Baked	1 (2.7 oz)	260	3	13	34
Chocolate Chip Cookie	1 (1.2 oz)	170	2	10	22
Cinnamon Roll	1	390	6	18	50
Danish Apple	1	340	5	15	47
Danish Cheese	1	400	7	21	45
Lowfat Muffin Apple Bran	1 (4 oz)	300	6	3	61
McDonaldland Cookies	1 pkg (1.5 oz)	180	3	5	32
beverages					
Coca-Cola Classic	1 sm (16 oz)	150	0	0	40
Diet Coke	1 sm (16 oz)	1	0	0	0
Hi-C Orange	1 sm (16 oz)	160	0	0	44
Orange Juice	1 serv (6 oz)	80	0	0	20
Shake Chocolate	1 sm (14.5 oz)	360	11	9	60
Shake Strawberry	1 sm (14.5 oz)	360	11	9	60
Shake Vanilla	1 sm (14.5 oz)	360	11	9	59
Sprite	1 sm (16 fl oz)	150	0	0	39
breakfast selections					
Bacon Egg & Cheese Biscuit	1	540	21	34	36
Bagel Ham & Egg Cheese	1	550	26	23	58
Bagel Steak & Egg Cheese	1	660	27	31	59
Biscuit	1 (2.9 oz)	290	5	15	34
Breakfast Burrito	1 (4.1 oz)	320	13	20	21
Egg McMuffin	1 (4.8 oz)	290	17	14	27
English Muffin	1 (1.9 oz)	140	4	2	25
Hash Browns	1 serv (1.9 oz)	130	1	8	14
Hotcakes Margarine & Syrup	1 serv	600	9	17	104
Hotcakes Plain	1 serv	340	9	8	58
Sausage	1 (1.5 oz)	170	6	16	0
Sausage Biscuit	1 (4.5 oz)	470	11	31	35
Sausage Biscuit w/ Egg	1 (6.2 oz)	550	18	37	35
Sausage McMuffin	1 (3.9 oz)	360	13	23	26
Sausage McMuffin w/ Egg	1 (5.7 oz)	440	19	28	27
Scrambled Eggs	2 (3.6 oz)	160	13	11	1

FOOD	PORTION	CALS	PROT	FAT	CARB
desserts					
McFlurry Butterfinger	1	620	16	22	90
McFlurry M&M	1	630	16	23	90
McFlurry Nestle Crunch	1	630	16	24	89
McFlurry Oreo	1	570	15	20	82
Nuts For Sundaes	1 serv (7 g)	40	2	4	2
Reduced Fat Ice Cream Cone Vanilla	1 (3.2 oz)	150	4	5	23
Sundae Hot Caramel	1 (6.4 oz)	360	7	10	61
Sundae Hot Fudge	1 (6.3 oz)	340	8	12	52
Sundae Strawberry	1 (6.2 oz)	290	7	7	50
main menu selections					
Barbeque Sauce	1 pkg (1 oz)	45	0	0	10
Big Mac	1	570	26	32	45
Big Xtra!	1	710	24	46	51
Big Xtra! w/ Cheese	1	810	29	55	52
Cheeseburger	1 (4.2 oz)	320	16	13	35
Chicken McNuggets	6 pieces (3.7 oz)	290	15	17	20
Chicken McNuggets	4 pieces (2.5 oz)	190	10	11	13
Chicken McNuggets	9 pieces	430	23	25	29
Crispy Chicken Deluxe	1 (7.8 oz)	500	26	25	43
Filet-O-Fish	1	470	15	26	45
French Fries	1 sm (2.4 oz)	210	3	10	26
French Fries	1 lg	540	8	26	68
French Fries	1 med	450	6	22	57
French Fries	1 super	610	9	29	77
Grilled Chicken Deluxe	1 (7.8 oz)	440	27	20	38
Grilled Chicken Deluxe Plain w/o Mayonnaise	1 (7.2 oz)	300	27	5	38
Grilled Chicken Salad Deluxe	1 serv (9 oz)	120	21	2	7
Hamburger	1	270	13	9	35
Honey	1 pkg (0.5 oz)	45	0	0	12
Honey Mustard	1 pkg (0.5 oz)	50	0	5	3
Hot Mustard	1 pkg (1 oz)	60	1	4	7
Light Mayonnaise	1 pkg (0.4 oz)	40	0	4	tr
Quarter Pounder	1	430	23	21	37
Quarter Pounder w/ Cheese	1 (7 oz)	530	28	30	38
Sweet 'N Sour Sauce	1 pkg (1 oz)	50	0	0	11
salad dressings					
Caesar	1 pkg (2.1 oz)	160	2	14	7
Fat Free Herb Vinaigrette	1 pkg (2.1 oz)	50	0	0	11
Ranch	1 pkg (2.1 oz)	230	1	21	10
Reduced Calorie Red French	1 pkg (2.1 oz)	160	0	8	23
salads and salad bars					
Croutons	1 pkg	50	1	1	9
Garden Salad	1 serv (6.2 oz)	35	2	0	7

FOOD	PORTION	CALS	PROT	FAT	CARB
MRS. FIELDS					
Brownie Double Fudge	1 (3.1 oz)	420	5	20	56
Brownie Fudge Walnut	1 (3.4 oz)	500	7	29	54
Brownie Pecan Fudge	1 (2.8 oz)	390	4	21	48
Brownie Pecan Pie	1 (3 oz)	400	5	21	48
Cookie Chewy Fudge	1 (1.7 oz)	230	3	12	32
Cookie Coconut Macadamia	1 (1.7 oz)	250	3	15	28
Cookie Milk Chocolate Chip	1 (1.7 oz)	240	3	12	32
Cookie Milk Chocolate Macadamia	1 (1.7 oz)	250	3	14	29
Cookie Milk Chocolate w/ Walnuts	1 (1.7 oz)	250	3	13	30
Cookie Oatmeal Raisin	1 (1.7 oz)	220	3	10	31
Cookie Peanut Butter	1 (1.7 oz)	240	4	13	27
Cookie Semi-Sweet Chocolate	1 (1.7 oz)	230	3	12	32
Cookie Semi-Sweet Chocolate w/ Walnuts	1 (1.8 oz)	240	3	13	30
Cookie Triple Chocolate	1 (1.7 oz)	230	3	12	31
Cookie White Chunk Macadamia	1 (1.7 oz)	260	3	15	29
Muffin Banana Walnut	1 (3.9 oz)	460	9	24	53
Muffin Blueberry	1 (4 oz)	390	6	15	58
Muffin Chocolate Chip	1 (4 oz)	450	7	19	65
Muffin Mandarin Orange	1 (4 oz)	420	6	17	59
Peanut Butter Dream Bar	1 (5 oz)	750	11	40	85
Stokabunga Energy Cookie	1 (5 oz)	750	11	48	74
NEWPORT CREAMERY					
ice cream					
Reduced Fat No Sugar Added Chocolate	½ cup (2.6 oz)	110	4	3	22
Reduced Fat No Sugar Added Coffee	½ cup (2.6 oz)	100	4	4	18
OLIVE GARDEN					
Garden Fare Apple Carmellina	1 serv (12.2 oz)	560	6	2	131
Garden Fare Dinner Capellini Pomodoro	1 serv (21.1 oz)	610	19	16	98
Garden Fare Dinner Capellini Primavera	1 serv (20.1 oz)	400	18	7	68
Garden Fare Dinner Capellini Primavera w/ Chicken	1 serv (23.8 oz)	560	47	10	71
Garden Fare Dinner Chicken Giardino	1 serv (20.6 oz)	550	42	11	71

FOOD	PORTION	CALS	PROT	FAT	CARB
Garden Fare Dinner Linguine Alla Marinara	1 serv (16.3 oz)	500	16	9	89
Garden Fare Dinner Penne Fra Diavolo	1 serv (14.3 oz)	420	13	7	77
Garden Fare Dinner Shrimp Primavera	1 serv (28.4 oz)	740	48	15	104
Garden Fare Lunch Capellini Pamodoro	1 serv (11.7 oz)	360	12	9	57
Garden Fare Lunch Capellini Primavera	1 serv (11.2 oz)	260	12	5	42
Garden Fare Lunch Capellini Primavera w/ Chicken	1 serv (14.9 oz)	420	41	8	45
Garden Fare Lunch Chicken Giardino	1 serv (12.8 oz)	360	23	9	47
Garden Fare Lunch Linguine Alla Marinara	1 serv (10.2 oz)	310	10	6	54
Garden Fare Lunch Penne Fra Diavolo	1 serv (10.2 oz)	300	9	5	57
Garden Fare Lunch Shrimp Primavera	1 serv (15.2 oz)	410	25	8	60
Minestrone Soup	1 serv (6 oz)	80	4	1	15
PIZZA HUT					
desserts					
Apple Pizza	1 slice (2.8 oz)	250	3	5	48
Cherry Pizza	1 slice (2.8 oz)	250	3	5	47
main menu selections					
Bread Stick	1 (1.3 oz)	130	3	4	20
Buffalo Wings Hot	4 pieces (2.1 oz)	210	22	12	4
Buffalo Wings Mild	5 pieces (2.9 oz)	200	23	12	tr
Cavatini Pasta	1 serv (12.5 oz)	480	21	14	66
Cavatini Supreme Pasta	1 serv (13.9 oz)	560	24	19	73
Garlic Bread	1 slice (1.3 oz)	150	3	8	16
Ham & Cheese Sandwich	1 (9.7 oz)	550	33	21	57
Spaghetti Marinara	1 serv (16.6 oz)	490	18	6	91
Spaghetti Meat Sauce	1 serv (16.4 oz)	600	23	13	98
Spaghetti Meatballs	1 serv (18.8 oz)	850	37	24	120
Supreme Sandwich	1 (10.2 oz)	640	34	28	62
pizza					
Edge Chicken Supreme	1 sq (2.5 oz)	90	7	4	9
Edge Meat Lover's	1 sq (2 oz)	160	7	11	8
Edge The Works	1 sq (2.2 oz)	110	5	6	9
Edge Veggie Lover's	1 sq (1.9 oz)	70	4	3	9
Hand Tossed Beef Topping	1 slice	330	16	17	29
Hand Tossed Cheese	1 slice	240	12	10	28
Hand Tossed Chicken Supreme	1 slice	230	13	7	29

FOOD	PORTION	CALS	PROT	FAT	CARB
Hand Tossed Ham	1 slice	260	14	10	28
Hand Tossed Italian Sausage	1 slice	340	16	18	28
Hand Tossed Meat Lover's	1 slice	320	14	17	28
Hand Tossed Pepperoni	1 slice	280	13	13	28
Hand Tossed Pepperoni Lover's	1 slice	250	11	11	27
Hand Tossed Pork Topping	1 slice	320	16	16	29
Hand Tossed Super Supreme	1 slice	290	13	14	29
Hand Tossed Supreme	1 slice	270	13	12	29
Hand Tossed Veggie Lover's	1 slice	220	9	8	29
Insider Cheese	1 med slice (4.9 oz)	370	17	16	41
Pan Beef Topping	1 med slice (4.3 oz)	330	14	18	29
Pan Cheese	1 med slice (3.9 oz)	290	12	14	28
Pan Chicken Supreme	1 med slice (4.5 oz)	270	13	12	29
Pan Ham	1 med slice (3.8 oz)	260	11	12	28
Pan Italian Sausage	1 med slice (4.3 oz)	340	13	20	29
Pan Meat Lover's	1 med slice (4.7 oz)	360	14	21	29
Pan Pepperoni	1 med slice (3.7 oz)	280	11	14	28
Pan Pepperoni Lover's	1 med slice (4.3 oz)	330	14	18	29
Pan Pork Topping	1 med slice (3.7 oz)	320	13	17	29
Pan Super Supreme	1 med slice (5 oz)	340	14	18	30
Pan Supreme	1 med slice (4.7 oz)	320	13	17	29
Pan Veggie Lover's	1 med slice (4.6 oz)	270	10	12	30
Personal Pan Beef Topping	1 pie (10.2 oz)	710	31	35	71
Personal Pan Cheese	1 pie (9.2 oz)	630	23	28	71
Personal Pan Ham	1 pie (9.1 oz)	580	27	23	70
Personal Pan Italian Sausage	1 pie (10.2 oz)	740	31	39	71
Personal Pan Pepperoni	1 pie (9 oz)	620	26	28	70
Personal Pan Pork Topping	1 pie (10.2 oz)	700	31	34	71
Sicilian Beef Topping	1 slice (4 oz)	260	11	11	31
Sicilian Cheese	1 slice (4 oz)	290	12	13	31
Sicilian Chicken Supreme	1 slice (4.6 oz)	270	12	11	32
Sicilian Ham	1 slice (3.8 oz)	257	11	10	30
Sicilian Italian Sausage	1 slice (4.4 oz)	333	13	18	31
Sicilian Meat Lover's	1 slice (4.7 oz)	350	14	19	31
Sicilian Pepperoni	1 slice (3.9 oz)	280	10	13	31
Sicilian Pepperoni Lover's	1 slice (4.4 oz)	320	13	16	31
Sicilian Pork Topping	1 slice (4.4 oz)	320	13	16	31
Sicilian Super Supreme	1 slice (5 oz)	340	13	18	32
Sicilian Supreme	1 slice (4.7 oz)	310	12	15	32
Sicilian Veggies Lover's	1 slice (4.6 oz)	270	12	11	32
Stuffed Crust Beef Topping	1 lg slice (5.8 oz)	390	19	18	40
Stuffed Crust Cheese	1 lg slice (5.5 oz)	360	18	16	39
Stuffed Crust Chicken Supreme	1 lg slice (6.5 oz)	350	21	13	41

FOOD	PORTION	CALS	PROT	FAT	CARB
Stuffed Crust Ham	1 lg slice (5.5 oz)	330	18	13	39
Stuffed Crust Italian Sausage	1 lg slice (5.8 oz)	400	19	20	40
Stuffed Crust Meat Lover's	1 lg slice (6.7 oz)	470	22	25	13
Stuffed Crust Pepperoni	1 lg slice (5.4 oz)	360	17	16	39
Stuffed Crust Pepperoni Lover's	1 lg slice (6.2 oz)	420	21	21	40
Stuffed Crust Pork Topping	1 lg slice (5.7 oz)	380	19	18	40
Stuffed Crust Super Supreme	1 lg slice (7.2 oz)	430	21	22	41
Stuffed Crust Supreme	1 lg slice (6.7 oz)	410	20	20	41
Stuffed Crust Veggie Lover's	1 lg slice (6.6 oz)	340	16	14	42
The Big New Yorker Beef Topping	1 slice (7.2 oz)	480	24	26	42
The Big New Yorker Cheese	1 slice (6.1 oz)	380	19	17	41
The Big New Yorker Ham	1 slice (5.9 oz)	340	18	13	41
The Big New Yorker Pepperoni	1 slice (5.6 oz)	370	17	16	41
The Big New Yorker Pork Topping	1 slice (7.2 oz)	470	23	25	42
The Big New Yorker Sausage	1 slice (8 oz)	570	27	33	42
The Big New Yorker Supreme	1 slice (7.8 oz)	450	22	23	43
The Big New Yorker Veggie Lover's	1 slice (12 oz)	450	18	22	52
Thin'N Crispy Cheese	1 med slice (3 oz)	200	10	9	22
Thin'N Crispy Chicken Supreme	1 med slice (4 oz)	200	12	7	23
Thin'N Crispy Ham	1 med slice (2.9 oz)	170	9	7	21
Thin'N Crispy Italian Sausage	1 med slice (3.7 oz)	290	12	17	22
Thin'N Crispy Meat Lover's	1 med slice (4.1 oz)	310	14	19	22
Thin'N Crispy Pepperoni	1 med slice (2.8 oz)	190	9	9	21
Thin'N Crispy Pepperoni Lover's	1 med slice (3.4 oz)	250	12	13	22
Thin'N Crispy Pork Topping	1 med slice (3.7 oz)	270	13	14	22
Thin'N Crispy Super Supreme	1 med slice (4.6 oz)	280	13	15	23
Thin'N Crispy Supreme	1 med slice (4.1 oz)	250	12	13	23
Thin'N Crispy Veggie Lover's	1 med slice (4 oz)	190	8	7	22
Thin'N Crispy Beef Topping	1 med slice (3.7 oz)	270	13	15	22
Twist Crust Cheese	1 lg slice (6.7 oz)	450	20	16	58
Twist Crust Marinara Sauce	1 serv (3 oz)	60	2	1	12
Twist Crust Ranch Sauce	1 serv (3 oz)	440	2	48	4
Twist Crust Supreme	1 lg slice (7.5 oz)	470	20	18	59

FOOD	PORTION	CALS	PROT	FAT	CARB
QUINCY'S					
baked selections					
Banana Nut Bread	1 serv (2 oz)	165	2	7	22
Biscuit	1 (2.5 oz)	270	5	15	29
Cornbread	1 serv (2 oz)	140	3	5	19
Yeast Roll	1 (2 oz)	160	1	4	29
breakfast selections					
Bacon	1 serv (0.25 oz)	35	2	3	0
Corned Beef Hash	1 serv (4.5 oz)	210	10	15	11
Country Ham	1 serv (1.5 oz)	90	9	6	1
Escalloped Apples	1 serv (3.5 oz)	120	0	2	26
Oatmeal	1 serv (1 oz)	175	4	2	18
Pancakes	1 (1.5 oz)	95	3	3	12
Sausage Gravy	1 serv (4 oz)	70	2	6	3
Sausage Links	1 (2 oz)	225	7	22	0
Sausage Patties	1 (2 oz)	230	7	23	0
Scrambled Eggs	1 serv (2 oz)	95	7	7	1
Steak Fingers	1 serv (3.5 oz)	360	16	25	18
Syrup	1 oz	75	0	0	20
desserts					
Banana Pudding	1 serv (5 oz)	240	3	12	30
Brownie Pudding Cake	1 serv (4 oz)	310	4	5	66
Caramel Topping	1 serv (1 oz)	105	0	1	24
Chocolate Chip Cookies	1 (0.5 oz)	60	1	8	8
Cobbler Apple	1 serv (6 oz)	255	1	8	49
Cobbler Cherry	1 serv (6 oz)	410	1	8	55
Cobbler Peach	1 serv (6 oz)	305	1	8	50
Frozen Yogurt	1 serv (4 oz)	135	5	2	25
Fudge Topping	1 serv (1 oz)	105	1	4	15
main menu selections					
⅓ Pound Hamburger	1 serv (8 oz)	565	32	33	32
BBQ Beans	1 serv (4 oz)	114	4	1	21
Bacon Cheese Burger	1 (9 oz)	663	37	41	33
Baked Potato	1 (6 oz)	115	5	0	30
Broccoli	1 serv (4 oz)	34	3	0	5
Cheese Sauce	1 serv (1 oz)	58	2	5	1
Chopped Steak Steak	1 serv (8 oz)	499	31	42	0
Cinnamon Apples	1 serv (4 oz)	172	0	5	34
Corn	1 serv (4 oz)	96	3	1	24
Country Steak w/ Gravy	1 serv (8 oz)	530	32	25	44
Cowboy Steak	1 serv (14 oz)	580	61	33	9
Filet w/ Bacon	1 serv (8 oz)	340	48	17	2
Green Beans	1 serv (4 oz)	61	1	4	6
Grilled Chicken	1 reg serv (5 oz)	120	25	2	1
Grilled Chicken Sandwich	1 (9 oz)	324	33	4	39
Grilled Salmon	1 serv (7 oz)	228	46	4	1
Homestyle Chicken Fillet	1 serv (3 oz)	217	13	9	21
Junior Sirloin Steak	1 serv (5.5 oz)	194	25	10	0

FOOD	PORTION	CALS	PROT	FAT	CARB
Large Sirloin Steak	1 serv (10 oz)	368	46	20	2
Mashed Potatoes	1 serv (4 oz)	54	1	6	11
NY Strip Steak	1 serv (10 oz)	450	53	26	1
Philly Cheese Steak	1 serv (11 oz)	588	37	30	38
Porterhouse Steak	1 serv (17 oz)	683	67	46	0
Regular Sirloin Steak	1 serv (8 oz)	285	34	16	0
Ribeye Steak	1 serv (10 oz)	452	48	29	0
Rice Pilaf	1 serv (4 oz)	119	2	2	23
Roasted BBQ Chicken	1 serv (14 oz)	941	70	65	21
Roasted Herb Chicken	1 serv (14 oz)	875	70	65	4
Sirloin Tips w/ Mushroom Gravy	1 serv (6 oz)	196	28	7	5
Sirloin Tips w/ Peppers & Onions	1 serv (5 oz)	203	27	8	4
Smothered Steak Sandwich	1 (9 oz)	429	34	15	36
Smothered Strip Steak	1 serv (10 oz)	622	55	41	12
Southern Breaded Shrimp	1 serv (7 oz)	546	19	31	47
Spicy BBQ Chicken Sandwich	1 (10 oz)	368	34	1	45
Steak & Shrimp	1 serv (9 oz)	677	48	39	33
Steak Fries	1 serv (4 oz)	358	5	19	45
T-Bone Steak	1 serv (13 oz)	521	51	35	0
salad dressings					
Blue Cheese	1 serv (1 oz)	155	2	16	2
French	1 serv (1 oz)	125	0	12	4
Honey Mustard	1 serv (1 oz)	100	2	6	10
Italian	1 serv (1 oz)	135	0	14	3
Light Creamy Italian	1 serv (1 oz)	65	2	4	8
Light French	1 serv (1 oz)	85	2	4	13
Light Italian	1 serv (1 oz)	20	2	2	2
Light Thousand Island	1 serv (1 oz)	65	2	4	8
Parmesan Peppercorn	1 serv (1 oz)	150	1	14	4
Ranch	1 serv (1 oz)	110	1	11	1
soups					
Chili w/ Beans	1 serv (6 oz)	235	13	11	21
Clam Chowder	1 serv (6 oz)	180	3	9	21
Cream Of Broccoli	1 serv (6 oz)	170	2	10	18
Vegetable Beef	1 serv (6 oz)	90	5	2	14
QUIZNO'S					
Sub Honey Burbon Chicken	1 sm	329	24	6	45
Sub Turkey Lite	1 sm	334	17	6	52
Sub Tuscan Chicken Salad	1 sm	326	21	6	45
RALLY'S					
beverages					
Coke	1 serv (16 oz)	132	0	0	35
Diet Coke	1 serv (20 oz)	1	0	0	0
Fanta Orange	1 serv (16 oz)	150	0	0	38
Mr. Pibb	1 serv (16 oz)	113	0	0	29

FOOD	PORTION	CALS	PROT	FAT	CARB
Root Beer	1 serv (16 oz)	146	0	0	38
Shake Banana	1 serv	399	9	11	70
Shake Chocolate	1 serv	411	10	12	73
Shake Strawberry	1 serv	399	9	11	70
Shake Vanilla	1 serv	320	9	11	49
Sprite	1 serv (16 oz)	132	0	0	33
main menu selections					
Big Buford	1	743	41	46	35
Chicken Fillet Sandwich	1	399	21	15	43
Chili w/ Cheese & Onion	1 serv (13 oz)	669	43	41	37
Chili w/ Cheese & Onion	1 serv (7 oz)	360	23	22	20
French Fries	1 extra lg (8 oz)	423	7	21	52
French Fries	1 reg (4 oz)	211	3	11	26
French Fries	1 lg (6 oz)	317	5	16	39
Onion Rings	1 serv	210	6	2	45
Rallyburger	1	433	20	22	35
Rallyburger w/ Cheese	1	488	23	35	35
Spicy Chicken Sandwich	1	437	18	18	50
Super Barbecue Bacon	1	593	29	31	49
Super Double Cheeseburger	1	762	41	48	37
SBARRO					
Pizza Veggie Slice	1 serv (10 oz)	490	20	12	75
SEE'S CANDIES					
Bridge Mix	14 pieces (1.4 oz)	200	2	12	24
Dark Chocolates	2 (1.2 oz)	160	2	10	19
Lollypop Butterscotch	1	90	0	3	17
Lollypop Cafe Latte	1	90	0	3	16
Lollypop Peanut Butter	1	90	2	4	14
Milk Chocolate Bordeaux	2 (1.4 oz)	170	1	8	27
Milk Chocolate Butter	2 (1.4 oz)	190	1	9	27
Milk Chocolate Buttercreams	2 (1.4 oz)	180	1	8	27
Milk Chocolate California Brittle	2 (1.3 oz)	220	3	16	19
Milk Chocolate Nuts & Chews	3 (1.7 oz)	250	4	16	26
Milk Chocolate Peanuts	3 (1.5 oz)	230	6	17	18
Milk Chocolate Soft Centers	2 (1.4 oz)	170	1	9	25
Milk Chocolates	2 (1.2 oz)	160	2	9	20
Nuts & Chews	3 (1.6 oz)	240	4	16	25
P-Nut Crunch	2 (1.4 oz)	220	4	15	21
Peanut Brittle	1.5 oz	230	4	16	21
Pecan Buds	3 (1.7 oz)	270	3	21	22
Soft Centers	2 (1.4 oz)	170	1	9	25
Truffles Black or Gold	2 (1.4 oz)	180	2	11	22
Truffles Mint	3 (1.6 oz)	200	2	11	26
Victoria Toffee	1.5 oz	250	4	19	19

FOOD	PORTION	CALS	PROT	FAT	CARB
SMOOTHIE KING					
Activator Banana	1 (20 oz)	429	19	1	90
Activator Chocolate	1 (20 oz)	429	19	1	90
Activator Strawberry	1 (20 oz)	559	20	1	123
Activator Vanilla	1 (20 oz)	429	19	1	90
Angel Food	1 (20 oz)	330	6	1	79
Blackberry Dream	1 (20 oz)	343	2	tr	86
Caribbean Way	1 (20 oz)	392	2	tr	96
Celestial Cherry High	1 (20 oz)	285	1	tr	69
Coconut Surprise	1 (20 oz)	457	8	6	99
Cranberry Supreme	1 (20 oz)	577	3	1	139
Cranberry Cooler	1 (20 oz)	538	1	tr	132
GoGuava	1 (20 oz)	300	1	0	72
Grape Expectations	1 (20 oz)	399	3	tr	96
Grape Expectations II	1 (20 oz)	529	4	tr	129
Hawaiian Cafe Au Lei	1 (20 oz)	286	10	tr	62
High Protein Almond Mocha	1 (20 oz)	402	31	13	45
High Protein Banana	1 (20 oz)	412	34	14	44
High Protein Chocolate	1 (20 oz)	401	31	13	45
High Protein Lemon	1 (20 oz)	390	29	13	41
High Protein Pineapple	1 (20 oz)	380	31	13	41
Hulk Chocolate	1 (20 oz)	846	23	29	129
Hulk Strawberry	1 (20 oz)	953	24	29	156
Hulk Vanilla	1 (20 oz)	846	23	29	129
Immune Builder	1 (20 oz)	333	5	1	80
Instant Vigor	1 (20 oz)	359	2	1	87
Island Treat	1 (20 oz)	334	2	1	81
Lemon Twist Banana	1 (20 oz)	339	3	tr	82
Lemon Twist Strawberry	1 (20 oz)	399	3	tr	97
Light & Fluffy	1 (20 oz)	389	2	tr	98
Malt	1 (20 oz)	887	17	41	119
Mangofest	1 (20 oz)	320	1	0	78
Mo'cuccino	1 (20 oz)	440	9	12	71
Muscle Punch	1 (20 oz)	339	6	1	80
Muscle Punch Plus	1 (20 oz)	340	6	1	80
Peach Slice	1 (20 oz)	341	5	tr	80
Peach Slice Plus	1 (20 oz)	471	5	tr	113
Peanut Power	1 (20 oz)	502	15	21	72
Peanut Power Plus Grape	1 (20 oz)	703	16	21	119
Peanut Power Plus Strawberry	1 (20 oz)	632	15	21	104
Pep Upper	1 (20 oz)	334	3	1	80
Pineapple Pleasure	1 (20 oz)	313	2	tr	76
Power Punch	1 (20 oz)	430	6	1	102
Power Punch Plus	1 (20 oz)	499	10	2	113
Raspberry Sunrise	1 (20 oz)	335	3	1	85
Shake	1 (20 oz)	875	16	41	117

FOOD	PORTION	CALS	PROT	FAT	CARB
Slim & Trim Chocolate	1 (20 oz)	270	12	2	55
Slim & Trim Strawberry	1 (20 oz)	357	7	1	79
Slim & Trim Vanilla	1 (20 oz)	227	6	1	51
Super Punch	1 (20 oz)	425	2	tr	95
Super Punch Plus	1 (20 oz)	516	2	tr	118
Yogurt D'Lite	1 (20 oz)	341	13	4	65
Youth Fountain	1 (20 oz)	267	3	tr	65
STARBUCKS					
ice cream					
Biscotte Bliss	½ cup	240	4	12	30
Caffe Almond Fudge	½ cup	260	5	13	30
Caffe Almond Roast	1 bar	280	4	18	26
Dark Roast Expresso Swirl	½ cup	220	4	10	29
Frappuccino Coffee	1 bar	110	4	2	20
Italian Roast Coffee	½ cup	230	5	12	26
Javachip	½ cup	250	4	13	29
Low Fat Latte	½ cup	170	5	3	31
Low Fat Mocha Mambo	½ cup	170	5	3	32
Vanilla Mochachip	½ cup	270	5	16	27
snacks					
Crunchy Honey Bar	1 (1.06 oz)	150	3	7	18
Lively Lemon Bar	1 (1.23 oz)	140	3	4	23
Tangy Apple Bar	1 (1.23 oz)	140	3	4	23
SUBWAY					
beverages					
Fruizle Smoothie Berry Lishus	1 sm (13 oz)	113	1	0	28
Fruizle Smoothie Berry Lishus w/ Banana	1 sm (17 oz)	221	1	1	56
Fruizle Smoothie Peach Pizazz	1 sm (12 oz)	103	1	0	26
Fruizle Smoothie Pineapple Delight w/ Banana	1 sm (17 oz)	241	1	1	61
Fruizle Smoothie Pineapple Delite	1 sm (13 oz)	133	1	0	33
Fruizle Smoothie Sunrise Refresher	1 sm (12 oz)	119	1	0	29
cookies					
Chocolate Chip	1	215	2	10	30
Chocolate Chunk	1	217	2	10	30
Double Chocolate	1	209	2	10	30
M&M	1	215	2	10	30
Oatmeal Raisin	1	210	3	8	30
Peanut Butter	1	221	4	12	26
Sugar	1	227	2	12	28
White Macadamia Nut	1	221	2	11	28

FOOD	PORTION	CALS	PROT	FAT	CARB
salad dressings					
Fat Free French	1 serv (2 oz)	70	0	0	17
Fat Free Italian	1 serv (2 oz)	20	0	0	4
Fat Free Ranch	1 serv (2 oz)	60	0	0	14
salads and salad bars					
BMT	1 serv	275	16	19	11
Cold Cut Trio	1 serv	234	14	15	11
Ham	1 serv	112	11	3	11
Meatball	1 serv	320	17	20	17
Roast Beef	1 serv	117	12	3	10
Roasted Chicken Breast	1 serv	130	18	3	9
Seafood & Crab	1 serv	197	9	11	17
Steak & Cheese	1 serv	181	17	8	12
Subway Club	1 serv	146	17	4	12
Subway Melt	1 serv	203	17	10	11
Tuna	1 serv	238	13	16	10
Turkey Breast	1 serv	105	11	2	11
Turkey Breast & Ham	1 serv	117	13	3	11
Veggie Delight	1 serv	50	2	1	9
sandwiches					
6 Inch Steak & Cheese	1	362	23	13	41
6 Inch Subway Melt	1	384	23	15	40
6 Inch Sub BMT	1	456	21	24	40
6 Inch Sub Cold Cut Trio	1	415	19	20	40
6 Inch Sub Ham	1	261	17	5	39
6 Inch Sub Meatball	1	501	23	25	46
6 Inch Sub Roast Beef	1	267	17	5	39
6 Inch Sub Roasted Chicken Breast	1	291	21	5	40
6 Inch Sub Seafood & Crab	1	378	14	16	46
6 Inch Sub Subway Club	1	296	22	5	40
6 Inch Sub Tuna	1	419	18	21	39
6 Inch Sub Turkey Breast	1	254	17	4	39
6 Inch Sub Turkey Breast & Ham	1	267	18	5	40
6 Inch Sub Veggie Delight	1	200	7	3	37
American Cheese Triangles	2	41	2	4	0
Asiago Caesar Sauce	1.5 tbsp	110	1	11	2
Bacon Strips	2	45	3	4	0
Breakfast Bacon & Egg	1	321	14	16	34
Breakfast Cheese & Egg	1	317	14	15	34
Breakfast Ham & Egg	1	338	21	14	34
Breakfast Western Egg	1	300	14	12	36
Cheddar Triangles	2	59	4	5	0
Cucumber Slices	3	2	0	0	0
Deli Ham	1	210	11	4	35
Deli Roast Beef	1	223	13	5	35

FOOD	PORTION	CALS	PROT	FAT	CARB
Deli Tuna	1	325	13	16	36
Deli Turkey Breast	1	215	13	4	36
Deli Style Roll	1	165	6	3	32
Dijon Horseradish	1.5 tbsp	91	0	10	1
Dijon Horseradish Melt	6 inch	465	25	22	47
Fat Free Red Wine Vinaigrette	1.5 tbsp	29	0	0	6
Fat Free Sweet Onion	1.5 tbsp	38	0	0	9
Green Pepper Strips	3 (0.2 oz)	2	0	0	0
Hearty Italian Bread	6 inch	207	8	3	41
Honey Mustard	1.5 tbsp	28	0	0	7
Honey Mustard Ham	6 inch	311	18	5	52
Honey Oat Bread	6 inch	249	10	4	48
Italian Bread	6 inch	178	7	2	33
Lettuce	1 serv (0.7 oz)	3	0	0	0
Mayonnaise	1 tbsp	111	0	12	0
Mayonnaise Light	1 tbsp	46	0	5	1
Monterey Cheddar Bread	6 inch	235	10	6	39
Mustard	2 tsp	7	0	0	1
Olive Oil Blend	1 tsp	45	0	5	0
Olive Rings	3 (3 g)	3	0	tr	0
Onions	1 serv (0.5 oz)	5	0	0	1
Parmesan Oregano Bread	6 inch	211	8	4	40
Pepperjack Cheese Triangles	2	40	2	4	0
Pickle Chips	3 pieces (0.3 oz)	1	0	0	0
Provolone Circles	2 halves	51	4	4	0
Red Wine Vinaigrette Club	6 inch	350	24	6	53
Roasted Garlic Bread	6 inch	225	8	3	45
Sourdough Bread	6 inch	208	8	3	41
Southwest Sauce	1.5 tbsp	86	0	9	2
Southwest Turkey Bacon	6 inch	407	21	17	48
Sweet Onion Chicken Teriyaki	6 inch	374	26	5	59
Swiss Triangles	2	53	4	4	0
Tomato Slices	3 (1.2 oz)	7	0	0	2
Vinegar	1 tsp	1	0	0	0
Wheat Sub	6 inch	186	7	2	36
soups					
Black Bean	1 cup	180	9	5	27
Brown & Wild Rice w/ Chicken	1 cup	190	6	11	17
Cheese w/ Ham & Bacon	1 cup	230	8	16	13
Chicken & Dumplings	1 cup	130	7	5	16
Cream Of Broccoli	1 cup	130	4	7	12
Cream Of Potato w/ Bacon	1 cup	210	5	12	20
Golden Broccoli Cheese	1 cup	180	6	12	12
Hearty Chili Beef	1 cup	250	15	7	31

FOOD	PORTION	CALS	PROT	FAT	CARB
Minestrone	1 cup	70	3	1	11
New England Clam Chowder	1 cup	140	5	5	19
Potato Cheese Chowder	1 cup	210	7	10	22
Roasted Chicken Noodle	1 cup	90	7	4	7
Tomato Bisque	1 cup	90	1	3	15
Vegetable Beef	1 cup	90	5	2	14
TACO BELL					
beverages					
Coffee Black	1 serv (12 oz)	5	0	0	1
Diet Pepsi	1 serv (16 oz)	0	0	0	0
Dr. Pepper	1 serv (16 oz)	208	0	0	52
Lipton Iced Tea Sweetened	1 serv (16 oz)	140	0	0	40
Lipton Iced Tea Unsweetened	1 serv (16 oz)	0	0	0	0
Mountain Dew	1 serv (16 oz)	227	0	0	61
Orange Juice	1 serv (6 oz)	80	1	0	18
Pepsi Cola	1 serv (16 oz)	200	0	0	51
Slice	1 serv (16 oz)	200	0	0	53
breakfast selections					
Breakfast Quesadilla Cheese	1 (5.5 oz)	380	15	21	33
Breakfast Quesadilla w/ Bacon	1 (6 oz)	450	19	27	33
Breakfast Quesadilla w/ Sausage	1 (6 oz)	430	17	25	33
Country Breakfast Burrito	1 (4 oz)	270	8	14	26
Double Bacon & Egg Burrito	1 (6.25 oz)	480	18	27	39
Fiesta Breakfast Burrito	1 (3.5 oz)	280	9	16	25
Grande Breakfast Burrito	1 (6.25 oz)	420	13	22	43
Hash Brown Nuggets	1 serv (3.5 oz)	280	2	18	29
main menu selections					
7-Layer Burrito	1 (10 oz)	530	16	23	66
BLT Soft Taco	1 (4.5 oz)	340	11	23	22
Bacon Cheeseburger Burrito	1 (8.5 oz)	570	27	31	46
Bean Burrito	1 (7 oz)	380	13	12	55
Big Beef Burrito Supreme	1 (10.5 oz)	520	24	23	54
Big Beef MexiMelt	1 (4.75 oz)	290	16	15	23
Big Chicken Burrito Supreme	1 (9 oz)	510	23	24	52
Border Sauce Fire	1 serv (0.3 oz)	0	0	0	0
Border Sauce Hot	1 serv (0.3 oz)	0	0	0	0
Border Sauce Mild	1 serv (0.3 oz)	0	0	0	0
Burger Sauce	1 serv (0.5 oz)	60	0	5	2
Burrito Supreme	1 (9 oz)	440	17	19	51
Cheddar Cheese	1 serv (0.25 oz)	30	2	2	0
Cheese Quesadilla	1 (4.25 oz)	350	16	18	32

FOOD	PORTION	CALS	PROT	FAT	CARB
Chicken Fajita Wrap	1 (8 oz)	470	17	22	51
Chicken Fajita Wrap Supreme	1 (9 oz)	520	18	25	53
Chicken Quesadilla	1 (6 oz)	410	23	21	34
Chicken Club Burrito	1 (8 oz)	540	20	32	43
Chili Cheese Burrito	1 (5 oz)	330	14	13	37
Choco Taco Ice Cream Dessert	1 serv (4 oz)	310	3	17	37
Cinnamon Twists	1 serv (1 oz)	140	1	6	19
Club Sauce	1 serv (0.5 oz)	80	0	8	1
Double Decker Taco	1 (5.75 oz)	340	14	15	38
Double Decker Taco Supreme	1 (7 oz)	390	15	19	40
Fajita Sauce	1 serv (0.5 oz)	70	0	7	1
Green Sauce	1 serv (1 oz)	5	0	0	1
Grilled Chicken Burrito	1 (7 oz)	410	17	15	50
Grilled Chicken Soft Taco	1 (4.5 oz)	240	12	12	21
Grilled Steak Soft Taco	1 (4.5 oz)	230	15	10	20
Grilled Steak Soft Taco Supreme	1 (5.75 oz)	290	16	14	24
Guacamole	1 serv (0.75 oz)	35	0	3	1
Mexican Pizza	1 serv (7.75 oz)	570	21	35	42
Mexican Rice	1 serv (4.75 oz)	190	5	9	23
Nacho Cheese Sauce	2 serv (2 oz)	120	2	10	5
Nachos	1 serv (3.5 oz)	320	5	18	34
Nachos Beef Beef Supreme	1 serv (7 oz)	450	14	24	45
Nachos Bellgrande	1 serv (11 oz)	770	21	39	84
Picante Sauce	1 serv (0.3 oz)	0	0	0	0
Pico De Gallo	1 serv (0.75 oz)	5	0	0	1
Pintos 'n Cheese	1 serv (4.5 oz)	190	9	9	18
Red Sauce	1 serv (1 oz)	10	0	0	2
Soft Taco	1 (3.5 oz)	220	11	10	21
Soft Taco Supreme	1 (5 oz)	260	12	14	23
Sour Cream	1 serv (0.75 oz)	40	1	4	1
Steak Fajita Wrap	1 (8 oz)	470	20	21	50
Steak Fajita Wrap Supreme	1 (9 oz)	510	21	25	52
Taco	1 (2.75 oz)	180	9	10	12
Taco Supreme	1 (4 oz)	220	10	14	14
Taco Salad w/ Salsa	1 (19 oz)	850	30	52	65
Taco Salad w/ Salsa w/o Shell	1 (16.5 oz)	420	24	22	32
Three Cheese Blend	1 serv (0.25 oz)	25	2	2	0
Tostada	1 (6.25 oz)	300	10	15	31
Veggie Fajita Wrap	1 (8 oz)	420	10	19	53
Veggie Fajita Wrap Supreme	1 (9 oz)	470	11	22	55

FOOD	PORTION	CALS	PROT	FAT	CARB
TACO JOHN'S					
children's menu selections					
Kid's Meal Softshell Taco	1 serv (8.5 oz)	617	15	33	64
Kid's Meal Crispy Taco	1 serv (8 oz)	579	13	34	54
desserts					
Choco Taco	1 serv (3.5 oz)	320	3	17	38
Churro	1 serv (1.5 oz)	147	2	8	17
Flauta Apple	1 serv (2 oz)	84	1	1	19
Flauta Cherry	1 serv (2 oz)	143	2	4	27
Flauta Cream Cheese	1 serv (2 oz)	181	2	8	27
Italian Ice	1 serv (4 oz)	80	0	0	19
main menu selections					
Bean Burrito	1 (6.5 oz)	387	15	11	57
Beans Refried	1 serv (9.5 oz)	357	18	9	53
Beef Burrito	1 (6.5 oz)	449	23	20	44
Chicken Fajita Burrito	1 (6.25 oz)	370	22	12	45
Chicken Fajita Salad w/o Dressing	1 serv (12.25 oz)	557	22	33	44
Chicken Fajita Softshell	1 (4.5 oz)	200	13	7	21
Chili	1 serv (9.25 oz)	350	20	21	19
Chimichanga Platter	1 serv (18 oz)	979	32	38	127
Combination Burrito	1 (6.5 oz)	418	19	16	50
Crispy Tacos	1 serv (3.25 oz)	182	9	11	12
Double Enchilada Platter	1 serv (18.25 oz)	967	42	42	106
Meat & Potato Burrito	1 (7.75 oz)	503	17	24	53
Mexi Rolls w/ Nacho Cheese	1 serv (9.75 oz)	863	30	48	72
Mexican Rice	1 serv (8 oz)	567	8	18	40
Nacho Cheese	1 serv (2 oz)	300	5	10	0
Nachos	1 serv (3.5 oz)	333	7	21	27
Potato Oles	1 lg serv (6.12 oz)	484	4	30	50
Potato Oles	1 serv (4.63 oz)	363	3	23	38
Potato Oles Bravo	1 serv (8.88 oz)	579	11	38	47
Potato Oles w/ Nacho Cheese	1 serv (6.63 oz)	483	8	33	38
Ranch Burrito	1 (7 oz)	447	18	23	44
Sampler Platter	1 serv (25.5 oz)	1406	61	61	156
Sierra Chicken Fillet Sandwich	1 (8.5 oz)	534	30	29	40
Smothered Burrito Platter	1 serv (19.5 oz)	1031	39	40	132
Softshell Tacos	1 serv (4.25 oz)	230	14	10	23
Sour Cream	1 oz	60	1	5	1
Super Burrito	1 (8.5 oz)	465	20	19	53
Super Nachos	1 serv (13 oz)	919	26	56	72
Taco Bravo	1 serv (6.25 oz)	346	15	14	39
Taco Burger	1 (5 oz)	280	15	12	28
Taco Salad w/o Dressing	1 (12.4 oz)	584	20	38	43

FOOD	PORTION	CALS	PROT	FAT	CARB
TACOTIME					
Casita Burrito Meat	1 serv (12 oz)	647	40	31	54
Cheddar Cheese	1 serv (0.75 oz)	86	5	7	0
Chicken	1 serv (2.5 oz)	109	11	6	2
Chips	1 serv (2 oz)	266	4	12	35
Crisp Burrito Bean	1 (5.25 oz)	427	15	18	53
Crisp Burrito Chicken	1 (4.75 oz)	422	17	25	32
Crisp Burrito Meat	1 (5.25 oz)	552	34	30	39
Crisp Taco	1 (4 oz)	295	22	17	16
Crustos	1 serv (3.5 oz)	373	9	15	47
Double Soft Bean Burrito	1 (9.5 oz)	506	23	12	77
Double Soft Combination Burrito	1 (9.5 oz)	617	39	23	66
Double Soft Meat Burrito	1 serv (6.5 oz)	726	57	33	55
Empanada Cherry	1 (4 oz)	250	5	9	37
Enchilada Sauce	1 serv (1 oz)	12	0	0	3
Flour Tortilla 10 in	1 (2.75 oz)	213	6	4	31
Flour Tortilla 7 in	1 (1.75 oz)	88	4	1	16
Flour Tortilla 8 in	1 (1.25 oz)	107	5	3	16
Fried Flour Tortilla 10 in	1 (2.75 oz)	318	6	16	37
Fried Flour Tortilla 8 in	1 (1.35 oz)	205	4	11	24
Guacamole	1 serv (1 oz)	29	0	2	2
Hot Sauce	1 serv (1 oz)	10	0	0	2
Lettuce	1 serv (0.5 oz)	2	0	0	0
Mexi Fries	1 lg (8 oz)	532	6	34	54
Mexi Fries	1 reg (4 oz)	266	3	17	27
Mexican Rice	1 serv (4 oz)	159	3	2	30
Nachos	1 serv (10.5 oz)	680	26	38	61
Nachos Deluxe	1 serv (15.25 oz)	1048	46	57	91
Natural Super Taco Meat	1 (11.25 oz)	627	41	27	60
Quesadilla Cheese	1 serv (3.25 oz)	205	11	11	17
Ranchero Salsa	1 serv (2 oz)	21	1	1	3
Refritos	1 serv (2.5 oz)	97	6	0	18
Refritos	1 serv (7 oz)	326	18	10	44
Rolled Soft Flour Taco	1 (7 oz)	512	33	23	46
Shredded Beef	1 serv (2.5 oz)	70	1	7	1
Soft Taco Chicken	1 (7 oz)	387	21	16	41
Sour Cream	1 serv (1 oz)	55	1	5	1
Sour Cream Dressing	1 serv (1.5 oz)	137	1	14	2
Super Shredded Beef Soft Taco	1 (8 oz)	368	12	11	38
Taco Cheeseburger	1 (7.5 oz)	633	31	36	48
Taco Meat	1 serv (2.5 oz)	208	22	11	7
Taco Salad Chicken w/o Dressing	1 serv (9 oz)	370	19	21	27
Taco Salad w/o Dressing	1 serv (7.75 oz)	479	30	28	30
Taco Shell 6 in	1 (1.25 oz)	110	2	6	14
Thousand Island Dressing	1 serv (1 oz)	160	0	16	4

FOOD	PORTION	CALS	PROT	FAT	CARB
Tomato	1 serv (0.5 oz)	3	0	0	1
Tostada Delight Salad Meat	1 (9.75 oz)	628	36	33	48
Value Soft Bean Burrito	1 (6.75 oz)	380	16	10	58
Value Soft Meat Burrito	1 (6.75 oz)	491	31	21	48
Value Soft Taco	1 (5.25 oz)	316	24	15	23
Veggie Burrito	1 (11 oz)	491	21	16	70
Wheat Tortilla 11 in	1 (3.5 oz)	175	8	3	33
TCBY					
Hand Dipped All Flavors 96% Fat Free	½ cup (3 oz)	140	3	3	26
Hand Dipped All Flavors Nonfat	½ cup (2.9 oz)	120	4	0	25
Lowfat Ice Cream All Flavors No Sugar Added	½ cup (2.6 oz)	110	3	3	19
Nonfat Ice Cream All Flavors	½ cup (2.9 oz)	120	3	0	26
Soft Serve All Flavors 96% Fat Free	½ cup (3.4 fl oz)	140	4	3	23
Soft Serve All Flavors No Sugar Added Nonfat	½ cup (2.8 oz)	80	4	0	20
Soft Serve All Flavors Nonfat	½ cup (3.4 oz)	110	4	0	23
Sorbet All Flavors Nonfat & Nondairy	½ cup (3.4 oz)	100	0	0	24
WENDY'S					
beverages					
Cola	11 oz	130	0	0	36
Diet Cola	11 oz	0	0	0	0
Frosty Junior	6 oz	170	4	4	26
Frosty Medium	16 oz	440	11	11	73
Frosty Small	12 oz	330	8	8	56
Lemon-Lime Soda	11 oz	130	0	0	34
children's menu selections					
French Fries Kid's Meal	1 serv (3.2 oz)	270	4	13	35
Kid's Meal Cheeseburger	1 (4.2 oz)	310	17	12	33
Kid's Meal Hamburger	1 (3.9 oz)	270	14	9	33
Kid's Meal Chicken Nuggets	4 pieces (2.1 oz)	190	9	13	9
main menu selections					
¼ lb Hamburger Patty	1 (2.6 oz)	200	19	14	0
2 oz Hamburger Patty	1 (1.3 oz)	100	9	7	0
American Cheese	1 slice (0.6 oz)	70	4	6	0
American Cheese Jr.	1 slice (0.4 oz)	45	3	4	0
Bacon	1 strip (4 g)	20	1	2	0
Big Bacon Classic	1 (9.9 oz)	580	34	30	46
Breaded Chicken Fillet	1 (3.5 oz)	230	22	11	13
Cheddar Shredded	2 tbsp (0.6 oz)	70	4	6	1
Chicken Breast Filet Sandwich	1 (7.3 oz)	430	27	16	46

FOOD	PORTION	CALS	PROT	FAT	CARB
Chicken Club Sandwich	1 (7.6 oz)	470	30	20	47
Chicken Nuggets	5 pieces (2.6 oz)	230	11	16	11
Chili	1 lg (12 oz)	310	23	10	32
Chili	1 sm (8 oz)	210	15	7	21
Classic Single w/ Everything	1 (7.6 oz)	410	25	19	37
French Fries	1 Great Biggie	570	8	27	73
French Fries	1 med (5 oz)	420	6	20	50
French Fries	1 Biggie (5.6 oz)	470	7	23	61
Grilled Chicken Fillet	1 (2.9 oz)	110	19	3	1
Grilled Chicken Sandwich	1 (6.6 oz)	300	24	7	36
Honey Mustard Reduced Calorie	1 tsp (7 g)	25	0	2	2
Hot Stuffed Bake Potato Plain	1 (10 oz)	310	7	0	72
Hot Stuffed Baked Potato Bacon & Cheese	1 (12.6 oz)	530	16	18	78
Hot Stuffed Baked Potato Broccoli & Cheese	1 (14.4 oz)	470	9	14	80
Jr. Bacon Cheeseburger	1 (5.8 oz)	380	20	19	34
Jr. Cheeseburger	1 (4.5 oz)	310	17	12	34
Jr. Cheeseburger Deluxe	1 (6.3 oz)	360	18	16	36
Kaiser Bun	1 (2.5 oz)	200	6	3	38
Ketchup	1 tsp (7 g)	10	0	0	2
Lettuce	1 leaf (0.5 oz)	0	0	0	0
Mayonnaise	1½ tsp (9 g)	30	0	3	1
Mustard	½ tsp (5 g)	5	0	0	0
Nuggets Sauce Barbeque	1 pkg (1 oz)	45	1	0	10
Nuggets Sauce Honey Mustard	1 pkg (1 oz)	130	0	12	6
Nuggets Sauce Sweet & Sour	1 pkg (1 oz)	50	0	0	12
Onion	4 rings (0.5 oz)	5	0	0	1
Pickles	4 slices (0.4 oz)	0	0	0	0
Saltines	2 (0.2 oz)	25	1	1	4
Sandwich Bun	1 (2 oz)	160	5	2	31
Spicy Chicken Fillet	1 (3.6 oz)	210	22	9	10
Spicy Chicken Sandwich	1 (7.5 oz)	410	28	14	43
Tomatoes	1 slice (0.9 oz)	5	0	0	1
Whipped Margarine	1 pkg (0.5 oz)	70	0	7	0
salad dressings					
Blue Cheese	1 pkg (2 oz)	360	2	36	1
French	1 pkg (2 oz)	250	0	21	13
Hidden Valley Ranch	1 pkg (2 oz)	200	1	20	3
Hidden Valley Ranch Reduced Fat Reduced Calorie	1 pkg (2 oz)	120	1	11	4
Italian Reduced Fat Reduced Calorie	1 pkg (2 oz)	80	0	7	6

FOOD	PORTION	CALS	PROT	FAT	CARB
Italian Caesar	1 pkg (1.5 oz)	230	1	24	1
Thousand Island	1 pkg (2 oz)	260	1	25	7
salads and salad bars					
Ceasar Side Salad w/o Dressing	1 (3.2 oz)	110	9	5	6
Deluxe Garden Salad w/o Dressing	1 (9.5 oz)	110	7	6	10
Grilled Chicken Salad w/o Dressing	1 (11.9 oz)	200	27	7	10
Side Salad w/o Dressing	1 (5.4 oz)	60	4	3	5
Soft Breadstick	1 (1.5 oz)	130	4	3	23
Taco Chips	15 (1.5 oz)	210	3	9	28
Taco Salad w/o Dressing	1 (16.4 oz)	380	26	19	28
WHATABURGER					
baked selections					
Biscuit	1	280	5	13	37
Blueberry Muffin	1	239	6	8	36
Cinnamon Roll	1	320	4	16	39
Cookie Chocolate Chunk	1	247	4	16	28
Cookie White Chocolate Macadamia Nut	1	269	3	16	31
Fried Apple Turnover	1	215	2	11	27
beverages					
Cherry Coke	1 reg	227	0	0	60
Coke Classic	1 reg	211	0	0	56
Creamer	1 pkg	10	0	1	1
Diet Coke	1 reg	2	0	0	1
Dr. Pepper	1 reg	207	0	1	52
Iced Tea	1 reg	5	0	0	2
Lemon Juice	1 pkg	1	0	0	tr
Orange Juice	1 serv (10 oz)	140	2	0	33
Root Beer	1 reg	237	0	0	63
Shake Chocolate	1 junior	364	9	9	61
Shake Strawberry	1 junior	352	9	9	60
Shake Vanilla	1 junior	325	9	10	51
Sprite	1 reg	211	0	0	48
breakfast selections					
Biscuit w/ Bacon	1	359	10	20	37
Biscuit w/ Bacon Egg & Cheese	1	511	18	33	38
Biscuit w/ Egg & Cheese	1	434	14	26	38
Biscuit w/ Sausage	1	446	12	29	37
Biscuit w/ Sausage Egg & Cheese	1	601	21	42	38
Biscuit w/ Sausage Gravy	1	479	9	27	48
Breakfast Platter w/ Bacon	1 serv	695	22	44	54
Breakfast Platter w/ Sausage	1 serv	785	25	53	54

FOOD	PORTION	CALS	PROT	FAT	CARB
Breakfast On A Bun w/ Bacon	1	365	18	19	29
Breakfast On A Bun w/ Sausage	1	455	20	28	30
Butter	1 pkg	36	0	4	0
Egg Omelette Sandwich	1	288	13	13	29
Grape Jelly	1 pkg	45	0	0	10
Hashbrown	1 serv	150	1	9	16
Honey	1 pkg	25	0	0	7
Margarine	1 pkg	25	0	3	0
Pancake Syrup	1 pkg	180	0	0	42
Pancakes	3	259	11	6	40
Pancakes w/ Bacon	1 serv	335	15	12	40
Pancakes w/ Sausage	1 serv	426	18	21	40
Srambled Eggs	2	189	11	15	2
Strawberry Jam	1 pkg	40	0	0	9
Taquito Bacon & Egg	1	335	15	16	32
main menu selections					
Bacon	1 slice	38	2	3	0
Cheese Slice	1 lg	89	5	7	tr
Cheese Slice	1 sm	46	3	4	tr
Chicken Strips	2	120	7	5	10
Club Crackers	1 pkg	30	1	2	4
Croutons	1 pkg	30	1	1	5
Fajita Beef	1	326	22	12	34
Fajita Grilled Chicken	1	272	18	7	35
French Fries	1 lg	442	7	24	49
French Fries	1 reg	332	5	18	37
French Fries	1 junior	221	4	12	25
Garden Salad	1	56	3	1	11
Grilled Chicken Salad	1 serv	150	23	1	14
Grilled Chicken Sandwich	1	442	34	14	48
Grilled Chicken Sandwich w/o Bun Oil w/ Mustard	1	300	33	3	35
Grilled Chicken Sandwich w/o Bun Oil & Dressing	1	358	34	6	46
Grilled Chicken Sandwich w/o Dressing	1	385	34	9	46
Justaburger	1	276	13	11	30
Ketchup	1 pkg	30	0	0	7
Onion Rings	1 lg	493	8	29	51
Onion Rings	1 reg	329	5	19	34
Peppered Gravy	1 serv (3 oz)	75	0	5	8
Taquito Potato & Egg	1	446	14	22	48
Taquito Sausage & Egg	1	443	20	26	32
Texas Toast	1 slice	147	4	5	22
Whataburger	1	598	30	26	61
Whataburger Double Meat	1	823	49	42	62

FOOD	PORTION	CALS	PROT	FAT	CARB
Whataburger Jr.	1	300	14	12	35
Whataburger w/o bun oil	1	407	25	19	34
Whatacatch Sandwich	1	467	18	25	43
Whatachick'n Sandwich	1	501	27	23	51
salad dressings					
Low Fat Ranch	1 pkg	66	1	3	9
Low Fat Vinaigrette	1 pkg	37	0	2	6
Ranch	1 pkg	320	0	33	4
Thousand Island	1 pkg	160	0	12	12

Visit the
Simon & Schuster Web site:
www.SimonSays.com

and sign up for our
mystery e-mail updates!

Keep up on the latest
new releases, author appearances,
news, chats, special offers, and more!
We'll deliver the information
right to your inbox — if it's new,
you'll know about it.

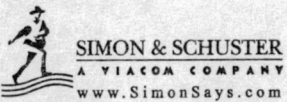

SIMON & SCHUSTER
A VIACOM COMPANY
www.SimonSays.com

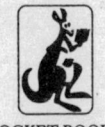

POCKET BOOKS   POCKET STAR BOOKS